GORDON'S FUNCTION

*Modified by Marjory Gordon, 2007, with permission.

Nurse's Pocket Guide

Diagnoses, Prioritized Interventions, and Rationales

Nurse's Pocket Guide

Diagnoses, Prioritized Interventions, and Rationales

EDITION 11

Marilynn E. Doenges, APRN, BC–retired
Clinical Specialist—Adult Psychiatric/Mental Health Nursing
Adjunct Faculty
Beth-El College of Nursing and Health Sciences, UCCS
Colorado Springs, Colorado

Mary Frances Moorhouse, RN, MSN, CRRN, LNC
Nurse Consultant
TNT-RN Enterprises
Adjunct Faculty
Pikes Peak Community College
Colorado Springs, Colorado

Alice C. Murr, RN, BSN, LNC
Nurse Consultant/Author
Collins, Mississippi

 F. A. Davis Company • Philadelphia

F. A. Davis Company
1915 Arch Street
Philadelphia, PA 19103
www.fadavis.com

Printed in the United States of America

Last digit indicates print number: 10 9 8 7 6 5 4 3 2 1

Publisher, Nursing: Joanne Patzek DaCunha, RN, MSN
Director of Content Development: Darlene D. Pedersen, MSN, APRN, BC
Project Editors: Padraic J. Maroney and Meghan K. Ziegler
Design and Illustration Manager: Carolyn O'Brien

As new scientific information becomes available through basic and clinical research, recommended treatments and drug therapies undergo
changes. The author(s) and publisher have done everything possible to
make this book accurate, up to date, and in accord with accepted standards at the time of publication. The author(s), editors, and publisher
are not responsible for errors or omissions or for consequences from
application of the book, and make no warranty, expressed or implied, in
regard to the contents of the book. Any practice described in this book
should be applied by the reader in accordance with professional standards of care used in regard to the unique circumstances that may apply
in each situation. The reader is advised always to check product information (package inserts) for changes and new information regarding
dose and contraindications before administering any drug. Caution is
especially urged when using new or infrequently ordered drugs.

ISBN-13: 978-0-8036-1857-2
ISBN-10: 0-8036-1857-3

Dedication

This book is dedicated to:

Our families, who helped with the mundane activities of daily living that allowed us to write this book and who provide us with love and encouragement in all our endeavors.

Our friends, who support us in our writing, put up with our memory lapses, and love us still.

Bob Martone, Publisher, Nursing, who asks questions that stimulate thought and discussion, and who maintains good humor throughout. Joanne DaCunha and Danielle Barsky who supported us and kept us focused. The F.A. Davis production staff who coordinated and expedited the project through the editing and printing processes, meeting unreal deadlines, and sending pages to us with bated breath.

Robert H. Craven, Jr., and the F.A. Davis family.

And last and most important:

The nurses we are writing for, to those who have found the previous editions of the Pocket Guide helpful, and to other nurses who are looking for help to provide quality nursing care in a period of transition and change, we say, "Nursing Diagnosis is the way."

CONTRIBUTOR

Sheila Marquez
Executive Director
Vice President/Chief Operating Officer
The Colorado SIDS Program, Inc.
Denver, Colorado

ACKNOWLEDGMENTS

A special acknowledgment to Marilynn's friend, the late Diane Camillone, who provoked an awareness of the role of the patient and continues to influence our thoughts about the importance of quality nursing care, and to our late colleague, Mary Jeffries, who introduced us to nursing diagnosis.

To our colleagues in NANDA International who continue to formulate and refine nursing diagnoses to provide nursing with the tools to enhance and promote the growth of the profession.

Marilynn E. Doenges
Mary Frances Moorhouse
Alice C. Murr

Contents

Health Conditions and Client Concerns with Associated Nursing Diagnoses appear on pages 781–908.

Taxonomy II, Domain, Class, Code, Year Submitted/revised
Diagnostic Division
Definition
Related/Risk Factors, Defining Characteristics:
Subjective/Objective
Desired Outcomes/Evaluation Criteria
Actions/Interventions
Nursing Priorities
Documentation Focus
Sample Nursing Outcomes & Interventions Classifications
(NOC/NIC)

How to Use the Nurse's Pocket Guide

The American Nurses Association (ANA) Social Policy Statement of 1980 was the first to define nursing as the diagnosis and treatment of human responses to actual and potential health problems. This definition, when combined with the ANA Standards of Practice, has provided impetus and support for the use of nursing diagnosis. Defining nursing and its effect on client care supports the growing awareness that nursing care is a key factor in client survival and in the maintenance, rehabilitative, and preventive aspects of healthcare. Changes and new developments in healthcare delivery in the last decade have given rise to the need for a common framework of communication to ensure continuity of care for the client moving between multiple healthcare settings and providers. Evaluation and documentation of care are important parts of this process.

This book is designed to aid the practitioner and student nurse in identifying interventions commonly associated with specific nursing diagnoses as proposed by NANDA International/NANDA-I (formerly the North American Nursing Diagnosis Association). These interventions are the activities needed to implement and document care provided to the individual client and can be used in varied settings from acute to community/home care.

Chapters 1 and 2 present brief discussions of the nursing process, data collection, and care plan construction. Chapter 3 contains the Diagnostic Divisions, Assessment Tool, a sample plan of care, mind map, and corresponding documentation/charting examples. For more in-depth information and inclusive plans of care related to specific medical/psychiatric conditions (with rationale and the application of the diagnoses), the nurse is referred to the larger works, all published by the F.A. Davis Company: *Nursing Care Plans Across the Life Span*, ed. 7 (Doenges, Moorhouse, Geissler-Murr, 2006); *Psychiatric Care Plans: Guidelines for Individualizing Care*, ed. 3 (Doenges, Townsend, Moorhouse, 1998); and *Maternal/Newborn Plans of Care: Guidelines for Individualizing Care*, ed. 3 (Doenges, Moorhouse, 1999) with updated versions included on the CD-ROM provided with *Nursing Care Plans*.

Nursing diagnoses are listed alphabetically in Chapter 4 for ease of reference and include the diagnoses accepted for use by

NANDA-I through 2007–2008. Each diagnosis approved for testing includes its definition and information divided into the NANDA-I categories of Related or Risk Factors and Defining Characteristics. Related/Risk Factors information reflects causative or contributing factors that can be useful for determining whether the diagnosis is applicable to a particular client. Defining Characteristics (signs and symptoms or cues) are listed as subjective and/or objective and are used to confirm actual diagnoses, aid in formulating outcomes, and provide additional data for choosing appropriate interventions. The authors have not deleted or altered NANDA-I's listings; however, on occasion, they have added to their definitions or suggested additional criteria to provide clarification and direction. These additions are denoted with brackets [ ].

With the development and acceptance of Taxonomy II following the biennial conference in 2000, significant changes were made to better reflect the content of the diagnoses within the taxonomy. Taxonomy II was designed to reduce miscalculations, errors, and redundancies. The framework has been changed from the Human Response Patterns and is organized in Domains and Classes, with 13 domains, 47 classes, and 188 diagnoses. Although clinicians will use the actual diagnoses, understanding the taxonomic structure will help the nurse to find the desired information quickly. Taxonomy II is designed to be multiaxial with 7 axes (see Appendix 2). An axis is defined as a dimension of the human response that is considered in the diagnostic process. Sometimes an axis may be included in the diagnostic concept, such as ineffective community Coping, in which the unit of care (e.g., community) is named. Some are implicit, such as Activity Intolerance, in which the individual is the unit of care. Sometimes an axis may not be pertinent to a particular diagnosis and will not be a part of the nursing diagnosis label or code. For example, the time axis may not be relevant to each diagnostic situation. The Taxonomic Domain and Class are noted under each nursing diagnosis heading. An Axis 6 descriptor is included in each nursing diagnosis label.

The ANA, in conjunction with NANDA, proposed that specific nursing diagnoses currently approved and structured according to Taxonomy I Revised be included in the International Classification of Diseases (ICD) within the section "Family of Health-Related Classifications." While the World Health Organization did not accept this initial proposal because of lack of documentation of the usefulness of nursing diagnoses at the international level, the NANDA-I list has been accepted by SNOMED (Systemized Nomenclature of Medicine) for inclusion in its international coding system and is included in the Unified Medical Language System of the National Library of

Medicine. Today, researchers from around the world are validating nursing diagnoses in support for resubmission and acceptance in future editions of ICD.

The authors have chosen to categorize the list of nursing diagnoses approved for clinical use and testing into Diagnostic Divisions, which is the framework for an assessment tool (Chapter 3) designed to assist the nurse to readily identify an appropriate nursing diagnosis from data collected during the assessment process. The Diagnostic Division label follows the Taxonomic label under each nursing diagnosis heading.

Desired Outcomes/Evaluation Criteria are identified to assist the nurse in formulating individual client outcomes and to support the evaluation process.

Interventions in this pocket guide are primarily directed to adult care settings (although general age span considerations are included) and are listed according to nursing priorities. Some interventions require collaborative or interdependent orders (e.g., medical, psychiatric), and the nurse will need to determine when this is necessary and take the appropriate action. In general, interventions that address specialty areas outside the scope of this book are not routinely presented (e.g., obstetrics). For example, when addressing deficient [isotonic] Fluid Volume, (hemorrhage), the nurse is directed to stop blood loss; however, specific direction to perform fundal massage is not listed.

The inclusion of Documentation Focus suggestions is to remind the nurse of the importance and necessity of recording the steps of the nursing process.

Finally, in recognition of the ongoing work of numerous researchers over the past 15 years, the authors have referenced the Nursing Interventions and Outcomes labels developed by the Iowa Intervention Projects (Bulechek & McCloskey; Johnson, Mass & Moorhead). These groups have been classifying nursing interventions and outcomes to predict resource requirements and measure outcomes, thereby meeting the needs of a standardized language that can be coded for computer and reimbursement purposes. As an introduction to this work in progress, sample NIC and NOC labels have been included under the heading Sample Nursing Interventions & Outcomes Classifications at the conclusion of each nursing diagnosis section. The reader is referred to the various publications by Joanne C. McCloskey and Marion Johnson for more in-depth information.

Chapter 5 presents over 400 disorders/health conditions reflecting all specialty areas, with associated nursing diagnoses written as client diagnostic statements that include the "related to" and "evidenced by" components. This section will facilitate and help validate the assessment and problem/need identification steps of the nursing process.

As noted, with few exceptions, we have presented NANDA-I's recommendations as formulated. We support the belief that practicing nurses and researchers need to study, use, and evaluate the diagnoses as presented. Nurses can be creative as they use the standardized language, redefining and sharing information as the diagnoses are used with individual clients. As new nursing diagnoses are developed, it is important that the data they encompass are added to the current database. As part of the process by clinicians, educators, and researchers across practice specialties and academic settings to define, test, and refine nursing diagnosis, nurses are encouraged to share insights and ideas with NANDA-I at the following address: NANDA International, 100 N. 20th Street, 4th Floor, Philadelphia, PA 19103, USA; e-mail: info@nanda.org

CHAPTER 1

The Nursing Process

Nursing is both a science and an art concerned with the physical, psychological, sociological, cultural, and spiritual concerns of the individual. The science of nursing is based on a broad theoretical framework; its art depends on the caring skills and abilities of the individual nurse. In its early developmental years, nursing did not seek or have the means to control its own practice. In more recent times, the nursing profession has struggled to define what makes nursing unique and has identified a body of professional knowledge unique to nursing practice. In 1980, the American Nurses Association (ANA) developed the first *Social Policy Statement* defining nursing as "the diagnosis and treatment of human responses to actual or potential health problems." Along with the definition of nursing came the need to explain the method used to provide nursing care.

Years before, nursing leaders had developed a problem-solving process consisting of three steps—assessment, planning, and evaluation—patterned after the scientific method of observing, measuring, gathering data, and analyzing findings. This method, introduced in the 1950s, was called *nursing process*. Shore (1988) described the nursing process as "combining the most desirable elements of the art of nursing with the most relevant elements of systems theory, using the scientific method." This process incorporates an interactive/interpersonal approach with a problem-solving and decision-making process (Peplau, 1952; King, 1971; Yura & Walsh, 1988).

Over time, the nursing process expanded to five steps and has gained widespread acceptance as the basis for providing effective nursing care. Nursing process is now included in the conceptual framework of all nursing curricula, is accepted in the legal definition of nursing in the *Nurse Practice Acts* of most states, and is included in the ANA *Standards of Clinical Nursing Practice*.

The five steps of the nursing process consist of the following:

1. **Assessment** is an organized dynamic process involving three basic activities: a) systematically gathering data, b) sorting and organizing the collected data, and c) documenting the data in a retrievable fashion. Subjective and objective data are collected from various sources, such as

the client interview and physical assessment. Subjective data are what the client or significant others report, believe, or feel, and objective data are what can be observed or obtained from other sources, such as laboratory and diagnostic studies, old medical records, or other healthcare providers. Using a number of techniques, the nurse focuses on eliciting a profile of the client that supplies a sense of the client's overall health status, providing a picture of the client's physical, psychological, sociocultural, spiritual, cognitive, and developmental levels; economic status; functional abilities; and lifestyle. The profile is known as the *client database.*

2. *Diagnosis/need identification* involves the analysis of collected data to identify the client's needs or problems, also known as the nursing diagnosis. The purpose of this step is to draw conclusions regarding the client's specific needs or human responses of concern so that effective care can be planned and delivered. This process of data analysis uses diagnostic reasoning (a form of clinical judgment) in which conclusions are reached about the meaning of the collected data to determine whether or not nursing intervention is indicated. The end product is the *client diagnostic statement* that combines the specific client need with the related factors or risk factors (etiology), and defining characteristics (or cues) as appropriate. The status of the client's needs are categorized as *actual* or currently existing diagnoses and potential or *risk* diagnoses that could develop due to specific vulnerabilities of the client. Ongoing changes in healthcare delivery and computerization of the client record require a commonality of communication to ensure continuity of care for the client moving from one setting/level of healthcare to another. The use of standardized terminology or NANDA International (NANDA-I) nursing diagnosis labels provides nurses with a common language for identifying client needs. Furthermore, the use of standardized nursing diagnosis labels also promotes identification of appropriate goals, provides acuity information, is useful in creating standards for nursing practice, provides a base for quality improvement, and facilitates research supporting evidence-based nursing practices.

3. *Planning* includes setting priorities, establishing goals, identifying desired client outcomes, and determining specific nursing interventions. These actions are documented as the *plan of care.* This process requires input from the client/significant others to reach agreement regarding the plan to facilitate the client taking responsibility for his or

her own care and the achievement of the desired outcomes and goals. Setting priorities for client care is a complex and dynamic challenge that helps ensure that the nurse's attention and subsequent actions are properly focused. What is perceived today to be the number one client care need or appropriate nursing intervention could change tomorrow, or, for that matter, within minutes, based on changes in the client's condition or situation. Once client needs are prioritized, goals for treatment and discharge are established that indicate the general direction in which the client is expected to progress in response to treatment. The goals may be short-term—those that usually must be met before the client is discharged or moved to a lesser level of care—and/or long-term, which may continue even after discharge. From these goals, desired outcomes are determined to measure the client's progress toward achieving the goals of treatment or the discharge criteria. To be more specific, outcomes are client responses that are achievable and desired by the client that can be attained within a defined period, given the situation and resources. Next, nursing interventions are chosen that are based on the client's nursing diagnosis, the established goals and desired outcomes, the ability of the nurse to successfully implement the intervention, and the ability and the willingness of the client to undergo or participate in the intervention, and they reflect the client's age/situation and individual strengths, when possible. Nursing interventions are direct-care activities or prescriptions for behaviors, treatments, activities, or actions that assist the client in achieving the measurable outcomes. Nursing interventions, like nursing diagnoses, are key elements of the knowledge of nursing and continue to grow as research supports the connection between actions and outcomes (McCloskey & Bulechek, 2000). Recording the planning step in a written or computerized plan of care provides for continuity of care, enhances communication, assists with determining agency or unit staffing needs, documents the nursing process, serves as a teaching tool, and coordinates provision of care among disciplines. A valid plan of care demonstrates individualized client care by reflecting the concerns of the client and significant others, as well as the client's physical, psychosocial, and cultural needs and capabilities.

4. *Implementation* occurs when the plan of care is put into action, and the nurse performs the planned interventions. Regardless of how well a plan of care has been constructed, it cannot predict everything that will occur with a particular client on a daily basis. Individual knowledge and

expertise and agency routines allow the flexibility that is necessary to adapt to the changing needs of the client. Legal and ethical concerns related to interventions also must be considered. For example, the wishes of the client and family/significant others regarding interventions and treatments must be discussed and respected. Before implementing the interventions in the plan of care, the nurse needs to understand the reason for doing each intervention, its expected effect, and any potential hazards that can occur. The nurse must also be sure that the interventions are: a) consistent with the established plan of care, b) implemented in a safe and appropriate manner, c) evaluated for effectiveness, and d) documented in a timely manner.

5. *Evaluation* is accomplished by determining the client's progress toward attaining the identified outcomes and by monitoring the client's response to/effectiveness of the selected nursing interventions for the purpose of altering the plan as indicated. This is done by direct observation of the client, interviewing the client/significant other, and/or reviewing the client's healthcare record. Although the process of evaluation seems similar to the activity of assessment, there are important differences. Evaluation is an ongoing process, a constant measuring and monitoring of the client status to determine: a) appropriateness of nursing actions, b) the need to revise interventions, c) development of new client needs, d) the need for referral to other resources, and e) the need to rearrange priorities to meet changing demands of care. Comparing overall outcomes and noting the effectiveness of specific interventions are the clinical components of evaluation that can become the basis for research for validating the nursing process and supporting evidenced-based practice. The external evaluation process is the key for refining standards of care and determining the protocols, policies, and procedures necessary for the provision of quality nursing care for a specific situation or setting.

When a client enters the healthcare system, whether as an acute care, clinic, or homecare client, the steps of the process noted above are set in motion. Although these steps are presented as separate or individual activities, the nursing process is an interactive method of practicing nursing, with the components fitting together in a continuous cycle of thought and action.

To effectively use the nursing process, the nurse must possess, and be able to apply, certain skills. Particularly important is a thorough knowledge of science and theory, as applied not only in nursing but also in other related disciplines, such as medicine and psychology. A sense of caring, intelligence, and competent technical skills are also essential. Creativity is needed in the application of nursing knowledge as well as adaptability for handling constant change in healthcare delivery and the many unexpected happenings that occur in the everyday practice of nursing.

Because decision making is crucial to each step of the process, the following assumptions are important for the nurse to consider:

- The client is a human being who has worth and dignity. This entitles the client to participate in his or her own healthcare decisions and delivery. It requires a sense of the personal in each individual and the delivery of competent healthcare.
- There are basic human needs that must be met, and when they are not, problems arise that may require interventions by others until and if the individual can resume responsibility for self. This requires healthcare providers to anticipate and initiate actions necessary to save another's life or to secure the client's return to health and independence.
- The client has the right to quality health and nursing care delivered with interest, compassion, competence, and a focus on wellness and prevention of illness. The philosophy of caring encompasses all of these qualities.
- The therapeutic nurse-client relationship is important in this process, providing a milieu in which the client can feel safe to disclose and talk about his or her deepest concerns.

In 1995, ANA acknowledged that since the release of the original statement, nursing has been influenced by many social and professional changes as well as by the science of caring. Nursing integrated these changes with the 1980 definition to include treatment of human responses to health and illness (*Nursing's Social Policy Statement,* ANA, 1995). The revised statement provided four essential features of today's contemporary nursing practice:

- Attention to the full range of human experiences and responses to health and illness without restriction to a problem-focused orientation (in short, clients may have needs for wellness or personal growth that are not "problems" to be corrected)
- Integration of objective data with knowledge gained from an understanding of the client's or group's subjective experience
- Application of scientific knowledge to the process of diagnosis and treatment
- Provision of a caring relationship that facilitates health and healing

In 2003, the definition of nursing was further expanded to reflect nursings' role in wellness promotion and responsibility to its clients, wherever they may be found. Therefore, "nursing is the protection, promotion, and optimization of health and abilities, prevention of illness and injury, alleviation of suffering through the diagnosis and treatment of human response, and advocacy in the care of individuals, families, communities, and populations" (*Social Policy Statement,* ANA, 2003, p 6).

Today our understanding of what nursing is and what nurses do continues to evolve. Whereas nursing actions were once based on variables such as diagnostic tests and medical diagnoses, use of the nursing process and nursing diagnoses provide a uniform method of identifying and dealing with specific client needs/responses in which the nurse can intervene. The nursing diagnosis is thus helping to set standards for nursing practice and should lead to improved care delivery.

Nursing and medicine are interrelated and have implications for each other. This interrelationship includes the exchange of data, the sharing of ideas/thinking, and the development of plans of care that include all data pertinent to the individual client as well as the family/significant others. Although nurses work within medical and psychosocial domains, nursing's phenomena of concern are the patterns of human response, not disease processes. Thus, the written plan of care should contain more than just nursing actions in response to medical orders and may reflect plans of care encompassing all involved disciplines to provide holistic care for the individual/family.

Summary

Because the nursing process is the basis of all nursing action, it is the essence of nursing. It can be applied in any healthcare or educational setting, in any theoretical or conceptual framework, and within the context of any nursing philosophy. In using nursing diagnosis labels as an integral part of the nursing process, the nursing profession has identified a body of knowledge that contributes to the prevention of illness as well as the maintenance/restoration of health (or the relief of pain and discomfort when a return to health is not possible). Subsequent chapters help the nurse applying the nursing process to review the current NANDA-I list of nursing diagnoses, their definition, related/risk factors (etiology), and defining characteristics. Aware of desired outcomes and commonly used interventions, the nurse can develop, implement, and document an individualized plan of care.

CHAPTER 2

Application of the Nursing Process

Because of their hectic schedules, many nurses believe that time spent writing a plan of care is time taken away from client care. Plans of care have been viewed as "busy work" to satisfy accreditation requirements or the whims of supervisors. In reality, however, quality client care must be planned and coordinated. Properly written and used plans of care can save time by providing direction and continuity of care and by facilitating communication among nurses and other caregivers. They also provide guidelines for documentation and tools for evaluating the care provided.

The components of a plan of care are based on the nursing process presented in the first chapter. Creating a plan of care begins with the collection of data (assessment). The client database consists of subjective and objective information encompassing the various concerns reflected in the current NANDA International (NANDA-I, formerly the North American Nursing Diagnosis Association) list of nursing diagnoses (NDs) (Table 2–1). Subjective data are those that are reported by the client (and significant others [SOs]) in the individual's own words. This information includes the individual's perceptions and what he or she wants to share. It is important to accept what is reported because the client is the "expert" in this area. Objective data are those that are observed or described (quantitatively or qualitatively) and include findings from diagnostic testing and physical examination and information from old medical records and other healthcare providers.

Analysis of the collected data leads to the identification or diagnosis of problems or areas of concern/need (including health promotion) specific to the client. These problems or needs are expressed as nursing diagnoses. The diagnosis of client needs has been determined by nurses on an informal basis since the beginning of the profession. The term *nursing diagnosis* came into formal use in the nursing literature during the 1950s (Fry, 1953), although its meaning continued to be seen in the context of medical diagnosis. In 1973, a national conference was held to identify client needs that fall within the scope of nursing, label them, and develop a classification system that

Table 2-1. NURSING DIAGNOSES ACCEPTED FOR USE AND RESEARCH (2007–2008)

Activity Intolerance [specify level]
Activity Intolerance, risk for
Airway Clearance, ineffective
*Allergy Response, latex
*Allergy Response, risk for latex
Anxiety [specify level]
*Anxiety, death
Aspiration, risk for
Attachment, risk for impaired parent/child
Autonomic Dysreflexia
Autonomic Dysreflexia, risk for

*Behavior, risk-prone health (previously Adjustment, impaired)
Body Image, disturbed
Body Temperature, risk for imbalanced
Bowel Incontinence
Breastfeeding, effective
Breastfeeding, ineffective
Breastfeeding, interrupted
Breathing Pattern, ineffective

Cardiac Output, decreased
Caregiver Role Strain
Caregiver Role Strain, risk for
+Comfort, readiness for enhanced
Communication, impaired verbal
Communication, readiness for enhanced
*Conflict, decisional (specify)
Conflict, parental role
*Confusion, acute
+Confusion, risk for acute
Confusion, chronic
Constipation
Constipation, perceived
Constipation, risk for
+Contamination
+Contamination, risk for
Coping, compromised family
Coping, defensive
Coping, disabled family
Coping, ineffective
Coping, ineffective community
Coping, readiness for enhanced
Coping, readiness for enhanced community
Coping, readiness for enhanced family

+New to the 4th NANDA/NIC/NOC (NNN) Conference
*Revised ND

Table 2–1. *(Continued)*

Death Syndrome, risk for sudden infant
+Decision Making, readiness for enhanced
*Denial, ineffective
Dentition, impaired
Development, risk for delayed
Diarrhea
+Dignity, risk for compromised human
+Distress, moral
Disuse Syndrome, risk for
Diversional Activity, deficient

Energy Field, disturbed
Environmental Interpretation Syndrome, impaired

Failure to Thrive, adult
Falls, risk for
Family Processes: alcoholism, dysfunctional
Family Processes, interrupted
Family Processes, readiness for enhanced
Fatigue
Fear [specify focus]
Fluid Balance, readiness for enhanced
[Fluid Volume, deficient hyper/hypotonic]
Fluid Volume, deficient [isotonic]
Fluid Volume, excess
Fluid Volume, risk for deficient
Fluid Volume, risk for imbalanced

Gas Exchange, impaired
+Glucose, risk for unstable blood
*Grieving (previously Grieving, anticipatory)
*Grieving, complicated (previously Grieving, dysfunctional)
*Grieving, risk for complicated (previously Grieving, risk for
   dysfunctional)
Growth, risk for disproportionate
Growth and Development, delayed

Health Maintenance, ineffective
Health-Seeking Behaviors (specify)
Home Maintenance, impaired
+Hope, readiness for enhanced
Hopelessness
Hyperthermia
Hypothermia

Identity, disturbed personal
+Immunization Status, readiness for enhanced

(Continued)

+New to the 4th NANDA/NIC/NOC (NNN) Conference
*Revised ND

Infant Behavior, disorganized
Infant Behavior, readiness for enhanced organized
Infant Behavior, risk for disorganized
*Infant Feeding Pattern, ineffective
Infection, risk for
Injury, risk for
*Injury, risk for perioperative positioning
*Insomnia (replaced Sleep Pattern, disturbed)
Intracranial Adaptive Capacity, decreased

Knowledge, deficient [Learning Need] (specify)
Knowledge (specify), readiness for enhanced

Lifestyle, sedentary
+Liver Function, risk for impaired
*Loneliness, risk for

Memory, impaired
*Mobility, impaired bed
Mobility, impaired physical
*Mobility, impaired wheelchair

Nausea
*Neglect, unilateral
Noncompliance [ineffective Adherence] [specify]
Nutrition: less than body requirements, imbalanced
Nutrition: more than body requirements, imbalanced
Nutrition: more than body requirements, risk for imbalanced
Nutrition, readiness for enhanced

Oral Mucous Membrane, impaired

Pain, acute
Pain, chronic
Parenting, impaired
Parenting, readiness for enhanced
Parenting, risk for impaired
Peripheral Neurovascular Dysfunction, risk for
*Poisoning, risk for
Post-Trauma Syndrome [specify stage]
Post-Trauma Syndrome, risk for
+Power, readiness for enhanced
Powerlessness [specify level]
Powerlessness, risk for
Protection, ineffective

Rape-Trauma Syndrome

+New to the 4th NANDA/NIC/NOC (NNN) Conference
*Revised ND

Table 2–1. *(Continued)*

Rape-Trauma Syndrome: compound reaction
Rape-Trauma Syndrome: silent reaction
Religiosity, impaired
Religiosity, readiness for enhanced
Religiosity, risk for impaired
Relocation Stress Syndrome
Relocation Stress Syndrome, risk for
Role Performance, ineffective

+Self-Care, readiness for enhanced
Self-Care Deficit, bathing/hygiene
Self-Care Deficit, dressing/grooming
Self-Care Deficit, feeding
Self-Care Deficit, toileting
Self-Concept, readiness for enhanced
Self-Esteem, chronic low
Self-Esteem, situational low
Self-Esteem, risk for situational low
Self-Mutilation
Self-Mutilation, risk for
Sensory Perception, disturbed (specify: visual, auditory, kinesthetic,
    gustatory, tactile, olfactory)
*Sexual Dysfunction
*Sexuality Pattern, ineffective
Skin Integrity, impaired
Skin Integrity, risk for impaired
Sleep, readiness for enhanced
Sleep Deprivation
Social Interaction, impaired
Social Isolation
Sorrow, chronic
Spiritual Distress
Spiritual Distress, risk for
Spiritual Well-Being, readiness for enhanced
+Stress Overload
Suffocation, risk for
Suicide, risk for
*Surgical Recovery, delayed
Swallowing, impaired

Therapeutic Regimen Management, effective
Therapeutic Regimen Management, ineffective community
Therapeutic Regimen Management, ineffective family
Therapeutic Regimen Management, ineffective
Therapeutic Regimen Management, readiness for enhanced

(*Continued*)

    +New to the 4th NANDA/NIC/NOC (NNN) Conference
    *Revised ND

Thermoregulation, ineffective
Thought Processes, disturbed
Tissue Integrity, impaired
Tissue Perfusion, ineffective (specify type: renal, cerebral, cardiopul-
 monary, gastrointestinal, peripheral)
*Transfer Ability, impaired
Trauma, risk for

*Urinary Elimination, impaired
Urinary Elimination, readiness for enhanced
Urinary Incontinence, functional
+Urinary Incontinence, overflow
Urinary Incontinence, reflex
*Urinary Incontinence, stress
Urinary Incontinence, total
*Urinary Incontinence, urge
Urinary Incontinence, risk for urge
Urinary Retention [acute/chronic]

Ventilation, impaired spontaneous
Ventilatory Weaning Response, dysfunctional
Violence, [actual/] risk for other-directed
Violence, [actual/] risk for self-directed

*Walking, impaired
Wandering [specify sporadic or continuous]

+New to the 4th NANDA/NIC/NOC (NNN) Conference
*Revised ND
 Used with permission from NANDA International: Definitions
and Classification, 2007–2008. NANDA, Philadelphia, 2007.
 Information in brackets added by authors to clarify and enhance
the use of nursing diagnoses.
 Please also see the NANDA diagnoses grouped according to
Gordon's Functional Health Patterns on the inside front cover.

could be used by nurses throughout the world. They called the labels *nursing diagnoses,* which represent clinical judgments about an individual's, family's, or community's responses to actual or potential health problems/life processes. Therefore, a nursing diagnosis (ND) is a decision about a need/problem that requires nursing intervention and management. The need may be anything that interferes with the quality of life the client is used to and/or desires. It includes concerns of the client, SOs, and/or nurse. The ND focuses attention on a physical or behavioral response, either a current need or a problem at risk for developing.

The identification of client needs and selection of an ND label involve the use of experience, expertise, and intuition. A six-step diagnostic reasoning/critical thinking process facilitates an accurate analysis of the client assessment data to determine specific client needs. First, data are reviewed to identify cues (signs and symptoms) reflecting client needs that can be described by ND labels. This is called *problem-sensing.* Next, alternative explanations are considered for the identified cues to determine which ND label may be the most appropriate. As the relationships among data are compared, etiological factors are identified based on the nurse's understanding of the biological, physical, and behavioral sciences, and the possible ND choices are *ruled out* until the most appropriate label remains. Next, a comprehensive picture of the client's past, present, and future health status is *synthesized,* and the suggested nursing diagnosis label is combined with the identified related (or risk) factors and cues to create a hypothesis. *Confirming the hypothesis* is done by reviewing the NANDA definition, defining characteristics (cues), and determining related factors (etiology) for the chosen ND to ensure the accuracy and objectivity in this diagnostic process. Now, based on the synthesis of the data (step 3) and evaluation of the hypothesis (step 4), the *client's needs are listed* and the correct ND label is combined with the assessed etiology and signs/symptoms to finalize the client diagnostic statement. Once all the NDs are identified, the problem list is *re-evaluated,* assessment data are reviewed again, and the client is consulted to ensure that all areas of concern have been addressed.

When the ND label is combined with the individual's specific related/risk factors and defining characteristics (as appropriate), the resulting client diagnostic statement provides direction for nursing care. It is important to remember that the affective tone of the ND can shape expectations of the client's response and/or influence the nurse's behavior toward the client.

The development and classification of NDs have continued through the years on a regular basis spurred on by the need to describe what nursing does in conjunction with changes in healthcare delivery and reimbursement, the expansion of nursing's role, and the dawning of the computer age. The advent of alternative healthcare settings (e.g., outpatient surgery centers, home health, rehabilitation or sub-acute units, extended or long-term care facilities) increases the need for a commonality of communication to ensure continuity of care for the client, who moves from one setting or level of care to another. The efficient documentation of the client encounter, whether that is a single office visit or a lengthy hospitalization, and the movement toward a paperless (computerized or electronic) client record have strengthened the need for standardizing nursing language to better demonstrate what nursing is and what nursing does.

NANDA-I nursing diagnosis is one of the standardized nursing languages recognized by the American Nurses Association (ANA) as providing clinically useful terminology that supports nursing practice. NANDA-I has also established a liaison with the International Council of Nursing to support and contribute to the global effort to standardize the language of healthcare with the goal that NANDA-I NDs will be included in the International Classification of Diseases. In the meantime, they are included in the United States version of International Classification of Diseases-Clinical Modifications (ICD-10CM). The NANDA nursing diagnosis labels have also been combined with Nursing Interventions Classification (NIC) and Nursing Outcomes Classification (NOC) to create a complete nursing language that has been coded into the Systematized Nomenclature of Medicine (SNOMED). Inclusion in an international coded terminology such as SNOMED is essential if nursing's contribution to healthcare is to be recognized in the computer database. Indexing of the entire medical record supports disease management activities, research, and analysis of outcomes for quality improvement for all healthcare disciplines. Coding also supports telehealth (the use of telecommunications technology to provide healthcare information and services over distance) and facilitates access to healthcare data across care settings and various computer systems.

The key to accurate diagnosis is collection and analysis of data. In Chapter 3, the NDs have been categorized into divisions (Diagnostic Divisions: Nursing Diagnoses Organized According to a Nursing Focus, Section 2), and a sample assessment tool designed to assist the nurse to identify appropriate NDs as the data are collected is provided. Nurses may feel at risk in committing themselves to documenting an ND for fear they might be wrong. However, unlike medical diagnoses, NDs can change as the client progresses through various stages of illness/maladaptation to resolution of the condition/situation.

Desired outcomes are then formulated to give direction to, as well as to evaluate, the care provided. These outcomes emerge from the diagnostic statement and are what the client hopes to achieve. They serve as the guidelines to evaluate progress toward resolution of needs/problems, providing impetus for revising the plan as appropriate. In this book, outcomes are stated in general terms to permit the practitioner to individualize them by adding timelines and other data according to specific client circumstances. Outcome terminology needs to be concise, realistic, measurable, and stated in words the client can understand, because they indicate what the client is expected to do or accomplish. Beginning the outcome statement with an action verb provides measurable direction, for example, "Verbalizes relationship between diabetes mellitus and circulatory changes in feet within 2 days" or "Correctly performs procedure of home glucose monitoring within 48 hours."

Interventions are the activities taken to achieve the desired outcomes and, because they are communicated to others, they must be clearly stated. A solid nursing knowledge base is vital to this process because the rationale for interventions needs to be sound and feasible with the intention of providing effective, individualized care. The actions may be independent or collaborative and may encompass specific orders from nursing, medicine, and other disciplines. Written interventions that guide ongoing client care need to be dated and signed. To facilitate the planning process, specific nursing priorities have been identified in this text to provide a general ranking of interventions. This ranking would be altered according to individual client situations. The seasoned practitioner may choose to use these as broad-based interventions. The student or beginning practitioner may need to develop a more detailed plan of care by including the appropriate interventions listed under each nursing priority. It is important to remember that because each client usually has a perception of individual needs or problems he or she faces and an expectation of what could be done about the situation, the plan of care must be congruent with the client's reality or it will fail. In short, the nurse needs to plan care with the client, because both are accountable for that care and for achieving the desired outcomes.

The plan of care is the end product of the nursing process and documents client care in areas of accountability, quality assurance, and liability. Therefore, the plan of care is a permanent part of the client's healthcare record. The format for recording the plan of care is determined by agency policy and may be handwritten, standardized forms or clinical pathways, or computer-generated documentation. Before implementing the plan of care, it should be reviewed to ensure that:

- It is based on accepted nursing practice, reflecting knowledge of scientific principles, nursing standards of care, and agency policies.

- It provides for the safety of the client by ensuring that the care provided will do no harm.
- The client diagnostic statements are supported by the client data.
- The goals and outcomes are measurable/observable and can be achieved.
- The interventions can benefit the client/family/significant others in a predictable way in achieving the identified outcomes, and they are arranged in a logical sequence.
- It demonstrates individualized client care by reflecting the concerns of the client and significant others, as well as their physical, psychosocial, and cultural needs and capabilities.

Once the plan of care is put into action, changes in the client's needs must be continually monitored because care is provided in a dynamic environment, and flexibility is required to allow changing circumstances. Periodic review of the client's response to nursing interventions and progress toward attaining the desired outcomes helps determine the effectiveness of the plan of care. Based on the findings, the plan may need to be modified or revised, referrals to other resources made, or the client may be ready for discharge from the care setting.

Summary

Healthcare providers have a responsibility for planning with the client and family for continuation of care to the eventual outcome of an optimal state of wellness or a dignified death. Today, the act of diagnosing client problems/needs is well-established and the use of standardized nursing language to describe what nursing does is rapidly becoming an integral part of an effective system of nursing practice. Although not yet comprehensive, the current NANDA-I list of diagnostic labels defines/refines professional nursing activity. With repeated use of NANDA-I NDs, strengths and weaknesses of the NDs can be identified, promoting research and further development.

Planning, setting goals, and choosing appropriate interventions are essential to the construction of a plan of care and delivery of quality nursing care. These nursing activities constitute the planning phase of the nursing process and are documented in the plan of care for a particular client. As a part of the client's permanent record, the plan of care not only provides a means for the nurse who is actively caring for the client to be aware of the client's needs (NDs), goals, and actions to be taken, but also substantiates the care provided for review by third-party payers and accreditation agencies, while meeting legal requirements.

CHAPTER 3

Putting Theory into Practice: Sample Assessment Tools, Plan of Care, Mind Mapping, and Documentation

The client assessment is the foundation on which identification of individual needs, responses, and problems is based. To facilitate the steps of assessment and diagnosis in the nursing process, an assessment tool (Assessment Tools for Choosing Nursing Diagnoses, Section 1) has been constructed using a nursing focus instead of the medical approach of "review of systems." This has the advantage of identifying and validating nursing diagnoses (NDs) as opposed to medical diagnoses.

To achieve this nursing focus, we have grouped the NANDA International (formerly the North American Nursing Diagnosis Association) NDs into related categories titled Diagnostic Divisions (Section 2), which reflect a blending of theories, primarily Maslow's Hierarchy of Needs and a self-care philosophy. These divisions serve as the framework or outline for data collection/clustering that focuses attention on the nurse's phenomena of concern—the human responses to health and illness—and directs the nurse to the most likely corresponding NDs.

Because the divisions are based on human responses and needs and not specific "systems," information may be recorded in more than one area. For this reason, the nurse is encouraged to keep an open mind, to pursue all leads, and to collect as much data as possible before choosing the ND label that best reflects the client's situation. For example, when the nurse identifies the cue of restlessness in a client, the nurse may infer that the client is anxious, assuming that the restlessness is psychologically based and overlook the possibility that it is physiologically based.

From the specific data recorded in the database, an individualized client diagnostic statement can be formulated using the problem, etiology, signs/symptoms (PES) format to accurately represent the client's situation. Whereas a medical diagnosis of diabetes mellitus is the same label used for all indivduals with this condition, the diagnostic statement developed by the nurse is individualized to reflect a specific client need. For example, the diagnostic statement may read, "deficient Knowledge regarding diabetic care, related to misinterpretation of information and/or lack of recall, evidenced by inaccurate follow-through of instructions and failure to recognize signs and symptoms of hyperglycemia."

Desired client outcomes are identified to facilitate choosing appropriate interventions and to serve as evaluators of both nursing care and client response. These outcomes also form the framework for documentation.

Interventions are designed to specify the action of the nurse, the client, and/or SOs. Interventions need to promote the client's movement toward health/independence in addition to achievement of physiological stability. This requires involvement of the client in his or her own care, including participation in decisions about care activities and projected outcomes.

Section 3, Client Situation and Prototype Plan of Care, contains a sample plan of care formulated on data collected in the nursing model assessment tool. Individualized client diagnostic statements and desired client outcomes (with timelines added to reflect anticipated length of stay and individual client/nurse expectations) have been identified. Interventions have been chosen based on concerns/needs identified by the client and nurse during data collection, as well as by physician orders.

Although not normally included in a written plan of care, rationales are included in this sample for the purpose of explaining or clarifying the choice of interventions to enhance the nurse's learning.

Another way to conceptualize the client's care needs is to create a *Mind Map*. This new technique or learning tool has been developed to help visualize the linkages or interconnections between various client symptoms, interventions, or problems as they impact each other. The parts that are great about traditional care plans (problem solving and categorizing) are retained, but the linear/columnar nature of the plan is changed to a design that uses the whole brain—a design that brings left-brained, linear problem-solving thinking together with the free-wheeling, interconnected, creative right brain. Joining mind mapping and care planning enables the nurse to create a holistic view of a client, strengthening critical thinking skills, and facilitating the creative process of planning client care.

Finally, to complete the learning experience, samples of documentation based on the client situation are presented in Section 4, Documentation Techniques. The plan of care provides documentation of the planning process and serves as a frame-work/outline for charting of administered care. The primary nurse needs to periodically review the client's progress and the effectiveness of the treatment plan. Other care providers then are able to read the notes and have a clear picture of what occurred with the client and make appropriate judgments regarding client management. The best way to ensure the clarity of progress notes is through the use of descriptive (or observa-tional) statements. Observations of client behavior and response to therapy provide invaluable information. Through this communication it can be determined if the client's current desired outcomes or interventions can be eliminated or need to be altered and if the development of new outcomes or interven-tions is warranted. Progress notes are an integral component of the overall medical record and should include all significant events that occur in the daily life of the client. They reflect implementation of the treatment plan and document that appropriate actions have been carried out, precautions taken, and so forth. It is important that both the implementation of interventions and progress toward the desired outcomes be doc-umented. The notes need to be written in a clear and objective fashion, specific as to date and time, and signed by the person making the entry.

Use of clear documentation helps the nurse to individualize client care. Providing a picture of what has happened and is happening promotes continuity of care and facilitates evalua-tion. This reinforces each person's accountability and responsi-bility for using the nursing process to provide individually appropriate and cost-effective client care.

ASSESSMENT TOOLS FOR CHOOSING NURSING DIAGNOSES

The following are suggested guidelines/tools for creating assessment databases reflecting Doenges & Moorhouse's Diagnostic Divisions of Nursing Diagnoses. They are intended to provide a nursing focus and should help the nurse think about planning care with the client at the center (following mind-mapping theory, see page 64) Although the divisions are alphabetized here for ease of presentation, they can be prioritized or rearranged to meet individual needs. In addition, the assessment tool can be adapted to meet the needs of specific client populations. Excerpts of assessment tools adapted for psychiatric and obstetric settings are included at the end of this section.

ADULT MEDICAL/SURGICAL ASSESSMENT TOOL

General Information

Name: _____ Age: _____ DOB: _____
Gender: _____
Race: _____
Admission: Date: _____ Time: _____ From: _____
Reason for this visit (primary concern): _____
Cultural concerns (relating to healthcare decisions, religious concerns, pain, childbirth, family involvement, communication, etc): _____
Source of information: _____ Reliability (1–4 with 4 = very reliable): _____

Activity/Rest

SUBJECTIVE (REPORTS)

Occupation: _____ Able to participate in usual activities/hobbies: _____
Leisure time/diversional activities: _____
Ambulatory: _____ Gait (describe): _____
Activity level (sedentary to very active): _____
    Daily exercise/type: _____
Muscle mass/tone/strength (e.g., normal, increased, decreased):
_____

History of problems/limitations imposed by condition (e.g., immobility, can't transfer, weakness, breathlessness):
_____

Feelings (e.g., exhaustion, restlessness, can't concentrate, dissatisfaction): _____
Developmental factors (e.g., delayed/age): _____
Sleep: Hours: _____ Naps: _____
Insomnia: _____ Related to: _____ Difficulty falling asleep: _____
Difficulty staying asleep: _____ Rested on awakening: _____
    Excessive grogginess: _____
Bedtime rituals: _____
Relaxation techniques: _____
Sleeps on more than one pillow: _____
Oxygen use (type): _____ When used:
_____
Medications or herbals for/affecting sleep: _____

Observed response to activity: Heart rate: _____
   Rhythm (reg/irreg): _____ Blood pressure: _____
   Respiration rate: _____ Pulse oximetry: _____
Mental status (i.e., cognitive impairment, withdrawn/lethargic):
_____

Muscle mass/tone: _____ Posture (e.g., normal,
   stooped, curved spine): _____
   Tremors: _____ (location): _____
   ROM: _____
   Strength: _____ Deformity: _____
Uses mobility aid (list): _____

Circulation

SUBJECTIVE (REPORTS)

History of/treatment for (date): High blood pressure: _____
   Brain injury: _____ Stroke: _____
   Heart problems/surgery: _____
   Palpitations: _____ Syncope: _____
   Cough/hemoptysis: _____Blood clots: _____
   Bleeding tendencies/episodes: _____ Pain in legs
   w/activity: _____
Extremities: Numbness: _____ (location): _____
   Tingling: _____ (location): _____
Slow healing/describe: _____
Change in frequency/amount of urine: _____
History of spinal cord injury/dysreflexia episodes: _____
Medications/herbals: _____

OBJECTIVE (EXHIBITS)

Color (e.g., pale, cyanotic, jaundiced, mottled, ruddy):
   Skin _____
   Mucous membranes: _____ Lips: _____
   Nail beds: _____ Conjunctiva: _____
   Sclera: _____
Skin moisture: (e.g., dry, diaphoretic): _____
BP: Lying: **R**_____ **L**_____ Sitting: **R**_____ **L**_____
   Standing: **R**_____ **L**_____ Pulse pressure: _____
   Auscultatory gap: _____
Pulses (palpated 1–4 strength): Carotid: _____ Temporal: _____
   Jugular: _____
   Radial: _____ Femoral: _____ Popliteal: _____
   Post-tibial: _____ Dorsalis pedis: _____
Cardiac (palpation): Thrill: _____ Heaves: _____

Heart sounds (auscultation): Rate: _____ Rhythm: _____
    Quality: _____ Friction rub: _____
    Murmur (describe location/sounds): _____
Vascular bruit (location): _____
Jugular vein distention: _____
Breath sounds (location/describe): _____
Extremities: Temperature: _____ Color: _____
    Capillary refill (1–3 sec): _____
    Homan's sign: _____ Varicosities (location): _____
    Nail abnormalities: _____
    Edema (location/severity +1–+4): _____
    Distribution/quality of hair: _____
    Trophic skin changes: _____

Ego Integrity

SUBJECTIVE (REPORTS)

Relationship status: _____ _____
Expression of concerns (e.g., financial, lifestyle, or role changes):

_____
Stress factors: _____
Usual ways of handling stress: _____
Expression of feelings: Anger: _____ Anxiety: _____
    Fear: _____ Grief: _____
    Helplessness: _____ Hopelessness: _____
    Powerlessness: _____
Cultural factors/ethnic ties: _____
Religious affiliation: _____ Active/practicing: _____
Practices prayer/meditation: _____
Religious/spiritual concerns: _____ Desires clergy visit: _____
Expression of sense of connectedness/harmony with self and
    others: _____
Medications/herbals: _____

OBJECTIVE (EXHIBITS)

Emotional status (<u>check</u> those that apply): Calm: _____
    Anxious: _____ Angry: _____
    Withdrawn: _____ Fearful: _____ Irritable: _____
    Restive: _____ Euphoric: _____
Observed body language: _____
Observed physiological responses (e.g., palpitations, crying,
    change in voice quality/volume): _____
Changes in energy field: Temperature: _____
    Color: _____ Distribution: _____
    Movement: _____
    Sounds: _____

Elimination

Usual bowel elimination pattern _____ Character
of stool (e.g., hard, soft, liquid): _____ Stool color
(e.g., brown, black, yellow, clay colored, tarry): _____
Date of last BM and character of stool: _____
History of bleeding: _____ Hemorrhoids/fistula: _____
Constipation acute: _____ or chronic: _____
Diarrhea: acute: _____ or chronic: _____
Bowel incontinence: _____
Laxative: _____ (how often): _____
   Enema/suppository: _____ (how often): _____
Usual voiding pattern and character of urine: _____
   Difficulty voiding: _____ Urgency: _____
   Frequency: _____
   Retention: _____ Bladder spasms: _____ Burning: _____
Urinary incontinence (type/time of day usually occurs):
_____
History of kidney/bladder disease: _____
Diuretic use: _____ Herbals: _____

OBJECTIVE (EXHIBITS)

Abdomen (palpation): Soft/firm: _____
   Tenderness/pain (quadrant location): _____
   Distention: _____ Palpable mass/location: _____
   Size/girth: _____
   Abdomen (auscultation): Bowel sounds (location/type):
_____
   CVA tenderness: _____
Bladder palpable: _____ Overflow voiding: _____
Rectal sphincter tone (describe): _____
Hemorrhoids/fistulas: _____ Stool in rectum: _____
   Impaction: _____ Occult blood (+ or −): _____
Presence/use of catheter or continence devices: _____
Ostomy appliances (describe appliance and location):
_____

Food/Fluid

SUBJECTIVE (REPORTS)

Usual diet (type): _____
Calorie/carbohydrate/protein/fat intake-g/day: _____
# of meals daily: _____
   snacks (number/time consumed): _____
Dietary pattern/content:
   B: _____ L: _____ D: _____
   Snacks: _____

Last meal consumed/content: _____
Food preferences: _____
Food allergies/intolerances: _____
Cultural or religious food preparation concerns/prohibitions:
_____
Usual appetite: _____ Change in appetite: _____
Usual weight: _____
Unexpected/undesired weight loss or gain: _____
Nausea/vomiting: _____ (related to) _____ Heartburn,
    indigestion: _____ (related to): ___ _____
    (relieved by): _____
Chewing/swallowing problems: _____
    Gag/swallow reflex present: _____
    Facial injury/surgery: _____
    Stroke/other neurological deficit: _____
Teeth: Normal: _____ Dentures (full/partial): _____
    Loose/absent teeth/poor dental care: _____
    Sore mouth/gums: _____
Diabetes: ____ Controlled with diet/pills/insulin: _____
Vitamin/food supplements: _____
Medications/herbals: _____

OBJECTIVE (EXHIBITS)

Current weight: _____ Height: _____ Body build: _____
    Body fat %: _____
Skin turgor (e.g., firm, supple, dehydrated): _____ Mucous
    membranes (moist/dry): _____
Edema: Generalized: ____ Dependent: ____ Feet/ankles: ____
    Periorbital: ____ Abdominal/ascites: _____
Jugular vein distention: _____
Breath sounds (auscultate)/location: Faint/distant: _____
    Crackles: _____
    Wheezes: _____
Condition of teeth/gums: _____
Appearance of tongue: _____
Mucous membranes: _____
Abdomen: Bowel sounds (quadrant location/type): _____
    Hernia/masses: _____
Urine S/A or Chemstix: _____
Serum glucose (Glucometer): _____

Hygiene

SUBJECTIVE (REPORTS)

Ability to carry out activities of daily living: Independent/
    dependent (level 1 = no assistance needed to 4 = completely
    dependent): _____

Mobility: _____ Assistance needed (describe): _____
   Assistance provided by: _____
   Equipment/prosthetic devices required: _____
Feeding: _____ Help with food preparation: _____
   Help with eating utensils: _____
Hygiene: _____ Get supplies: _____
   Wash body or body parts: _____
   Can regulate bath water temperature: _____
   Get in and out alone: _____
   Preferred time of personal care/bath: _____
Dressing: _____ Can select clothing and dress self: _____
   Needs assistance with (describe): _____
Toileting: _____ Can get to toilet or commode alone: _____
   Needs assistance with (describe): _____

OBJECTIVE (EXHIBITS)

General appearance: Manner of dress: _____
   Grooming/personal habits: _____ Condition of hair/scalp:
   _____ Body odor: _____
   Presence of vermin (e.g., lice, scabies):_____

Neurosensory

SUBJECTIVE (REPORTS)

History of brain injury, trauma, stroke (residual effects):
_____
Fainting spells/dizziness: _____
Headaches (location/type/frequency): _____
Tingling/numbness/weakness (location): _____
Seizures: _____ History or new onset seizures: _____
   Type (e.g., grand mal, partial): _____
   Frequency: _____ Aura: _____ Postictal state: _____
   How controlled: _____
Vision: Loss or changes in vision: _____
   Date last exam: _____ Glaucoma: _____
   Cataract: _____ Eye surgery (type/date): _____
Hearing loss: _____ Sudden or gradual: _____
   Date last exam: _____
Sense of smell (changes): _____
Sense of taste (changes): _____ Epistaxis: _____
Other: _____

OBJECTIVE (EXHIBITS)

Mental status: (note duration of change): _____
   Oriented/disoriented: Person: _____ Place: ____ Time: ____
Situation: _____
Check all that apply: Alert: ____ Drowsy: ____ Lethargic: ____
   Stuporous: _____ Comatose: _____

Cooperative: _____ Agitated/Restless: _____ Combative: _____
Follows commands: _____
Delusions (describe): _____ Hallucinations (describe):
_____

Affect (describe): _____ Speech: _____
Memory: Recent: _____ Remote: _____
Pupil shape: _____ Size/reaction: R/L: _____
Facial droop: _____ Swallowing: _____
Handgrasp/release: R: _____ L: _____
Coordination: _____ Balance: _____
Walking: _____
Deep tendon reflexes (present/absent/location): _____
Tremors: _____ Paralysis (R/L): _____
Posturing: _____
Wears glasses: _____ Contacts: _____ Hearing aids: _____

Pain/Discomfort

SUBJECTIVE (REPORTS)

Primary focus: _____ Location: _____
Intensity (use pain scale or pictures): _____
Quality (e.g., stabbing, aching, burning): _____
Radiation:_____ Duration: _____
Frequency: _____
Precipitating factors:_____
Relieving factors (including nonpharmaceuticals/therapies):
_____

Associated symptoms (e.g., nausea, sleep problems, crying):
_____

Effect on daily activities: _____
Relationships: _____ Job: _____ Enjoyment of life: _____
Additional pain focus/describe: _____
Medications: _____ Herbals: _____

OBJECTIVE (EXHIBITS)

Facial grimacing: _____ Guarding affected area: _____
Emotional response (e.g., crying, withdrawal, anger): _____
Narrowed focus: _____
Vitals sign changes (acute pain): BP: _____ Pulse: _____
Respirations: _____

Respiration

SUBJECTIVE (REPORTS)

Dyspnea/related to: _____
Precipitating factors: _____
Relieving factors: _____

Airway clearance (e.g., spontaneous/device): _____
Cough/describe (e.g., hard, persistent, croupy): _____
   Produces sputum (describe color/character): _____
   Requires suctioning: _____
History of (year): Bronchitis: _____ Asthma: _____
   Emphysema: _____ Tuberculosis: _____
   Recurrent pneumonia: _____
   Exposure to noxious fumes/allergens, infectious agents/
   diseases, poisons/pesticides: _____
Smoker: _____ packs/day: _____ # of years: _____
Use of respiratory aids: _____
   Oxygen (type/frequency):_____
Medications/herbals: _____

OBJECTIVE (EXHIBITS)

Respirations (spontaneous/assisted): _____ Rate: _____
   Depth: _____
   Chest excursion (e.g., equal/unequal): _____
   Use of accessory muscles: _____
   Nasal flaring: _____ Fremitus: _____
Breath sounds (presence/absence; crackle, wheezes): _____
   Egophony: _____
Skin/mucous membrane color (e.g., pale, cyanotic): _____
Clubbing of fingers: _____
   Sputum characteristics: _____
Mentation (e.g., calm, anxious, restless): _____
Pulse oximetry:_____

Safety

SUBJECTIVE (REPORTS)

Allergies/sensitivity (medications, foods, environment, latex):
_____
   Type of reaction: _____
Exposure to infectious diseases (e.g., measles, influenza, pink eye):
_____
Exposure to pollution, toxins, poisons/pesticides, radiation
   (describe reactions): _____
Geographic areas lived in/visited:_____
Immunization history: Tetanus: _____ Pneumonia: _____
   Influenza: _____ MMR: _____ Polio: _____ Hepatitis: _____
   HPV: _____
Altered/suppressed immune system (list cause): _____
History of sexually transmitted disease (date/type): _____
   Testing: _____
High risk behaviors: _____
Blood transfusion/number: _____ Date: _____
   Reaction (describe): _____

Uses seat belt regularly: _____ Bike helmets: _____
  Other safety devices:_____
Work place safety/health issues (describe): _____
  Currently working: _____
  Rate working conditions (e.g., safety, noise, heating, water,
  ventilation): _____
History of accidental injuries: _____
Fractures/dislocations: _____
Arthritis/unstable joints: _____
  Back problems: _____
Skin problems (e.g., rashes, lesions, moles, breast lumps,
  enlarged nodes)/describe:_____
Delayed healing (describe): _____
Cognitive limitations (e.g., disorientation, confusion):

_____
Sensory limitations (e.g., impaired vision/hearing, detecting
  heat/cold, taste, smell, touch): _____
Prostheses: _____ Ambulatory devices: _____
Violence (episodes or tendencies):_____

OBJECTIVE (EXHIBITS)

Body temperature/method: (e.g., oral, rectal, tympanic):

_____
Skin integrity (e.g., scars, rashes, lacerations, ulcerations,
  bruises, blisters, burns [degree/%], drainage)/mark location
  on diagram: _____
Musculoskeletal: General strength: _____
  Muscle tone: _____ Gait: _____
  ROM: _____ Paresthesia/paralysis: _____
Results of testing (e.g., cultures, immune function, TB, hepatitis):

_____

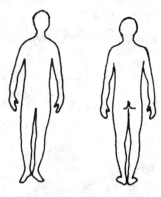

Sexuality [Component of Social Interaction]

SUBJECTIVE (REPORTS)

Sexually active: _____ Birth control method: _____
  Use of condoms: _____
Sexual concerns/difficulties (e.g., pain, relationship, role):
_____
Recent change in frequency/interest: _____

FEMALE: SUBJECTIVE (REPORTS)

Menstruation: Age at menarche: _____
  Length of cycle: _____ Duration: _____
  Number of pads/tampons used/day: _____
  Last menstrual period: _____ Bleeding between periods: _____
Reproductive: Infertility concerns: _____
  Type of therapy: _____
  Pregnant now: _____ Para: _____ Gravida: _____
  Due date: _____
Menopause: _____ Last period: _____
  Hysterectomy (type/date): _____
  Problem with: Hot flashes: _____
  Vaginal lubrication: _____ Vaginal discharge: _____
Hormonal therapies: _____
Osteoporosis medications: _____
Breasts: Practices breast self-exam: _____
  Last mammogram: _____
Last PAP smear: _____ Results: _____

OBJECTIVE (EXHIBITS)

Breast examination: _____
Genitalia: Warts/lesions: _____
Vaginal bleeding/discharge: _____
STD test results: _____

MALE: SUBJECTIVE (REPORTS)

Circumcised: _____ Vasectomy (date): _____
Prostate disorder: _____
Practice self-exam: Breast: _____ Testicles: _____
Last proctoscopic/prostate exam: _____
  Last PSA/date: _____
Medications/herbals: _____

OBJECTIVE (EXHIBITS)

Genitalia: Penis: Circumcised: _____ Warts/lesions _____
  Bleeding/discharge: _____
Testicles (e.g., lumps): _____ Vasectomy: _____
Breast examination: _____ STD test results: _____

Social Interactions

SUBJECTIVE (REPORTS)

Relationship status (check): Single _____ Married _____
  Living with partner: ____ Divorced: _____ Widowed: ____
  Years in relationship: _____ Perception of
  relationship: _____
  Concerns/stresses: _____
  Role within family structure: _____
  Number/age of children: _____
  Perception of relationship with family members:
  _____
Extended family: _____ Other support person(s): _____
Ethnic/cultural affiliations: _____
  Strength of ethnic identity: _____
  Lives in ethnic community: _____
Feelings of (describe): Mistrust: _____
  Rejection: _____ Unhappiness: _____
  Loneliness/isolation: _____
Problems related to illness/condition: _____
Problems with communication (e.g., speech, another language,
  brain injury): _____
  Use of speech/communication aids (list): _____
  Is interpreter needed: _____
  Primary language: _____
Genogram: Diagram on separate page

OBJECTIVE (EXHIBITS)

Communication/speech: Clear: _____ Slurred: _____
  Unintelligible: _____
  Aphasic: _____
  Unusual speech pattern/impairment: _____
  Laryngectomy present: _____
Verbal/nonverbal communication with family/SO(s):
  _____
  Family interaction (behavioral) pattern: _____
  _____

Teaching/Learning

SUBJECTIVE (REPORTS)

Communication: Dominant language (specify): _____
  Second language: _____ Literate (reading/writing): _____
  Education level: _____
  Learning disabilities (specify): _____
  Cognitive limitations: _____
Culture/ethnicity: Where born: _____
  If immigrant, how long in this country: _____

Health and illness beliefs/practices/customs: _____

Which family member makes healthcare decisions/is spokesperson for client: _____

Presence of Advance Directives: _____ Code status: _____
  Durable Medical Power of Attorney: ___ Designee: _____

Health goals: _____

Current health problem: Client understanding of problem:
_____

Special healthcare concerns (e.g., impact of religious/cultural
  practices): _____

Familial risk factors (indicate relationship):
  Diabetes: _____ Thyroid (specify): _____
  Tuberculosis: _____ Heart disease: _____
  Stroke: _____ Hypertension: _____
  Epilepsy/seizures: _____ Kidney disease: _____
  Cancer: _____ Mental illness/depression: _____
  Other: _____

Prescribed medications:
  Drug: _____ Dose: _____
  Times (circle last dose): _____
  Take regularly: _____ Purpose: _____
  Side effects/problems: _____

Nonprescription drugs/frequency: OTC drugs: _____
  Vitamins: _____ Herbals: _____
  Street drugs: _____
  Alcohol (amount/frequency): _____
  Tobacco: _____ Smokeless tobacco: _____

Admitting diagnosis per provider: _____

Reason for hospitalization per client: _____

History of current complaint: _____

Expectations of this hospitalization: _____

Will admission cause any lifestyle changes (describe):
_____

Previous illnesses and/or hospitalizations/surgeries:
_____

Evidence of failure to improve: _____

Last complete physical exam: _____

Discharge Plan Considerations

Projected length of stay (days or hours): _____
Anticipated date of discharge: _____
Date information obtained: _____
Resources available: Persons: _____
  Financial: _____ Community supports: _____
  Groups: _____

Areas that may require alteration/assistance:

Food preparation: _____ Shopping: _____

Transportation: _____ Ambulation: _____

Medication/IV therapy: _____

Treatments: _____

Wound care: _____

Supplies: _____

Self-care (specify): _____

Homemaker/maintenance (specify): _____

Socialization: _____

Physical layout of home (specify): _____

Anticipated changes in living situation after discharge:

_____

Living facility other than home (specify): _____

Referrals (date/source/services): Social services: _____

Rehab services: _____ Dietary: _____

Home care: _____ Resp/O_2: _____

Equipment: _____

Supplies: _____

Other: _____

EXCERPT FROM PSYCHIATRIC NURSING ASSESSMENT TOOL

Ego Integrity

SUBJECTIVE (REPORTS)

What kind of person are you (positive/negative, etc.)?_____
What do you think of your body? _____
How would you rate your self-esteem (1–10; with 10 the
    highest)? _____
What are your problematic moods? Depressed: _____
    Guilty: _____ Unreal: _____
    Ups/downs: _____ Apathetic: _____
    Separated from the world: _____
    Detached: _____
Are you a nervous person? ___ Are your feelings easily hurt? ___
Report of stress factors: _____
    Previous patterns of handling stress: _____
Financial concerns: _____
Relationship status: _____
Work history/military service: _____
Cultural/ethnic factors: _____
Religion: _____ Practicing: _____
Lifestyle: _____ Recent changes: _____
    Significant losses/changes (dates): _____
Stages of grief/manifestations of loss: _____
Feelings of (check those that apply): Helplessness: _____
    Hopelessness: _____
    Powerlessness: _____ Restive: _____ Passive: _____
    Dependent: _____ Euphoric: _____
    Angry/hostile: _____ Other (specify): _____

OBJECTIVE (EXHIBITS)

Emotional status (check those that apply): Calm: _____
    Friendly: _____ Cooperative: _____
    Evasive: __ Fearful: __ Anxious: __ Irritable: __Withdrawn: __
Defense mechanisms:
    Projection: _____ Denial: _____ Undoing: _____
    Rationalization: _____ Repression: _____
    Regression: _____
    Passive/aggressive: _____ Sublimation: _____
    Intellectualization: _____ Somatization: _____
    Identification: _____ Introjection: _____
    Reaction formation: _____
    Isolation: _____ Displacement: _____
    Substitution: _____

Consistency of behavior: Verbal _____ Nonverbal: _____
Characteristics of speech: _____
   Slow/rapid: _____ Pressured: _____
   Volume: _____ Impairments: _____
   Aphasia: _____
Motor behaviors: _____ Posturing: _____
   Restless:_____
   Underactive/overactive: _____
   Stereotypic: _____Tics/tremors: _____
   Gait patterns: _____
Observed physiological response(s): _____

Neurosensory

SUBJECTIVE (REPORTS)

Dreamlike states: _____ Walking in sleep: _____
   Automatic writing: _____
Believe/feel you are another person:_____
Perception different than others: _____
Ability to follow directions: _____
   Perform calculations: _____
   Accomplish ADL: _____
Fainting spells/dizziness: _____Blackouts: _____
   Seizures: _____

OBJECTIVE (EXHIBITS)

Mental status (note duration of change):_____
Oriented: Person: _____ Place: _____ Time: _____
Check all that apply: Alert: ____ Drowsy: ____ Lethargic: ____
   Stuporous: _____ Comatose: _____
   Cooperative: __ Combative: __ Delusions: __ Hallucinations: __
Memory: Immediate: _____ Recent: _____ Remote: _____
   Comprehension: _____
Thought processes (assessed through speech): Patterns of
   speech (e.g., spontaneous/sudden silences):_____
   Content: _____ Change in topic: _____
   Delusions: _____ Hallucinations: _____
   Illusions: _____
   Rate or flow: _____ Clear, logical progression: _____
   Expression: _____ Flight of ideas: _____
   Ability to concentrate: _____ Attention span: _____
Mood: Affect: _____ Appropriateness: _____
   Intensity: _____
   Range: _____
Insight: _____ Misperceptions: _____
Attention/calculation skills: _____
   Judgment:_____

Ability to follow directions: _____

Problem solving: _____

Impulse control: Aggression: _____ Hostility: _____

Affection: _____

Sexual feelings: _____

EXCERPT FROM PRENATAL ASSESSMENT TOOL

Safety

SUBJECTIVE (REPORTS)

Allergies/sensitivity: _____

  Reaction: _____

Previous alteration of immune system: _____

  Cause: _____

History of sexually transmitted diseases/gynecologic infections

  (date/type): _____

  Testing/date: _____

High-risk behaviors:_____

Blood transfusion/number: _____ When: _____

  Reaction: _____

  Describe: _____

Childhood diseases: _ _____

  Immunization history/date: Tetanus: _____

  Pneumonia: _____

  Influenza: _____ Hepatitis: _____ MMR: _____

  Polio: _____ HPV: _____

Recent exposure to German measles: _____

  Other viral infections: _____

  X-ray/radiation: _____ House pets: _____

Previous obstetric problems: PIH: _____ Kidney: _____

  Hemorrhage: _____ Cardiac: _____

  Diabetes: ___ Infection/UTI: ___ ABO/Rh sensitivity: ___

  Uterine surgery: _____

  Anemia: ___ Explain "yeses": _____

Length of time since last pregnancy: _____

  Type of previous delivery: _____

History of accidental injuries: Fractures/dislocations: _____

  Physical abuse: _____

  Arthritis/unstable joints: _____

  Back problems:_____

Changes in moles: _____ Enlarged nodes: _____

Impaired vision: _____ Hearing: _____

Prostheses: _____ Ambulatory devices:_____

OBJECTIVE (EXHIBITS)

Temperature: _____ Diaphoresis: _____

Skin integrity: _____ Scars: _____ Rashes: _____

  Ecchymosis: _____ Genital warts/lesions: _____

General strength: _____ Muscle tone: _____

  Gait: _____

  ROM: _____ Paresthesia/paralysis: _____

Fetal: Heart rate: _____ Location: _____
    Method of auscultation: _____ Fundal height: _____
    Estimated gestation (weeks): _____ Movement: _____
    Ballottement: _____
Fetal testing: Date: _____ Test: _____ Result: _____
    AFT: _____
Screenings: Serology: _____ Syphilis: _____
    Sickle cell: _____ Rubella: _____
    Hepatitis: _____ HIV: _____ AFP: _____
Results of cultures (cervical/rectal): _____
    Immune system testing: _____
Blood type: Maternal: _____ Paternal: _____

Sexuality (Component of Social Interactions)

SUBJECTIVE (REPORTS)

Sexual concerns: _____
Menarche: _____ Length of cycle (days): _____
    Duration (days): _____
First day of last menstrual period: _____ Amount:_____
    Bleeding/cramping since LMP: _____
    Vaginal discharge:_____
Client's belief of when conception occurred: _____
Estimated date of delivery: _____
Last PAP smear: _____ Practices breast self-examination: ____
Recent contraceptive method: _____
OB history (GPTPAL): Gravida: _____ Para: ____ Term: _____
    Preterm: ___ Abortions: ___ Living: ___ Multiple births: ___
Delivery history: Year: _____ Place of delivery:_____
    Length of gestation (weeks): _____
    Length of labor (hours): _____ Type of delivery: ____
    Born (alive): ____ Weight: _____ Apgar scores: _____
Complications (maternal/fetal): _____

OBJECTIVE (EXHIBITS)

Pelvic: Vulva: _____ Perineum: _____ Vagina: _____
    Cervix: _____ Uterus: _____ Adnexal:_____
    Diagonal conjugate: _____
    Transverse: _____ Diameter: _____ Outlet (cm): _____
    Shape of sacrum: _____ Arch: _____ Coccyx: _____
    SS notch: _____
    Ischial spines: _____
    Adequacy of inlet: _____ Mid: _____ Outlet: _____
Prognosis for delivery: _____
Breast exam: _____ Nipples: _____
Pregnancy test: _____ Serology test (date): _____
PAP smear results: _____

EXCERPT FROM INTRAPARTAL ASSESSMENT TOOL

Pain/Discomfort

SUBJECTIVE (REPORTS)

Uterine contractions began: _____ Became regular: _____
  Character: _____ Frequency (minutes): _____ Duration:_____
Location of contractile pain (check): Front: __ Sacral area: _____
Degree of discomfort (check): Mild: __ Moderate: __ Severe: _____
How relieved: Breathing/relaxation techniques: _____
  Positioning: _____Sacral rubs: _____ Effleurage: _____
  Other: _____

OBJECTIVE (EXHIBITS)

Facial expression: _____ Narrowed focus: _____
Body movement: _____ Change in BP: _____ Pulse: _____

Safety

SUBJECTIVE (REPORTS)

Allergies/sensitivity: _____
  Reaction (specify): _____
History of STD (date/type): _____
Month of first prenatal visit: _____
Previous/current obstetric problems/treatment:
  PIH: _____ Kidney: _____ Hemorrhage: _____Cardiac:_____
  Diabetes: _____ Infection/UTI: _____
  ABO/Rh sensitivity: _____
  Uterine surgery: _____ Anemia: _____
Length of time since last pregnancy: _____
Type of previous delivery: _____
Health status of living children: _____
Blood transfusion: _____ When: _____
  Reaction (describe): _____
Maternal stature/build: _____
Pelvis: _____
Fractures/dislocations: _____ Arthritis/unstable joints: _____
Spinal problems/deformity: Kyphosis: _____ Scoliosis: _____
  Trauma: _____
  Surgery: _____
Prosthesis: _____ Ambulatory devices: _____

Temperature: _____

Skin integrity: _____ Rashes: _____ Sores: _____

   Bruises: _____

   Scars: _____

Paresthesia/paralysis: _____

Fetal status: Heart rate: _____ Location: _____

   Method of auscultation: _____

   Fundal height: _____ Estimated gestation (weeks): _____

   Activity/movement: _____

   Fetal assessment/testing: Test: _____

   Date: _____ Results: _____

Labor status: Cervical dilation: _____ Effacement: _____

   Fetal descent: _____ Engagement: _____

   Presentation: _____ Lie: _____ Position: _____

Membranes: Intact: _____ Ruptured/time: _____

   AM/PM Nitrazine test $(+/-)$: _____

   Amount of drainage: _____ Character: _____

Blood type/Rh: Maternal: _____ Paternal: _____

Screens (check): Sickle cell: __ Rubella: __ Hepatitis: __ HIV: __

   Tuberculosis: _____ HPV: _____

   Serology: Syphilis $(+/-)$: _____

   Cervical/rectal culture $(+/-)$: _____

Vaginal warts/lesions: _____ Perineal varicosities: _____

DIAGNOSTIC DIVISIONS: NURSING DIAGNOSES ORGANIZED ACCORDING TO A NURSING FOCUS

After data are collected and areas of concern/need identified, the nurse is directed to the Diagnostic Divisions to review the list of nursing diagnoses that fall within the individual categories. This will assist the nurse in choosing the specific diagnostic label to accurately describe the data. Then, with the addition of etiology or related/risk factors (when known) and signs and symptoms or cues (defining characteristics), the client diagnostic statement emerges.

ACTIVITY/REST—Ability to engage in necessary/desired activities of life (work and leisure) and to obtain adequate sleep/rest

Activity Intolerance
Activity Intolerance, risk for
Disuse Syndrome, risk for
Diversional Activity, deficient
Fatigue
Insomnia
Lifestyle, sedentary
Mobility, impaired bed
Mobility, impaired wheelchair
Sleep, readiness for enhanced
Sleep Deprivation
Transfer Ability, impaired
Walking, impaired

CIRCULATION—Ability to transport oxygen and nutrients necessary to meet cellular needs

Autonomic Dysreflexia
Autonomic Dysreflexia, risk for
Cardiac Output, decreased
Intracranial Adaptive Capacity, decreased

Please also see the NANDA diagnoses grouped according to Gordon's Functional Health Patterns on the inside front cover.

Tissue Perfusion, ineffective (specify type: renal, cerebral, cardiopulmonary, gastrointestinal, peripheral)

EGO INTEGRITY—Ability to develop and use skills and behaviors to integrate and manage life experiences*

Anxiety [specify level]
Anxiety, death
Behavior, risk-prone health
Body Image, disturbed
Conflict, decisional [specify]
Coping, defensive
Coping, ineffective
Coping, readiness for enhanced
Decision Making, readiness for enhanced
Denial, ineffective
Dignity, risk for compromised human
Distress, moral
Energy Field, disturbed
Fear
Grieving
Grieving, complicated
Grieving, risk for complicated
Hope, readiness for enhanced
Hopelessness
Identity, disturbed personal
Post-Trauma Syndrome
Post-Trauma Syndrome, risk for
Power, readiness for enhanced
Powerlessness
Powerlessness, risk for
Rape-Trauma Syndrome
Rape-Trauma Syndrome: compound reaction
Rape-Trauma Syndrome: silent reaction
Religiosity, impaired
Religiosity, readiness for enhanced
Religiosity, risk for impaired
Relocation Stress Syndrome
Relocation Stress Syndrome, risk for
Self-Concept, readiness for enhanced
Self-Esteem, chronic low
Self-Esteem, situational low
Self-Esteem, risk for situational low
Sorrow, chronic
Spiritual Distress

*Information that appears in brackets has been added by authors to clarify and enhance the use of nursing diagnoses.

Spiritual Distress, risk for
Spiritual Well-Being, readiness for enhanced

ELIMINATION—Ability to excrete waste products*

Bowel Incontinence
Constipation
Constipation, perceived
Constipation, risk for
Diarrhea
Urinary Elimination, impaired
Urinary Elimination, readiness for enhanced
Urinary Incontinence, functional
Urinary Incontinence, overflow
Urinary Incontinence, reflex
Urinary Incontinence, risk for urge
Urinary Incontinence, stress
Urinary Incontinence, total
Urinary Incontinence, urge
Urinary Retention [acute/chronic]

FOOD/FLUID—Ability to maintain intake of and utilize nutri-ents and liquids to meet physiological needs*

Breastfeeding, effective
Breastfeeding, ineffective
Breastfeeding, interrupted
Dentition, impaired
Failure to Thrive, adult
Fluid Balance, readiness for enhanced
[Fluid Volume, deficient hyper/hypotonic]
Fluid Volume, deficient [isotonic]
Fluid Volume, excess
Fluid Volume, risk for deficient
Fluid Volume, risk for imbalanced
Glucose, risk for unstable blood
Infant Feeding Pattern, ineffective
Liver Function, risk for impaired
Nausea
Nutrition: less than body requirements, imbalanced
Nutrition: more than body requirements, imbalanced
Nutrition: more than body requirements, risk for imbalanced
Nutrition, readiness for enhanced
Oral Mucous Membrane, impaired
Swallowing, impaired

---

*Information that appears in brackets has been added by authors to clarify and enhance the use of nursing diagnoses.

HYGIENE—Ability to perform activities of daily living

Self-Care, readiness for enhanced
Self-Care Deficit, bathing/hygiene
Self-Care Deficit, dressing/grooming
Self-Care Deficit, feeding
Self-Care Deficit, toileting

NEUROSENSORY—Ability to perceive, integrate, and respond to internal and external cues

Confusion, acute
Confusion, risk for acute
Confusion, chronic
Infant Behavior, disorganized
Infant Behavior, readiness for enhanced organized
Infant Behavior, risk for disorganized
Memory, impaired
Neglect, unilateral
Peripheral Neurovascular Dysfunction, risk for
Sensory Perception, disturbed (specify: visual, auditory, kines-
    thetic, gustatory, tactile, olfactory)
Stress Overload
Thought Processes, disturbed

PAIN/DISCOMFORT—Ability to control internal/external environment to maintain comfort

Comfort, readiness for enhanced
Pain, acute
Pain, chronic

RESPIRATION—Ability to provide and use oxygen to meet physiological needs

Airway Clearance, ineffective
Aspiration, risk for
Breathing Pattern, ineffective
Gas Exchange, impaired
Ventilation, impaired spontaneous
Ventilatory Weaning Response, dysfunctional

SAFETY—Ability to provide safe, growth-promoting environment

Allergy Response, latex
Allergy Response, risk for latex
Body Temperature, risk for imbalanced
Contamination
Contamination, risk for

Death Syndrome, risk for sudden infant
Environmental Interpretation Syndrome, impaired
Falls, risk for
Health Maintenance, ineffective
Home Maintenance, impaired
Hyperthermia
Hypothermia
Immunization Status, readiness for enhanced
Infection, risk for
Injury, risk for
Injury, risk for perioperative positioning
Mobility, impaired physical
Poisoning, risk for
Protection, ineffective
Self-Mutilation
Self-Mutilation, risk for
Skin Integrity, impaired
Skin Integrity, risk for impaired
Suffocation, risk for
Suicide, risk for
Surgical Recovery, delayed
Thermoregulation, ineffective
Tissue Integrity, impaired
Trauma, risk for
Violence, [actual/] risk for other-directed
Violence, [actual/] risk for self-directed
Wandering [specify sporadic or continual]

SEXUALITY—[Component of Ego Integrity and Social Inter-action] Ability to meet requirements/characteristics of male/female role*

Sexual Dysfunction
Sexuality Pattern, ineffective

SOCIAL INTERACTION—Ability to establish and maintain relationships*

Attachment, risk for impaired parent/child
Caregiver Role Strain
Caregiver Role Strain, risk for
Communication, impaired verbal
Communication, readiness for enhanced
Conflict, parental role
Coping, ineffective community
Coping, readiness for enhanced community

---

*Information that appears in brackets has been added by authors to clarify and enhance the use of nursing diagnoses.

Coping, compromised family
Coping, disabled family
Coping, readiness for enhanced family
Family Processes: alcoholism, dysfunctional
Family Processes, interrupted
Family Processes, readiness for enhanced
Loneliness, risk for
Parenting, impaired
Parenting, readiness for enhanced
Parenting, risk for impaired
Role Performance, ineffective
Social Interaction, impaired
Social Isolation

TEACHING/LEARNING—Ability to incorporate and use information to achieve healthy lifestyle/optimal wellness*

Development, risk for delayed
Growth, risk for disproportionate
Growth and Development, delayed
Health-Seeking Behaviors (specify)
Knowledge (specify), deficient
Knowledge, readiness for enhanced
Noncompliance [ineffective Adherence] [specify]
Therapeutic Regimen Management, effective
Therapeutic Regimen Management, ineffective
Therapeutic Regimen Management, ineffective community
Therapeutic Regimen Management, ineffective family
Therapeutic Regimen Management, readiness for enhanced

---

*Information that appears in brackets has been added by authors to clarify and enhance the use of nursing diagnoses.

SECTION 3

CLIENT SITUATION AND PROTOTYPE PLAN OF CARE

Client Situation

Mr. R.S., a client with type 2 diabetes (non–insulin-dependent) for 8 years, presented to his physician's office with a nonhealing ulcer of 3 weeks' duration on his left foot. Screening studies done in the doctor's office revealed blood glucose of 356/fingerstick and urine Chemstix of 2%. Because of distance from medical provider and lack of local community services, he is admitted to the hospital.

ADMITTING PHYSICIAN'S ORDERS

Culture/sensitivity and Gram's stain of foot ulcer
Random blood glucose on admission and fingerstick BG qid
CBC, electrolytes, serum lipid profile, glycosylated Hb in AM
Chest x-ray and ECG in AM
DiaBeta 10 mg, PO BID
Glucophage 500 mg, PO daily to start—will increase gradually
Humulin N 10 U SC q AM and HS. Begin insulin instruction for post-discharge self-care if necessary
Dicloxacillin 500 mg PO q6h, start after culture obtained
Darvocet-N 100 mg PO q4h prn pain
Diet—2400 calories, 3 meals with 2 snacks
Up in chair ad lib with feet elevated
Foot cradle for bed
Irrigate lesion L foot with NS tid, then cover with wet to dry sterile dressing
Vital signs qid

CLIENT ASSESSMENT DATABASE

Name: R.S.   Informant: Client
Reliability (Scale 1–4): 3
Age: 70   DOB: 5/3/36   Race: White   Gender: M
Adm. date: 6/28/2007   Time: 7 PM   From: home

Activity/Rest

SUBJECTIVE (REPORTS)

Occupation: farmer
Usual activities/hobbies: reading, playing cards. "Don't have

time to do much. Anyway, I'm too tired most of the time to do anything after the chores."

Limitations imposed by illness: "Have to watch what I order if I eat out."

Sleep: Hours: 6 to 8 hr/night   Naps: no   Aids: no

Insomnia: "Not unless I drink coffee after supper."

Usually feels rested when awakens at 4:30 AM

OBJECTIVE (EXHIBITS)

Observed response to activity: limps, favors L foot when walking

Mental status: alert/active

Neuro/muscular assessment: Muscle mass/tone: bilaterally equal/firm Posture: erect

ROM: full Strength: equal 4 extremities/(favors L foot currently)

Circulation

SUBJECTIVE (REPORTS)

History of slow healing: lesion L foot, 3 weeks' duration

Extremities: Numbness/tingling: "My feet feel cold and tingly like sharp pins poking the bottom of my feet when I walk the quarter mile to the mailbox."

Cough/character of sputum: occ./white

Change in frequency/amount of urine: yes/voiding more lately

OBJECTIVE (EXHIBITS)

Peripheral pulses: radials 3+; popliteal, dorsalis, post-tibial/pedal, all 1+

BP: R: Lying: 146/90   Sitting: 140/86   Standing: 138/90
    L: Lying: 142/88   Sitting: 138/88   Standing: 138/84

Pulse: Apical: 86   Radial: 86   Quality: strong
    Rhythm: regular

Chest auscultation: few wheezes clear with cough, no murmurs/rubs

Jugular vein distention: 0

Extremities:

    Temperature: feet cool bilaterally/legs warm

    Color: Skin: legs pale

    Capillary refill: slow both feet (approx. 4 seconds)

    Homans' sign: 0

    Varicosities: few enlarged superficial veins both calves

    Nails: toenails thickened, yellow, brittle

    Distribution and quality of hair: coarse hair to midcalf, none on ankles/toes

Color:

    General: ruddy face/arms

    Mucous membranes/lips: pink

Nailbeds: pink
Conjunctiva and sclera: white

Ego Integrity

SUBJECTIVE (REPORTS)

Report of stress factors: "Normal farmer's problems: weather, pests, bankers, etc."

Ways of handling stress: "I get busy with the chores and talk things over with my livestock. They listen pretty good."

Financial concerns: medicare only needs to hire someone to do chores while here

Relationship status: married

Cultural factors: rural/agrarian, eastern European descent, "American," no ethnic ties

Religion: Protestant/practicing

Lifestyle: middle class/self-sufficient farmer

Recent changes: no

Feelings: "I'm in control of most things, except the weather and this diabetes now."

Concerned re possible therapy change "from pills to shots."

OBJECTIVE (EXHIBITS)

Emotional status: generally calm, appears frustrated at times

Observed physiological response(s): occasionally sighs deeply/frowns, fidgeting with coin, shoulders tense/shrugs shoulders, throws up hands

Elimination

SUBJECTIVE (REPORTS)

Usual bowel pattern: almost every PM

Last BM: last night   Character of stool: firm/brown
   Bleeding: 0   Hemorrhoids: 0   Constipation: occ.

Laxative used: hot prune juice on occ.

Urinary: no problems   Character of urine: pale yellow

OBJECTIVE (EXHIBITS)

Abdomen tender: no   Soft/firm: soft   Palpable mass: 0
Bowel sounds: active all 4 quads

Food/Fluid

SUBJECTIVE (REPORTS)

Usual diet (type): 2400 calorie (occ. "cheats" with dessert; "My wife watches it pretty closely.")

No. of meals daily: 3/1 snack

Dietary pattern:
    B: fruit juice/toast/ham/decaf coffee
    L: meat/potatoes/veg/fruit/milk
    D: ½ meat sandwich/soup/fruit/decaf coffee
    Snack: milk/crackers at HS. Usual beverage: skim milk, 2 to
        3 cups decaf coffee, drinks "lots of water"—several
        quarts
Last meal/intake: Dinner: roast beef sandwich, vegetable soup,
    pear with cheese, decaf coffee
Loss of appetite: "Never, but lately I don't feel as hungry as
    usual."
Nausea/vomiting: 0   Food allergies: none
Heartburn/food intolerance: cabbage causes gas, coffee after
    supper causes heartburn
Mastication/swallowing problems: 0
    Dentures: partial upper plate—fits well
Usual weight: 175 lb Recent changes: has lost about 6 lb this month
Diuretic therapy: no

OBJECTIVE (EXHIBITS)

Wt: 171 lb   Ht: 5 ft 10 in   Build: stocky
Skin turgor: good/leathery Mucous membranes: moist
Condition of teeth/gums: good, no irritation/bleeding noted
    Appearance of tongue: midline, pink
    Mucous membranes: pink, intact
Breath sounds: few wheezes cleared with cough
Bowel sounds: active all 4 quads
Urine Chemstix: 2%   Fingerstick: 356 (Dr. office) 450 random
    BG on adm

Hygiene

SUBJECTIVE (REPORTS)

Activities of daily living: independent in all areas
Preferred time of bath: PM

OBJECTIVE (EXHIBITS)

General appearance: clean, shaven, short-cut hair; hands rough
    and dry; skin on feet dry, cracked, and scaly
Scalp and eyebrows: scaly white patches
No body odor

Neurosensory

SUBJECTIVE (REPORTS)

Headache: "Occasionally behind my eyes when I worry too much."
Tingling/numbness: feet, 4 or 5 times/week (as noted)

Eyes: Vision loss, farsighted, "Seems a little blurry now." Examination: 2 yrs ago
Ears: Hearing loss R: "Some" L: no Has not been tested
Nose: Epistaxis: 0   Sense of smell: "No problem"

OBJECTIVE (EXHIBITS)

Mental status: alert, oriented to person, place, time, situation
Affect: concerned   Memory: Remote/recent: clear and intact
Speech: clear/coherent, appropriate
Pupil reaction: PERRLA/small
Glasses: reading   Hearing aid: no
Handgrip/release: strong/equal

Pain/Discomfort

SUBJECTIVE (REPORTS)

Primary focus: left foot   Location: medial aspect, L heel
Intensity (0–10): 4 to 5   Quality: dull ache with occ. sharp
    stabbing sensation
Frequency/duration: "Seems like all the time."   Radiation: no
Precipitating factors: shoes, walking   How relieved: ASA, not
    helping
Other complaints: sometimes has back pain following
    chores/heavy lifting, relieved by ASA/liniment rubdown

OBJECTIVE (EXHIBITS)

Facial grimacing: when lesion border palpated
Guarding affected area: pulls foot away
Narrowed focus: no
Emotional response: tense, irritated

Respiration

SUBJECTIVE (REPORTS)

Dyspnea: 0   Cough: occ. morning cough, white sputum
Emphysema: 0   Bronchitis: 0 Asthma: 0   Tuberculosis: 0
Smoker: filters pk/day: 1/2   No. yrs: 25+
Use of respiratory aids: 0

OBJECTIVE (EXHIBITS)

Respiratory rate: 22 Depth: good Symmetry: equal, bilateral
Auscultation: few wheezes, clear with cough
Cyanosis: 0   Clubbing of fingers: 0
Sputum characteristics: none to observe
Mentation/restlessness: alert/oriented/relaxed

Safety

Allergies: 0   Blood transfusions: 0
Sexually transmitted disease: 0
Wears seat belt
Fractures/dislocations: L clavicle, 1960's, fell getting off tractor
Arthritis/unstable joints: "some in my knees."
Back problems: occ. lower back pain
Vision impaired: requires glasses for reading
Hearing impaired: slightly (R), compensates by turning "good
   ear" toward speaker
Immunizations: current flu/pneumonia 3 yrs ago/tetanus
   maybe 8 yrs ago

Temperature: 99.4°F (37.4°C) Tympanic
Skin integrity: impaired L foot   Scars: R inguinal, surgical
Rashes: 0   Bruises: 0   Lacerations: 0   Blisters: 0
Ulcerations: medial aspect L heel, 2.5-cm diameter, approx.
   3 mm deep, wound edges inflamed, draining small amount
   cream-color/pink-tinged matter, slight musty odor noted
Strength (general): equal all extremities   Muscle tone: firm
ROM: good   Gait: favors L foot   Paresthesia/paralysis:
   tingling, prickly sensation in feet after walking ¼ mile

Sexuality: Male

Sexually active: yes   Use of condoms: no (monogamous)
Recent changes in frequency/interest: "I've been too tired lately."
Penile discharge: 0   Prostate disorder: 0   Vasectomy: 0
Last proctoscopic examination: 2 yrs ago   Prostate examina-
   tion: 1 yr ago
Practice self-examination: Breasts/testicles: No
Problems/complaints: "I don't have any problems, but you'd
   have to ask my wife if there are any complaints."

Examination: Breasts: no masses   Testicles: deferred
   Prostate: deferred

Social Interactions

Marital status: married 45 yr   Living with: wife
Report of problems: none

Extended family: 1 daughter lives in town (30 miles away); 1
   daughter married/grandson, living out of state
Other: several couples, he and wife play cards/socialize with 2 to
   3 times/mo
Role: works farm alone; husband/father/grandfather
Report of problems related to illness/condition: none until now
Coping behaviors: "My wife and I have always talked things out.
   You know the 11th commandment is 'Thou shalt not go to
   bed angry.'"

OBJECTIVE (EXHIBITS)

Speech: clear, intelligible
Verbal/nonverbal communication with family/SO(s): speaks
   quietly with wife, looking her in the eye; relaxed posture
Family interaction patterns: wife sitting at bedside, relaxed, both
   reading paper, making occasional comments to each other

Teaching/Learning

SUBJECTIVE (REPORTS)

Dominant language: English   Second language: 0   Literate: yes
Education level: 2-yr college
Health and illness/beliefs/practices/customs: "I take care of the
   minor problems and see the doctor only when something's
   broken."
Presence of Advance Directives: yes—wife to bring in
Durable Medical Power of Attorney: wife
Familial risk factors/relationship:
   Diabetes: maternal uncle
   Tuberculosis: brother died, age 27
   Heart disease: father died, age 78, heart attack
   Strokes: mother died, age 81
   High BP: mother
Prescribed medications:
   Drug: Diabeta Dose: 10 mg bid
   Schedule: 8 AM/6 PM, last dose 6 PM today
   Purpose: control diabetes
   Takes medications regularly? yes
   Home urine/glucose monitoring: "Only using TesTape,
      stopped some months ago when I ran out. It was always
      negative, anyway."
Nonprescription (OTC) drugs: occ. ASA
Use of alcohol (amount/frequency): socially, occ. beer
Tobacco: 1/2 pk/day
Admitting diagnosis (physician): hyperglycemia with nonheal-
   ing lesion L foot

Reason for hospitalization (client): "Sore on foot and the doctor is concerned about my blood sugar, and says I'm supposed to learn this fingerstick test now."

History of current complaint: "Three weeks ago I got a blister on my foot from breaking in my new boots. It got sore so I lanced it but it isn't getting any better."

Client's expectations of this hospitalization: "Clear up this infection and control my diabetes."

Other relevant illness and/or previous hospitalizations/surgeries: 1960's, R inguinal hernia repair

Evidence of failure to improve: lesion L foot, 3 wk

Last physical examination: complete 1 yr ago, office follow-up 5 mo ago

Discharge Considerations (as of 6/28)

Anticipated discharge: 7/1/07 (3 days)

Resources: self, wife

Financial: "If this doesn't take too long to heal, we got some savings to cover things."

Community supports: diabetic support group (has not participated)

Anticipated lifestyle changes: become more involved in management of condition

Assistance needed: may require farm help for several days

Teaching: learn new medication regimen and wound care; review diet; encourage smoking cessation

Referral: Supplies: Downtown Pharmacy or AARP

Equipment: Glucometer-AARP

Follow-up: primary care provider 1 wk after discharge to evaluate wound healing and potential need for additional changes in diabetic regimen

PLAN OF CARE FOR CLIENT WITH DIABETES MELLITUS

Client Diagnostic Statement:

impaired Skin Integrity related to pressure, altered metabolic state, circulatory impairment, and decreased sensation, as evidenced by draining wound L foot.

Outcome: Wound Healing: Secondary Intention (NOC) Indicators: Client Will:

Be free of purulent drainage within 48 hr (6/30 1900).
Display signs of healing with wound edges clean/pink within 60 hr (discharge) (7/1 0700).

ACTIONS/INTERVENTIONS	RATIONALE
Wound Care (NIC)	
Irrigate wound with room temperature sterile NS tid.	Cleans wound without harming delicate tissues.
Assess wound with each dressing change. Obtain wound tracing on adm and at discharge.	Provides information about effectiveness of therapy, and identifies additional needs.
Apply wet to dry sterile dressing.	Keeps wound clean/minimizes cross contamination.
Use paper tape.	Adhesive tape may be abrasive to fragile tissues.
Infection Control (NIC)	
Follow wound precautions.	Use of gloves and proper handling of contaminated dressings reduces likelihood of spread of infection.
Obtain sterile specimen of wound drainage on admission.	Culture/sensitivity identifies pathogens and therapy of choice.
Administer dicloxacillin 500 mg PO q6h, starting 10 PM. Observe for signs of hypersensitivity (i.e., pruritus, urticaria, rash).	Treatment of infection/prevention of complications. Food interferes with drug absorption, requiring scheduling around meals. Although no history of penicillin reaction, it may occur at any time.

Client Diagnostic Statement:

unstable blood Glucose related to lack of adherence to diabetes management and inadequate blood glucose monitoring as evidenced by fingerstick 450/adm.

Outcome: Blood Glucose Control (NOC)
Indicators: Client Will:

Demonstrate correction of metabolic state as evidenced by FBS less than 120 mg/dL within 36 hr (6/30 0700).

ACTIONS/INTERVENTIONS	RATIONALE
Hyperglycemia Management (NIC)	
Perform fingerstick BG qid	Bedside analysis of blood glucose levels is a more timely method for monitoring effectiveness of therapy and provides direction for alteration of medications.
Administer antidiabetic medications:	Treats underlying metabolic dysfunction, reducing hyperglycemia and promoting healing.
10 U Humulin N insulin SC q am/HS after fingerstick BG;	Intermediate-acting preparation with onset of 2–4 hr, peak 4–10 hr, and duration 10–16 hr. Increases transport of glucose into cells and promotes the conversion of glucose to glycogen.
DiaBeta 10 mg PO BID;	Lowers blood glucose by stimulating the release of insulin from the pancreas and increasing the sensitivity to insulin at the receptor sites.
Glucophage 500 mg PO qday. Note onset of side effects.	Glucophage lowers serum glucose levels by decreasing hepatic glucose production and intestinal glucose absorption, and increasing sensitivity to insulin. By using in conjunction with Diabeta, client may be able to discontinue insulin once target dosage is achieved (e.g., 2000 mg/day). Increase of 1 tablet per week is necessary to limit side effects of diarrhea, abdominal cramping, vomiting, possibly leading to

ACTIONS/INTERVENTIONS	RATIONALE
	dehydration and prerenal azotemia.
Provide diet 2400 cals—3 meals/2 snacks.	Proper diet decreases glucose levels/insulin needs, prevents hyperglycemic episodes, can reduce serum cholesterol levels, and promote satiation.
Schedule consultation with dietitian to restructure meal plan and evaluate food choices.	Calories are unchanged on new orders but have been redistributed to 3 meals and 2 snacks. Dietary choices (e.g., increased vitamin C) may enhance healing.

Client Diagnostic Statement:

acute Pain related to physical agent (open wound L foot), as evidenced by verbal report of pain and guarding behavior.

Outcome: Pain Control (NOC)
Indicators: Client Will:

Report pain is minimized/relieved within 1 hr of analgesic administration (ongoing).
Report absence or control of pain by discharge (7/1).

Outcome: Pain Disruptive Effects (NOC) Indicators: Client Will:

Ambulate normally, full weight bearing by discharge (7/1).

ACTIONS/INTERVENTIONS	RATIONALE
Pain Management (NIC)	
Determine pain characteristics through client's description.	Establishes baseline for assessing improvement/changes.
Place foot cradle on bed; encourage use of loose-fitting slipper when up.	Avoids direct pressure to area of injury, which could result in vasoconstriction/increased pain.
Administer Darvocet-N 100 mg PO q4h as needed. Document effectiveness.	Provides relief of discomfort when unrelieved by other measures.

Client Diagnostic Statement:

ineffective peripheral Tissue Perfusion related to decreased arterial flow evidenced by decreased pulses, pale/cool feet; thick, brittle nails; numbness/tingling of feet "when walks 1/4 mile."

Outcome: Knowledge: Diabetes Management (NOC) Indicators: Client Will:

Verbalize understanding of relationship between chronic disease (diabetes mellitus) and circulatory changes within 48 hr (6/30 1900).

Demonstrate awareness of safety factors/proper foot care within 48 hr (6/30 1900).

Maintain adequate level of hydration to maximize perfusion, as evidenced by balanced intake/output, moist skin/mucous membranes, adequate capillary refill less than 3 seconds (ongoing).

ACTIONS/INTERVENTIONS	RATIONALE
Circulatory Care: Arterial Insufficiency (NIC)	
Elevate feet when up in chair.	
Avoid long periods with feet dependent.	Minimizes interruption of blood flow, reduces venous pooling.
Assess for signs of dehydration. Monitor intake/output. Encourage oral fluids.	Glycosuria may result in dehydration with consequent reduction of circulating volume and further impairment of peripheral circulation.
Instruct client to avoid constricting clothing/socks and ill-fitting shoes.	Compromised circulation and decreased pain sensation may precipitate or aggravate tissue breakdown.
Reinforce safety precautions regarding use of heating pads, hot water bottles/soaks.	Heat increases metabolic demands on compromised tissues. Vascular insufficiency alters pain sensation, increasing risk of injury.
Recommend cessation of smoking.	Vascular constriction associated with smoking and diabetes impairs peripheral circulation.
Discuss complications of disease that result from	Although proper control of diabetes mellitus may not

ACTIONS/INTERVENTIONS	RATIONALE
vascular changes (i.e., ulceration, gangrene, muscle or bony structure changes).	prevent complications, severity of effect may be minimized. Diabetic foot complications are the leading cause of nontraumatic lower extremity amputations. **Note:** Skin dry, cracked, scaly; feet cool; pain when walking a distance suggest mild to moderate vascular disease (autonomic neuropathy) that can limit response to infection, impair wound healing, and increase risk of bony deformities.
Review proper foot care as outlined in teaching plan.	Altered perfusion of lower extremities may lead to serious/persistent complications at the cellular level.

Client Diagnostic Statement:

Learning Need regarding diabetic condition related to misinterpretation of information and/or lack of recall as evidenced by inaccurate follow-through of instructions regarding home glucose monitoring and foot care, and failure to recognize signs/symptoms of hyperglycemia.

Outcome: Knowledge: Diabetes Management (NOC) Indicators: Client Will:

Perform procedure of home glucose monitoring correctly within 36 hr (6/30 0700).
Verbalize basic understanding of disease process and treatment within 38 hr (6/30 0900).
Explain reasons for actions within 28 hr (6/30 0900).
Perform insulin administration correctly within 60 hr (7/1 0700).

ACTIONS/INTERVENTIONS	RATIONALE

Teaching: Disease Process (NIC)

Determine client's level of knowledge, priorities of learning needs, desire/need for including wife in instruction.	Establishes baseline and direction for teaching/planning. Involvement of wife, if desired, will provide additional resource for recall/understanding and may enhance client's follow through.
Provide teaching guide, "Understanding Your Diabetes," 6/29 AM. Show film "Living with Diabetes" 6/29 4 PM, when wife is visiting. Include in group teaching session 6/30 AM. Review information and obtain feedback from client/wife.	Provides different methods for accessing/reinforcing information and enhances opportunity for learning/understanding.
Discuss factors related to/altering diabetic control (e.g., stress, illness, exercise).	Drug therapy/diet may need to be altered in response to both short-term and long-term stressors.
Review signs/symptoms of hyperglycemia (e.g., fatigue, nausea/vomiting, polyuria/polydipsia). Discuss how to prevent and evaluate this situation and when to seek medical care. Have client identify appropriate interventions.	Recognition/understanding of these signs/symptoms and timely intervention will aid client in avoiding recurrences and preventing complications.
Review and provide information about necessity for routine examination of feet and proper foot care (e.g., daily inspection for injuries, pressure areas, corns, calluses; proper nail cutting; daily washing, application of good moisturizing lotion [e.g., Eucerin, Keri, Nivea] BID). Recommend wearing loose-fitting socks and properly fitting shoes (break new shoes in gradually)	Reduces risk of tissue injury; promotes understanding and prevention of stasis ulcer formation and wound healing difficulties.

ACTIONS/INTERVENTIONS	RATIONALE
and avoiding going barefoot. If foot injury/skin break occurs, wash with soap/dermal cleanser and water, cover with sterile dressing, inspect wound and change dressing daily; report redness, swelling, or presence of drainage.	
Instruct regarding prescribed insulin therapy:	May be a temporary treatment of hyperglycemia with infection or may be permanent replacement of oral hypoglycemic agent.
Humulin N Insulin, SC.	Intermediate-acting insulin generally lasts 18–28 hr, with peak effect 6–12 hr.
Keep vial in current use at room temperature (if used within 30 days).	Cold insulin is poorly absorbed.
Store extra vials in refrigerator.	Refrigeration prevents wide fluctuations in temperature, prolonging the drug shelf life.
Roll bottle and invert to mix, or shake gently, avoiding bubbles.	Vigorous shaking may create foam, which can interfere with accurate dose withdrawal and may damage the insulin molecule. **Note:** New research suggests that shaking the vial may be more effective in mixing suspension.
Choice of injection sites (e.g., across lower abdomen in Z pattern).	Provides for steady absorption of medication. Site is easily visualized and accessible by client, and Z pattern minimizes tissue damage.
Demonstrate, then observe client drawing insulin into syringe, reading syringe markings, and administering dose. Assess for accuracy.	May require several instruction sessions and practice before client/wife feel comfortable drawing up and injecting medication.

Actions/Interventions	Rationale
Instruct in signs/symptoms of insulin reaction/ hypoglycemia (i.e., fatigue, nausea, headache, hunger, sweating, irritability, shakiness, anxiety, difficulty concentrating).	Knowing what to watch for and appropriate treatment (such as 1/2 cup of grape juice for immediate response and snack within 1/2 hr [e.g., 1 slice bread with peanut butter or cheese, fruit and slice of cheese for sustained effect]) may prevent/ minimize complications.
Review "Sick Day Rules" (e.g., call the doctor if too sick to eat normally/stay active), take insulin as ordered. Keep record as noted in Sick Day Guide.	Understanding of necessary actions in the event of mild/severe illness promotes competent self-care and reduces risk of hyper/hypoglycemia.
Instruct client/wife in fingerstick glucose monitoring to be done qid until stable, then BID rotating times (e.g., FBS and before dinner; before lunch and HS). Observe return demonstrations of the procedure.	Fingerstick monitoring provides accurate and timely information regarding diabetic status. Return demonstration verifies correct learning.
Recommend client maintain record/log of fingerstick testing, antidiabetic medication, and insulin dosage/site, unusual physiological response, dietary intake. Outline desired goals (e.g., FBS 80–110, premeal 80–130).	Provides accurate record for review by caregivers for assessment of therapy effectiveness/needs.
Discuss other healthcare issues, such as smoking habits, self-monitoring for cancer (breasts/testicles), and reporting changes in general well-being.	Encourages client involve- ment, awareness, and responsibility for own health; promotes wellness. **Note:** Smoking tends to increase client's resistance to insulin.

ANOTHER APPROACH TO PLANNING CLIENT CARE—MIND MAPPING

Mind mapping starts in the center of the page with a representation of the main concept—the client. (This helps keep in mind that the client is the focus of the plan, not the medical diagnosis or condition.) From that central thought, other main ideas that relate to the client are added. Different concepts can be grouped together by geometric shapes, color-coding, or by placement on the page. Connections and interconnections between groups of ideas are represented by the use of arrows or lines with defining phrases added that explain how the interconnected thoughts relate to one another. In this manner, many different pieces of information *about* the client can be connected directly *to* the client.

Whichever piece is chosen becomes the first layer of connections—clustered assessment data, nursing diagnoses, or outcomes. For example, a map could start with nursing diagnoses featured as the first "branches," each one being listed separately in some way on the map. Next, the signs and symptoms or data supporting the diagnoses could be added, or the plan could begin with the client outcomes to be achieved with connections then to nursing diagnoses. When the plan is completed, there should be a nursing diagnosis (supported by subjective and objective assessment data), nursing interventions, desired client outcomes and any evaluation data, all connected in a manner that shows there is a relationship between them. It is critical to understand that there is no pre-set order for the pieces, because one cluster is not more or less important than another (or one is not "subsumed" under another). It is important, however, that those pieces within a branch be in the same order in each branch.

Figure 3-1 shows a mind map for Mr. R.S., the client with type 2 diabetes in our Client Situation at the beginning of this section of the chapter.

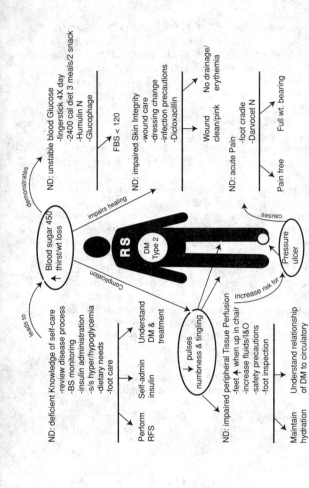

ND: unstable blood Glucose
-fingerstick 4X day
-2400 cal diet 3 meals/2 snack
-Humulin N
-Glucophage

→ FBS < 120

ND: impaired Skin Integrity
-wound care
-dressing change
-infection precautions
-Dicloxacillin

Wound clean/pink → No drainage/erythemia

ND: acute Pain
-foot cradle
-Darvocet N

Pain free → Full wt. bearing

demonstrates

Blood sugar 450 thirst/wt loss

impairs healing

Complication

RS

DM Type 2

causes

Pressure ulcer

increase risk for

leads to

ND: deficient Knowledge of self-care
-review disease process
-BS monitoring
-insulin administration
-s/s hyper/hypoglycemia
-dietary needs
-foot care

Perform RFS

Self-admin insulin

Understand DM & treatment

pulses numbness & tingling

ND: impaired peripheral Tissue Perfusion
-feet ← when up in chair
-increase fluids/I&O
-safety precautions
-foot inspection

Maintain hydration

Understand relationship of DM to circulatory changes

Figure 3-1. Mind map for Mr. R.S.

DOCUMENTATION TECHNIQUES: SOAP AND FOCUS CHARTING®

Several charting formats are currently used for documentation. These include block notes, with a single entry covering an entire shift (e.g., 7 AM to 3 PM); narrative timed notes (e.g., "8:30 AM, ate breakfast well"); and the problem-oriented medical record system (POMR or PORS) using SOAP/SOAPIER approach, to name a few. The latter can provide thorough documentation; however, the SOAP/SOAPIER charting system was designed by physicians for episodic care and requires that the entries be tied to a problem identified from a problem list. (See Example 1.)

The Focus Charting® system (see Example 2) has been designed by nurses for documentation of frequent/repetitive care and to encourage viewing the client from a positive rather than a negative (problem only) perspective. Charting is focused on client and nursing concerns, with the focal point of client status and the associated nursing care. A Focus is usually a client problem/concern or nursing diagnosis but is not a medical diagnosis or a nursing task/treatment (e.g., wound care, indwelling catheter insertion, tube feeding).

Recording of assessment, interventions, and evaluation using Data, Action, and Response (DAR) categories facilitates tracking what is happening to the client at any given moment. Thus, the four components of this charting system are:

(1) **Focus:** Nursing diagnosis, client problem/concern, signs/symptoms of potential importance (e.g., fever, dysrhythmia, edema), a significant event or change in status or specific standards of care/agency policy.

(2) **Data:** Subjective/objective information describing and/or supporting the Focus.

(3) **Action:** Immediate/future nursing actions based on assessment and consistent with/complementary to the goals and nursing action recorded in the client plan of care.

(4) **Response:** Describes the effects of interventions and whether the goal was met.

The following charting examples are based on the data within the client situation of Mr. R.S. in Chapter 3, Section 3, pages 47–64.

Example 1. SAMPLE SOAP/IER CHARTING FOR
PROTOTYPE PLAN OF CARE

**S = Subjective O = Objective A = Analysis P = Plan
I = Implementation   E = Evaluation   R = Revision**

DATE	TIME	NUMBER/ PROBLEM*	NOTE
6/29/07	1900	No. 1 (impaired Skin Integrity)*	S: "That hurts" (when tissue surrounding wound palpated). O: Scant amount serous drainage on dressing. Wound borders pink. No odor present. A: Wound shows early signs of healing, free of infection. P: Continue skin care per plan of care.

To document more of the nursing process, some institutions have added the following: Implementation, Evaluation, and Revision (if plan was ineffective).

DATE	TIME	NUMBER/ PROBLEM*	NOTE
			I: NS irrig. as ordered. Applied sterile wet dressing with paper tape. E: Wound clean, no drainage present. R: None required. Signed: E. Moore, RN
6/29/07	2100	No. 2 (acute Pain)*	S: "Dull, throbbing pain in left foot." 4/10 States there is no radiation to other areas. O: Muscles tense. Moving about bed, appears uncomfortable. A: Persistent pain. P: Per plan of care. I: Foot cradle on bed. Darvocet-N given PO. Signed: M. Siskin, RN
	2200		E: Reports pain relieved 0/10. Appears relaxed. Signed: M. Siskin, RN
6/30/07	1100	No. 3 (Learning Need, Diabetic Care)*	S: "My wife and I have some questions and concerns we wish to discuss."

*As noted on Plan of Care.

(*Continued*)

S = Subjective O = Objective A = Analysis P = Plan
I = Implementation   E = Evaluation   R = Revision

DATE	TIME	NUMBER/ PROBLEM*	NOTE
			O: Copy of list of questions attached to teaching plan.
			A: R.S. and wife need review of information and practice for insulin administration.
			P: Attended group teaching session with wife and read "Understanding Your Diabetes." To meet with dietitian.
			I: R.S. demonstrated insulin administration techniques for wife to observe. Procedure handout sheet for future reference provided to couple. Scheduled meeting for them with dietitian at 1300 today to discuss remaining questions
			E: R.S. more confident in demonstration, performed activity correctly without hesitation or hand tremors. R.S. explained steps of procedure and reasons for actions to wife. Couple identified resources to contact if questions/ problems arise. Signed: B. Briner, RN

Example 2. SAMPLE OF FOCUS CHARTING®
FOR PROTOTYPE PLAN OF CARE

D = Data	A = Action	R = Response

DATE	TIME	FOCUS®	
6/29/07	1900	Skin integrity	D: Scant amount serous drainage on dressing, wound borders pink, no odor present, denies discomfort except with direct palpation of surrounding tissue. A: NS irrig. as ordered. Sterile wet dressing applied with paper tape. R: Wound clean—no drainage present. Signed: E. Moore, RN
6/29/07	2100	Pain L foot	D: Reports dull/throbbing ache L foot 4/10—no radiation. Muscles tense, restless in bed. A: Foot cradle on bed. Darvocet-N 100 mg given PO. Signed: M. Siskin, RN
	2200	Pain L foot	R: Reports pain relieved 0/10. Appears relaxed. Signed: M. Siskin, RN
6/30/07	1100	Learning Need, Diabetic Teaching	D: Attended group teaching session with wife. Both have read "Understanding Your Diabetes." A: Reviewed list of questions/concerns from R.S. and wife. (Copy attached to teaching plan.) R.S. demonstrated insulin administration technique for wife to observe. Procedure handout sheet for future reference provided to couple. Meeting scheduled with dietitian for 1300 today to discuss remaining questions.

(*Continued*)

D = Data	A = Action	R = Response

DATE	TIME	FOCUS®

| | | | R: | R.S. more confident in demonstration, performed activity correctly without hesitation or hand tremors. He explained steps of procedure and reasons for actions to wife. Couple identified resources to contact if questions/problems arise. |

The following is an example of documentation of a client need/concern that currently does not require identification as a client problem (nursing diagnosis) or inclusion in the plan of care and therefore is not easily documented in the SOAP format:

6/28/07	2120	Gastric distress	D:	Awakened from light sleep by "indigestion/burning sensation." Places hand over epigastrie area. Skin warm/dry, color pink, vital signs unchanged.
			A:	Given Mylanta 30 mL PO. Head of bed elevated approximately 15 degrees.
			R:	Reports pain relieved. Appears relaxed, resting quietly. Signed: E. Moore, RN

FOCUS Charting®, Susan Lampe, RN, MS: Creative Nursing Management, Inc., 614 East Grant Street, Minneapolis, MN 55404.

CHAPTER 4

Nursing Diagnoses in Alphabetical Order

Activity Intolerance
[Specify Level]

Taxonomy II: Activity/Rest—Class 4 Cardiovascular/
   Pulmonary Responses (00092)
[Diagnostic Division: Activity/Rest]
Submitted 1982

Definition: Insufficient physiological or psychological
energy to endure or complete required or desired daily
activities

Related Factors

Generalized weakness
Sedentary lifestyle
Bedrest/immobility
Imbalance between oxygen supply and demand; [anemia]
[Cognitive deficits/emotional status; secondary to underlying
   disease process/depression]
[Pain, vertigo, dysrhythmias, extreme stress]

Defining Characteristics

SUBJECTIVE

Verbal report of fatigue/weakness
Exertional discomfort/dyspnea
[Verbalizes no desire and/or lack of interest in activity]

OBJECTIVE

Abnormal heart rate/blood pressure response to activity
Electrocardiographic changes reflecting arrhythmias/or ischemia
[Pallor, cyanosis]

Information in brackets added by the authors to clarify and enhance
the use of nursing diagnoses.

Functional Level Classification (Gordon, 1987):

Level I: Walk, regular pace, on level indefinitely; one flight or more but more short of breath than normally

Level II: Walk one city block [or] 500 ft on level; climb one flight slowly without stopping

Level III: Walk no more than 50 ft on level without stopping; unable to climb one flight of stairs without stopping

Level IV: Dyspnea and fatigue at rest

Desired Outcomes/Evaluation Criteria—Client Will:

- Identify negative factors affecting activity tolerance and eliminate or reduce their effects when possible.
- Use identified techniques to enhance activity tolerance.
- Participate willingly in necessary/desired activities.
- Report measurable increase in activity tolerance.
- Demonstrate a decrease in physiological signs of intolerance (e.g., pulse, respirations, and blood pressure remain within client's normal range).

Actions/Interventions

NURSING PRIORITY NO. 1. To identify causative/precipitating factors:

- Note presence of factors contributing to fatigue (e.g., age, frail, acute or chronic illness, heart failure, hypothyroidism, cancer, and cancer therapies). **Fatigue affects both the client's actual and perceived ability to participate in activities.** (Refer to ND Fatigue.)
- Evaluate client's actual and perceived limitations/degree of deficit in light of usual status. **Provides comparative baseline and provides information about needed education/ interventions regarding quality of life.**
- Note client reports of weakness, fatigue, pain, difficulty accomplishing tasks, and/or insomnia. **Symptoms may be result of/or contribute to intolerance of activity.**
- Assess cardiopulmonary response to physical activity, including vital signs before, during, and after activity. Note progression/accelerating degree of fatigue.
- Ascertain ability to stand and move about and degree of assistance necessary/use of equipment **to determine current status and needs associated with participation in needed/ desired activities.**

Information in brackets added by the authors to clarify and enhance the use of nursing diagnoses.

 Diagnostic Studies 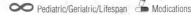 Pediatric/Geriatric/Lifespan Medications

- Identify activity needs versus desires (e.g., is barely able to walk upstairs but would like to play racquetball).
- Assess emotional/psychological factors affecting the current situation (**e.g., stress and/or depression may be increasing the effects of an illness, or depression might be the result of being forced into inactivity**).

- Note treatment-related factors, such as side effects/interactions of medications.

NURSING PRIORITY NO. 2. To assist client to deal with contributing factors and manage activities within individual limits:

- Monitor vital/cognitive signs, watching for changes in blood pressure, heart and respiratory rate; note skin pallor and/or cyanosis and presence of confusion.
- Adjust activities **to prevent overexertion**. Reduce intensity level or discontinue activities that cause undesired physiological changes.
- Provide/monitor response to supplemental oxygen and medications and changes in treatment regimen.
- Increase exercise/activity levels gradually; teach methods **to conserve energy**, such as stopping to rest for 3 minutes during a 10-minute walk or sitting down to brush hair instead of standing.
- Plan care to carefully balance rest periods with activities **to reduce fatigue**.
- Provide positive atmosphere, while acknowledging difficulty of the situation for the client. **Helps to minimize frustration and rechannel energy.**
- Encourage expression of feelings contributing to/resulting from condition.
- Involve client/SO(s) in planning of activities as much as possible.
- Assist with activities and provide/monitor client's use of assistive devices (e.g., crutches, walker, wheelchair, or oxygen tank) **to protect client from injury**.
- Promote comfort measures and provide for relief of pain **to enhance ability to participate in activities.** (Refer to NDs acute Pain; chronic Pain.)
- Provide referral to other disciplines, such as exercise physiologist, psychological counseling/therapy, occupational/ physical therapists, and recreation/leisure specialists, as indicated, **to develop individually appropriate therapeutic regimens.**

NURSING PRIORITY NO. 3. To promote wellness (Teaching/ Discharge Considerations):

Information in brackets added by the authors to clarify and enhance the use of nursing diagnoses.

  Cultural Collaborative Community/Home Care

- Plan for maximal activity within the client's ability. **Promotes the idea of need for/normalcy of progressive abilities in this area.**
- Review expectations of client/SO(s)/providers **to establish individual goals.** Explore conflicts/differences **to reach agreement for the most effective plan.**
- Instruct client/SO(s) in monitoring response to activity and in recognizing signs/symptoms that **indicate need to alter activity level.**
- Plan for progressive increase of activity level/participation in exercise training, as tolerated by client. **Both activity tolerance and health status may improve with progressive training.**
- Give client information that provides evidence of daily/weekly progress **to sustain motivation.**
- Assist client in learning and demonstrating appropriate safety measures **to prevent injuries.**
- Provide information about the effect of lifestyle and overall health factors on activity tolerance (e.g., nutrition, adequate fluid intake, smoking cessation, and mental health status).
- Encourage client to maintain positive attitude; suggest use of relaxation techniques, such as visualization/guided imagery, as appropriate, **to enhance sense of well-being.**
- Encourage participation in recreation/social activities and hobbies appropriate for situation. (Refer to ND deficient Diversional Activity.)

Documentation Focus

ASSESSMENT/REASSESSMENT

- Level of activity as noted in Functional Level Classification.
- Causative/precipitating factors.
- Client reports of difficulty/change.
- Vital signs before/during/following activity.

PLANNING

- Plan of care and who is involved in planning.

IMPLEMENTATION/EVALUATION

- Response to interventions/teaching and actions performed.
- Implemented changes to plan of care based on assessment/reassessment findings.
- Teaching plan and response/understanding of material presented.
- Attainment/progress toward desired outcome(s).

Information in brackets added by the authors to clarify and enhance the use of nursing diagnoses.

Diagnostic Studies   Pediatric/Geriatric/Lifespan   Medications

- Referrals to other resources.
- Long-term needs and who is responsible for actions.

SAMPLE NURSING OUTCOMES & INTERVENTIONS CLASSIFICATIONS (NOC/NIC)

NOC—Activity Tolerance
NIC—Energy Management

risk for Activity Intolerance

Taxonomy II: Activity/Rest—Class 4 Cardiovascular/
  Pulmonary Response (00094)
[Diagnostic Division: Activity/Rest]
Submitted 1982

Definition: At risk of experiencing insufficient
physiological or psychological energy to endure or
complete required or desired daily activities

Risk Factors

History of previous intolerance
Presence of circulatory/respiratory problems; [dysrhythmias]
Deconditioned status; [aging]
Inexperience with the activity
[Diagnosis of progressive disease state/debilitating condition,
  anemia]
[Verbalized reluctance/inability to perform expected activity]

> NOTE: A risk diagnosis is not evidenced by signs and symptoms, as
> the problem has not occurred and nursing interventions are
> directed at prevention.

Desired Outcomes/Evaluation
Criteria—Client Will:

- Verbalize understanding of potential loss of ability in relation
  to existing condition.
- Participate in conditioning/rehabilitation program to
  enhance ability to perform.
- Identify alternative ways to maintain desired activity level
  (e.g., if weather is bad, walking in a shopping mall).

Information in brackets added by the authors to clarify and enhance
the use of nursing diagnoses.

 Cultural Collaborative 🏠 Community/Home Care

- Identify conditions/symptoms that require medical reevaluation.

Actions/Interventions

NURSING PRIORITY NO. 1. To assess factors affecting current situation:

- Note presence of medical diagnosis and/or therapeutic regimens (e.g., acquired immunodeficiency syndrome [AIDS], chronic obstructive pulmonary disease [COPD], cancer, heart failure/other cardiac problems, anemia, multiple medications/treatment modalaties, extensive surgical interventions, musculoskeletal trauma, neurological disorders, or renal failure) **that have potential for interfering with client's ability to perform at a desired level of activity.**
- Ask client/SO about usual level of energy **to identify potential problems and/or client's/SO's perception of client's energy and ability to perform needed/desired activities.**

- Identify factors, such as age, functional decline, painful conditions, breathing problems, client who is resistive to efforts, vision or hearing impairments, climate or weather, unsafe areas to exercise, and need for mobility assistance, **that could block/affect desired level of activity.**
- Determine current activity level and physical condition with observation, exercise tolerance testing, or use of functional level classification system (e.g., Gordon's), as appropriate. **Provides baseline for comparison and opportunity to track changes.**

NURSING PRIORITY NO. 2. To develop/investigate alternative ways to remain active within the limits of the disabling condition/situation:

- Implement physical therapy/exercise program in conjunction with the client and other team members (e.g., physical and/or occupational therapist, exercise/rehabilitation physiologist). **Coordination of program enhances likelihood of success.**
- Promote/implement conditioning program and support inclusion in exercise/activity groups **to prevent/limit deterioration.**
- Instruct client in unfamiliar activities and in alternate ways of doing familiar activities **to conserve energy and promote safety.**

NURSING PRIORITY NO. 3. To promote wellness (Teaching/Discharge Considerations):

- Discuss with client/SO the relationship of illness/debilitating condition to inability to perform desired activities.

Information in brackets added by the authors to clarify and enhance the use of nursing diagnoses.

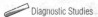 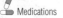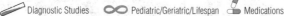

Understanding these relationships can help with acceptance of limitations or reveal opportunity for changes of practical value.

- Provide information regarding potential interfering factors with activity, such as smoking when one has respiratory problems or lack of motivation/interest in exercise, **which may be amenable to modification.**

 - Assist client/SO(s) with planning for changes that may become necessary, such as use of supplemental oxygen **to improve client's ability to participate in desired activities.**

 - Identify and discuss symptoms for which client needs to seek medical assistance/evaluation, **providing for timely intervention.**

 - Refer to appropriate resources for assistance and/or equipment, as needed, **to sustain activity level.**

Documentation Focus

ASSESSMENT/REASSESSMENT

- Identified/potential risk factors for individual.
- Current level of activity tolerance and blocks to activity.

PLANNING

- Treatment options, including physical therapy/exercise program, other assistive therapies and devices.
- Lifestyle changes that are planned, who is to be responsible for each action, and monitoring methods.

IMPLEMENTATION/EVALUATION

- Responses to interventions/teaching and actions performed.
- Attainment/progress toward desired outcome(s).
- Modification of plan of care.

DISCHARGE PLANNING

- Referrals for medical assistance/evaluation.

SAMPLE NURSING OUTCOMES & INTERVENTIONS CLASSIFICATIONS (NOC/NIC)

NOC—Endurance
NIC—Energy Management

Information in brackets added by the authors to clarify and enhance the use of nursing diagnoses.

  Cultural Collaborative Community/Home Care

ineffective Airway Clearance

Taxonomy II: Safety/Protection—Class 2 Physical Injury (00031)
[Diagnostic Division: Respiration]
Submitted 1980; Revised 1996, and Nursing Diagnosis Extension and Classification (NDEC) 1998

Definition: Inability to clear secretions or obstructions from the respiratory tract to maintain a clear airway

Related Factors

ENVIRONMENTAL

Smoking; second-hand smoke; smoke inhalation

OBSTRUCTED AIRWAY

Retained secretions; secretions in the bronchi; exudate in the alveoli; excessive mucus; airway spasm; foreign body in airway; presence of artificial airway

PHYSIOLOGICAL

Chronic obstructive pulmonary disease [COPD]; asthma; allergic airways; hyperplasia of the bronchial walls
Neuromuscular dysfunction
Infection

Defining Characteristics

SUBJECTIVE

Dyspnea

OBJECTIVE

Diminished/adventitious breath sounds [rales, crackles, rhonchi, wheezes]
Cough ineffective/absent; excessive sputum
Changes in respiratory rate/rhythm
Difficulty vocalizing
Wide-eyed; restlessness
Orthopnea
Cyanosis

Information in brackets added by the authors to clarify and enhance the use of nursing diagnoses.

 Diagnostic Studies 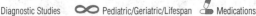 Pediatric/Geriatric/Lifespan   Medications

Desired Outcomes/Evaluation Criteria—Client Will:

- Maintain airway patency.
- Expectorate/clear secretions readily.
- Demonstrate absence/reduction of congestion with breath sounds clear, respirations noiseless, improved oxygen exchange (e.g., absence of cyanosis, ABG/pulse oximetry results within client norms).
- Verbalize understanding of cause(s) and therapeutic management regimen.
- Demonstrate behaviors to improve or maintain clear airway.
- Identify potential complications and how to initiate appropriate preventive or corrective actions.

Actions/Interventions

NURSING PRIORITY NO. 1. To maintain adequate, patent airway:

- Identify client populations at risk. **Persons with impaired ciliary function (e.g., cystic fibrosis); those with excessive or abnormal mucus production (e.g., asthma, emphysema, pneumonia, dehydration, mechanical ventilation); those with impaired cough function (e.g., neuromuscular diseases/conditions such as muscular dystrophy, Guillain-Barre); those with swallowing abnormalities (e.g., stroke, seizures, coma/sedation, head/neck cancer, facial burns/trauma/surgery); immobility (e.g., spinal cord injury, developmental delay, fractures); infant/child feeding difficulties (e.g., congenital malformations, developmental delays, abdominal distention) are all at risk for problems with maintenance of open airways.**
- Monitor respirations and breath sounds, noting rate and sounds (e.g., tachypnea, stridor, crackles, wheezes) **indicative of respiratory distress and/or accumulation of secretions.**
- Evaluate client's cough/gag reflex and swallowing ability **to determine ability to protect own airway.**
- Position head appropriate for age/condition **to open or maintain open airway in at-rest or compromised individual.**
- Assist with appropriate testing (e.g., pulmonary function/sleep studies) **to identify causative/precipitating factors.**
- Suction naso/tracheal/oral prn **to clear airway when excessive or viscous secretions are blocking airway or client is unable to swallow or cough effectively.**
- Elevate head of bed/change position every 2 hours and prn **to take advantage of gravity decreasing pressure on the**

Information in brackets added by the authors to clarify and enhance the use of nursing diagnoses.

  Cultural Collaborative Community/Home Care

diaphragm and enhancing drainage of/ventilation to different lung segments.

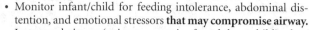

- Monitor infant/child for feeding intolerance, abdominal distention, and emotional stressors **that may compromise airway.**
- Insert oral airway (using correct size for adult or child) when needed, **to maintain anatomic position of tongue and natural airway, especially when tongue/laryngeal edema or thick secretions may block airway.**
- Assist with procedures (e.g., bronchoscopy, tracheostomy) **to clear/maintain open airway.**
- Keep environment allergen free (e.g., dust, feather pillows, smoke) according to individual situation.

NURSING PRIORITY NO. 2. To mobilize secretions:
- Encourage deep-breathing and coughing exercises; splint chest/incision **to maximize effort.**
- Administer analgesics **to improve cough when pain is inhibiting effort. (Caution: Overmedication can depress respirations and cough effort.)**
- Give expectorants/bronchodilators as ordered.
- Increase fluid intake to at least 2000 mL/day within cardiac tolerance (may require IV in acutely ill, hospitalized client). Encourage/provide warm versus cold liquids as appropriate. Provide supplemental humidification, if needed (ultrasonic nebulizer, room humidifier). **Hydration can help liquefy viscous secretions and improve secretion clearance.** Monitor for signs/symptoms of congestive heart failure (crackles, edema, weight gain) when client is at risk.
- Perform/assist client with postural drainage and percussion as indicated if not contraindicated by condition, such as asthma.
- Assist with use of respiratory devices and treatments (e.g., intermittent positive-pressure breathing [IPPB]; incentive spirometer [IS]; positive expiratory pressure [PEP] mask; mechanical ventilation; oscillatory airway device [flutter]; assisted and directed cough techniques, etc.). **Various therapies/modalities may be required to acquire/maintain adequate airways, improve respiratory function and gas exchange.** (Refer to NDs ineffective Breathing Pattern; impaired Gas Exchange; impaired spontaneous Ventilation.)
- Support reduction/cessation of smoking **to improve lung function.**
- Position appropriately (e.g., head of bed elevated, side lying) and discourage use of oil-based products around nose **to prevent vomiting with aspiration into lungs.** (Refer to NDs risk for Aspiration; impaired Swallowing.)

Information in brackets added by the authors to clarify and enhance the use of nursing diagnoses.

 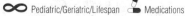
ineffective AIRWAY CLEARANCE

NURSING PRIORITY NO. 3. To assess changes, note complications:

- Auscultate breath sounds and assess air movement **to ascertain status and note progress.**
- Monitor vital signs, noting blood pressure/pulse changes.
- Observe for signs of respiratory distress (increased rate, restlessness/anxiety, use of accessory muscles for breathing).
- Evaluate changes in sleep pattern, noting insomnia or daytime somnolence.
- Document response to drug therapy and/or development of adverse side effects or interactions with antimicrobials, steroids, expectorants, bronchodilators.
- Observe for signs/symptoms of infection (e.g., increased dyspnea with onset of fever, change in sputum color, amount, or character) **to identify infectious process/promote timely intervention.**
- Obtain sputum specimen, preferably before antimicrobial therapy is initiated, **to verify appropriateness of therapy.**
- Monitor/document serial chest x-rays/ABGs/pulse oximetry readings.

NURSING PRIORITY NO. 4. To promote wellness (Teaching/Discharge Considerations):

- Assess client's/SO's knowledge of contributing causes, treatment plan, specific medications, and therapeutic procedures. **Modalities to manage secretions and improve airflow vary according to client's diagnosis.**
- Provide information about the necessity of raising and expectorating secretions versus swallowing them, **to report changes in color and amount in the event that medical intervention may be needed to prevent/treat infection.**
- Demonstrate/assist client/SO in performing specific airway clearance techniques (e.g., forced expiratory breathing [also called huffing] or respiratory muscle strength training, chest percussion), as indicated.
- Review breathing exercises, effective coughing, and use of adjunct devices (e.g., IPPB or incentive spirometer) in preoperative teaching.
- Encourage/provide opportunities for rest; limit activities to level of respiratory tolerance. (**Prevents/reduces fatigue.**)
- Refer to appropriate support groups (e.g., stop-smoking clinic, COPD exercise group, weight reduction).
- Determine that client has equipment and is informed in use of nocturnal continuous positive airway pressure (CPAP) **for**

Information in brackets added by the authors to clarify and enhance the use of nursing diagnoses.

  Cultural Collaborative 🏠 Community/Home Care

treatment of obstructive sleep apnea, when indicated. (Refer to NDs Insomnia; Sleep Deprivation.)

Documentation Focus

ASSESSMENT/REASSESSMENT

- Related Factors for individual client.
- Breath sounds, presence/character of secretions, use of accessory muscles for breathing.
- Character of cough/sputum.
- Respiratory rate, pulse oximetry/O_2 saturation, vital signs.

PLANNING

- Plan of care and who is involved in planning.
- Teaching plan.

IMPLEMENTATION/EVALUATION

- Client's response to interventions/teaching and actions performed.
- Use of respiratory devices/airway adjuncts.
- Response to medications administered.
- Attainment/progress toward desired outcome(s).
- Modifications to plan of care.

DISCHARGE PLANNING

- Long-term needs and who is responsible for actions to be taken.
- Specific referrals made.

SAMPLE NURSING OUTCOMES & INTERVENTIONS CLASSIFICATIONS (NOC/NIC)

NOC—Respiratory Status: Airway Patency
NIC—Airway Management

latex Allergy Response

Taxonomy II: Safety/Protection—Class 5 Defensive
    Processes (00041)
[Diagnostic Division: Safety]
Submitted 1998; Revised 2006

Definition: A hypersensitive reaction to natural latex
rubber products

Information in brackets added by the authors to clarify and enhance the use of nursing diagnoses.

 Diagnostic Studies 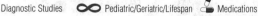 Pediatric/Geriatric/Lifespan Medications

Related Factors

Hypersensitivity to natural latex rubber protein

Defining Characteristics

SUBJECTIVE

Life-threatening reactions occurring <1 hour after exposure to latex proteins:
Tightness in chest [feeling breathless]
Gastrointestinal characteristics: Abdominal pain; nausea
Orofacial characteristics: Itching of the eyes; nasal/facial/oral itching; nasal congestion
Generalized characteristics: Generalized discomfort; increasing complaint of total body warmth
Type 1V reactions occurring >1 hour after exposure to latex protein: Discomfort reaction to additives such as thiurams and carbamates

OBJECTIVE

Life-threatening reactions occurring <1 hour after exposure to latex proteins:
Contact urticaria progressing to generalized symptoms
Edema of the lips/tongue/uvula/throat
Dyspnea; wheezing; bronchospasm; respiratory arrest
Hypotension; syncope; cardiac arrest
Orofacial characteristics: Edema of sclera/eyelids; erythema/tearing of the eyes; nasal facial/erythema; rhinorrhea
Generalized characteristics: Flushing; generalized edema; restlessness
Type IV reactions occurring >1 hour after exposure to latex protein: Eczema; irritation; redness

Desired Outcomes/Evaluation Criteria—Client Will:

- Be free of signs of hypersensitive response.
- Verbalize understanding of individual risks/responsibilities in avoiding exposure.
- Identify signs/symptoms requiring prompt intervention.

Actions/Interventions

NURSING PRIORITY NO. 1. To assess contributing factors:
- Identify persons in high-risk categories such as those with history of certain food allergies (e.g., banana, avocado, chestnut,

---

Information in brackets added by the authors to clarify and enhance the use of nursing diagnoses.

  Cultural Collaborative 🏠 Community/Home Care

kiwi, papya, peach, nectarine), prior allergies, asthma, and skin conditions (e.g., eczema and other dermatitis), those occupationaly exposed to latex products (e.g., healthcare workers, police/firefighters, emergency medical technicians [EMTs], food handlers, hairdressers, cleaning staff, factory workers in plants that manufacture latex-containing products), those with neural tube defects (e.g., spina bifida), or congenital urological conditions requiring frequent surgeries and/or catheterizations (e.g., extrophy of the bladder). **The most severe reactions tend to occur with latex proteins contacting internal tissues during invasive procudures and when they touch mucous membranes of the mouth, vagina, urethra, or rectum.**

- Discuss history of recent exposure; for example, blowing up balloons or using powdered gloves (this might be an acute reaction to the powder); use of latex diaphragm/condoms (may affect either partner).
- Note positive skin-prick test (SPT) when client is skin-tested with latex extracts. **Sensitive, specific, and rapid test, and should be used with caution in persons with suspected sensitivity as it carries risk of anaphylaxis.**
- Perform challenge/patch test, if appropriate, **to identify specific allergens in client with known type IV hypersensitivity.**
- Note response to radioallergosorbent test (RAST) or enzyme-linked assasys of latex-specific IgE (ELISA). **This is the only safe test for the client with a history of life-threatening reaction.**

NURSING PRIORITY NO. 2. To take measures to reduce/limit allergic response/avoid exposure to allergens:
- Ascertain client's current symptoms, noting reports of rash, hives, itching, eye symptoms, edema, diarrhea, nausea, feeling of faintness.
- Determine time since exposure (e.g., immediate or delayed onset, such as 24–48 hours).
- Assess skin (usually hands but may be anywhere) for dry, crusty, hard bumps, scaling, lesions, and horizontal cracks. **May be *irritant contact dermatitis* (the least serious type/most common type of hypersensitivity reaction) or evidence of *allergic contact dermatitis* (a delayed-onset and more severe form of skin/other tissue reaction).**
- Assist with treatment of dermatitis/type IV reaction (e.g., washing affected skin with mild soap and water, possible application of topical steroid ointment, avoidance of further exposure to latex).

Information in brackets added by the authors to clarify and enhance the use of nursing diagnoses.

- Monitor closely for signs of systemic reactions (e.g., difficulty breathing, wheezing, hypotension, tremors, chest pain, tachycardia, dysrhythmias). **Indicative of anaphylactic reaction and can lead to cardiac arrest.**
- Administer treatment, as appropriate, if severe/life-threatening reaction occurs, including antihistamines, epinephrine, IV fluids, corticosteroids, and oxygen/mechanical ventilation, if indicated.
- Ascertain that latex-safe environment (e.g., surgery/hospital room) and products are available according to recommended guidelines and standards, including equipment and supplies (e.g., powder-free, low-protein latex products and latex-free items: gloves, syringes, catheters, tubings, tape, thermometers, electrodes, oxygen cannulas, underpads, storage bags, diapers, feeding nipples, etc.), as appropriate.
- Educate all care providers in ways to prevent inadvertent exposure (e.g., post latex precaution signs in client's room, document allergy to latex in chart), and emergency treatment measures should they be needed.

NURSING PRIORITY NO. **3.** To promote wellness (Teaching/Learning):

- Instuct client/SO(s) to survey and routinely monitor environment for latex-containing products, and replace as needed.
- Provide lists of products that can replace latex (e.g., rubber grip utensils/toys/hoses, rubber-containing pads, undergarments, carpets, shoe soles, computer mouse pad, erasers, rubber bands).
- Emphasize necessity of wearing medical ID bracelet and informing all new care providers of hypersensitivity **to reduce preventable exposures.**
- Advise client to be aware of potential for related food allergies.
- Instruct client/family/SO about signs of reaction as well as how to implement emergency treatment. **Promotes awareness of problem and facilitates timely intervention.**
- Provide worksite review/recommendations to prevent exposure.
- Refer to resources (e.g., *Latex Allergy News*, National Institute for Occupational Safety and Health—NIOSH) **for further information and assistance.**

Documentation Focus

ASSESSMENT/REASSESSMENT

- Assessment findings/pertinent history of contact with latex products/frequency of exposure.

Information in brackets added by the authors to clarify and enhance the use of nursing diagnoses.

  Cultural Collaborative Community/Home Care

- Type/extent of symptomatology.

PLANNING

- Plan of care and interventions and who is involved in planning.
- Teaching plan.

IMPLEMENTATION/EVALUATION

- Response to interventions/teaching and actions performed.
- Attainment/progress toward desired outcome(s).
- Modifications to plan of care.

DISCHARGE PLANNING

- Discharge needs/referrals made, additional resources available.

SAMPLE NURSING OUTCOMES & INTERVENTIONS CLASSIFICATIONS (NOC/NIC)

NOC—Immune Hypersensitivity Control
NIC—Latex Precautions

risk for latex Allergy Response

Taxonomy II: Safety/Protection—Class 5 Defensive
Processes (00042)
[Diagnostic Division: Safety]
Submitted 1998; Revised 2006

Definition: Risk of hypersensitivity to natural latex
rubber products

Risk Factors

History of reactions to latex
Allergies to bananas, avocados, tropical fruits, kiwi, chestnuts,
poinsettia plants
History of allergies/asthma
Professions with daily exposure to latex
Multiple surgical procedures, especially from infancy

NOTE: A risk diagnosis is not evidenced by signs and symptoms, as
the problem has not occurred and nursing interventions are
directed at prevention.

Information in brackets added by the authors to clarify and enhance
the use of nursing diagnoses.

 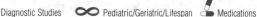

Desired Outcomes/Evaluation Criteria—Client Will:

- Identify and correct potential risk factors in the environment.
- Demonstrate appropriate lifestyle changes to reduce risk of exposure.
- Identify resources to assist in promoting a safe environment.
- Recognize need for/seek assistance to limit response/complications.

Actions/Interventions

NURSING PRIORITY NO. 1. To assess causative/contributing factors:

- Identify persons in high-risk categories such as those with history of certain food allergies (e.g., banana, avocado, chestnut, kiwi, papya, peach, nectarine); asthma; skin conditions (e.g., eczema); those occupationally exposed to latex products (e.g., healthcare workers, police/firefighters, emergency medical technicians [EMTs], food handlers, hairdressers, cleaning staff, factory workers in plants that manufacture latex-containing products); those with neural tube defects (e.g., spina bifida); or congenital urological conditions requiring frequent surgeries and/or catheterizations (e.g., extrophy of the bladder). **The most severe reactions tend to occur when latex proteins contact internal tissues during invasive procedures and when they touch mucous membranes of the mouth, vagina, urethra, or rectum.**
- Ascertain if client could be exposed through catheters, IV tubing, dental/other procedures in healthcare setting. **Although many healthcare facilities and providers use latex-safe equipment, latex is present in many medical supplies and/or in the healthcare environment, with possible risk to client and healthcare provider.**

NURSING PRIORITY NO. 2. To assist in correcting factors that could lead to latex allergy:

- Discuss necessity of avoiding/limiting latex exposure if sensitivity is suspected.
- Recommend that client/family survey environment and remove any medical or household products containing latex.
- Create latex-safe environments (e.g., substitute nonlatex products, such as natural rubber gloves, PCV IV tubing, latex-free tape, thermometers, electrodes, oxygen cannulas) **to enhance client safety by reducing exposure.**

Information in brackets added by the authors to clarify and enhance the use of nursing diagnoses.

 Cultural Collaborative Community/Home Care

- Obtain lists of latex-free products and supplies for client/care provider if appropriate **in order to limit exposure.**
- Ascertain that facilities and/or employers have established policies and procedures to address safety and reduce risk to workers and clients.
- Promote good skin care when latex gloves may be preferred for barrier protection in specific disease conditions such as HIV or during surgery. Use powder-free gloves, wash hands immediately after glove removal; refrain from use of oil-based hand cream. **Reduces dermal and respiratory exposure to latex proteins that bind to the powder in gloves.**

NURSING PRIORITY NO. 3. To promote wellness (Teaching/Discharge Considerations):

- Discuss ways to avoid exposure to latex products with client/SO/caregiver.
- Instruct client/care providers about potential for sensitivity reactions, how to recognize symptoms of latex allergy (e.g., skin rash; hives; flushing; itching; nasal, eye, or sinus symptoms; asthma; and [rarely] shock).
- Identify measures to take if reactions occur.
- Refer to allergist **for testing, as appropriate.** Perform challenge/patch test with gloves to skin **(hives, itching, and reddened areas indicate sensitivity).**

Documentation Focus

ASSESSMENT/REASSESSMENT

- Assessment findings/pertinent history of contact with latex products/frequency of exposure.

PLANNING

- Plan of care, interventions, and who is involved in planning.
- Teaching plan.

IMPLEMENTATION/EVALUATION

- Response to interventions/teaching and actions performed.

DISCHARGE PLANNING

- Discharge needs/referrals made.

SAMPLE NURSING OUTCOMES & INTERVENTIONS CLASSIFICATIONS (NOC/NIC)

NOC—Immune Hypersensitivity Control
NIC—Latex Precautions

Information in brackets added by the authors to clarify and enhance the use of nursing diagnoses.

 Diagnostic Studies   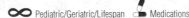 Pediatric/Geriatric/Lifespan   Medications   **87**

Anxiety
[Specify Level: Mild, Moderate, Severe, Panic]

Taxonomy II: Coping/Stress Tolerance—Class 2 Coping
    Responses (00146)
[Diagnostic Division: Ego Integrity]
Submitted 1973; Revised 1982, 1998 (by small group
    work 1996)

Definition: Vague uneasy feeling of discomfort or dread
accompanied by an autonomic response (the source
often nonspecific or unknown to the individual); a
feeling of apprehension caused by anticipation of
danger. It is an altering signal that warns of impending
danger and enables the individual to take measures to
deal with threat.

Related Factors

Unconscious conflict about essential [beliefs]/goals/values
    of life
Situational/maturational crises
Stress
Familial association; heredity
Interpersonal transmission/contagion
Threat to self-concept [perceived or actual]; [unconscious
    conflict]
Threat of death [perceived or actual]
Threat to/change in: health status [progressive/debilitating dis-
    ease, terminal illness]; interaction patterns; role function/
    status; environment [safety]; economic status
Unmet needs
Exposure to toxins; substance abuse
[Positive or negative self-talk]
[Physiological factors, such as hyperthyroidism, pulmonary
    embolism, dysrhythmias, pheochromocytoma, drug therapy,
    including steroids]

Defining Characteristics

SUBJECTIVE

Behavioral
Expressed concerns due to change in life events; insomnia

Information in brackets added by the authors to clarify and enhance
the use of nursing diagnoses.

 Cultural Collaborative   Community/Home Care

Affective

Regretful; scared; rattled; distressed; apprehensive; fearful; feelings of inadequacy; uncertainty; jittery; worried; painful/persistent increased helplessness; [sense of impending doom]; [hopelessness]

Cognitive

Fear of unspecified consequences; awareness of physiological symptoms

Physiological

Shakiness

Sympathetic

Dry mouth; heart pounding; weakness; respiratory difficulties; anorexia; diarrhea

Parasympathetic

Tingling in extremities; nausea; abdominal pain; diarrhea; urinary frequency/hesitancy; faintness; fatigue; sleep disturbance; [chest, back, neck pain]

OBJECTIVE

Behavioral

Poor eye contact; glancing about; scanning; vigilance; extraneous movement [e.g., foot shuffling, hand/arm movements, rocking motion]; fidgeting; restlessness; diminished productivity; [crying/tearfulness]; [pacing/purposeless activity]; [immobility]

Affective

Increased wariness; focus on self; irritability; overexcited; anguish

Cognitive

Preoccupation; impaired attention; difficulty concentrating; forgetfulness; diminished ability to problem solve; diminished ability to learn; rumination; tendency to blame others; blocking of thought; confusion; decreased perceptual field

Physiological

Voice quivering; trembling/hand tremors; increased tension; facial tension; increased perspiration

Sympathetic

Cardiovascular excitation; facial flushing; superficial vasoconstriction; increased pulse/respiration; increased blood pressure; pupil dilation; twitching; increased reflexes

---

Information in brackets added by the authors to clarify and enhance the use of nursing diagnoses.

 Diagnostic Studies ∞ Pediatric/Geriatric/Lifespan Medications

Parasympathetic
Urinary urgency; decreased blood pressure/pulse

Desired Outcomes/Evaluation Criteria—Client Will:

- Appear relaxed and report anxiety is reduced to a manageable level.
- Verbalize awareness of feelings of anxiety.
- Identify healthy ways to deal with and express anxiety.
- Demonstrate problem-solving skills.
- Use resources/support systems effectively.

Actions/Interventions

NURSING PRIORITY NO. 1. To assess level of anxiety:
- Review familial/physiological factors, such as genetic depressive factors; psychiatric illness; active medical conditions (e.g., thyroid problems, metabolic imbalances, cardiopulmonary disease, anemia, or dysrhythmias); recent/ongoing stressors (e.g., family member illness/death, spousal conflict/abuse, or loss of job). **These factors can cause/exacerbate anxiety/ anxiety disorders.**

- Determine current prescribed medications and recent drug history of prescribed or OTC medications (e.g., steroids, thyroid preparations, weight loss pills, or caffeine). **These medications can heighten feelings/sense of anxiety.**
- Identify client's perception of the threat represented by the situation.
- Monitor vital signs (e.g., rapid or irregular pulse, rapid breathing/hyperventilation, changes in blood pressure, diaphorsesis, tremors, or restlessness) **to identify physical responses associated with both medical and emotional conditions.**
- Observe behaviors, **which can point to the client's level of anxiety:**

Mild
Alert; more aware of environment; attention focused on environment and immediate events
Restless; irritable; wakeful; reports of insomnia
Motivated to deal with existing problems in this state

Moderate
Perception narrower; concentration increased; able to ignore distractions in dealing with problem(s)

Information in brackets added by the authors to clarify and enhance the use of nursing diagnoses.

  Cultural Collaborative Community/Home Care

Voice quivers or changes pitch
Trembling; increased pulse/respirations

Severe

Range of perception is reduced; anxiety interferes with effective functioning

Preoccupied with feelings of discomfort/sense of impending doom

Increased pulse/respirations with reports of dizziness, tingling sensations, headache, and so forth

Panic

Ability to concentrate is disrupted; behavior is disintegrated; client distorts the situation and does not have realistic perceptions of what is happening. Client may be experiencing terror or confusion or be unable to speak or move (paralyzed with fear)

- Note reports of insomnia or excessive sleeping, limited/avoidance of interactions with others, use of alcohol or other drugs of abuse, **which may be behavioral indicators of use of withdrawal to deal with problems.**

- Review results of diagnostic tests (e.g., drug screens, cardiac testing, complete blood count, and chemistry panel), **which may point to physiological sources of anxiety.**
- Be aware of defense mechanisms being used (e.g., denial or regression) **that interfere with ability to deal with problem.**
- Identify coping skills the individual is currently using, such as anger, daydreaming, forgetfulness, overeating, smoking, or lack of problem solving.
- Review coping skills used in past **to determine those that might be helpful in current circumstances.**

NURSING PRIORITY NO. 2. To assist client to identify feelings and begin to deal with problems:

- Establish a therapeutic relationship, conveying empathy and unconditional positive regard. *Note:* Nurse needs to be aware of own feelings of anxiety or uneasiness, exercising care **to avoid the contagious effect/transmission of anxiety.**
- Be available to client for listening and talking.
- Encourage client to acknowledge and to express feelings; for example, crying (sadness), laughing (fear, denial), or swearing (fear, anger).
- Assist client to develop self-awareness of verbal and nonverbal behaviors.
- Clarify meaning of feelings/actions by providing feedback and checking meaning with the client.

Information in brackets added by the authors to clarify and enhance the use of nursing diagnoses.

- Acknowledge anxiety/fear. Do not deny or reassure client that everything will be all right.
- Provide accurate information about the situation. **Helps client to identify what is reality based.**
- With a child, be truthful, avoid bribing, and provide physical contact (e.g., hugging or rocking) **to soothe fears and provide assurance.**
- Provide comfort measures (e.g., calm/quiet environment, soft music, warm bath, or back rub).
- Modify procedures as much as possible (e.g., substitute oral for intramuscular medications or combine blood draws/use fingerstick method) **to limit degree of stress and avoid over-whelming child or anxious adult.**
- Manage environmental factors, such as harsh lighting and high traffic flow, which may be confusing/stressful to older individuals.
- Accept client as is. (**The client may need to be where he or she is at this point in time, such as in denial after receiving the diagnosis of a terminal illness.**)
- Allow the behavior to belong to the client; do not respond personally. (**The nurse may respond inappropriately, escalating the situation to a nontherapeutic interaction.**)
- Assist client to use anxiety for coping with the situation, if helpful. (**Moderate anxiety heightens awareness and permits the client to focus on dealing with problems.**)

Panic State

- Stay with client, maintaining a calm, confident manner.
- Speak in brief statements using simple words.
- Provide for nonthreatening, consistent environment/atmosphere. Minimize stimuli. Monitor visitors and interactions **to lessen effect of transmission of feelings.**
- Set limits on inappropriate behavior and help client to develop acceptable ways of dealing with anxiety.

> NOTE: Staff may need to provide safe controls/environment until client regains control.

- Gradually increase activities/involvement with others as anxiety is decreased.
- Use cognitive therapy **to focus on/correct faulty catastrophic interpretations of physical symptoms.**
- Administer medications (antianxiety agents/sedatives), as ordered.

Information in brackets added by the authors to clarify and enhance the use of nursing diagnoses.

  Cultural Collaborative 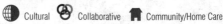 Community/Home Care

NURSING PRIORITY NO. **3.** To promote wellness (Teaching/ Discharge Considerations):

- Assist client to identify precipitating factors and new methods of coping with disabling anxiety.
- Review happenings, thoughts, and feelings preceding the anxiety attack.
- Identify actions/activities the client has previously used to cope successfully when feeling nervous/anxious.
- List helpful resources/people, including available "hotline" or crisis managers **to provide ongoing/timely support.**
- Encourage client to develop an exercise/activity program, **which may serve to reduce level of anxiety by relieving tension.**
- Assist in developing skills (e.g., awareness of negative thoughts, saying "Stop," and substituting a positive thought) **to eliminate negative self-talk. Mild phobias tend to respond well to behavioral therapy.**
- Review strategies, such as role playing, use of visualizations to practice anticipated events, prayer/meditation; **useful for being prepared for/dealing with anxiety-provoking situations.**
- Review medication regimen and possible interactions, especially with over-the-counter drugs/alcohol, and so forth. Discuss appropriate drug substitutions, changes in dosage, or time of dose **to minimize side effects.**
- Refer to physician for drug management program/alteration of prescription regimen. (**Drugs often causing symptoms of anxiety include aminophylline/theophylline, anticholinergics, dopamine, levodopa, salicylates, and steroids.**)
- Refer to individual and/or group therapy, as appropriate, **to deal with chronic anxiety states.**

Documentation Focus

ASSESSMENT/REASSESSMENT

- Level of anxiety and precipitating/aggravating factors.
- Description of feelings (expressed and displayed).
- Awareness/ability to recognize and express feelings.
- Related substance use, if present.

PLANNING

- Treatment plan and individual responsibility for specific activities.
- Teaching plan.

Information in brackets added by the authors to clarify and enhance the use of nursing diagnoses.

Diagnostic Studies   ∞ Pediatric/Geriatric/Lifespan   Medications

IMPLEMENTATION/EVALUATION

- Client involvement and response to interventions/teaching and actions performed.
- Attainment/progress toward desired outcome(s).
- Modifications to plan of care.

DISCHARGE PLANNING

- Referrals and follow-up plan.
- Specific referrals made.

SAMPLE NURSING OUTCOMES & INTERVENTIONS CLASSIFICATIONS (NOC/NIC)

NOC—Anxiety Control
NIC—Anxiety Reduction

death Anxiety

Taxonomy II: Coping/Stress Tolerance—Class 2 Coping Response (00147)
[Diagnostic Division: Ego Integrity]
Submitted 1998; Revised 2006

Definition: Vague uneasy feeling of discomfort or dread generated by perceptions of a real or imagined threat to one's existence

Related Factors

Anticipating: pain; suffering; adverse consequences of general anesthesia; impact of death on others
Confronting reality of terminal disease; experiencing dying process; perceived proximity of death
Discussions on topic of death; observations related to death; near death experience
Uncertainty of prognosis; nonacceptance of own mortality
Uncertainty about: the existence of a higher power; life after death; an encounter with a higher power

Defining Characteristics

SUBJECTIVE

Fear of: developing a terminal illness; the process of dying; pain/suffering related to dying; loss of mental [/physical] abilities when dying; premature death; prolonged dying

---

Information in brackets added by the authors to clarify and enhance the use of nursing diagnoses.

 Cultural Collaborative Community/Home Care

Negative thoughts related to death and dying

Feeling powerlessness over dying

Worrying about the impact of one's own death on significant others

Concerns of overworking the caregiver; [about meeting one's creator or feeling doubtful about the existence of God or higher being]

Deep sadness

(Refer to ND Grieving)

Desired Outcomes/Evaluation Criteria—Client Will:

• Identify and express feelings (e.g., sadness, guilt, fear) freely/effectively.
• Look toward/plan for the future one day at a time.
• Formulate a plan dealing with individual concerns and eventualities of dying as appropriate.

Actions/Interventions

NURSING PRIORITY NO. 1. To assess causative/contributing factors:

• Determine how client sees self in usual lifestyle role functioning and perception and meaning of anticipated loss to him or her and SO(s).
• Ascertain current knowledge of situation **to identify misconceptions, lack of information, other pertinent issues.**
• Determine client's role in family constellation. Observe patterns of communication in family and response of family/SO to client's situation and concerns. **In addition to identifying areas of need/concern, also reveals strengths useful in addressing the concerns.**
• Assess impact of client reports of subjective experiences and past experience with death (or exposure to death); for example, witnessed violent death or as a child viewed body in casket, and so on.
• Identify cultural factors/expectations and impact on current situation/feelings.
• Note physical/mental condition, complexity of therapeutic regimen.
• Determine ability to manage own self-care, end-of-life and other affairs, awareness/use of available resources.
• Observe behavior indicative of the level of anxiety present (mild to panic) **as it affects client's/SO's ability to process information/participate in activities.**

Information in brackets added by the authors to clarify and enhance the use of nursing diagnoses.

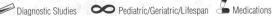

- Identify coping skills currently used and how effective they are. Be aware of defense mechanisms being used by the client.
- Note use of alcohol or other drugs of abuse, reports of insomnia, excessive sleeping, avoidance of interactions with others **which may be behavioral indicators of use of withdrawal to deal with problems.**
- Note client's religious/spiritual orientation, involvement in religious/church activities, presence of conflicts regarding spiritual beliefs.
- Listen to client/SO reports/expressions of anger/concern, alienation from God, belief that impending death is a punishment for wrongdoing, and so on.
- Determine sense of futility; feelings of hopelessness, helplessness; lack of motivation to help self. **May indicate presence of depression and need for intervention.**
- Active-listen comments regarding sense of isolation.
- Listen for expressions of inability to find meaning in life or suicidal ideation.

NURSING PRIORITY NO. 2. To assist client to deal with situation:
- Provide open and trusting relationship.
- Use therapeutic communication skills of active-listening, silence, acknowledgment. Respect client's desire/request not to talk. Provide hope within parameters of the individual situation.
- Encourage expressions of feelings (anger, fear, sadness, etc.). Acknowledge anxiety/fear. Do not deny or reassure client that everything will be all right. Be honest when answering questions/providing information. **Enhances trust and therapeutic relationship.**
- Provide information about normalcy of feelings and individual grief reaction.
- Make time for nonjudgmental discussion of philosophic issues/questions about spiritual impact of illness/situation.
- Review life experiences of loss and use of coping skills, noting client's strengths and successes.
- Provide calm, peaceful setting and privacy as appropriate. **Promotes relaxation and ability to deal with situation.**
- Assist client to engage in spiritual growth activities, experience prayer/meditation and forgiveness to heal past hurts. Provide information that anger with God is a normal part of the grieving process. **Reduces feelings of guilt/conflict, allowing client to move forward toward resolution.**
- Refer to therapists, spiritual advisors, counselors **to facilitate grief work.**

Information in brackets added by the authors to clarify and enhance the use of nursing diagnoses.

  Cultural Collaborative Community/Home Care

- Refer to community agencies/resources **to assist client/SO for planning for eventualities (legal issues, funeral plans, etc.).**

NURSING PRIORITY NO. 3. To promote independence:

- Support client's efforts to develop realistic steps to put plans into action.
- Direct client's thoughts beyond present state to enjoyment of each day and the future when appropriate.
- Provide opportunities for the client to make simple decisions. **Enhances sense of control.**
- Develop individual plan using client's locus of control **to assist client/family through the process.**
- Treat expressed decisions and desires with respect and convey to others as appropriate.
- Assist with completion of Advance Directives, cardiopulmonary resuscitation (CPR) instructions, and durable medical power of attorney.

Documentation Focus

ASSESSMENT/REASSESSMENT

- Assessment findings, including client's fears and signs/symptoms being exhibited.
- Responses/actions of family/SO(s).
- Availability/use of resources.

PLANNING

- Plan of care and who is involved in planning.

IMPLEMENTATION/EVALUATION

- Client's response to interventions/teaching and actions performed.
- Attainment/progress toward desired outcome(s).
- Modifications to plan of care.

DISCHARGE PLANNING

- Identified needs and who is responsible for actions to be taken.
- Specific referrals made.

SAMPLE NURSING OUTCOMES & INTERVENTIONS CLASSIFICATIONS (NOC/NIC)

NOC—Dignified Dying
NIC—Dying Care

Information in brackets added by the authors to clarify and enhance the use of nursing diagnoses.

 Diagnostic Studies   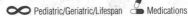 Pediatric/Geriatric/Lifespan   Medications   **97**

risk for Aspiration

Taxonomy II: Safety/Protection—Class 2 Physical Injury (00039)
[Diagnostic Division: Respiration]
Submitted 1988

Definition: At risk for entry of gastrointestinal secretions, oropharyngeal secretions, or [exogenous food] solids or fluids into tracheobronchial passages

Risk Factors

Reduced level of consciousness [sedation/anesthesia]

Depressed cough/gag reflexes

Impaired swallowing [inability of the epiglottis and true vocal cords to move to close off trachea]

Facial/oral/neck surgery or trauma; wired jaws; [congenital malformations]

Situation hindering elevation of upper body [weakness, paralysis]

Incomplete lower esophageal sphincter [hiatal hernia or other esophageal disease affecting stomach valve function]; delayed gastric emptying; decreased gastrointestinal motility; increased intragastric pressure; increased gastric residual

Presence of tracheostomy or endotracheal (ET) tube [inadequate or overinflation of tracheostomy/ET tube cuff]

[Presence of] gastrointestinal tubes; tube feedings; medication administration

---

NOTE: A risk diagnosis is not evidenced by signs and symptoms, as the problem has not occurred and nursing interventions are directed at prevention.

Desired Outcomes/Evaluation Criteria—Client Will:

• Experience no aspiration as evidenced by noiseless respirations; clear breath sounds; clear, odorless secretions.
• Identify causative/risk factors.
• Demonstrate techniques to prevent and/or correct aspiration.

Actions/Interventions

NURSING PRIORITY NO. **1.** To assess causative/contributing factors:

• Identify at-risk client according to condition/disease process,

---

Information in brackets added by the authors to clarify and enhance the use of nursing diagnoses.

  Cultural Collaborative 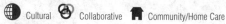 Community/Home Care as listed in Risk Factors, **to determine when observation and/or interventions may be required.**

- Note client's level of consciousness, awareness of surroundings, and cognitive function, **as impairments in these areas increase client's risk of aspiration.**
- Determine presence of neuromuscular disorders, noting muscle groups involved, degree of impairment, and whether they are of an acute or progressive nature (e.g., stroke, Parkinson's disease, Guillain-Barré syndrome, or amyotrophic lateral sclerosis [ALS]).
- Assess client's ability to swallow and strength of gag/cough reflex and evaluate amount/consistency of secretions. **Helps to determine presence/effectiveness of protective mechanisms.**
- Observe for neck and facial edema. **Client with head/neck surgery, tracheal/bronchial injury (e.g., upper torso burns or inhalation/chemical injury) is at particular risk for airway obstruction and inability to handle secretions.**
- Note administration of enteral feedings **because of potential for regurgitation and/or misplacement of tube.**
- Ascertain lifestyle habits; for example, use of alcohol, tobacco, and other CNS-suppressant drugs, **which can affect awareness and muscles of gag/swallow.**
- Assist with/review diagnostic studies (e.g., video-fluoroscopy or fiberoptic endoscopy), **which may be done to assess for presence/degree of impairment.**

NURSING PRIORITY NO. 2. To assist in correcting factors that can lead to aspiration:

- Monitor use of oxygen masks in clients at risk for vomiting. Refrain from using oxygen masks for comatose individuals.
- Keep wire cutters/scissors with client at all times when jaws are wired/banded **to facilitate clearing airway in emergency situations.**
- Maintain operational suction equipment at bedside/chairside.
- Suction (oral cavity, nose, and ET/tracheostomy tube), as needed, and avoid triggering gag mechanism when performing suction or mouth care **to clear secretions while reducing potential for aspiration of secretions.**
- Avoid keeping client supine/flat when on mechanical ventilation (especially when also receiving enteral feedings). **Supine positioning and enteral feedings have been shown to be independent risk factors for the development of aspiration pneumonia.**

Information in brackets added by the authors to clarify and enhance the use of nursing diagnoses.

Diagnostic Studies   Pediatric/Geriatric/Lifespan   Medications

- Assist with postural drainage **to mobilize thickened secretions that may interfere with swallowing.**
- Auscultate lung sounds frequently, especially in client who is coughing frequently or not coughing at all, or in client on ventilator being tube-fed, **to determine presence of secretions/silent aspiration**.
- Elevate client to highest or best possible position (e.g., sitting upright in chair) for eating and drinking and during tube feedings.
- Provide a rest period prior to feeding time. **The rested client may have less difficulty with swallowing**.
- Feed slowly, using small bites, instructing client to chew slowly and thoroughly.
- Vary placement of food in client's mouth according to type of deficit (e.g., place food in right side of mouth if facial weakness is present on left side).
- Provide soft foods that stick together/form a bolus (e.g., casseroles, puddings, or stews) **to aid swallowing effort**.
- Determine liquid viscosity best tolerated by client. Add thickening agent to liquids, as appropriate. **Some individuals may swallow thickened liquids better than thin liquids**.
- Offer very warm or very cold liquids. **Activates temperature receptors in the mouth that help to stimulate swallowing**.
- Avoid washing solids down with liquids.
- Ascertain that feeding tube (when used) is in correct position. Ask client about feeling of fullness and/or measure residuals (just prior to feeding and several hours after feeding), when appropriate, **to reduce risk of aspiration**.
- Determine best resting position for infant/child (e.g., with the head of bed elevated 30 degrees and infant propped on right side after feeding). **Upper airway patency is facilitated by upright position and turning to right side decreases likelihood of drainage into trachea**.
- Provide oral medications in elixir form or crush, if appropriate.
- Minimize use of sedatives/hypnotics whenever possible. **These agents can impair coughing and swallowing.**
- Refer to physician/speech therapist for medical/surgical interventions and/or exercises **to strengthen muscles and learn techniques to enhance swallowing/reduce potential aspiration**.

NURSING PRIORITY NO. 3. To promote wellness (Teaching/Discharge Considerations):

- Review with client/SO individual risk/potentiating factors.

Information in brackets added by the authors to clarify and enhance the use of nursing diagnoses.

 Cultural Collaborative 🏠 Community/Home Care

- Provide information about the effects of aspiration on the lungs. **Note: Severe coughing and cyanosis associated with eating or drinking or changes in vocal quality after swallowing indicates onset of respiratory symptoms associated with aspiration and requires immediate intervention.**
- Instruct in safety concerns regarding oral or tube feeing. (Refer to ND impaired Swallowing.)
- Train client how to self-suction or train family members in suction techniques (especially if client has constant or copious oral secretions) **to enhance safety/self-sufficiency.**
- Instruct individual/family member to avoid/limit activities after eating that increase intra-abdominal pressure (straining, strenuous exercise, or tight/constrictive clothing), **which may slow digestion/increase risk of regurgitation.**

Documentation Focus

ASSESSMENT/REASSESSMENT

- Assessment findings/conditions that could lead to problems of aspiration.
- Verification of tube placement, observations of physical findings.

PLANNING

- Interventions to prevent aspiration or reduce risk factors and who is involved in the planning.
- Teaching plan.

IMPLEMENTATION/EVALUATION

- Client's responses to interventions/teaching and actions performed.
- Foods/fluids client handles with ease/difficulty.
- Amount/frequency of intake.
- Attainment/progress toward desired outcome(s).
- Modifications to plan of care.

DISCHARGE PLANNING

- Long-term needs and who is responsible for actions to be taken.

SAMPLE NURSING OUTCOMES & INTERVENTIONS CLASSIFICATIONS (NOC/NIC)

NOC—Risk Control
NIC—Aspiration Precautions

Information in brackets added by the authors to clarify and enhance the use of nursing diagnoses.

 Diagnostic Studies ∞ Pediatric/Geriatric/Lifespan 💊 Medications **101**

risk for impaired parent/child Attachment

Taxonomy II: Role Relationships—Class 2 Family
  Relationships (00058)
[Diagnostic Division: Social Interaction]
Submitted 1994

Definition: Disruption of the interactive process between
parent/SO and child/infant that fosters the development
of a protective and nurturing reciprocal relationship

Risk Factors

Inability of parents to meet personal needs
Anxiety associated with the parent role; [parents who them-
  selves experienced altered attachment]
Premature infant or ill infant/child who is unable to effectively
  initiate parental contact due to altered behavioral organiza-
  tion; parental conflict due to altered behavioral organization
Separation; physical barriers; lack of privacy
Substance abuse
[Difficult pregnancy and/or birth (actual or perceived)]
[Uncertainty of paternity; conception as a result of rape/sexual
  abuse]

> NOTE: A risk diagnosis is not evidenced by signs and symptoms, as
> the problem has not occurred and nursing interventions are
> directed at prevention.

Desired Outcomes/Evaluation Criteria—Parent Will:

• Identify and prioritize family strengths and needs.
• Exhibit nurturant and protective behaviors toward child.
• Identify and use resources to meet needs of family members.
• Demonstrate techniques to enhance behavioral organization
  of the infant/child.
• Engage in mutually satisfying interactions with child.

Actions/Interventions

NURSING PRIORITY NO. 1. To identify causative/contributing factors:
• Interview parents, noting their perception of situation and
  individual concerns.
 • Assess parent/child interactions.

Information in brackets added by the authors to clarify and enhance
the use of nursing diagnoses.

 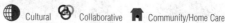

- Ascertain availability/use of resources to include extended family, support groups, and financial resources.
- Evaluate parents' ability to provide protective environment and participate in reciprocal relationship.

NURSING PRIORITY NO. 2. To enhance behavioral organization of child:
- Identify infant's strengths and vulnerabilities. **Each child is born with his or her own temperament that affects interactions with caregivers.**
- Educate parents regarding child growth and development, addressing parental perceptions. **Helps clarify realistic or unrealistic expectations.**
- Assist parents in modifying the environment **to provide appropriate stimulation.**
- Model caregiving techniques that best support behavioral organization.
- Respond consistently with nurturing to infant/child.

NURSING PRIORITY NO. 3. To enhance best functioning of parents:
- Develop therapeutic nurse-client relationship. Provide a consistently warm, nurturing, and nonjudgmental environment.
- Assist parents in identifying and prioritizing family strengths and needs. **Promotes positive attitude by looking at what they already do well and using those skills to address needs.**
- Support and guide parents in process of assessing resources.
- Involve parents in activities with the child that they can accomplish successfully. **Promotes sense of confidence, thus enhancing self-concept.**
- Recognize and provide positive feedback for nurturing and protective parenting behaviors. **Reinforces continuation of desired behaviors.**
- Minimize number of professionals on team with whom parents must have contact **to foster trust in relationships.**

NURSING PRIORITY NO. 4. To support parent/child attachment during separation:
- Provide parents with telephone contact, as appropriate.
- Establish a routine time for daily phone calls/initiate calls, as indicated. **Provides sense of consistency and control; allows for planning of other activities.**
- Invite parents to use Ronald McDonald House or provide them with a listing of a variety of local accommodations/restaurants when child is hospitalized out of town.
- Arrange for parents to receive photos/progress reports from the child.

Information in brackets added by the authors to clarify and enhance the use of nursing diagnoses.

- Suggest parents provide a photo and/or audiotape of themselves for the child.
- Consider use of contract with parents **to clearly communicate expectations of both family and staff.**
- Suggest parents keep a journal of infant/child progress.
- Provide "homelike" environment for situations requiring supervision of visits.

NURSING PRIORITY NO. 5. To promote wellness (Teaching/Discharge Considerations):

- Refer to individual counseling, family therapies, or addiction counseling/treatment, as indicated.
- Identify services for transportation, financial resources, housing, and so forth.
- Develop support systems appropriate to situation (e.g., extended family, friends, social worker).
- Explore community resources (e.g., church affiliations, volunteer groups, day/respite care).

Documentation Focus

ASSESSMENT/REASSESSMENT

- Identified behaviors of both parents and child.
- Specific risk factors, individual perceptions/concerns.
- Interactions between parent and child.

PLANNING

- Plan of care and who is involved in planning.
- Teaching plan.

IMPLEMENTATION/EVALUATION

- Parents'/child's responses to interventions/teaching and actions performed.
- Attainment/progress toward desired outcomes.
- Modifications to plan of care.

DISCHARGE PLANNING

- Long-term needs and who is responsible.
- Plan for home visits to support parents and to ensure infant/child safety and well-being.
- Specific referrals made.

SAMPLE NURSING OUTCOMES & INTERVENTIONS CLASSIFICATIONS (NOC/NIC)

NOC—Parent-Infant Attachment
NIC—Attachment Promotion

Information in brackets added by the authors to clarify and enhance the use of nursing diagnoses.

 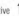

Autonomic Dysreflexia

Taxonomy II: Coping/Stress Tolerance—Class 3
   Neurobehavioral Stress (00009)
[Diagnostic Division: Circulation]
Submitted 1988

Definition: Life-threatening, uninhibited sympathetic
response of the nervous system to a noxious stimulus
after a spinal cord injury [SCI] at T7 or above

Related Factors

Bladder/bowel distention; [catheter insertion, obstruction,
   irrigation; constipation]
Skin irritation
Deficient patient/caregiver knowledge
[Sexual excitation; menstruation; pregnancy; labor and delivery]
[Environmental temperature extremes]

Defining Characteristics

SUBJECTIVE

Headache (a diffuse pain in different portions of the head and
   not confined to any nerve distribution area)
Paresthesia; chilling; blurred vision; chest pain; metallic taste in
   mouth; nasal congestion

OBJECTIVE

Paroxysmal hypertension [sudden periodic elevated blood
   pressure in which systolic pressure >140 mm Hg and dias-
   tolic pressure >90 mm Hg]
Bradycardia/tachycardia
Diaphoresis (above the injury), red splotches on skin (above the
   injury), pallor (below the injury)
Horner's syndrome [contraction of the pupil, partial ptosis of
   the eyelid, enophthalmos and sometimes loss of sweating
   over the affected side of the face]; conjunctival congestion
Pilomotor reflex [gooseflesh formation when skin is cooled]

Desired Outcomes/Evaluation
Criteria—Client/Caregiver Will:

• Identify risk factors.
• Recognize signs/symptoms of syndrome.

Information in brackets added by the authors to clarify and enhance
the use of nursing diagnoses.

 Diagnostic Studies   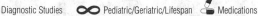 Pediatric/Geriatric/Lifespan   Medications   **105**

- Demonstrate corrective techniques.
- Experience no episodes of dysreflexia or will seek medical intervention in a timely manner.

Actions/Interventions

NURSING PRIORITY NO. 1. To assess precipitating risk factors:

- Monitor for bladder distention, presence of bladder spasms/stones, or infection. **The most common stimulus for autonomic dysreflexia (AD) is bladder irritation or over-stretch associated with urinary retention or infection, blocked catheter, overfilled collection bag, or noncompliance with intermittent catheterization.**
- Assess for bowel distention, fecal impaction, problems with bowel management program. **Bowel irritation or overstretch is associated with constipation or impaction; digital stimulation, suppository/enema use during bowel program; hemorrhoids/fissures; and/or infection of gastrointestinal tract, such as might occur with ulcers, appendicitis.**
- Observe skin/tissue pressure areas, especially following prolonged sitting. **Skin/tissue irritants include direct pressure (e.g., object in chair or shoe, leg straps, abdominal support, orthotics), wounds (e.g., bruise, abrasion, laceration, pressure ulcer), ingrown toenail, tight clothing, sunburn/other burn.**
- Inquire about sexual activity and/or determine if reproductive issues are involved. **Overstimulation/vibration, sexual intercouse/ejaculation, scrotal compression, menstrual cramps, and/or pregnancy (especially labor and delivery) are known stimulants.**
- Inform client/care providers of additional precipitators during course of care. **Client is prone to physical conditions/treatments (e.g., intolerance to temperature extremes; deep vein thrombosis [DVT]; kidney stones; fractures/other truama; surgical, dental, and diagnostic procedures), any of which can precipitate AD.**

NURSING PRIORITY NO. 2. To provide for early detection and immediate intervention:

- Investigate associated complaints/symptoms (e.g., sudden severe headache, chest pains, blurred vision, facial flushing, nausea, metallic taste). **AD is a potentially life-threatening condition which requires immediate intervention**.
- Correct/eliminate causative stimulus immediately when possible (e.g., perform immediate catheterization or restore

---

Information in brackets added by the authors to clarify and enhance the use of nursing diagnoses.

  Cultural   Collaborative   Community/Home Care

urine flow if blocked; remove bowel impaction or stop digital stimulation; reduce skin pressure by changing position or removing restrictive clothing; protect from temperature extremes).

- Elevate head of bed as high as tolorated or place client in sitting position with legs dangling **to lower blood pressure.**
- Monitor vital signs frequently during acute episode. Continue to monitor blood pressure at intervals after symptoms subside **to evaluate effectiveness of interventions.**
- Administer medications as required **to block excessive autonomic nerve transmission, normalize heart rate, and reduce hypertension.**
- Carefully adjust dosage of antihypertensive medications for children, the elderly, or pregnant women. (**Assists in preventing seizures and maintaining blood pressure within desired range.**)

NURSING PRIORITY NO. 3. To promote wellness (Teaching/Discharge Considerations):

- Discuss warning signs and how to avoid onset of syndrome with client/SO(s). **Knowledge can support adherence to preventative measures and promote prompt intervention when required. Note: If cause cannot be detected, or situation quickly resolved, contact physician immediately for further interventions to reduce risk of serious complications.**
- Instruct client/caregivers in preventative care (e.g., safe and timely bowel and bladder care; prevention of skin breakdown; care of existing skin breaks; prevention of infection).
- Instruct family member/caregiver in blood pressure monitoring and discuss plan for monitoring and treatment of high blood pressure during acute episodes.
- Review proper use/administration of medication if indicated. **Client may have medication(s) both for emergent situations and/or prevention of AD.**
- Assist client/family in identifying emergency referrals (e.g., physician, rehabilitation nurse/home care supervisor). Place phone number(s) in prominent place.
- Recommend wearing Medical Alert bracelet/necklace and carrying information card reviewing client's typical signs/symptoms and usual methods of treatment. **Provides vital information to care providers in emergent situation.**
- Refer for advice/treatment of sexual and reproductive concerns as indicated.
- Refer to ND risk for Autonomic Dysreflexia.

Information in brackets added by the authors to clarify and enhance the use of nursing diagnoses.

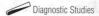

Diagnostic Studies   Pediatric/Geriatric/Lifespan   Medications   **107**

Documentation Focus

ASSESSMENT/REASSESSMENT

- Individual findings, noting previous episodes, precipitating factors, and individual signs/symptoms.

PLANNING

- Plan of care and who is involved in planning.
- Teaching plan.

IMPLEMENTATION/EVALUATION

- Client's responses to interventions and actions performed, understanding of teaching.
- Attainment/progress toward desired outcome(s).
- Modifications to plan of care.

DISCHARGE PLANNING

- Long-term needs and who is responsible for actions to be taken.

SAMPLE NURSING OUTCOMES & INTERVENTIONS CLASSIFICATIONS (NOC/NIC)

NOC—Neurological Status: Autonomic
NIC—Dysreflexia Management

risk for Autonomic Dysreflexia

Taxonomy II: Coping/Stress Tolerance—Class 3 Neurobehavioral Stress (00010)
[Diagnostic Division: Circulation]
Nursing Diagnosis Extension and Classification (NDEC) Submission 1998/Revised 2000

Definition: At risk for life-threatening, uninhibited response of the sympathetic nervous system post-spinal shock, in an individual with a spinal cord injury [SCI] or lesion at T6 or above (has been demonstrated in patients with injuries at T7 and T8)

Risk Factors

An injury at T6 or above or a lesion at T6 or above AND at least one of the following noxious stimuli:

Information in brackets added by the authors to clarify and enhance the use of nursing diagnoses.

 Cultural Collaborative Community/Home Care

MUSCULOSKELETAL—INTEGUMENTARY STIMULI

Cutaneous stimulations (e.g., pressure ulcer, ingrown toenail, dressing, burns, rash); sunburns; wounds

Pressure over bony prominences/genitalia; range-of-motion exercises; spasms

Fractures; heterotrophic bone

GASTROINTESTINAL STIMULI

Constipation; difficult passage of feces; fecal impaction; bowel distention; hemorrhoids

Digital stimulation; suppositories; enemas

GI system pathology; esophageal reflux; gastric ulcers; gallstones

UROLOGICAL STIMULI

Bladder distention/spasm

Detrusor sphincter dyssynergia

Catheterization; instrumentation; surgery; calculi

Urinary tract infection; cystitis; urethritis; epididymitis

REGULATORY STIMULI

Temperature fluctuations; extreme environmental temperatures

SITUATIONAL STIMULI

Positioning; surgical procedure; [diagnostic procedures]

Constrictive clothing (e.g., straps, stockings, shoes)

Drug reactions (e.g., decongestants, sympathomimetics, vasoconstrictors, narcotic withdrawal)

[Surgical or diagnostic procedures]

NEUROLOGICAL STIMULI

Painful or irritating stimuli below the level of injury

CARDIAC/PULMONARY STIMULI

Pulmonary emboli; deep vein thrombosis

REPRODUCTIVE [AND SEXUALITY] STIMULI

Sexual intercourse; ejaculation; [vibrator overstimulation; scrotal compression]

Menstruation; pregnancy; labor and delivery; ovarian cyst

NOTE: A risk diagnosis is not evidenced by signs and symptoms as the problem has not occurred; rather, nursing interventions are directed at prevention.

Information in brackets added by the authors to clarify and enhance the use of nursing diagnoses.

 Diagnostic Studies   ∞ Pediatric/Geriatric/Lifespan   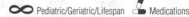 Medications   **109**

Desired Outcomes/Evaluation Criteria—Client Will:

- Identify risk factors present.
- Demonstrate preventive/corrective techniques.
- Be free of episodes of dysreflexia.

Actions/Interventions

NURSING PRIORITY NO. 1. To assess risk factors present:
- Monitor for potential precipitating factors, including urological (e.g., bladder distention, urinary tract infections, kidney stones); gastrointestinal (e.g., bowel overdistention, hemorrhoids, digital stimulation); cutaneous (e.g., pressure ulcers, extreme external temperatures, dressing changes); reproductive (e.g., sexual activity, menstruation, pregnancy/delivery); and miscellaneous (e.g., pulmonary emboli, drug reaction, deep vein thrombosis).

NURSING PRIORITY NO. 2. To prevent occurrence:
- Monitor vital signs, noting elevation in blood pressure, heart rate, and temperature, especially during times of physical stress, **to identify trends and intervene in a timely manner.**
- Instruct in appropriate interventions (e.g., regularly timed catheter and bowel care, appropriate padding for skin and tissues, proper positioning with frequent pressure relief actions, checking frequently for tight clothes/leg straps, routine foot/toenail care, temperature control, sunburn/other burn prevention, compliance with preventative medications when used) **to prevent occurrence/limit severity.**
- Instruct all caregivers in safe bowel and bladder care, and immediate and long-term care for the prevention of skin stress/breakdown. **These problems are associated most frequently with dysreflexia.**
- Administer antihypertensive medications when at-risk client is placed on routine "maintenance dose," **as might occur when noxious stimuli cannot be removed (presence of chronic sacral pressure sore, fracture, or acute postoperative pain).**
- Refer to ND Autonomic Dysreflexia.

NURSING PRIORITY NO. 3. To promote wellness (Teaching/Discharge Considerations):
- Discuss warning signs of autonomic dysreflexia with client/caregiver (i.e., sudden, severe pounding headache; flushed red face; increased blood pressure/acute hypertension; nasal congestion; anxiety; blurred vision; metallic taste in mouth; sweating and/or flushing above the level of SCI;

Information in brackets added by the authors to clarify and enhance the use of nursing diagnoses.

    Cultural   Collaborative   Community/Home Care

goosebumps; bradycardia; cardiac irregularities). **AD can develop rapidly (in minutes), requiring quick intervention.**

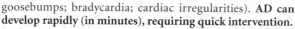

- Review proper use/administration of medication if preventive medications are anticipated.
- Assist client/family in identifying emergency referrals (e.g., healthcare provider number in prominent place).

Documentation Focus

ASSESSMENT/REASSESSMENT

- Individual risk factors.
- Previous episodes, precipitating factors, and individual signs/symptoms.

PLANNING

- Plan of care and who is involved in planning.
- Teaching plan.

IMPLEMENTATION/EVALUATION

- Client's responses to interventions and actions performed; understanding of teaching.
- Attainment/progress toward desired outcome(s).
- Modifications to plan of care.

DISCHARGE PLANNING

- Long-term needs and who is responsible for actions to be taken.

SAMPLE NURSING OUTCOMES & INTERVENTIONS CLASSIFICATIONS (NOC/NIC)

NOC—Risk Control
NIC—Dysreflexia Management

risk-prone health Behavior

Taxonomy II: Coping/Stress Tolerance—Class 2 Coping Responses (00188)
[Diagnostic Division: Ego Integrity]
Submitted as impaired Adjustment 1986; Nursing Diagnosis Extension and Classification (NDEC) Revision 1998; Revised/Renamed 2006

Definition: Inability to modify lifestyle/behaviors in a manner consistent with a change in health status

---

Information in brackets added by the authors to clarify and enhance the use of nursing diagnoses.

 Diagnostic Studies   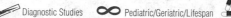 Pediatric/Geriatric/Lifespan

risk-prone health BEHAVIOR *(vertical side text)*

Related Factors

Inadequate comprehension; low self-efficacy
Multiple stressors
Inadequate social support; low socioeconomic status
Negative attitude toward healthcare

Defining Characteristics

SUBJECTIVE

Minimizes health status change
Failure to achieve optimal sense of control

OBJECTIVE

Failure to take action that prevents health problems
Demonstrates nonacceptance of health status change

> NOTE: A risk diagnosis is not evidenced by signs and symptoms as the problem has not occurred; rather, nursing interventions are directed at prevention.

Desired Outcomes/Evaluation Criteria—Client Will:

- Demonstrate increasing interest/participation in self-care.
- Develop ability to assume responsibility for personal needs when possible.
- Identify stress situations leading to difficulties in adapting to change in health status and specific actions for dealing with them.
- Initiate lifestyle changes that will permit adaptation to current life situations.
- Identify and use appropriate support systems.

Actions/Interventions

NURSING PRIORITY NO. 1. To assess degree of impaired function:
- Perform a physical and/or psychosocial assessment **to determine the extent of the limitation(s) of the current condition.**
- Listen to the client's perception of inability/reluctance to adapt to situations that are currently occurring.
- Survey (with the client) past and present significant support systems (e.g., family, church, groups, and organizations) **to identify helpful resources.**

Information in brackets added by the authors to clarify and enhance the use of nursing diagnoses.

 Cultural   Collaborative   Community/Home Care

- Explore the expressions of emotions signifying impaired adjustment by client/SO(s) (e.g., overwhelming anxiety, fear, anger, worry, passive and/or active denial).
 • Note child's interaction with parent/caregiver (**development of coping behaviors is limited at this age, and primary caregivers provide support for the child and serve as role models**).
 • Determine whether child displays problems with school performance, withdraws from family/peers, or demonstrates aggressive behavior toward others/self.

NURSING PRIORITY NO. 2. To identify the causative/contributing factors relating to the change in health behavior:
- Listen to client's perception of the factors leading to the present dilemma, noting onset, duration, presence/absence of physical complaints, and social withdrawal.
- Review previous life situations and role changes with client **to determine coping skills used.**
- Determine lack of/inability to use available resources.
- Review available documentation and resources to determine actual life experiences (e.g., medical records, statements by SO[s], consultants' notes). **In situations of great stress, physical and/or emotional, the client may not accurately assess occurrences leading to the present situation.**

NURSING PRIORITY NO. 3. To assist client in coping/dealing with impairment:
- Organize a team conference (including client and ancillary services) **to focus on contributing factors effecting adjustment and plan for management of the situation.**
- Acknowledge client's efforts to adjust: "Have done your best." **Lessens feelings of blame/guilt and defensive response.**
- Share information with adolescent's peers as indicated when illness/injury affects body image (**peers are primary support for this age group**).
- Explain disease process/causative factors and prognosis, as appropriate, and promote questioning **to enhance understanding.**
- Provide an open environment encouraging communication **so that expression of feelings concerning impaired function can be dealt with realistically and openly.**
- Use therapeutic communication skills (active-listening, acknowledgment, silence, I-statements).
- Discuss/evaluate resources that have been useful to the client in adapting to changes in other life situations (e.g., vocational

Information in brackets added by the authors to clarify and enhance the use of nursing diagnoses.

rehabilitation, employment experiences, psychosocial support services).

• Develop a plan of action with client to meet immediate needs (e.g., physical safety and hygiene, emotional support of professionals and SO[s]) and assist in implementation of the plan. **Provides a starting point to deal with current situation for moving ahead with plan and for evaluation of progress.**

• Explore previously used coping skills and application to current situation. Refine/develop new strategies, as appropriate.

 • Identify and problem solve with the client frustration in daily care. **(Focusing on the smaller factors of concern gives the individual the ability to perceive the impaired function from a less-threatening perspective, one-step-at-a-time concept.)**

 • Involve SO(s) in long-range planning for emotional, psychological, physical, and social needs.

NURSING PRIORITY NO. 4. To promote wellness (Teaching/Discharge Considerations):

 • Identify strengths the client perceives in current life situation. Keep focus on the present, **as unknowns of the future may be too overwhelming.**

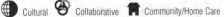 • Refer to other resources in the long-range plan of care (e.g., occupational therapy, vocational rehabilitation) as indicated.

 • Assist client/SO(s) to see appropriate alternatives and potential changes in locus of control.

 • Assist SO(s) to learn methods for managing present needs. (Refer to NDs specific to client's deficits.)

 • Pace and time learning sessions **to meet client's needs.** Provide feedback during and after learning experiences (e.g., self-catheterization, range-of-motion exercises, wound care, therapeutic communication) **to enhance retention, skill, and confidence.**

Documentation Focus

ASSESSMENT/REASSESSMENT

• Reasons for/degree of impaired adaptation.
• Client's/SO's perception of the situation.
• Effect of behavior on health status/condition.

PLANNING

• Plan for adjustments and interventions for achieving the plan and who is involved.
• Teaching plan.

Information in brackets added by the authors to clarify and enhance the use of nursing diagnoses.

      Cultural   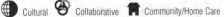 Collaborative   Community/Home Care

IMPLEMENTATION/EVALUATION

- Client responses to the interventions/teaching and actions performed.
- Attainment/progress toward desired outcome(s).
- Modifications to plan of care.

DISCHARGE PLANNING

- Resources that are available for the client and SO(s) and referrals that are made.

SAMPLE NURSING OUTCOMES & INTERVENTIONS CLASSIFICATIONS (NOC/NIC)

NOC—Acceptance: Health Status
NIC—Coping Enhancement

disturbed Body Image

Taxonomy II: Self-Perception—Class 3
    Body Image (00118)
[Diagnostic Division: Ego Integrity]
Submitted 1973; Revised 1998 (by small group work 1996)

Definition: Confusion [and/or dissatisfaction] in mental picture of one's physical self

Related Factors

Biophysical; illness; trauma; injury; surgery; [mutilation, pregnancy]
Illness treatment [change caused by biochemical agents (drugs), dependence on machine]
Psychosocial
Cultural; spiritual
Cognitive; perceptual
Developmental changes [maturational changes]
[Significance of body part or functioning with regard to age, gender, developmental level, or basic human needs]

Defining Characteristics

SUBJECTIVE

Verbalization of feelings that reflect an altered view of one's body (e.g., appearance, structure, function)

Information in brackets added by the authors to clarify and enhance the use of nursing diagnoses.

Diagnostic Studies   Pediatric/Geriatric/Lifespan   Medications   **115**

Verbalization of perceptions that reflect an altered view of one's body in appearance

Verbalization of change in lifestyle

Fear of rejection/reaction by others

Focus on past strength/function/appearance

Negative feelings about body (e.g., feelings of helplessness, hopelessness, or powerlessness); [depersonalization/grandiosity]

Preoccupation with change/loss

Refusal to verify actual change

Emphasis on remaining strengths; heightened achievement

Personalization of part/loss by name

Depersonalization of part/loss by impersonal pronouns

OBJECTIVE

Behaviors of: acknowledgment of one's body; avoidance of one's body; monitoring one's body

Nonverbal response to actual/perceived change in body (e.g., appearance, structure, function)

Missing body part

Actual change in structure/function

Not looking at/not touching body part

Trauma to nonfunctioning part

Change in ability to estimate spatial relationship of body to environment

Extension of body boundary to incorporate environmental objects

Intentional/unintentional hiding/overexposing of body part

Change in social involvement

[Aggression; low frustration tolerance level]

Desired Outcomes/Evaluation Criteria—Client Will:

- Verbalize understanding of body changes.
- Recognize and incorporate body image change into self-concept in accurate manner without negating self-esteem.
- Verbalize acceptance of self in situation (e.g., chronic progressive disease, amputee, decreased independence, weight as is, effects of therapeutic regimen).
- Verbalize relief of anxiety and adaptation to actual/altered body image.
- Seek information and actively pursue growth.

Information in brackets added by the authors to clarify and enhance the use of nursing diagnoses.

🌐 Cultural   Collaborative   🏠 Community/Home Care

- Acknowledge self as an individual who has responsibility for self.
- Use adaptive devices/prosthesis appropriately.

Actions/Interventions

NURSING PRIORITY NO. 1. To assess causative/contributing factors:

- Discuss pathophysiology present and/or situation affecting the individual and refer to additional NDs as appropriate. For example, when alteration in body image is related to neurological deficit (e.g., cerebrovascular accident—CVA), refer to ND unilateral Neglect; in the presence of severe, ongoing pain, refer to ND chronic Pain; or in loss of sexual desire/ability, refer to ND Sexual Dysfunction.
- Determine whether condition is permanent/no expectation for resolution. (May be associated with other NDs, such as Self-Esteem [specify] or risk for impaired parent/child Attachment, when child is affected.) **There is always something that can be done to enhance acceptance and it is important to hold out the possibility of living a good life with the disability.**
- Assess mental/physical influence of illness/condition on the client's emotional state (e.g., diseases of the endocrine system, use of steroid therapy, and so on).
- Evaluate level of client's knowledge of and anxiety related to situation. Observe emotional changes **which may indicate acceptance or nonacceptance of situation.**
- Recognize behavior indicative of overconcern with body and its processes.
- Have client describe self, noting what is positive and what is negative. Be aware of how client believes others see self.
- Discuss meaning of loss/change to client. **A small (seemingly trivial) loss may have a big impact (such as the use of a urinary catheter or enema for continence). A change in function (such as immobility in elderly) may be more difficult for some to deal with than a change in appearance. Permanent facial scarring of child may be difficult for parents to accept.**
- Use developmentally appropriate communication techniques for determining exact expression of body image in child (e.g., puppet play or constructive dialogue for toddler). **Developmental capacity must guide interaction to gain accurate information.**
- Note signs of grieving/indicators of severe or prolonged depression **to evaluate need for counseling and/or medications.**
- Determine ethnic background and cultural/religious perceptions and considerations. **May influence how individual deals with what has happened.**

Information in brackets added by the authors to clarify and enhance the use of nursing diagnoses.

 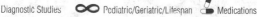

- Identify social aspects of illness/disease (e.g., sexually transmitted diseases, sterility, chronic conditions).
- Observe interaction of client with SO(s). **Distortions in body image may be unconsciously reinforced by family members and/or secondary gain issues may interfere with progress.**

NURSING PRIORITY NO. 2. To determine coping abilities and skills:
- Assess client's current level of adaptation and progress.
- Listen to client's comments and responses to the situation. **Different situations are upsetting to different people, depending on individual coping skills and past experiences.**
- Note withdrawn behavior and the use of denial. **May be normal response to situation or may be indicative of mental illness (e.g., schizophrenia).** (Refer to ND ineffective Denial.)

- Note use of addictive substances/alcohol; **may reflect dysfunctional coping.**
- Identify previously used coping strategies and effectiveness.
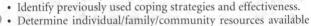
- Determine individual/family/community resources available to client.

NURSING PRIORITY NO. 3. To assist client and SO(s) to deal with/accept issues of self-concept related to body image:
- Establish therapeutic nurse-client relationship, conveying an attitude of caring and developing a sense of trust.
- Visit client frequently and acknowledge the individual as someone who is worthwhile. **Provides opportunities for listening to concerns and questions.**
- Assist in correcting underlying problems **to promote optimal healing/adaptation.**
- Provide assistance with self-care needs/measures as necessary while promoting individual abilities/independence.
- Work with client's self-concept avoiding moral judgments regarding client's efforts or progress (e.g., "You should be progressing faster; You're weak/lazy/not trying hard enough"). Positive reinforcement encourages client to continue efforts/strive for improvement.
- Discuss concerns about fear of mutilation, prognosis, rejection when client is facing surgery or potentially poor outcome of procedure/illness, **to address realities and provide emotional support.**
- Acknowledge and accept feelings of dependency, grief, and hostility.
- Encourage verbalization of and role play anticipated conflicts **to enhance handling of potential situations.**
- Encourage client and SO(s) to communicate feelings to each other.

Information in brackets added by the authors to clarify and enhance the use of nursing diagnoses.

  Cultural Collaborative Community/Home Care

- Assume all individuals are sensitive to changes in appearance but avoid stereotyping.
- Alert staff to monitor own facial expressions and other non-verbal behaviors **because they need to convey acceptance and not revulsion when the client's appearance is affected.**
- Encourage family members to treat client normally and not as an invalid.
- Encourage client to look at/touch affected body part **to begin to incorporate changes into body image.**
- Allow client to use denial without participating (e.g., client may at first refuse to look at a colostomy; the nurse says "I am going to change your colostomy now" and proceeds with the task). **Provides individual time to adapt to situation.**
- Set limits on maladaptive behavior and assist client to identify positive behaviors **to aid in recovery.**
- Provide accurate information as desired/requested. Reinforce previously given information.
- Discuss the availability of prosthetics, reconstructive surgery, and physical/occupational therapy or other referrals as dictated by individual situation.
- Help client to select and use clothing/makeup **to minimize body changes and enhance appearance.**
- Discuss reasons for infectious isolation and procedures when used and make time to sit down and talk/listen to client while in the room **to decrease sense of isolation/loneliness.**

NURSING PRIORITY NO. 4. To promote wellness (Teaching/Discharge Considerations):

- Begin counseling/other therapies (e.g., biofeedback/relaxation) as soon as possible **to provide early/ongoing sources of support.**
- Provide information at client's level of acceptance and in small pieces **to allow easier assimilation.** Clarify misconceptions. Reinforce explanations given by other health team members.
- Include client in decision-making process and problem-solving activities.
- Assist client to incorporate therapeutic regimen into activities of daily living (ADLs) (e.g., including specific exercises, housework activities). **Promotes continuation of program.**
- Identify/plan for alterations to home and work environment/activities **to accommodate individual needs and support independence.**
- Assist client in learning strategies for dealing with feelings/venting emotions.

Information in brackets added by the authors to clarify and enhance the use of nursing diagnoses.

- Offer positive reinforcement for efforts made (e.g., wearing makeup, using prosthetic device).
- Refer to appropriate support groups.

Documentation Focus

ASSESSMENT/REASSESSMENT

- Observations, presence of maladaptive behaviors, emotional changes, stage of grieving, level of independence.
- Physical wounds, dressings; use of life-support–type machine (e.g., ventilator, dialysis machine).
- Meaning of loss/change to client.
- Support systems available (e.g., SOs, friends, groups).

PLANNING

- Plan of care and who is involved in planning.
- Teaching plan.

IMPLEMENTATION/EVALUATION

- Client's response to interventions/teaching and actions performed.
- Attainment/progress toward desired outcome(s).
- Modifications of plan of care.

DISCHARGE PLANNING

- Long-term needs and who is responsible for actions.
- Specific referrals made (e.g., rehabilitation center, community resources).

SAMPLE NURSING OUTCOMES & INTERVENTIONS CLASSIFICATIONS (NOC/NIC)

NOC—Body Image
NIC—Body Image Enhancement

risk for imbalanced Body Temperature

Taxonomy II: Safety/Protection—Class 6
   Thermoregulation (00005)
[Diagnostic division: Safety]
Submitted 1986; Revised 2000

Definition: At risk for failure to maintain body temperature within normal range

---

Information in brackets added by the authors to clarify and enhance the use of nursing diagnoses.

 Cultural Collaborative Community/Home Care

Risk Factors

Extremes of age/weight

Exposure to cold/cool or warm/hot environments; inappropriate clothing for environmental temperature

Dehydration

Inactivity; vigorous activity

Medications causing vasoconstriction/vasodilation; sedation [use or overdose of certain drugs or exposure to anesthesia]

Illness/trauma affecting temperature regulation [e.g., infections, systemic or localized; neoplasms, tumors; collagen/vascular disease]; altered metabolic rate

> NOTE: A risk diagnosis is not evidenced by signs and symptoms as the problem has not occurred; rather, nursing interventions are directed at prevention.

Desired Outcomes/Evaluation Criteria—Client WIll:

- Maintain body temperature within normal range.
- Verbalize understanding of individual risk factors and appropriate interventions.
- Demonstrate behaviors for monitoring and maintaining appropriate body temperature.

Actions/Interventions

NURSING PRIORITY NO. 1. To identify causative/risk factors present:

- Determine if present illness/condition results from exposure to environmental factors, surgery, infection, trauma. **Helps to determine the scope of interventions that may be needed (e.g., simple addition of warm blankets after surgery, or hypothermia therapy following brain trauma).**
- Monitor laboratory values (e.g., tests indicative of infection, thyroid/other endocrine tests, drug screens) **to identify potential internal causes of temperature imbalances.**
- Note client's age (e.g., premature neonate, young child, or aging individual), **as it can directly impact ability to maintain/regulate body temperature and respond to changes in environment.**
- Assess nutritional status **to determine metabolism effect on body temperature and to identify foods or nutrient deficits that affect metabolism.**

Information in brackets added by the authors to clarify and enhance the use of nursing diagnoses.

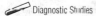 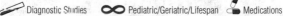

NURSING PRIORITY NO. 2. To prevent occurrence of temperature alteration:

- Monitor/maintain comfortable ambient environment (e.g., provide heating/cooling measures such as space heaters/fans) as indicated.
- Supervise use of heating pads, electric blankets, ice bags, and hypothermia blankets, especially in clients who cannot self-protect.
- Dress or discuss with client/caregiver(s) dressing appropriately (e.g., layering clothing, use of hat and gloves in cold weather, light loose clothing in warm weather, water-resistant outer gear).
- Cover infant's head with knit cap, place under adequate blankets. Place newborn infant under radiant warmer. **Heat loss in newborns/infants is greatest through head and by evaporation and convection.**
- Limit clothing/remove blanket from premature infant placed in incubator **to prevent overheating in climate-controlled environment.**
- Monitor core body temperature. (**Tympanic temperature may be preferred, as it is the most accurate noninvasive method, except in infants where skin electrode is preferred.**)
- Restore/maintain core temperature within client's normal range. **Client may require interventions to treat hypothermia or hyperthermia.** (Refer to NDs Hypothermia; Hyperthermia.)
- Recommend lifestyle changes, such as cessation of smoking/substance use, normalization of body weight, nutritious meals and regular exercise **to maximize metabolism to meet individual needs.**
- Refer at-risk persons to appropriate community resources (e.g., home care/social services, foster adult care, housing agencies) **to provide assistance to meet individual needs.**

NURSING PRIORITY NO. 3. To promote wellness (Teaching/Discharge Considerations):

- Discuss potential problem/individual risk factors with client/SO(s).
- Review age and gender issues, as appropriate. **Older/debilitated persons, babies, and young children typically feel more comfortable in higher ambient temperatures. Women notice feeling cooler quicker than men, which may be related to body size, or to differences in metabolism and the rate that blood flows to extremities to regulate body temperature.**
- Instruct in appropriate self-care measures (e.g., adding or removing clothing; adding or removing heat sources; reviewing

---

Information in brackets added by the authors to clarify and enhance the use of nursing diagnoses.

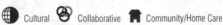

Cultural   Collaborative   Community/Home Care

medication regimen with physician to identify those which can affect thermoregulaton; evaluating home/shelter for ability to manage heat and cold; addressing nutritional and hydration status) **to protect from identified risk factors.**

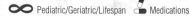 • Review ways to prevent accidental alterations, such as induced hypothermia as a result of overzealous cooling to reduce fever or maintaining too warm an environment for client who has lost the ability to perspire.

Documentation Focus

ASSESSMENT/REASSESSMENT

• Identified individual causative/risk factors.
• Record of core temperature, initially and prn.
• Results of diagnostic studies/laboratory tests.

PLANNING

• Plan of care and who is involved in planning.
• Teaching plan, including best ambient temperature, and ways to prevent hypothermia or hyperthermia.

IMPLEMENTATION/EVALUATION

• Response to interventions/teaching and actions performed.
• Attainment/progress toward desired outcome(s).
• Modifications to plan of care.

DISCHARGE PLANNING

• Long-term needs and who is responsible for actions.
• Specific referrals made.

SAMPLE NURSING OUTCOMES & INTERVENTIONS CLASSIFICATIONS (NOC/NIC)

NOC—Risk Control
NIC—Temperature Regulation

Bowel Incontinence

Taxonomy II: Elimination—Class 2 Gastrointestinal System (00014)
[Diagnostic Division: Elimination]
Submitted 1975; Nursing Diagnosis Extension and Classification (NDEC) Revision 1998

Definition: Change in normal bowel habits characterized by involuntary passage of stool

Information in brackets added by the authors to clarify and enhance the use of nursing diagnoses.

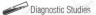 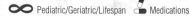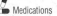

Related Factors

Toileting self-care deficit; environmental factors (e.g., inaccessible bathroom); impaired cognition; immobility

Dietary habits; medications; laxative abuse

Stress

Colorectal lesions; impaired reservoir capacity

Incomplete emptying of bowel; impaction; chronic diarrhea

General decline in muscle tone; abnormally high abdominal/intestinal pressure

Rectal sphincter abnormality; loss of rectal sphincter control; lower/upper motor nerve damage

Defining Characteristics

SUBJECTIVE

Recognizes rectal fullness, but reports inability to expel formed stool

Urgency; inability to delay defecation

Self-report of inability to feel rectal fullness

OBJECTIVE

Constant dribbling of soft stool

Fecal staining of clothing/bedding

Fecal odor

Red perianal skin

Inability to recognize/inattention to urge to defecate

Desired Outcomes/Evaluation Criteria—Client Will:

- Verbalize understanding of causative/controlling factors.
- Identify individually appropriate interventions.
- Participate in therapeutic regimen to control incontinence.
- Establish/maintain as regular a pattern of bowel functioning as possible.

Actions/Interventions

NURSING PRIORITY NO. 1. To assess causative/contributing factors:
- Identify pathophysiological factors present (e.g., multiple sclerosis [MS], acute/chronic cognitive and self-care impairments, spinal cord injury, stroke, ileus, ulcerative colitis).
- Determine historical aspects of incontinence with preceding/precipitating events. **The most common factors in incontinence include chronic constipation with leakage around**

Information in brackets added by the authors to clarify and enhance the use of nursing diagnoses.

  Cultural  Collaborative Community/Home Care

impacted stool; severe diarrhea; decreased awareness of bowel fullness due to nerve or muscle damage (e.g., stroke, trauma, tumor, radiation); injury to anal muscles (e.g., due to childbirth, sugery, rectal prolapse); chronic laxative abuse; and emotional/psychological disorders.

- Review medication regimen (e.g., sedatives/hypnotics, narcotics, muscle relaxants, antacids). **Use and/or side effects/interactions can increase potential for bowel problems.**
- Review results of diagnostic studies (e.g., abdominal x-rays, colon imaging, complete blood count, serum chemistries, stool for blood [guaiac]), as appropriate.
- Palpate abdomen **for distention, masses, tenderness.**

NURSING PRIORITY NO. 2. To determine current pattern of elimination:

- Note stool characteristics (color, odor, consistency, amount, shape, and frequency). **Provides comparative baseline.**
- Encourage client or SO to record times at which incontinence occurs, **to note relationship to meals, activity, client's behavior.**
- Auscultate abdomen **for presence, location, and characteristics of bowel sounds.**

NURSING PRIORITY NO. 3. To promote control/management of incontinence:

- Assist in treatment of causative/contributing factors (e.g., as listed in the Related Factors and Defining Characteristics).
- Establish bowel program with predictable time for defecation efforts; use suppositories and/or digital stimulation when indicated. Maintain daily program initially. Progress to alternate days dependent on usual pattern/amount of stool.
- Take client to the bathroom/place on commode or bedpan at specified intervals, taking into consideration individual needs and incontinence patterns **to maximize success of program.**
- Encourage and instruct client/caregiver in providing diet high in bulk/fiber and adequate fluids (minimum of 2000 to 2400 mL/day). Encourage warm fluids after meals.
- Identify/eliminate problem foods **to avoid diarrhea/constipation, gas formation.**
- Give stool softeners/bulk formers as indicated/needed.
- Provide pericare with frequent gentle cleansing and use of emollients **to avoid perineal excoriation.**
- Promote exercise program, as individually able, **to increase muscle tone/strength, including perineal muscles.**

Information in brackets added by the authors to clarify and enhance the use of nursing diagnoses.

Diagnostic Studies   Pediatric/Geriatric/Lifespan   Medications   **125**

• Provide incontinence aids/pads until control is obtained. *Note*: Incontinence pads should be changed frequently **to reduce incidence of skin rashes/breakdown**.

 • Demonstrate techniques (e.g., contracting abdominal muscles, leaning forward on commode, manual compression) **to increase intra-abdominal pressure during defecation, and left to right abdominal massage to stimulate peristalsis.**

• Refer to ND Diarrhea if incontinence is due to uncontrolled diarrhea; ND Constipation if incontinence is due to impaction.

NURSING PRIORITY NO. 4. To promote wellness (Teaching/Discharge Considerations):

• Review and encourage continuation of successful interventions as individually identified.

• Instruct in use of suppositories or stool softeners, if indicated, **to stimulate timed defecation.**

• Identify foods (e.g., daily bran muffins, prunes) that promote bowel regularity.

• Provide emotional support to client and SO(s), especially when condition is long-term or chronic. **Enhances coping with difficult situation**.

• Encourage scheduling of social activities within time frame of bowel program, as indicated (e.g., avoid a 4-hour excursion if bowel program requires toileting every 3 hours and facilities will not be available), **to maximize social functioning and success of bowel program.**

Documentation Focus

ASSESSMENT/REASSESSMENT

• Current and previous pattern of elimination/physical findings, character of stool, actions tried.

PLANNING

• Plan of care and who is involved in planning.
• Teaching plan.

IMPLEMENTATION/EVALUATION

• Client's/caregiver's responses to interventions/teaching and actions performed.
• Changes in pattern of elimination, characteristics of stool.
• Attainment/progress toward desired outcome(s).
• Modifications to plan of care.

Information in brackets added by the authors to clarify and enhance the use of nursing diagnoses.

  Cultural Collaborative Community/Home Care

DISCHARGE PLANNING

• Identified long-term needs, noting who is responsible for each action.
• Specific bowel program at time of discharge.

SAMPLE NURSING OUTCOMES & INTERVENTIONS CLASSIFICATIONS (NOC/NIC)

NOC—Bowel Continence
NIC—Bowel Incontinence Care

effective Breastfeeding [Learning Need]*

Taxonomy II: Role Relationships—Class 3 Role Performance (00106)
[Diagnostic Division: Food/Fluid]
Submitted 1990

Definition: Mother-infant dyad/family exhibits adequate proficiency and satisfaction with breastfeeding process

Related Factors

Basic breastfeeding knowledge
Normal breast structure
Normal infant oral structure
Infant gestational age greater than 34 weeks
Support sources [available]
Maternal confidence

Defining Characteristics

SUBJECTIVE

Maternal verbalization of satisfaction with the breastfeeding process

_____

*This ND is diffficult to address, as the Related Factors and Defining Characteristics are in fact the outcome/evaluation criteria that would be desired. We believe that normal breastfeeding behaviors need to be learned and supported, with interventions directed at learning activities for enhancement.

_____

Information in brackets added by the authors to clarify and enhance the use of nursing diagnoses.

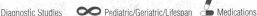

OBJECTIVE

Mother able to position infant at breast to promote a successful latch-on response

Infant content after feedings

Regular and sustained suckling/swallowing at the breast [e.g., 8 to 10 times/24 hr]

Appropriate infant weight patterns for age

Effective mother/infant communication patterns [infant cues, maternal interpretation and response]

Signs/symptoms of oxytocin release (let-down or milk ejection reflex)

Adequate infant elimination patterns for age [stools soft; more than 6 wet diapers/day of unconcentrated urine]

Eagerness of infant to nurse

Desired Outcomes/Evaluation Criteria—Client Will:

• Verbalize understanding of breastfeeding techniques.
• Demonstrate effective techniques for breastfeeding.
• Demonstrate family involvement and support.
• Attend classes/read appropriate materials/access resources as necessary.

Actions/Interventions

NURSING PRIORITY NO. 1. To assess individual learning needs:

• Assess mother's knowledge and previous experience with breastfeeding.
• Identify cultural beliefs/practices regarding lactation, let-down techniques, maternal food preferences.
• Note incorrect myths/misunderstandings especially in teenage mothers **who are more likely to have limited knowledge and concerns about body image issues.**
• Monitor effectiveness of current breastfeeding efforts.
• Determine support systems available to mother/family. **Infant's father and maternal grandmother, in addition to caring healthcare providers, are important factors in whether breastfeeding is successful.**

NURSING PRIORITY NO. 2. To promote effective breastfeeding behaviors:

• Initiate breastfeeding within first hour after birth.
• Demonstrate how to support and position infant.
• Observe mother's return demonstration.

Information in brackets added by the authors to clarify and enhance the use of nursing diagnoses.

- Encourage skin-to-skin contact.
- Keep infant with mother **for unrestricted breastfeeding duration and frequency.**
- Encourage mother to drink at least 2000 mL of fluid per day or 6 to 8 oz every hour.
- Provide information as needed about early infant feeding cues (e.g., rooting, lip smacking, sucking fingers/hand) versus late cue of crying. **Early recognition of infant hunger promotes timely/more rewarding feeding experience for infant and mother.**
- Discuss/demonstrate breastfeeding aids (e.g., infant sling, nursing footstool/pillows, breast pumps).
- Promote peer counseling for teen mothers. **Provides positive role model that teen can relate to and feel comfortable discussing concerns/feelings.**

NURSING PRIORITY NO. 3. To enhance optimum wellness (Teaching/Discharge Considerations):

- Provide for follow-up contact/home visit 48 hours after discharge; repeat visits as necessary **to provide support and assist with problem solving, if needed.**
- Recommend monitoring number of infant's wet diapers (**at least 6 wet diapers in 24 hours suggests adequate hydration**).
- Encourage mother/other family members to express feelings/concerns, and active-listen **to determine nature of concerns.**
- Educate father/SO about benefits of breastfeeding and how to manage common lactation challenges. **Enlisting support of father/SO is associated with higher ratio of successful breastfeeding at 6 months.**
- Review techniques for expression and storage of breast milk **to help sustain breastfeeding activity.**
- Problem solve return-to-work issues or periodic infant care requiring bottle/supplemental feeding.
- Recommend using expressed breast milk instead of formula or at least partial breastfeeding for as long as mother and child are satisfied.
- Explain changes in feeding needs/frequency. **Growth spurts require increased intake/more feedings by infant.**
- Review normal nursing behaviors of older breastfeeding infants/toddlers.
- Discuss importance of delaying introduction of solid foods until infant is at least 4 months, preferably 6 months old.
- Recommend avoidance of specific medications/substances (e.g., estrogen-containing contraceptives, bromocriptine, nicotine, alcohol) **that are known to decrease milk supply.**

Information in brackets added by the authors to clarify and enhance the use of nursing diagnoses.

Note: Small amounts of alcohol have not been shown to be detrimental.

 • Stress importance of client notifying healthcare providers/dentists/pharmacists of breastfeeding status.

 • Refer to support groups, such as La Leche League, as indicated.

• Refer to ND ineffective Breastfeeding for more specific information addressing challenges to breastfeeding, as appropriate.

Documentation Focus

ASSESSMENT/REASSESSMENT

• Identified assessment factors (maternal and infant).
• Number of wet diapers daily and periodic weight.

PLANNING

• Plan of care/interventions and who is involved in the planning.
• Teaching plan.

IMPLEMENTATION/EVALUATION

• Mother's response to actions/teaching plan and actions performed.
• Effectiveness of infant's efforts to feed.
• Attainment/progress toward desired outcome(s).
• Modifications to plan of care.

DISCHARGE PLANNING

• Long-term needs/referrals and who is responsible for follow-up actions.

SAMPLE NURSING OUTCOMES & INTERVENTIONS CLASSIFICATIONS (NOC/NIC)

NOC—Breastfeeding Maintenance
NIC—Lactation Counseling

ineffective Breastfeeding

Taxonomy II: Role Relationships—Class 3 Role Performance (00104)
[Diagnostic Division: Food/Fluid]
Submitted 1988

Definition: Dissatisfaction or difficulty a mother, infant, or child experiences with the breastfeeding process

---

Information in brackets added by the authors to clarify and enhance the use of nursing diagnoses.

 Cultural Collaborative Community/Home Care

Related Factors

Prematurity; infant anomaly; poor infant sucking reflex

Infant receiving [numerous or repeated] supplemental feedings with artificial nipple

Maternal anxiety/ambivalence

Knowledge deficit

Previous history of breastfeeding failure

Interruption in breastfeeding

Nonsupportive partner/family

Maternal breast anomaly; previous breast surgery

Defining Characteristics

SUBJECTIVE

Unsatisfactory breastfeeding process

Persistence of sore nipples beyond the first week of breastfeeding

Insufficient emptying of each breast per feeding

Inadequate/perceived inadequate milk supply

OBJECTIVE

Observable signs of inadequate infant intake [decrease in number of wet diapers, inappropriate weight loss/or inadequate gain]

Nonsustained/insufficient opportunity for suckling at the breast; infant inability [failure] to latch onto maternal breast correctly

Infant arching/crying at the breast; resistant latching on

Infant exhibiting fussiness/crying within the first hour after breastfeeding; unresponsive to other comfort measures

No observable signs of oxytocin release

Desired Outcomes/Evaluation Criteria—Client Will:

- Verbalize understanding of causative/contributing factors.
- Demonstrate techniques to improve/enhance breastfeeding experience.
- Assume responsibility for effective breastfeeding.
- Achieve mutually satisfactory breastfeeding regimen with infant content after feedings and gaining weight appropriately.

Actions/Interventions

NURSING PRIORITY NO. 1. To identify maternal causative/contributing factors:
- Assess client knowledge about breastfeeding and extent of instruction that has been given.

Information in brackets added by the authors to clarify and enhance the use of nursing diagnoses.

 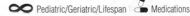

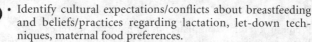

- Identify cultural expectations/conflicts about breastfeeding and beliefs/practices regarding lactation, let-down techniques, maternal food preferences.
- Note incorrect myths/misunderstandings especially in teenage mothers **who are more likely to have limited knowledge and more concerns about body image issues.**
- Encourage discussion of current/previous breastfeeding experience(s).
- Note previous unsatisfactory experience (including self or others) **because it may be affecting current situation.**
- Perform physical assessment, noting appearance of breasts/nipples, marked asymmetry of breasts, obvious inverted or flat nipples, minimal or no breast enlargement during pregnancy.
- Determine whether lactation failure is primary **(i.e., maternal prolactin deficiency/serum prolactin levels, inadequate mammary gland tissue, breast surgery that has damaged the nipple, areola enervation [irremediable])** or secondary **(i.e., sore nipples, severe engorgement, plugged milk ducts, mastitis, inhibition of let-down reflex, maternal/infant separation with disruption of feedings [treatable]). Note: Overweight/obese women are 2.5/3.6 times less successful, respectively, in initiating breastfeeding than the general population.**
- Note history of pregnancy, labor, and delivery (vaginal or cesarean section); other recent or current surgery; preexisting medical problems (e.g., diabetes, seizure disorder, cardiac diseases, or presence of disabilities); or adoptive mother.
- Identify maternal support systems; presence and response of SO(s), extended family, friends. **Infant's father and maternal grandmother (in addition to caring healthcare providers) are important factors that contribute to successful breastfeeding.**
- Ascertain mother's age, number of children at home, and need to return to work.
- Determine maternal feelings (e.g., fear/anxiety, ambivalence, depression).

NURSING PRIORITY NO. 2. To assess infant causative/contributing factors:

- Determine suckling problems, as noted in Related Factors/Defining Characteristics.
- Note prematurity and/or infant anomaly (e.g., cleft palate) **to determine special equipment/feeding needs.**
- Review feeding schedule **to note increased demand for feeding (at least 8 times/day, taking both breasts at each feeding**

Information in brackets added by the authors to clarify and enhance the use of nursing diagnoses.

    Cultural   Collaborative   Community/Home Care

for more than 15 minutes on each side) or use of supplements with artificial nipple.

• Evaluate observable signs of inadequate infant intake (e.g., baby latches onto mother's nipples with sustained suckling but minimal audible swallowing/gulping noted, infant arching and crying at the breasts with resistance to latching on, decreased urinary output/frequency of stools, inadequate weight gain).

• Determine whether baby is content after feeding, or exhibits fussiness and crying within the first hour after breastfeeding, **suggesting unsatisfactory breastfeeding process.**

• Note any correlation between maternal ingestion of certain foods and "colicky" response of infant.

NURSING PRIORITY NO. 3. To assist mother to develop skills of adequate breastfeeding:

• Provide emotional support to mother. Use 1:1 instruction with each feeding during hospital stay/clinic/home visit. Refer adoptive mothers choosing to breastfeed to a lactation consultant **to assist with induced lactation techniques.**

• Inform mother about early infant feeding cues (e.g., rooting, lip smacking, sucking fingers/hand) versus late cue of crying. **Early recognition of infant hunger promotes timely/more rewarding feeding experience for infant and mother.**

• Recommend avoidance or overuse of supplemental feedings and pacifiers (unless specifically indicated) **that can lessen infant's desire to breastfeed/increase risk of early weaning.** (Adoptive mothers may not develop a full breast milk supply, necessitating supplemental feedings.)

• Restrict use of breast shields (i.e., only temporarily to help draw the nipple out), then place baby directly on nipple.

• Demonstrate use of electric piston-type breast pump with bilateral collection chamber when necessary **to maintain or increase milk supply.**

• Discuss/demonstrate breastfeeding aids (e.g., infant sling, nursing footstool/pillows).

• Recommend using a variety of nursing positions **to find the most comfortable for mother and infant. Positions particularly helpful for "plus-sized" women or those with large breasts include the "football" hold with infant's head to mother's breast and body curved around behind mother, or lying down to nurse.**

• Encourage frequent rest periods, sharing household/childcare duties **to limit fatigue and facilitate relaxation at feeding times.**

Information in brackets added by the authors to clarify and enhance the use of nursing diagnoses.

Diagnostic Studies   Pediatric/Geriatric/Lifespan   Medications   **133**

ineffective BREASTFEEDING

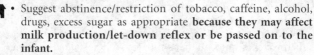

- Suggest abstinence/restriction of tobacco, caffeine, alcohol, drugs, excess sugar as appropriate **because they may affect milk production/let-down reflex or be passed on to the infant.**
- Promote early management of breastfeeding problems. For example:

Engorgement: Heat and/or cool applications to the breasts, massage from chest wall down to nipple; use synthetic oxytocin nasal spray **to enhance let-down reflex;** soothe "fussy baby" before latching on the breast; properly position baby on breast/nipple; alternate the side baby starts nursing on; nurse round-the-clock and/or pump with piston-type electric breast pump with bilateral collection chambers at least 8 to 12 times/day.

Sore nipples: Wear 100% cotton fabrics; do not use soap/alcohol/drying agents on nipples; avoid use of nipple shields or nursing pads that contain plastic; cleanse and then air dry; use thin layers of lanolin (if mother/baby not sensitive to wool); expose to sunlight/sunlamps with extreme caution; administer mild pain reliever as appropriate; apply ice before nursing; soak with warm water before attaching infant **to soften nipple and remove dried milk;** begin with least sore side or begin with hand expression **to establish let-down reflex;** properly position infant on breast/nipple; and use a variety of nursing positions.

Clogged ducts: Use larger bra or extender to avoid pressure on site; use moist or dry heat, gently massage from above plug down to nipple; nurse infant, hand express, or pump after massage; nurse more often on affected side.

Inhibited let-down: Use relaxation techniques before nursing (e.g., maintain quiet atmosphere, assume position of comfort, massage, apply heat to breasts, have beverage available); develop a routine for nursing, concentrate on infant; administer synthetic oxytocin nasal spray as appropriate.

Mastitis: Promote bedrest (with infant) for several days; administer antibiotics; provide warm, moist heat before and during nursing; empty breasts completely, continuing to nurse baby at least 8 to 12 times/day, or pumping breasts for 24 hours, then resuming breastfeeding as appropriate.

NURSING PRIORITY NO. 4. To condition infant to breastfeed:
- Scent breast pad with breast milk and leave in bed with infant along with mother's photograph when separated from mother for medical purposes (e.g., prematurity).
- Increase skin-to-skin contact.

Information in brackets added by the authors to clarify and enhance the use of nursing diagnoses.

   Cultural   Collaborative   Community/Home Care

- Provide practice times at breast.
- Express small amounts of milk into baby's mouth.
- Have mother pump breast after feeding to enhance milk production.
- Use supplemental nutrition system cautiously when necessary.
- Identify special interventions for feeding in presence of cleft lip/palate.

NURSING PRIORITY NO. 5. To promote wellness (Teaching/Discharge Considerations):

- Schedule follow-up visit with healthcare provider 48 hours after hospital discharge and 2 weeks after birth **for evaluation of milk intake/breastfeeding process.**
- Recommend monitoring number of infant's wet diapers (**at least 6 wet diapers in 24 hours suggests adequate hydration**).
- Weigh infant at least every third day initially as indicated and record (**to verify adequacy of nutritional intake**).
- Educate father/SO about benefits of breastfeeding and how to manage common lactation challenges. **Enlisting support of father/SO is associated with higher ratio of successful breastfeeding at 6 months.**
- Promote peer counseling for teen mothers. **Provides positive role model that teen can relate to and feel comfortable discussing concerns/feelings.**
- Review mother's need for rest, relaxation, and time with other children as appropriate.
- Discuss importance of adequate nutrition/fluid intake, prenatal vitamins, or other vitamin/mineral supplements, such as vitamin C, as indicated.
- Address specific problems (e.g., suckling problems, prematurity/anomalies).
- Inform mother that return of menses within first 3 months after infant's birth may indicate inadequate prolactin levels.
- Refer to support groups (e.g., La Leche League, parenting support groups, stress reduction, or other community resources, as indicated).
- Provide bibliotherapy/appropriate websites for further information.

Documentation Focus

ASSESSMENT/REASSESSMENT

- Identified assessment factors, both maternal and infant (e.g., engorgement present, infant demonstrating adequate weight gain without supplementation).

Information in brackets added by the authors to clarify and enhance the use of nursing diagnoses.

PLANNING

- Plan of care/interventions and who is involved in planning.
- Teaching plan.

IMPLEMENTATION/EVALUATION

- Mother's/infant's responses to interventions/teaching and actions performed.
- Changes in infant's weight.
- Attainment/progress toward desired outcome(s).
- Modifications to plan of care.

DISCHARGE PLANNING

- Referrals that have been made and mother's choice of participation.

SAMPLE NURSING OUTCOMES & INTERVENTIONS CLASSIFICATIONS (NOC/NIC)

NOC—Breastfeeding Establishment: Maternal [or] Infant
NIC—Breastfeeding Assistance

interrupted Breastfeeding

Taxonomy II: Role Relationships—Class 3 Role
  Performance (00105)
[Diagnostic Division: Food/Fluid]
Submitted 1992

Definition: Break in the continuity of the breastfeeding process as a result of inability or inadvisability to put baby to breast for feeding

Related Factors

Maternal/infant illness
Prematurity
Maternal employment
Contraindications to breastfeeding [e.g., drugs, true breast milk jaundice]
Need to abruptly wean infant

Defining Characteristics

SUBJECTIVE

Infant receives no nourishment at the breast for some or all of feedings

---

Information in brackets added by the authors to clarify and enhance the use of nursing diagnoses.

 Cultural Collaborative Community/Home Care

Maternal desire to maintain breastfeeding for infant/child's nutritional needs

Maternal desire to provide/eventually provide breast milk for infant/child's nutritional needs

Lack of knowledge regarding expression/storage of breast milk

OBJECTIVE

Separation of mother and infant

Desired Outcomes/Evaluation Criteria—Client Will:

- Identify and demonstrate techniques to sustain lactation until breastfeeding is reinitiated.
- Achieve mutually satisfactory feeding regimen with infant content after feedings and gaining weight appropriately.
- Achieve weaning and cessation of lactation if desired or necessary.

Actions/Interventions

NURSING PRIORITY NO. 1. To identify causative/contributing factors:

- Assess client knowledge and perceptions about breastfeeding and extent of instruction that has been given.
- Note incorrect myths/misunderstandings especially in teenage mothers **who are more likely to have limited knowledge and concerns about body image issues.**
- Ascertain cultural expectations/conflicts.
- Encourage discussion of current/previous breastfeeding experience(s).
- Determine maternal responsibilities, routines, and scheduled activities (e.g., caretaking of siblings, employment in/out of home, work/school schedules of family members, ability to visit hospitalized infant).
- Identify factors necessitating interruption, or occassionally cessation of breastfeeding (e.g., maternal illness, drug use); desire/need to wean infant. **In general, infants with chronic diseases benefit from breastfeeding and only a few maternal infections (e.g., HIV, active/untreated tuberculosis for initial 2 weeks of multidrug therapy, active herpes simplex of the breasts, development of chickenpox within 5 days prior to delivery or 2 days after delivery) are hazardous to breastfeeding infants. Also, use of antiretroviral medications/chemotherapy agents or maternal substance abuse usually**

Information in brackets added by the authors to clarify and enhance the use of nursing diagnoses.

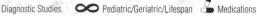

requires weaning of infant. Exposure to radiation therapy requires interruption of breastfeeding for length of time radioactivity is known to be present in breast milk and is therefore dependent on agent used. (However, feedings with stored breast milk may be an option.)

 • Determine support systems available to mother/family. **Infant's father and maternal grandmother, in addition to caring healthcare providers, are important factors that contribute to successful breastfeeding.**

NURSING PRIORITY NO. 2. To assist mother to maintain breastfeeding if desired:

 • Provide information as needed regarding need/decision to interrupt breastfeeding.

 • Promote peer counseling for teen mothers. **Provides positive role model that teen can relate to and feel comfortable with discussing concerns/feelings.**

• Educate father/SO about benefits of breastfeeding and how to manage common lactation challenges. **Enlisting support of father/SO is associated with higher ratio of successful breastfeeding at six months.**

 • Discuss/demonstrate breastfeeding aids (e.g., infant sling, nursing footstool/pillows, manual and/or electric piston-type breast pumps).

 • Suggest abstinence/restriction of tobacco, caffeine, alcohol, drugs, excess sugar, as appropriate when breastfeeding is reinitiated **because they may affect milk production/let-down reflex or be passed on to the infant**.

 • Review techniques for expression and storage of breast milk **to help sustain breastfeeding activity.**

 • Discuss proper techniques use of expressed breast milk **to provide optimal nutrition and promote continuation of breastfeeding process.**

 • Problem solve return-to-work issues or periodic infant care requiring bottle/supplemental feeding.

• Provide privacy/calm surroundings when mother breastfeeds in hospital/work setting.

• Determine if a routine visiting schedule or advance warning can be provided **so that infant will be hungry/ready to feed.**

 • Recommend using expressed breast milk instead of formula or at least partial breastfeeding for as long as mother and child are satisfied. **Prevents temporary interruption in breastfeeding, decreasing the risk of premature weaning.**

 • Encourage mother to obtain adequate rest, maintain fluid and nutritional intake, and schedule breast pumping every

---

Information in brackets added by the authors to clarify and enhance the use of nursing diagnoses.

   Cultural   Collaborative   Community/Home Care

3 hours while awake as indicated **to sustain adequate milk production and breastfeeding process.**

NURSING PRIORITY NO. 3. To assist mother in weaning process when desired:

- Provide emotional support to mother and accept decision regarding cessation of breastfeeding. **Feelings of sadness are common even if weaning is the mother's choice.**
- Discuss reducing frequency of daily feedings/breast pumping by one session every 2 to 3 days. **Preferred method of weaning, if circumstance permits, to reduce problems associated with engorgement.**
- Encourage wearing a snug, well-fitting bra, but refrain from binding breasts **because of increased risk of clogged milk ducts and inflammation.**
- Recommend expressing some milk from breasts regularly each day over 1–3 week period if necessary **to reduce discomfort associated with engorgement until milk production decreases.**
- Suggest holding infant differently during bottle feeding/interactions **to prevent infant rooting for breast and prevent stimulation of nipples.**
- Discuss use of ibuprofen/acetaminophen **for discomfort during weaning process.**
- Suggest use of ice packs to breast tissue (not nipples) for 15 to 20 minutes at least four times a day **to help reduce swelling during sudden weaning.**

NURSING PRIORITY NO. 4. To promote successful infant feeding:

- Recommend/provide for infant sucking on a regular basis, especially if gavage feedings are part of the therapeutic regimen. **Reinforces that feeding time is pleasurable and enhances digestion.**
- Discuss proper use and choice of supplemental nutrition and alternate feeding method (e.g., bottle/syringe) if desired.
- Review safety precautions (e.g., proper flow of formula from nipple, frequency of burping, holding bottle instead of propping, formula preparation, and sterilization techniques).

NURSING PRIORITY NO. 5. To promote wellness (Teaching/Discharge Considerations):

- Identify other means (other than breastfeeding) of nurturing/strengthening infant attachment (e.g., comforting, consoling, play activities).
- Explain anticipated changes in feeding needs/frequency. **Growth spurts require increased intake/more feedings by infant.**

Information in brackets added by the authors to clarify and enhance the use of nursing diagnoses.

interrupted BREASTFEEDING

- Refer to support groups (e.g., La Leche League, Lact-Aid), community resources (e.g., public health nurse, lactation specialist, Women/Infant/Children program [WIC]).

- Promote use of bibliotherapy/appropriate websites for further information.

Documentation Focus

ASSESSMENT/REASSESSMENT

- Baseline findings maternal/infant factors.
- Reason for interruption/cessation of breastfeeding.
- Number of wet diapers daily/periodic weight.

PLANNING

- Method of feeding chosen.
- Plan of care and who is involved in planning.
- Teaching plan.

IMPLEMENTATION/EVALUATION

- Maternal response to interventions/teaching and actions performed.
- Infant's response to feeding and method.
- Whether infant appears satisfied or still seems to be hungry.
- Attainment/progress toward desired outcome(s).
- Modifications to plan of care.

DISCHARGE PLANNING

- Plan for follow-up and who is responsible.
- Specific referrals made.

SAMPLE NURSING OUTCOMES & INTERVENTIONS CLASSIFICATIONS (NOC/NIC)

NOC—Breastfeeding Maintenance
NIC—Lactation Counseling

ineffective Breathing Pattern

Taxonomy II: Activity/Rest—Class 4 Cardiovascular/
  Pulmonary Responses (00032)
[Diagnostic Division: Respiration]
Submitted 1980; Revised 1996, and Nursing Diagnosis
  Extension and Classification (NDEC) 1998

Definition: Inspiration and/or expiration that does not provide adequate ventilation

---

Information in brackets added by the authors to clarify and enhance the use of nursing diagnoses.

 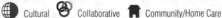

Related Factors

Neuromuscular dysfunction; spinal cord injury; neurological immaturity
Musculoskeletal impairment; bony/chest wall deformity
Anxiety; [panic attacks]
Pain
Perception/cognitive impairment
Fatigue; [deconditioning]; respiratory muscle fatigue
Body position; obesity
Hyperventilation; hypoventilation syndrome [alteration of client's normal O_2:CO_2 ratio (e.g., lung diseases, pulmonary hypertension, airway obstruction, O_2 therapy in COPD)]

Defining Characteristics

SUBJECTIVE

[Feeling breathless]

OBJECTIVE

Dyspnea; orthopnea
Bradypnea; tachypnea
Alterations in depth of breathing
Timing ratio; prolonged expiration phases; pursed-lip breathing
Decreased minute ventilation/vital capacity
Decreased inspiratory/expiratory pressure
Use of accessory muscles to breathe; assumption of three-point position
Altered chest excursion; [paradoxical breathing patterns]
Nasal flaring; [grunting]
Increased anterior-posterior diameter

Desired Outcomes/Evaluation Criteria—Client Will:

• Establish a normal/effective respiratory pattern as evidenced by absence of cyanosis and other signs/symptoms of hypoxia, with ABGs within client's normal/acceptable range.
• Verbalize awareness of causative factors.
• Initiate needed lifestyle changes.
• Demonstrate appropriate coping behaviors.

Actions/Interventions

NURSING PRIORITY NO. 1. To identify etiology/precipitating factors:
• Determine presence of factors/physical conditions as noted in Related Factors **that would cause breathing impairments.**

Information in brackets added by the authors to clarify and enhance the use of nursing diagnoses.

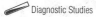 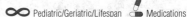

- Auscultate chest **to evaluate presence/character of breath sounds/secretions**.
- Note rate and depth of respirations, type of breathing pattern (e.g., tachypnea, grunting, Cheyne-Stokes, other irregular patterns).
- Evaluate cough (e.g., tight or moist); presence of secretions, **indicating possible obstruction**.
- Assist with/review results of necessary testing (e.g., chest x-rays, lung volumes/flow studies, pulmonary function/sleep studies) **to diagnose presence/severity of lung diseases.**
- Review laboratory data; for example, ABGs (**determines degree of oxygenation, CO_2 retention**); drug screens; and pulmonary function studies (**determines vital capacity/tidal volume**).
- Note emotional responses (e.g., gasping, crying, reports of tingling fingers). **Anxiety may be causing/exacerbating acute or chronic hyperventilation.**
- Assess for concomitant pain/discomfort **that may restrict/limit respiratory effort.**

NURSING PRIORITY NO. 2. To provide for relief of causative factors:

- 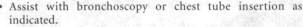 Administer oxygen at lowest concentration indicated and prescribed respiratory medications **for management of underlying pulmonary condition, respiratory distress, or cyanosis**.
- Suction airway, as needed, **to clear secretions.**
- Assist with bronchoscopy or chest tube insertion as indicated.
- Elevate HOB and/or have client sit up in chair, as appropriate, **to promote physiological/psychological ease of maximal inspiration.**
- Encourage slower/deeper respirations, use of pursed-lip technique, and so on **to assist client in "taking control" of the situation.**
- Have client breathe into a paper bag, if appropriate, **to correct hyperventilation. (Research suggests this may not be effective and could actually stress the heart/respiratory system, potentially lowering O_2 saturation, especially if the hyperventilation is not simply anxiety based.)**
- Monitor pulse oximetry, as indicated, **to verify maintenance/improvement in O_2 saturation.**
- Maintain calm attitude while dealing with client and SO(s) **to limit level of anxiety.**
- Assist client in the use of relaxation techniques.

Information in brackets added by the authors to clarify and enhance the use of nursing diagnoses.

  Cultural Collaborative Community/Home Care

- Deal with fear/anxiety that may be present. (Refer to NDs Fear; Anxiety.)
- Encourage position of comfort. Reposition client frequently if immobility is a factor.
- Splint rib cage during deep-breathing exercises/cough, if indicated.
- Medicate with analgesics, as appropriate, **to promote deeper respiration and cough.** (Refer to NDs acute Pain; chronic Pain.)
- Encourage ambulation/exercise, as individually indicated.
- Avoid overeating/gas-forming foods; **may cause abdominal distention.**
- Provide/encourage use of adjuncts, such as incentive spirometer, **to facilitate deeper respiratory effort.**
- Supervise use of respirator/diaphragmatic stimulator, rocking bed, apnea monitor, and so forth **when neuromuscular impairment is present.**
- Ascertain that client possesses and properly operates continuous positive airway pressure (CPAP) machine **when obstructive sleep apnea is causing breathing problems.**
- Maintain emergency equipment in readily accessible location and include age/size appropriate ET/trach tubes (e.g., infant, child, adolescent, or adult) **when ventilatory support might be needed.**

NURSING PRIORITY NO. 3. To promote wellness (Teaching/Discharge Considerations):

- Review etiology and possible coping behaviors.
- Stress importance of good posture and effective use of accessory muscles **to maximize respiratory effort.**
- Teach conscious control of respiratory rate, as appropriate.
- Assist client in breathing retraining (e.g., diaphragmatic, abdominal breathing, inspiratory resistive, and pursed-lip), as indicated.
- Recommend energy conservation techniques and pacing of activities.
- Refer for general exercise program (e.g., upper and lower extremity endurance and strength training), as indicated, **to maximize client's level of functioning.**
- Encourage adequate rest periods between activities **to limit fatigue.**
- Discuss relationship of smoking to respiratory function.
- Encourage client/SO(s) to develop a plan **for smoking cessation.** Provide appropriate referrals.

Information in brackets added by the authors to clarify and enhance the use of nursing diagnoses.

• Review environmental factors (e.g., exposure to dust, high pollen counts, severe weather, perfumes, animal dander, household chemicals, fumes, second-hand smoke; insufficient home support for safe care, etc.) **that may require avoidance/modification of lifestyle or environment to limit impact on client's breathing.**

 • Advise regular medical evaluation with primary care provider **to determine effectiveness of current therapeutic regimen and to promote general well-being.**

 • Instruct in proper use and safety concerns for home oxygen therapy, as indicated.

 • Make referral to support groups/contact with individuals who have encountered similar problems.

Documentation Focus

ASSESSMENT/REASSESSMENT

• Relevant history of problem.
• Respiratory pattern, breath sounds, use of accessory muscles.
• Laboratory values.
• Use of respiratory aids/supports, ventilator settings, and so forth.

PLANNING

• Plan of care/interventions and who is involved in the planning.
• Teaching plan.

IMPLEMENTATION/EVALUATION

• Response to interventions/teaching, actions performed, and treatment regimen.
• Mastery of skills, level of independence.
• Attainment/progress toward desired outcome(s).
• Modifications to plan of care.

DISCHARGE PLANNING

• Long-term needs, including appropriate referrals and action taken, available resources.
• Specific referrals provided.

SAMPLE NURSING OUTCOMES & INTERVENTIONS CLASSIFICATIONS (NOC/NIC)

NOC—Respiratory Status: Ventilation
NIC—Ventilation Assistances

Information in brackets added by the authors to clarify and enhance the use of nursing diagnoses.

 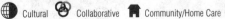  Cultural Collaborative Community/Home Care

decreased Cardiac Output

Taxonomy II: Activity/Rest—Class 4 Cardiovascular/
   Pulmonary Responses (00029)
[Diagnostic Division: Circulation]
Submitted 1975; Revised 1996, 2000

Definition: Inadequate blood pumped by the heart to
meet the metabolic demands of the body. [Note: In a
hypermetabolic state, although cardiac output may be
within normal range, it may still be inadequate to meet
the needs of the body's tissues. Cardiac output and tissue
perfusion are interrelated, although there are differences.
When cardiac output is decreased, tissue perfusion
problems will develop; however, tissue perfusion
problems can exist without decreased cardiac output.]

Related Factors

Altered heart rate/rhythm; [conduction]
Altered stroke volume: altered preload [e.g., decreased venous
   return]; altered afterload [e.g., systemic vascular resistance];
   altered contractility [e.g., ventricular-septal rupture, ventricular
   aneurysm, papillary muscle rupture, valvular disease]

Defining Characteristics

SUBJECTIVE

Altered Heart Rate/Rhythm: Palpitations
Altered Preload: Fatigue
Altered Afterload: [Feeling breathless]
Altered Contractility: Orthopnea/paroxysmal nocturnal dyspnea
   [PND]
Behavioral/Emotional: Anxiety

OBJECTIVE

Altered Heart Rate/Rhythm: [Dys]arrhythmias; tachycardia;
   bradycardia; EKG [ECG] changes
Altered Preload: Jugular vein distention (JVD); edema; weight
   gain; increased/decreased central venous pressure (CVP);
   increased/decreased pulmonary artery wedge pressure
   (PAWP); murmurs
Altered Afterload: Dyspnea; clammy skin; skin [and mucous
   membrane] color changes [cyanosis, pallor]; prolonged capillary refill; decreased peripheral pulses; variations in blood
   pressure readings; increased/decreased systemic vascular

Information in brackets added by the authors to clarify and enhance
the use of nursing diagnoses.

 Diagnostic Studies   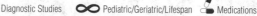 Pediatric/Geriatric/Lifespan   Medications   **145** resistance (SVR); increased/decreased pulmonary vascular resistance (PVR); oliguria; [anuria]

Altered Contractility: Crackles; cough; decreased cardiac output/cardiac index; decreased ejection fraction; decreased stroke volume index (SVI)/left ventricular stroke work index (LVSWI); S3 or S4 sounds [gallop rhythm]

Behavioral/Emotional: Restlessness

Desired Outcomes/Evaluation Criteria—Client Will:

- Display hemodynamic stability (e.g., blood pressure, cardiac output, renal perfusion/urinary output, peripheral pulses).
- Report/demonstrate decreased episodes of dyspnea, angina, and dysrhythmias.
- Demonstrate an increase in activity tolerance.
- Verbalize knowledge of the disease process, individual risk factors, and treatment plan.
- Participate in activities that reduce the workload of the heart (e.g., stress management or therapeutic medication regimen program, weight reduction, balanced activity/rest plan, proper use of supplemental oxygen, cessation of smoking).
- Identify signs of cardiac decompensation, alter activities, and seek help appropriately.

Actions/Interventions

NURSING PRIORITY NO. 1. To identify causative/contributing factors:
- Review clients at risk as noted in Related Factors and Defining Characteristics, as well as individuals with conditions that stress the heart. **Persons with acute/chronic conditions (e.g., multiple trauma, renal failure, brainstem trauma, spinal cord injures at T8 or above, alcohol or other drug abuse/overdose, pregnant women in hypertensive state) may compromise circulation and place excessive demands on the heart.**
- Assess potential for/type of developing shock states: hematogenic, septicemic, cardiogenic, vasogenic, and psychogenic.
- Review laboratory data (e.g., cardiac markers, complete blood cell [CBC] count, electrolytes, ABGs, blood urea nitrogen/creatinine (BUN/Cr), cardiac enzymes, and cultures, such as blood/wound/secretions).

NURSING PRIORITY NO. 2. To assess degree of debilitation:
- 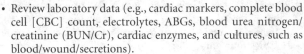 Evaluate client reports/evidence of extreme fatigue, intolerance for activity, sudden or progressive weight gain, swelling

---

Information in brackets added by the authors to clarify and enhance the use of nursing diagnoses.

of extremities, and progressive shortness of breath **to assess for signs of poor ventricular function and/or impending cardiac failure.**

- Determine vital signs/hemodynamic parameters including cognitive status. Note vital sign response to activity/procedures and time required to return to baseline. **Provides baseline for comparison to follow trends and evaluate response to interventions.**

- Review signs of impending failure/shock, noting decreased cognition and unstable/low blood pressure/invasive hemodynamic parameters; tachypnea; labored respirations; changes in breath sounds(e.g., crackles, wheezing); distant or altered heart sounds (e.g., murmurs, dysrythmias); and reduced urinary output. **Early detection of changes in these parameters promote timely intervention to limit degree of cardiac dysfunction.**

- Note presence of pulsus paradoxus, especially in the presence of distant heart sounds, **suggesting cardiac tamponade.**

- Review diagnostic studies (e.g., cardiac stress testing, ECG, scans, echocardiogram, heart catheterization, chest x-rays, electrolytes, CBC). **Helps determine underlying cause.**

NURSING PRIORITY NO. 3. To minimize/correct causative factors, maximize cardiac output:

ACUTE PHASE

- Keep client on bed or chair rest in position of comfort. In congestive state, semi-Fowler's position is preferred. May raise legs 20–30 degrees in shock situation. **Decreases oxygen consumption and risk of decompensation.**

- Administer high-flow oxygen via mask or ventilator, as indicated, **to increase oxygen available for cardiac function/tissue perfusion.**

- Monitor vital signs frequently **to note response to activities/interventions.**

- Perform periodic hemodynamic measurements, as indicated (e.g., arterial, CVP, pulmonary, and left atrial pressures; cardiac output).

- Monitor cardiac rhythm continuously **to note effectiveness of medications and/or assistive devices, such as implanted pacemaker/defibrillator.**

- Administer blood/fluid replacement, antibiotics, diuretics, inotropic drugs, antidysrhythmics, steroids, vasopressors, and/or dilators, as indicated. Evaluate response **to determine therapeutic, adverse, or toxic effects of therapy.**

Information in brackets added by the authors to clarify and enhance the use of nursing diagnoses.

 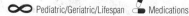

decreased CARDIAC OUTPUT

- Restrict or administer fluids (IV/PO), as indicated. Provide adequate fluid/free water, depending on client needs.
- Assess urine ouput hourly or periodically; weigh daily, noting total fluid balance **to allow for timely alterations in therapeutic regimen.**

- Monitor rate of IV drugs closely, using infusion pumps, as appropriate, **to prevent bolus/overdose.**
- Decrease stimuli; provide quiet environment **to promote adequate rest**.
- Schedule activities and assessments **to maximize sleep periods.**
- Assist with or perform self-care activities for client.
- Avoid the use of restraints whenever possible if client is confused. **May increase agitation and increase the cardiac workload.**

- Use sedation and analgesics, as indicated, with caution **to achieve desired effect without compromising hemodynamic readings.**
- Maintain patency of invasive intravascular monitoring and infusion lines. Tape connections **to prevent air embolus and/or exsanguination.**
- Maintain aseptic technique during invasive procedures. Provide site care, as indicated.

- Alter environment/bed linens and administer antipyretics or cooling measures, as indicated, **to maintain body temperature in near-normal range.**
- Instruct client to avoid/limit activities that may stimulate a Valsalva response (e.g., isometric exercises, rectal stimulation, bearing down during bowel movement, spasmodic coughing) **which can cause changes in cardiac pressures and/or impede blood flow.**

- Encourage client to breathe in/out during activities that increase risk for Valsalva effect; limit suctioning/stimulation of coughing reflex in intubated client; administer stool softeners, when indicated.
- Provide psychological support. Maintain calm attitude, but admit concerns if questioned by the client. **Honesty can be reassuring when so much activity and "worry" are apparent to the client.**
- Provide information about testing procedures and client participation.

- Assist with special procedures, as indicated (e.g., invasive line placement, intra-aortic balloon pump (IABP) insertion, pericardiocentesis, cardioversion, pacemaker insertion).
- Explain dietary/fluid restrictions.

Information in brackets added by the authors to clarify and enhance the use of nursing diagnoses.

 Cultural Collaborative 🏠 Community/Home Care

- Refer to NDs ineffective Tissue Perfusion; risk for Autonomic Dysreflexia.

NURSING PRIORITY NO. 4. To promote venous return:

POSTACUTE/CHRONIC PHASE

- Provide for adequate rest, positioning client for maximum comfort.
- Administer analgesics, as appropriate, **to promote comfort/rest**.
- Encourage relaxation techniques **to reduce anxiety.**
- Elevate legs when in sitting position; apply abdominal binder, if indicated, **to enhance venous return**; use tilt table, as needed, **to prevent orthostatic hypotension.**
- Give skin care, provide sheepskin or air/water/gel/foam mattress, and assist with frequent position changes **to avoid the development of pressure sores.**
- Elevate edematous extremities and avoid restrictive clothing. When support hose are used, be sure they are individually fitted and appropriately applied.
- Increase activity levels as permitted by individual condition/physiologic response.

NURSING PRIORITY NO. 5. To maintain adequate nutrition and fluid balance:
- Provide for diet restrictions (e.g., low-sodium, bland, soft, low-calorie/residue/fat diet, with frequent small feedings), as indicated.
- Note reports of anorexia/nausea and withhold oral intake, as indicated.
- Provide fluids/electrolytes, as indicated, **to minimize dehydration and dysrhythmias.**
- Monitor intake/output and calculate 24-hour fluid balance.

NURSING PRIORITY NO. 6. To promote wellness (Teaching/Discharge Considerations):
- Note individual risk factors present (e.g., smoking, stress, obesity) and specify interventions for reduction of identified factors.
- Review specifics of drug regimen, diet, exercise/activity plan. Emphasize necessity for long-term medical management of cardiac conditons.
- Discuss significant signs/symptoms that require prompt reporting to healthcare provider (e.g., muscle cramps, headaches, dizziness, skin rashes) **that may be signs of drug toxicity and/or mineral loss, especially potassium.**

Information in brackets added by the authors to clarify and enhance the use of nursing diagnoses.

decreased **CARDIAC OUTPUT**

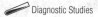 Diagnostic Studies   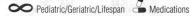 Pediatric/Geriatric/Lifespan   Medications   **149**

- Review "danger" signs requiring immediate physician notification (e.g., unrelieved or increased chest pain, functional decline, dyspnea, edema), **which may indicate deteriorating cardiac function, heart failure**.
- Encourage changing positions slowly, dangling legs before standing **to reduce risk for orthostatic hypotension.**
- Give information about positive signs of improvement, such as decreased edema, improved vital signs/circulation, **to provide encouragement.**
- Teach home monitoring of weight, pulse, and/or blood pressure, as appropriate, **to detect change and allow for timely intervention.**
- Arrange time with dietician **to determine/adjust individually appropriate diet plan**.
- Promote visits from family/SO(s) who provide positive social interaction.
- Encourage relaxing environment, using relaxation techniques, massage therapy, soothing music, quiet activities.
- Instruct in stress management techniques, as indicated, including appropriate exercise program.
- Identify resources for weight reduction, cessation of smoking, and so forth, **to provide support for change.**
- Refer to NDs Activity Intolerance; deficient Diversional Activity; ineffective Coping, compromised family Coping; Sexual Dysfunction; acute or chronic Pain; imbalanced Nutrition; deficient or excess Fluid Volume, as indicated.

Documentation Focus

ASSESSMENT/REASSESSMENT

- Baseline and subsequent findings and individual hemodynamic parameters, heart and breath sounds, ECG pattern, presence/strength of peripheral pulses, skin/tissue status, renal output, and mentation.

PLANNING

- Plan of care and who is involved in planning.
- Teaching plan.

IMPLEMENTATION/EVALUATION

- Client's responses to interventions/teaching and actions performed.
- Status and disposition at discharge.
- Attainment/progress toward desired outcome(s).
- Modifications to plan of care.

Information in brackets added by the authors to clarify and enhance the use of nursing diagnoses.

DISCHARGE PLANNING

- Discharge considerations and who will be responsible for carrying out individual actions.
- Long-term needs and available resources.
- Specific referrals made.

SAMPLE NURSING OUTCOMES & INTERVENTIONS CLASSIFICATIONS (NOC/NIC)

NOC—Cardiac Pump Effectiveness
NIC—Hemodynamic Regulations

Caregiver Role Strain

Taxonomy II: Role Relationships—Class 1 Caregiving
    Roles (00061)
[Diagnostic Division: Social Interaction]
Submitted 1992; Nursing Diagnosis Extension and
    Classification (NDEC) Revision 1998; 2000

Definition: Difficulty in performing caregiver role

Related Factors

CARE RECEIVER HEALTH STATUS

Illness severity/chronicity
Unpredictability of illness course; instability of care receiver's
    health
Increasing care needs; dependency
Problem behaviors; psychological or cognitive problems
Addiction; codependency

CAREGIVING ACTIVITIES

Discharge of family member to home with significant care
    needs [e.g., premature birth/congenital defect, frail elder
    post stroke]
Unpredictability of care situation; 24-hour care responsibilities;
    amount/complexity of activities; years of caregiving
Ongoing changes in activities

CAREGIVER HEALTH STATUS

Physical problems; psychological/cognitive problems
Inability to fulfill one's own/others' expectations; unrealistic
    expectations of self

Information in brackets added by the authors to clarify and enhance
the use of nursing diagnoses.

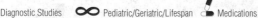

Marginal coping patterns
Addiction; codependency

SOCIOECONOMIC

Competing role commitments
Alienation/isolation from others
Insufficient recreation

CAREGIVER-CARE RECEIVER RELATIONSHIP

Unrealistic expectations of caregiver by care receiver
History of poor relationship
Mental status of elder inhibits conversation
Presence of abuse/violence

FAMILY PROCESSES

History of marginal family coping/family dysfunction

RESOURCES

Inadequate physical environment for providing care (e.g., housing, temperature, safety)
Inadequate equipment for providing care; inadequate transportation
Insufficient finances
Inexperience with caregiving; insufficient time; physical energy; emotional strength; lack of support
Lack of caregiver privacy
Deficient knowledge about/difficulty accessing community resources; inadequate community services (e.g., respite services, recreational resources)
Formal/informal assistance; formal/informal support
Caregiver is not developmentally ready for caregiver role

NOTE: The presence of this problem may encompass other numerous problems/high-risk concerns, such as deficient Diversional Activity, Insomnia, Fatigue, Anxiety, ineffective Coping, compromised family Coping, and disabled family Coping, decisional Conflict, ineffective Denial, Grieving, Hopelessness, Powerlessness, Spiritual Distress, ineffective Health Maintenance, impaired Home Maintenance, ineffective Sexuality Pattern, readiness for enhanced family Coping, interrupted Family Processes, Social Isolation. Careful attention to data gathering will identify and clarify the client's specific needs, which can then be coordinated under this single diagnostic label.

Information in brackets added by the authors to clarify and enhance the use of nursing diagnoses.

    Cultural   Collaborative   Community/Home Care

Defining Characteristics

SUBJECTIVE

CAREGIVING ACTIVITIES

Apprehension about: possible institutionalization of care receiver; the future regarding care receiver's health/caregiver's ability to provide care; care receiver's care if caregiver unable to provide care

CAREGIVER HEALTH STATUS—PHYSICAL

GI upset; weight change
Headaches; fatigue; rash
Hypertension; cardiovascular disease; diabetes

CAREGIVER HEALTH STATUS—EMOTIONAL

Feeling depressed; anger; stress; frustration; increased nervousness
Disturbed sleep
Lack of time to meet personal needs

CAREGIVER HEALTH STATUS—SOCIOECONOMIC

Changes in leisure activities; refuses career advancement

CAREGIVER-CARE RECEIVER RELATIONSHIP

Difficulty watching care receiver go through the illness
Grief/uncertainty regarding changed relationship with care receiver

FAMILY PROCESSES—CAREGIVING ACTIVITIES

Concerns about family members

OBJECTIVE

CAREGIVING ACTIVITIES

Difficulty performing/completing required tasks
Preoccupation with care routine
Dysfunctional change in caregiving activities

CAREGIVER HEALTH STATUS—EMOTIONAL

Impatience; increased emotional lability; somatization
Impaired individual coping

CAREGIVER HEALTH STATUS—SOCIOECONOMIC

Low work productivity; withdraws from social life

Information in brackets added by the authors to clarify and enhance the use of nursing diagnoses.

 Diagnostic Studies 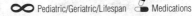 Pediatric/Geriatric/Lifespan Medications

FAMILY PROCESSES

Family conflict

Desired Outcomes/Evaluation Criteria—Client Will:

- Identify resources within self to deal with situation.
- Provide opportunity for care receiver to deal with situation in own way.
- Express more realistic understanding and expectations of the care receiver.
- Demonstrate behavior/lifestyle changes to cope with and/or resolve problematic factors.
- Report improved general well-being, ability to deal with situation.

Actions/Interventions

NURSING PRIORITY NO. 1. To assess degree of impaired function:

 • Inquire about/observe physical condition of care receiver and surroundings, as appropriate.
- Assess caregiver's current state of functioning (e.g., hours of sleep, nutritional intake, personal appearance, demeanor).
- Determine use of prescription/over-the-counter (OTC) drugs, alcohol to deal with situation.
- Identify safety issues concerning caregiver and receiver.
- Assess current actions of caregiver and how they are viewed by care receiver (e.g., caregiver may be trying to be helpful, but is not perceived as helpful; may be too protective or may have unrealistic expectations of care receiver). **May lead to misunderstanding and conflict.**
- Note choice/frequency of social involvement and recreational activities.
- Determine use/effectiveness of resources and support systems.

NURSING PRIORITY NO. 2. To identify the causative/contributing factors relating to the impairment:

∞ • Note presence of high-risk situations (e.g., elderly client with total self-care dependence, or family with several small children with one child requiring extensive assistance due to physical condition/developmental delays). **May necessitate role reversal, resulting in added stress or place excessive demands on parenting skills.**
- Determine current knowledge of the situation, noting misconceptions, lack of information. **May interfere with caregiver/care receiver response to illness/condition.**

Information in brackets added by the authors to clarify and enhance the use of nursing diagnoses.

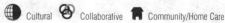 Cultural ⚕ Collaborative 🏠 Community/Home Care

- Identify relationship of caregiver to care receiver (e.g., spouse/lover, parent/child, sibling, friend).
- Ascertain proximity of caregiver to care receiver. **Caregiver could be living in the home of care receiver (e.g., spouse or parent of disabled child), or be adult child stopping by to check on elderly parent each day, providing support, food preparation/shopping, assistance in emergencies. Either situation can be taxing.**
- Note physical/mental condition, complexity of therapeutic regimen of care receiver. **Caregiving activities can be complex, requiring hands-on care, problem-solving skills, clinical judgment, and organizational and communication skills that can tax the caregiver.**
- Determine caregiver's level of involvement in/preparedness for the responsibilities of caring for the client, and anticipated length of care.
- Ascertain physical/emotional health and developmental level/abilities, as well as additional responsibilities of caregiver (e.g., job, raising family). **Provides clues to potential stressors and possible supportive interventions.**
- Use assessment tool, such as Burden Interview, when appropriate, **to further determine caregiver's coping abilities.**
- Identify individual cultural factors and impact on caregiver. **Helps clarify expectations of caregiver/receiver, family, and community.**
- Note codependency needs/enabling behaviors of caregiver.
- Determine availability/use of support systems and resources.
- Identify presence/degree of conflict between caregiver/care receiver/family.
- Determine pre-illness/current behaviors that may be interfering with the care/recovery of the care receiver.

NURSING PRIORITY NO. 3. To assist caregiver in identifying feelings and in beginning to deal with problems:
- Establish a therapeutic relationship, conveying empathy and unconditional positive regard. **A compassionate approach, blending the nurse's expertise in health care with the caregiver's first-hand knowledge of the care receiver can provide encouragement, especially in a long-term difficult situation.**
- Acknowledge difficulty of the situation for the caregiver/family. **Research shows that the two greatest predictors of caregiver strain are poor health and the feeling that there is no choice but to take on additional responsibilities.**
- Discuss caregiver's view of and concerns about situation.

Information in brackets added by the authors to clarify and enhance the use of nursing diagnoses.

- Encourage caregiver to acknowledge and express feelings. Discuss normalcy of the reactions without using false reassurance.
- Discuss caregiver's/family members' life goals, perceptions, and expectations of self **to clarify unrealistic thinking and identify potential areas of flexibility or compromise.**
- Discuss impact of and ability to handle role changes necessitated by situation.

NURSING PRIORITY NO. 4. To enhance caregiver's ability to deal with current situation:
- Identify strengths of caregiver and care receiver.
- Discuss strategies to coordinate caregiving tasks and other responsibilities (e.g., employment, care of children/dependents, housekeeping activities).
- Facilitate family conference, as appropriate, **to share information and develop plan for involvement in care activities.**
- Identify classes and/or needed specialists (e.g., first aid/CPR classes, enterostomal/physical therapist).
- Determine need for/sources of additional resources (e.g., financial, legal, respite care, social, spiritual).
- Provide information and/or demonstrate techniques for dealing with acting out/violent or disoriented behavior. **Enhances safety of caregiver and care receiver.**
- Identify equipment needs/resources, adaptive aids **to enhance the independence and safety of the care receiver.**
- Provide contact person/case manager **to partner with care provider(s) in coordinating care, providing physical/social support, and assisting with problem solving, as needed/desired.**

NURSING PRIORITY NO. 5. To promote wellness (Teaching/Discharge Considerations):
- Advocate for/assist caregiver to plan for and implement changes that may be necessary (e.g., home care providers, adult day care, eventual placement in long-term care facility/hospice).
- Support caregiver in setting practical goals for self (and care receiver) that are realistic for care receiver's condition/prognosis and caregiver's own abilities.
- Review signs of burnout (e.g., emotional/physical exaustion; changes in appetite and sleep; withdrawal from friends, family, life interests).
- Discuss/demonstrate stress management techniques (e.g., accepting own feelings/frustrations and limitations, talking with trusted friend, taking a break from situation) and

---

Information in brackets added by the authors to clarify and enhance the use of nursing diagnoses.

      Cultural   Collaborative   Community/Home Care

importance of self-nurturing (e.g., eating and sleeping regularly; pursuing self-development interests, personal needs, hobbies, social activities, spiritual enrichment). **May provide care provider with options to look after self.**

- Encourage involvement in caregiver support group.
- Refer to classes/other therapies, as indicated.
- Identify available 12-step program, when indicated, to provide tools **to deal with enabling/codependent behaviors that impair level of function.**
- Refer to counseling or psychotherapy, as needed.
- Provide bibliotherapy of appropriate references **for self-paced learning** and encourage discussion of information.

Documentation Focus

ASSESSMENT/REASSESSMENT

- Assessment findings, functional level/degree of impairment, caregiver's understanding/perception of situation.
- Identified risk factors.

PLANNING

- Plan of care and individual responsibility for specific activities.
- Needed resources, including type and source of assistive devices/durable equipment.
- Teaching plan.

IMPLEMENTATION/EVALUATION

- Caregiver/receiver response to interventions/teaching and actions performed.
- Identification of inner resources, behavior/lifestyle changes to be made.
- Attainment/progress toward desired outcome(s).
- Modifications to plan of care.

DISCHARGE PLANNING

- Plan for continuation/follow-through of needed changes.
- Referrals for assistance/evaluation.

SAMPLE NURSING OUTCOMES & INTERVENTIONS CLASSIFICATIONS (NOC/NIC)

NOC—Caregiver Lifestyle Disruption
NIC—Caregiver Support

Information in brackets added by the authors to clarify and enhance the use of nursing diagnoses.

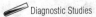 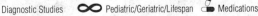

risk for Caregiver Role Strain

Taxonomy II: Role Relationships—Class 1 Caregiving Roles (00062)
[Diagnostic Division: Social Interaction]
Submitted 1992

Definition: Caregiver is vulnerable for felt difficulty in performing the family caregiver role

Risk Factors

Illness severity of the care receiver; psychological or cognitive problems in care receiver; addiction or codependency

Discharge of family member with significant home-care needs; premature birth/congenital defect

Unpredictable illness course or instability in the care receiver's health

Duration of caregiving required; inexperience with caregiving; complexity/amount of caregiving tasks; caregiver's competing role commitments

Caregiver health impairment

Caregiver is female/spouse

Caregiver not developmentally ready for caregiver role [e.g., a young adult needing to provide care for middle-aged parent]; developmental delay or retardation of the care receiver or caregiver

Presence of situational stressors that normally affect families (e.g., significant loss, disaster or crisis, economic vulnerability, major life events [e.g., birth, hospitalization, leaving home, returning home, marriage, divorce, change in employment, retirement, death])

Inadequate physical environment for providing care (e.g., housing, transportation, community services, equipment)

Family/caregiver isolation

Lack of respite/recreation for caregiver

Marginal family adaptation or dysfunction prior to the caregiving situation

Marginal caregiver coping patterns

Past history of poor relationship between caregiver and care receiver

Care receiver exhibits deviant, bizarre behavior

Presence of abuse or violence

> NOTE: A risk diagnosis is not evidenced by signs and symptoms, as the problem has not occurred and nursing interventions are directed at prevention.

Information in brackets added by the authors to clarify and enhance the use of nursing diagnoses.

  Cultural Collaborative Community/Home Care

Desired Outcomes/Evaluation Criteria—Client Will:

- Identify individual risk factors and appropriate interventions.
- Demonstrate/initiate behaviors or lifestyle changes to prevent development of impaired function.
- Use available resources appropriately.
- Report satisfaction with current situation.

Actions/Interventions

NURSING PRIORITY NO. 1. To assess factors affecting current situation:

- Note presence of high-risk situations (e.g., elderly client with total self-care dependence or several small children with one child requiring extensive assistance due to physical condition/developmental delays). **May necessitate role reversal, resulting in added stress or place excessive demands on parenting skills.**
- Identify relationship and proximity of caregiver to care receiver (e.g., spouse/lover, parent/child, friend).
- Note therapeutic regimen and physical/mental condition of care receiver **to ascertain potential areas of need (e.g., teaching, direct care support, respite).**
- Determine caregiver's level of responsibility, involvement in, and anticipated length of care.
- Ascertain physical/emotional health and developmental level/abilities, as well as additional responsibilities of caregiver (e.g., job, school, raising family). **Provides clues to potential stressors and possible supportive interventions.**
- Use assessment tool, such as Burden Interview, when appropriate, **to further determine caregiver's abilities.**
- Identify strengths/weaknesses of caregiver and care receiver.
- Verify safety of caregiver/receiver.
- Discuss caregiver's and care receiver's view of and concerns about situation.
- Determine available supports and resources currently used.
- Note any codependency needs of caregiver.

NURSING PRIORITY NO. 2. To enhance caregiver's ability to deal with current situation:

- Discuss strategies to coordinate care and other responsibilities (e.g., employment, care of children/dependents, housekeeping activities).

Information in brackets added by the authors to clarify and enhance the use of nursing diagnoses.

 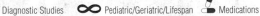

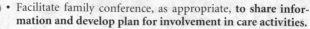

- Facilitate family conference, as appropriate, **to share information and develop plan for involvement in care activities.**
- Refer to classes and/or specialists (e.g., first aid/CPR classes, enterostomal/physical therapist) **for special training, as indicated.**
- Identify additional resources to include financial, legal, respite care.
- Identify equipment needs/resources, adaptive aids **to enhance the independence and safety of the care receiver.**
- Identify contact person/case manager as needed **to coordinate care, provide support, and assist with problem solving.**
- Provide information and/or demonstrate techniques for dealing with acting out/violent or disoriented behavior **to protect/prevent injury to caregiver and care receiver**.
- Assist caregiver to recognize codependent behaviors (i.e., doing things for others that others are able to do for themselves) and how these behaviors affect the situation.

NURSING PRIORITY NO. 3. To promote wellness (Teaching/Discharge Considerations):

- Stress importance of self-nurturing (e.g., pursuing self-development interests, personal needs, hobbies, and social activities*)* **to improve/maintain quality of life for caregiver.**
- Advocate for/assist caregiver to plan/implement changes that may be necessary (e.g., home care providers, adult day care, eventual placement in long-term care facility/hospice).
- Review signs of burnout (e.g., emotional/physical exaustion; changes in appetite and sleep; withdrawal from friends, family, life interests).
- Discuss/demonstrate stress management techniques and importance of self-nurturing (e.g., pursuing self-development interests, personal needs, hobbies, social activities, spiritual enrichment). **May provide care provider with options to protect self/promote well-wing.**
- Encourage involvement in caregiver/other specific support group(s).
- Provide bibliotherapy of appropriate references and encourage discussion of information.
- Refer to classes/therapists as indicated.
- Identify available 12-step program, when indicated, **to provide tools to deal with codependent behaviors that impair level of function.**
- Refer to counseling or psychotherapy as needed.

Information in brackets added by the authors to clarify and enhance the use of nursing diagnoses.

 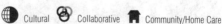

Documentation Focus

ASSESSMENT/REASSESSMENT

- Identified risk factors and caregiver perceptions of situation.
- Reactions of care receiver/family.
- Involvement of family members/others.

PLANNING

- Treatment plan and individual responsibility for specific activities.
- Teaching plan.

IMPLEMENTATION/EVALUATION

- Caregiver/receiver response to interventions/teaching and actions performed.
- Attainment/progress toward desired outcome(s).
- Modifications to plan of care.

DISCHARGE PLANNING

- Long-term needs and who is responsible for actions to be taken.
- Specific referrals provided for assistance/evaluation.

SAMPLE NURSING OUTCOMES & INTERVENTIONS CLASSIFICATIONS (NOC/NIC)

NOC—Caregiving Endurance Potential
NIC—Caregiver Support

readiness for enhanced Comfort

Taxonomy II: Comfort—Class 1 Physical Comfort/Class 2 Environmental Comfort (00183)
[Diagnostic Division: Pain/Discomfort]
Submitted 2006

Definition: A pattern of ease, relief, and transcendence in physical, psychospiritual, environmental, and/or social dimensions that can be strengthened

Related Factors

To be developed

Information in brackets added by the authors to clarify and enhance the use of nursing diagnoses.

 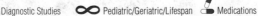

Defining Characteristics

SUBJECTIVE

- Expresses desire to enhance comfort/feeling of contentment
- Expresses desire to enhance relaxation
- Expresses desire to enhance resolution of complaints

OBJECTIVE

[Appears relaxed/calm]
[Participating in comfort measures of choice]

Desired Outcomes/Evaluation Criteria—Client Will:

- Verbalize sense of comfort/contentment.
- Demonstrate behaviors of optimal level of ease.
- Participate in desirable and realistic health-seeking behaviors.

Actions/Interventions

NURSING PRIORITY NO. 1. To determine current level of comfort/motivation for growth:

- Determine the type of comfort client is experiencing: 1) relief [as from pain]; 2) ease [a state of calm or contentment]; or 3) transcendence [state in which one rises above one's problems or pain]).
- Ascertain motivation/expectations for change.
- Establish context(s) in which comfort is realized: 1) physical (pertaining to bodily sensations); 2) psychospiritual (pertaining to internal awareness of self and meaning in one's life; relationship to a higher order or being); 3) environmental (pertaining to external surroundings, conditions, and influences; 4) sociocultural (pertaining to interpersonal, family, and societal relationships):

PHYSICAL

- Verify that client is managing pain and pain components effectively. Success in this arena usually addresses other issues/emotions (e.g., fear, loneliness, anxiety, noxious stimuli, anger).
- Ascertain what is used/required for comfort or rest (e.g., head of bed up/down, music on/off, white noise, rocking motion, certain person or thing).

PSYCHOSPIRITUAL

- Determine how psychological and spiritual indicators overlap (e.g., meaningfulness, faith, identity, self-esteem) for client **in enhancing comfort.**

Information in brackets added by the authors to clarify and enhance the use of nursing diagnoses.

  Cultural Collaborative 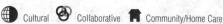 Community/Home Care

- Determine influence of cultural beliefs/values.
- Ascertain that client/SO has received desired support regarding spiritual enrichment, including prayer/meditation/access to spiritual counselor of choice.

ENVIRONMENTAL

- Determine that client's environment respects privacy and provides natural lighting and readily accessible view to outdoors **(an aspect that can be manipulated to enhance comfort).**

SOCIOCULTURAL

- Ascertain meaning of comfort in context of interpersonal, family, cultural values, and societal relationships.
- Validate client/SO understanding of client's diagnosis/prognosis and ongoing methods of managing condition, as appropriate and/or desired by client. **Considers client/family needs in this area and/or shows appreciation for their desires.**

NURSING PRIORITY NO. 2. To assist client in developing plan to improve comfort:

PHYSICAL

- Collaborate in treating/managing medical conditions involving oxygenation, elimination, mobility, cognitive abilities, electrolyte balance, thermoregulation, hydration, **to promote physical stability.**
- Work with client to prevent pain, nausea, itching, thirst/other physical discomforts.
- Suggest parent be present during procedures **to comfort child.**
- Provide age-appropriate comfort measures (e.g., back rub, change of position, cuddling, use of heat/cold) **to provide nonpharmacological pain management.**
- Review interventions/activities **to promote ease,** such as Therapeutic Touch (TT), biofeedback, self-hypnosis, guided imagery, breathing exercises, play therapy, and humor **to promote relaxation and refocus attention.**
- Assist client to use and modify medication regimen **to make best use of pharmacologic pain management.**
- Assist client/SO(s) to develop plan for activity and exercise within individual ability, emphasizing necessity of allowing sufficient time to finish activities.
- Maintain open/flexible visitation with client's desired persons.

Information in brackets added by the authors to clarify and enhance the use of nursing diagnoses.

• Encourage adequate rest periods **to prevent fatigue.**
• Plan care to allow individually adequate rest periods. Schedule activities for periods when client has the most energy **to maximize participation.**
 • Discuss routines to promote restful sleep.

PSYCHOSPIRITUAL

• Interact with client in therapeutic manner. **The nurse could be the most important comfort intervention for meeting client's needs. For example, assuring client that nausea can be treated successfully with both pharmacologic and non-pharmacologic methods may be more effective than simply administering antiemetic without reassurance and comforting presence.**
• Encourage verbalization of feelings and make time for listening/interacting.
• Identify ways (e.g., meditation, sharing oneself with others, being out in nature/garden, other spiritual activities) to achieve connectedness or harmony with self, others, nature, higher power.
 • Establish realistic activity goals with client. **Enhances commitment to promoting optimal outcomes.**
 • Involve client/SO(s) in schedule planning and decisions about timing and spacing of treatments **to promote relaxation/reduce sense of boredom.**
• Encourage client to do whatever possible (e.g., self-care, sit up in chair, walk). **Enhances self-esteem and independence.**
 • Use distraction with music, chatting/texting with family/friends, watching TV, playing video/computer games, **to limit dwelling on/transcend unpleasant sensations and situations.**
 • Encourage client to develop assertiveness skills, prioritizing goals/activities, and to make use of beneficial coping behaviors. **Promotes sense of control and improves self-esteem.**
 • Offer/identify opportunities for client to participate in experiences that enhance control and independence.

ENVIRONMENTAL

• Provide quiet environment, calm activities.
 • Provide for periodic changes in the personal surroundings when client is confined. Use the individual's input in creating the changes (e.g., seasonal bulletin boards, color changes, rearranging furniture, pictures).
 • Suggest activities, such as bird feeders/baths for bird-watching, a garden in a window box/terrarium, or a fish

---

Information in brackets added by the authors to clarify and enhance the use of nursing diagnoses.

   Cultural   Collaborative   Community/Home Care

bowl/aquarium, **to stimulate observation as well as involvement and participation in activity.**

SOCIOCULTURAL

 • Encourage age-appropriate diversional activities (e.g., TV/radio, playtime, socialization/outings with others).
• Avoid overstimulation/understimulation (cognitive and sensory).
 • Make appropriate referrals to available support groups, hobby clubs, service organizations.

NURSING PRIORITY NO. 3. To promote optimum wellness (Teaching/ Discharge Considerations):

PHYSICAL

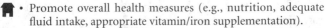 • Promote overall health measures (e.g., nutrition, adequate fluid intake, appropriate vitamin/iron supplementation).
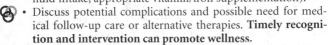 • Discuss potential complications and possible need for medical follow-up care or alternative therapies. **Timely recognition and intervention can promote wellness.**
• Assist client/SO(s) to identify and acquire necessary equipment (e.g., lifts, commode chair, safety grab bars, personal hygiene supplies) **to meet individual needs.**

PSYCHOSPIRITUAL

 • Collaborate with others when client expresses interest in lessons, counseling, coaching and/or mentoring **to meet/ enhance emotional and/or spiritual comfort.**
• Promote/encourage client's contributions toward meeting realistic goals.
• Encourage client to take time to be introspective in the search for contentment/transcendence.

ENVIRONMENTAL

 • Create a compassionate, supportive, and therapeutic environment incorporating client's cultural and age/developmental factors.
• Correct environmental hazards **that could influence safety/ negatively affect comfort.**
• Arrange for home visit/evaluation, as needed.
• Discuss long-term plan for taking care of environmental needs.

SOCIOCULTURAL

• Advocate for growth-promoting environment in conflict situations, and consider issues from client/family perspective.

Information in brackets added by the authors to clarify and enhance the use of nursing diagnoses.

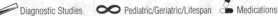

readiness for enhanced COMFORT

• Support client/SO access to resources (e.g., knowledge and skills; financial resources/assistance; personal/psychological support; social systems.)

Documentation Focus

ASSESSMENT/REASSESSMENT

• Individual findings, including client's description of current status/situation.
• Motivation and expectations for change.
• Medication use/nonpharmacological measures.

PLANNING

• Plan of care/interventions and who is involved in planning.
• Teaching plan.

IMPLEMENTATION/EVALUATION

• Responses to interventions/teaching and actions performed.
• Attainment/progress toward desired outcome(s).
• Modifications to plan of care.

DISCHARGE PLANNING

• Long-term needs and who is responsible for actions to be taken.
• Specific referrals made.

SAMPLE NURSING OUTCOMES & INTERVENTIONS CLASSIFICATIONS (NOC/NIC)

NOC—Comfort Level
NIC—Self-Modification Assistance

impaired verbal Communication

Taxonomy II: Perception/Cognition—Class 5
 Communication (00051)
[Diagnostic Division: Social Interaction]
Submitted 1983; Revised 1998 (by small group work 1996)

Definition: Decreased, delayed, or absent ability to receive, process, transmit, and/or use a system of symbols

Related Factors

Decrease in circulation to brain; brain tumor

Information in brackets added by the authors to clarify and enhance the use of nursing diagnoses.

      Cultural   Collaborative   Community/Home Care

Anatomical deficit (e.g., cleft palate, alteration of the neurovascular visual system, auditory system, or phonatory apparatus)
Difference related to developmental age
Physical barrier (tracheostomy, intubation)
Physiological conditions [e.g., dyspnea]; alteration of central nervous system (CNS); weakening of the musculoskeletal system
Psychological barriers (e.g., psychosis, lack of stimuli); emotional conditions [depression, panic, anger]; stress
Environmental barriers
Cultural difference
Lack of information
Side effects of medication
Alteration in self-esteem or self-concept
Altered perceptions
Absence of SO(s)

Defining Characteristics

SUBJECTIVE

[Reports of difficulty expressing self]

OBJECTIVE

Inability to speak dominant language
Speaks/verbalizes with difficulty; stuttering; slurring
Does not/cannot speak; willful refusal to speak
Difficulty forming words/sentences (e.g., aphonia, dyslalia, dysarthria)
Difficulty expressing thoughts verbally (e.g., aphasia, dysphasia, apraxia, dyslexia)
Inappropriate verbalization [incessant, loose association of ideas; flight of ideas]
Difficulty in comprehending/maintaining usual communication pattern
Absence of eye contact/difficulty in selective attending; partial/total visual deficit
Inability/difficulty in use of facial/body expressions
Dyspnea
Disorientation to person/space/time
[Inability to modulate speech]
[Message inappropriate to content]
[Use of nonverbal cues (e.g., pleading eyes, gestures, turning away)]
[Frustration, anger, hostility]

Information in brackets added by the authors to clarify and enhance the use of nursing diagnoses.

 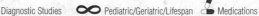

Desired Outcomes/Evaluation Criteria—Client Will:

- Verbalize or indicate an understanding of the communication difficulty and plans for ways of handling.
- Establish method of communication in which needs can be expressed.
- Participate in therapeutic communication (e.g., using silence, acceptance, restating, reflecting, active-listening, and I-messages).
- Demonstrate congruent verbal and nonverbal communication.
- Use resources appropriately.

Actions/Interventions

NURSING PRIORITY NO. 1. To assess causative/contributing factors:

- Review history for neurological conditions **that could affect speech, such as stroke, tumor, multiple sclerosis (MS), hearing or vision impairment.**
- Note results of neurological tests (e.g., electroencephalogram [EEG]; computed tomography [CT]/magnetic resonance imaging [MRI] scans; and language/speech tests [e.g., Boston Diagnostic Aphasia Examination, the Action Naming Test, etc.]).
- Note whether aphasia is motor (expressive: loss of images for articulated speech), sensory (receptive: unable to understand words and does not recognize the defect), conduction (slow comprehension: uses words inappropriately but knows the error), and/or global (total loss of ability to comprehend and speak). Evaluate the degree of impairment.
- Evaluate mental status, note presence of psychiatric conditions (e.g., manic-depressive, schizoid/affective behavior). Assess psychological response to communication impairment, willingness to find alternate means of communication.
- Note presence of ET tube/tracheostomy or other physical blocks to speech (e.g., cleft palate, jaws wired).
- Assess environmental factors that may affect ability to communicate (e.g., room noise level).
- Determine primary language spoken and cultural factors.
- Assess style of speech (as outlined in Defining Characteristics).
- Note level of anxiety present; presence of angry, hostile behavior; frustration.
- Interview parent to determine child's developmental level of speech and language comprehension.
- Note parent's speech patterns and manner of communicating with child, including gestures.

Information in brackets added by the authors to clarify and enhance the use of nursing diagnoses.

 Cultural Collaborative Community/Home Care

NURSING PRIORITY NO. 2. To assist client to establish a means of communication to express needs, wants, ideas, and questions:

- Ascertain that you have client's attention before communicating.
- Determine ability to read/write. Evaluate musculoskeletal states, including manual dexterity (e.g., ability to hold a pen and write).
- Advise other healthcare providers of client's communication deficits (e.g., deafness, aphasia, presence of mechanical ventilation strategies) and needed means of communication (e.g., writing pad, signing, yes/no responses, gestures, picture board) **to minimize client's frustration and promote understanding (aphasia).**
- Obtain a translator/written translation or picture chart **when writing is not possible or client speaks a different language than that spoken by healthcare provider.**
- Facilitate hearing and vision examinations **to obtain necessary aids.**
- Ascertain that hearing aid(s) are in place and batteries charged, and/or glasses are worn when needed **to facilitate/improve communication.** Assist client to learn to use and adjust to aids.
- Reduce environmental noise that can interfere with comprehension. Provide adequate lighting, especially if client is reading lips or attempting to write.
- Establish relationship with the client, listening carefully and attending to client's verbal/nonverbal expressions. **Conveys interest and concern.**
- Maintain eye contact, preferably at client's level. Be aware of cultural factors that may preclude eye contact (e.g., found in some American Indians, Indo-Chinese, Arabs, natives of Appalachia).
- Keep communication simple, speaking in short sentences, using appropriate words, and using all modes for accessing information: visual, auditory, and kinesthetic.
- Maintain a calm, unhurried manner. Provide sufficient time for client to respond. Downplay errors and avoid frequent corrections. **Individuals with expressive aphasia may talk more easily when they are rested and relaxed and when they are talking to one person at a time.**
- Determine meaning of words used by the client and congruency of communication and nonverbal messages.
- Validate meaning of nonverbal communication; do not make assumptions **because they may be wrong.** Be honest; if you do not understand, seek assistance from others.

Information in brackets added by the authors to clarify and enhance the use of nursing diagnoses.

 Diagnostic Studies   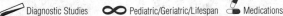 Pediatric/Geriatric/Lifespan   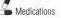 Medications   **169**

- Individualize techniques using breathing for relaxation of the vocal cords, rote tasks (such as counting), and singing or melodic intonation **to assist aphasic clients in relearning speech.**
- Anticipate needs and stay with client until effective communication is reestablished, and/or client feels safe/comfortable.
- Plan for alternative methods of communication (e.g., slate board, letter/picture board, hand/eye signals, typewriter/computer), incorporating information about type of disability present.
- Identify previous solutions tried/used if situation is chronic or recurrent.
- Provide reality orientation by responding with simple, straightforward, honest statements.
- Provide environmental stimuli, as needed, **to maintain contact with reality,** or reduce stimuli **to lessen anxiety that may worsen problem.**
- Use confrontation skills, when appropriate, within an established nurse-client relationship **to clarify discrepancies between verbal and nonverbal cues.**

NURSING PRIORITY NO. 3. To promote wellness (Teaching/Discharge Considerations):

- Review information about condition, prognosis, and treatment with client/SO(s).
- Reinforce that loss of speech does not imply loss of intelligence.
- Discuss individual methods of dealing with impairment.
- Recommend placing a tape recorder with a prerecorded emergency message near the telephone. Information to include: client's name, address, telephone number, type of airway, and a request for immediate emergency assistance.
- Use and assist client/SO(s) to learn therapeutic communication skills of acknowledgment, active-listening, and I-messages. **Improves general communication skills.**
- Involve family/SO(s) in plan of care as much as possible. **Enhances participation and commitment to communication with loved one.**
- Refer to appropriate resources (e.g., speech/language therapist, support groups such as stroke club, individual/family and/or psychiatric counseling).
- Refer to NDs ineffective Coping; disabled family Coping (as indicated); Anxiety; Fear.

Information in brackets added by the authors to clarify and enhance the use of nursing diagnoses.

    Cultural   Collaborative Community/Home Care

Documentation Focus

ASSESSMENT/REASSESSMENT

- Assessment findings/pertinent history information (i.e., physical/psychological/cultural concerns).
- Meaning of nonverbal cues, level of anxiety client exhibits.

PLANNING

- Plan of care and interventions (e.g., type of alternative communication/translator).
- Teaching plan.

IMPLEMENTATION/EVALUATION

- Response to interventions/teaching and actions performed.
- Attainment/progress toward desired outcome(s).
- Modifications to plan of care.

DISCHARGE PLANNING

- Discharge needs/referrals made; additional resources available.

SAMPLE NURSING OUTCOMES & INTERVENTIONS CLASSIFICATIONS (NOC/NIC)

NOC—Communication Ability
NIC—Communication Enhancement: Speech Deficit

readiness for enhanced Communication

Taxonomy II: Perception/Cognition—Class 4 Cognition (00161)
[Diagnostic Division: Teaching/Learning]
Submitted 2002

Definition: A pattern of exchanging information and ideas with others that is sufficient for meeting one's needs and life goals, and can be strengthened

Related Factors

To be developed

Defining Characteristics

SUBJECTIVE

Expresses willingness to enhance communication
Expresses thoughts/feelings

Information in brackets added by the authors to clarify and enhance the use of nursing diagnoses.

 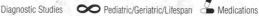

readiness for enhanced COMMUNICATION

Expresses satisfaction with ability to share information/ideas with others

OBJECTIVE

Able to speak/write a language
Forms words, phrases, sentences
Uses/interprets nonverbal cues appropriately

Desired Outcomes/Evaluation Criteria—Client/SO/Caregiver Will:

• Verbalize or indicate an understanding of the communication process.
• Identify ways to improve communication.

Actions/Interventions

NURSING PRIORITY NO. 1. To assess how client is managing communication/challenges:

• Ascertain circumstances that result in client's desire to improve communication. **Many factors are involved in communication, and identifying specific needs/expectations helps in developing realistic goals and determining likelihood of success.**
• Evaluate mental status. **Disorientation and psychotic conditions may be affecting speech and the communication of thoughts, needs, and desires.**
• Determine client's developmental level of speech and language comprehension. **Provides baseline information for developing plan for improvement.**
• Determine ability to both read/write preferred language. **Evaluating grasp of language as well as musculoskeletal states, including manual dexterity (e.g., ability to hold a pen and write), provides information about nature of client's situation. Educational plan can address language skills. Neuromuscular deficits will require individual program in order to improve.**
 • Determine country of origin, dominant language, whether client is recent immigrant and what cultural, ethnic group client identifies as own. **Recent immigrant may identify with home country and its people, language, beliefs, and health-care practices, thus affecting language skills and ability to improve interactions in new country.**
• Ascertain if interpreter is needed/desired. **Law mandates that interpretation services be made available. A trained,**

Information in brackets added by the authors to clarify and enhance the use of nursing diagnoses.

professional interpreter who translates precisely and possesses a basic understanding of medical terminology and healthcare ethics is preferred to enhance client and provider satisfaction.

- Determine comfort level in expression of feelings and concepts in nonproficient language. **Concern about language skills can impact perception of own ability to communicate.**
- Note any physical challenges to effective communication (e.g., talking tracheostomy, wired jaws) or physiological/neurological conditions (e.g., severe shortness of breath, neuromuscular weakness, stroke, brain trauma, hearing impairment, cleft palate, facial trauma). **Client may be dealing with speech/language comprehension or have voice production problems (pitch, loudness, or quality) that call attention to voice rather than what speaker is saying. These barriers may need to be addressed to enable client to improve communication skills.**
- Clarify meaning of words used by the client to describe important aspects of life and health/well-being (e.g., pain, sorrow, anxiety). **Words can easily be misinterpreted when sender and receiver have different ideas about their meanings. Restating what one has heard can clarify whether an expressed statement has been understood or misinterpreted.**
- Determine presence of emotional lability (e.g., anger outbursts) and frequency of unstable behaviors. **Emotional/psychiatric issues can affect communication and interfere with understanding.**
- Evaluate congruency of verbal and nonverbal messages. **Communication is enhanced when verbal and nonverbal messages are congruent.**
- Evaluate need/desire for pictures or written communications and instructions as part of treatment plan. **Alternative methods of communication can help client feel understood and promote feelings of satisfaction with interaction.**

NURSING PRIORITY NO. 2. To improve client's ability to communicate thoughts, needs, and ideas:

- Maintain a calm, unhurried manner. Provide sufficient time for client to respond. **An atmosphere in which client is free to speak without fear of criticism provides the opportunity to explore all the issues involved in making decisions to improve communication skills.**
- Pay attention to speaker. Be an active listener. **The use of active-listening communicates acceptance and respect for the client, establishing trust and promoting openness and**

Information in brackets added by the authors to clarify and enhance the use of nursing diagnoses.

 Diagnostic Studies   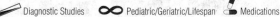 Pediatric/Geriatric/Lifespan   Medications   **173** honest expression. It communicates a belief that the client is a capable and competent person.

- Sit down, maintain eye contact as culturally appropriate, preferably at client's level, and spend time with the client. **Conveys message that the nurse has time and interest in communicating.**

- Observe body language, eye movements, and behavioral cues. **May reveal unspoken concerns; for example, when pain is present, client may react with tears, grimacing, stiff posture, turning away, or angry outbursts.**

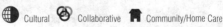 - Help client identify and learn to avoid use of nontherapeutic communication. **These barriers are recognized as detriments to open communication and learning to avoid them maximizes the effectiveness of communication between client and others.**

- Obtain interpreter with language or signing abilities, as needed. **May be needed to enhance understanding of words and language concepts or to ascertain that interpretation of communication is accurate.**

- Suggest use of pad and pencil, slate board, letter/picture board when interacting or to interface in new situations. **When client has physical impairments that challenge verbal communication, alternate means can provide clear concepts that are understandable to both parties.**

- Obtain/provide access to voice-enabled computer. **Use of these devices may be more helpful when communication challenges are long-standing and/or when client is used to working with them.**

- Respect client's cultural communication needs. **Different cultures can dictate beliefs of what is normal or abnormal (i.e., in some cultures, eye-to-eye contact is considered disrespectful, impolite, or an invasion of privacy; silence and tone of voice have various meanings, and slang words can cause confusion).**

- Encourage use of glasses, hearing aids, dentures, electronic speech devices, as needed. **These devices maximize sensory perception/speech formation and can improve understanding and enhance speech patterns.**

- Reduce distractions and background noises (e.g., close the door, turn down the radio/TV). **A distracting environment can interfere with communication, limiting attention to tasks and making speech and communication more difficult. Reducing noise can help both parties hear clearly, thus improving understanding.**

Information in brackets added by the authors to clarify and enhance the use of nursing diagnoses.

Cultural   Collaborative   Community/Home Care

- Associate words with objects—using repetition and redundancy—point to objects or demonstrate desired actions. **Speaker's own body language can be used to enhance client's understanding.**
- Use confrontation skills carefully, when appropriate, within an established nurse-client relationship. **Can be used to clarify discrepancies between verbal and nonverbal cues, enabling client to look at areas that may require change.**

NURSING PRIORITY NO. 3. To promote optimum communication:

- Discuss with family/SO and other caregivers effective ways in which the client communicates. **Identifying positive aspects of current communication skills enables family members to learn and move forward in desire to enhance ways of interacting.**
- Encourage client/SO(s) to familiarize themselves with and use new/developing communication technologies. **Enhances family relationships and promotes self-esteem for all members as they are able to communicate regardless of the problems (e.g., progressive disorder) that could interfere with ability to interact.**
- Reinforce client/SO(s) learning and using therapeutic communication skills of acknowledgment, active-listening, and I-messages. **Improves general communication skills, emphasizes acceptance, and conveys respect, enabling family relationships to improve.**
- Refer to appropriate resources (e.g., speech therapist, language classes, individual/family and/or psychiatric counseling). **May be needed to help overcome challenges as family strives toward desired goal of enhanced communication.**

Documentation Focus

ASSESSMENT/REASSESSMENT

- Assessment findings/pertinent history information (i.e., physical/psychological/cultural concerns).
- Meaning of nonverbal cues, level of anxiety client exhibits.

PLANNING

- Plan of care and interventions (e.g., type of alternative communication/translator).
- Teaching plan.

IMPLEMENTATION/EVALUATION

- Progress toward desired outcome(s).
- Modifications to plan of care.

Information in brackets added by the authors to clarify and enhance the use of nursing diagnoses.

DISCHARGE PLANNING

• Discharge needs/referrals made, additional resources available.

SAMPLE NURSING OUTCOMES & INTERVENTIONS CLASSIFICATIONS (NOC/NIC)

NOC—Communication Ability
NIC—Communication Enhancement [specify]

decisional Conflict
(Specify)

Taxonomy II: Life Principles—Class 3 Value/Belief/Action Congruence (00083)
[Diagnostic Division: Ego Integrity]
Submitted 1988; Revised 2006

Definition: Uncertainty about course of action to be taken when choice among competing actions involves risk, loss, or challenge to values and beliefs

Related Factors

Unclear personal values/beliefs; perceived threat to value system
Lack of experience or interference with decision making
Lack of relevant information; multiple or divergent sources of information
Moral obligations require performing/not performing actions
Moral principles/rules/values support mutually inconsistent courses of action
Support system deficit
[Age, developmental state]
[Family system, sociocultural factors]
[Cognitive, emotional, behavioral level of functioning]

Defining Characteristics

SUBJECTIVE

Verbalizes: uncertainty about choices; undesired consequences of alternative actions being considered
Verbalizes feeling of distress while attempting a decision
Questioning moral principles/rules/values or personal values/beliefs while attempting a decision

---

Information in brackets added by the authors to clarify and enhance the use of nursing diagnoses.

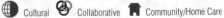 Cultural Collaborative Community/Home Care

Vacillation between alternative choices; delayed decision making
Self-focusing
Physical signs of distress or tension (e.g., increased heart rate, increased muscle tension, restlessness, etc.)

Desired Outcomes/Evaluation Criteria—Client Will:

- Verbalize awareness of positive and negative aspects of choices/alternative actions.
- Acknowledge/ventilate feelings of anxiety and distress associated with choice/related to making difficult decision.
- Identify personal values and beliefs concerning issues.
- Make decision(s) and express satisfaction with choices.
- Meet psychological needs as evidenced by appropriate expression of feelings, identification of options, and use of resources.
- Display relaxed manner/calm demeanor, free of physical signs of distress.

Actions/Interventions

NURSING PRIORITY NO. 1. To assess causative/contributing factors:

- Determine usual ability to manage own affairs. Clarify who has legal right to intervene on behalf of child/elder/impaired individual (e.g., parent/spouse, other relative, designee for durable medical power of attorney, or court appointed guardian/advocate). (Family disruption/conflicts can complicate decision process.)
- Note expressions of indecision, dependence on others, availability/involvement of support persons (e.g., lack of/conflicting advice). Ascertain dependency of other(s) on client and/or issues of codependency.
- Active-listen/identify reason for indecisiveness. Helps client to clarify problem and work toward a solution.
- Determine effectiveness of current problem-solving techniques.
- Note presence/intensity of physical signs of anxiety (e.g., increased heart rate, muscle tension).
- Listen for expressions of inability to find meaning in life/reason for living, feelings of futility, or alienation from God and others around them. (Refer to ND Spiritual Distress, as indicated.)
- Review information client has about the healthcare decision. Accurate and clearly understood information about situation will help the client make the best decision for self.

Information in brackets added by the authors to clarify and enhance the use of nursing diagnoses.

NURSING PRIORITY NO. 2. To assist client to develop/effectively use problem-solving skills:

• Promote safe and hopeful environment, as needed, while client regains inner control.

• Encourage verbalization of conflicts/concerns.

• Accept verbal expressions of anger/guilt, setting limits on maladaptive behavior **to promote client safety.**

 • Clarify and prioritize individual goals, noting where the subject of the "conflict" falls on this scale. **Choices may have risky, uncertain outcomes; may reflect a need to make value judgments or may generate anticipated regret over having to reject positive choice and acccept negative consequences.**

• Identify strengths and presence of positive coping skills (e.g., use of relaxation technique, willingness to express feelings).

 • Identify positive aspects of this experience and assist client to view it as a learning opportunity **to develop new and creative solutions.**

• Correct misperceptions client may have and provide factual information. **Provides for better decision making.**

• Provide opportunities for client to make simple decisions regarding self-care and other daily activities. Accept choice not to do so. Advance complexity of choices, as tolerated.

∞ • Encourage child to make developmentally appropriate decisions concerning own care. **Fosters child's sense of self-worth, enhances ability to learn/exercise coping skills.**

 • Discuss time considerations, setting time line for small steps and considering consequences related to not making/postponing specific decisions **to facilitate resolution of conflict.**

 • Have client list some alternatives to present situation or decisions, using a brainstorming process. Include family in this activity as indicated (e.g., placement of parent in long-term care facility, use of intervention process with addicted member). (Refer to NDs interrupted Family Processes; dysfunctional Family Processes: alcoholism; compromised family Coping; moral Distress.)

• Practice use of problem-solving process with current situation/decision.

 • Discuss/clarify cultural or spiritual concerns, accepting client's values in a nonjudgmental manner.

NURSING PRIORITY NO. 3. To promote wellness (Teaching/Discharge Considerations):

Information in brackets added by the authors to clarify and enhance the use of nursing diagnoses.

 Cultural   Collaborative   Community/Home Care

- Promote opportunities for using conflict-resolution skills, identifying steps as client does each one.
- Provide positive feedback for efforts and progress noted. **Promotes continuation of efforts.**
- Encourage involvement of family/SO(s), as desired/available, **to provide support for the client.**
- Support client for decisions made, especially if consequences are unexpected, difficult to cope with.
- Encourage attendance at stress reduction, assertiveness classes.
- Refer to other resources, as necessary (e.g., clergy, psychiatric clinical nurse specialist/psychiatrist, family/marital therapist, addiction support groups).

Documentation Focus

ASSESSMENT/REASSESSMENT

- Assessment findings/behavioral responses, degree of impairment in lifestyle functioning.
- Individuals involved in the conflict.
- Personal values/beliefs.

PLANNING

- Plan of care/interventions and who is involved in the planning process.
- Teaching plan.

IMPLEMENTATION/EVALUATION

- Client's and involved individual's responses to interventions/teaching and actions performed.
- Ability to express feelings, identify options; use of resources.
- Attainment/progress toward desired outcome(s).
- Modifications to plan of care.

DISCHARGE PLANNING

- Long-term needs/referrals, actions to be taken, and who is responsible for doing.
- Specific referrals made.

SAMPLE NURSING OUTCOMES & INTERVENTIONS CLASSIFICATIONS (NOC/NIC)

NOC—Decision Making
NIC—Decision-Making Support

Information in brackets added by the authors to clarify and enhance the use of nursing diagnoses.

 Diagnostic Studies 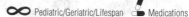 Pediatric/Geriatric/Lifespan Medications **179**

parental role Conflict

Taxonomy II: Role Relationships—Class 1 Role
   Performance (00064)
[Diagnostic Division: Social Interaction]
Submitted 1988

Definition: Parent experience of role confusion and
conflict in response to crisis

Related Factors

Separation from child due to chronic illness [/disability]
Intimidation with invasive modalities (e.g., intubation); restric-
   tive modalities (e.g., isolation); specialized care centers
Home care of a child with special needs [e.g., apnea monitoring,
   postural drainage, hyperalimentation]
Change in marital status; [conflicts of the role of the single parent]
Interruptions of family life due to home care regimen (e.g.,
   treatments, caregivers, lack of respite)

Defining Characteristics

SUBJECTIVE

Parent(s) express(es) concerns/feeling of inadequacy to provide
   for child's needs (e.g., physical and emotional)
Parent(s) express(es) concerns about changes in parental role;
   about family (e.g., functioning, communication, health)
Express(es) concern about perceived loss of control over decisions relating to their child
Verbaliz(es) feelings of guilt/frustration; anxiety; fear
[Verbalizes concern about role conflict of wanting to date while
   having responsibility of childcare]

OBJECTIVE

Demonstrates disruption in caretaking routines
Reluctant to participate in usual caretaking activities even with
   encouragement and support

Desired Outcomes/Evaluation
Criteria—Parent(s) Will:

- Verbalize understanding of situation and expected parent's/
  child's role.
- Express feelings about child's illness/situation and effect on
  family life.

Information in brackets added by the authors to clarify and enhance
the use of nursing diagnoses.

 Cultural Collaborative Community/Home Care

- Demonstrate appropriate behaviors in regard to parenting role.
- Assume caretaking activities as appropriate.
- Handle family disruptions effectively.

Actions/Interventions

NURSING PRIORITY NO. 1. To assess causative/contributory factors:

- Assess individual situation and parent's perception of/concern about what is happening and expectations of self as caregiver.
- Note parental status, including age and maturity, stability of relationship, single parent, other responsibilities. (Increasing numbers of elderly individuals are providing full-time care for young grandchildren whose parents are unavailable or unable to provide care.)
- Ascertain parent's understanding of child's developmental stage and expectations for the future **to identify misconceptions/strengths.**
- Note coping skills currently being used by each individual as well as how problems have been dealt with in the past. **Provides basis for comparison and reference for client's coping abilities.**
- Determine use of substances (e.g., alcohol, other drugs, including prescription medications). **May interfere with individual's ability to cope/problem solve.**
- Assess availability/use of resources, including extended family, support groups, and financial.
- Perform testing, such as Parent-Child Relationship Inventory (PCRI), for further evaluation as indicated.

NURSING PRIORITY NO. 2. To assist parents to deal with current crisis:

- Encourage free verbal expression of feelings (including negative feelings of anger and hostility), setting limits on inappropriate behavior.
- Acknowledge difficulty of situation and normalcy of feeling overwhelmed and helpless. Encourage contact with parents who experienced similar situation with child and had positive outcome.
- Provide information, including technical information when appropriate, **to meet individual needs/correct misconceptions.**
- Promote parental involvement in decision making and care as much as possible/desired. **Enhances sense of control.**

Information in brackets added by the authors to clarify and enhance the use of nursing diagnoses.

• Encourage interaction/facilitate communication between parent(s) and children.

 • Promote use of assertiveness, relaxation skills **to help individuals to deal with situation/crisis.**

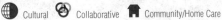 • Assist parent to learn proper administration of medications/treatments, as indicated.

 • Provide for/encourage use of respite care, parental time off **to enhance emotional well-being.**

• Help single parent distinguish between parent love and partner love. **Love is constant, but attention can be given to one or the other, as appropriate.**

NURSING PRIORITY NO. 3. To promote wellness (Teaching/Discharge Considerations):

 • Provide anticipatory guidance **to encourage making plans for future needs.**

 • Encourage parents to set realistic and mutually agreed-on goals.

 • Discuss attachment behaviors such as breastfeeding on cue, co-sleeping, and babywearing (carrying baby around on chest/back). **Dealing with ill child/home care pressures can strain the bond between parent/child. Activities such as these encourage secure relationships.**

 • Provide/identify learning opportunities specific to needs (e.g., parenting classes, healthcare equipment use/troubleshooting).

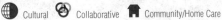 • Refer to community resources, as appropriate (e.g., visiting nurse, respite care, social services, psychiatric care/family therapy, well-baby clinics, special needs support services).

• Refer to ND impaired Parenting for additional interventions.

Documentation Focus

ASSESSMENT/REASSESSMENT

• Findings, including specifics of individual situation/parental concerns, perceptions, expectations.

PLANNING

• Plan of care and who is involved in the planning.
• Teaching plan.

IMPLEMENTATION/EVALUATION

• Parent's responses to interventions/teaching and actions performed.
• Attainment/progress toward desired outcome(s).
• Modifications to plan of care.

Information in brackets added by the authors to clarify and enhance the use of nursing diagnoses.

🌐 Cultural 🔃 Collaborative 🏠 Community/Home Care

DISCHARGE PLANNING

- Long-term needs and who is responsible for each action to be taken.
- Specific referrals made.

SAMPLE NURSING OUTCOMES & INTERVENTIONS CLASSIFICATIONS (NOC/NIC)

NOC—Parenting
NIC—Parenting Promotion

acute Confusion

Taxonomy II: Perception/Cognition—Class 4 Cognition (00128)
[Diagnostic Division: Neurosensory]
Submitted 1994; Revised 2006

Definition: Abrupt onset of reversible disturbances of consciousness, attention, cognition, and perception that develop over a short period of time

Related Factors

Alcohol abuse; drug abuse; [medication reaction/interaction; anesthesia/surgery; metabolic imbalances]
Fluctuation in sleep-wake cycle
Over 60 years of age
Delirium [including febrile epilepticum (following or instead of an epileptic attack), toxic and traumatic]
Dementia
[Exacerbation of a chronic illness; hypoxemia]
[Severe pain]

Defining Characteristics

SUBJECTIVE

Hallucinations [visual/auditory]
[Exaggerated emotional responses]

OBJECTIVE

Fluctuation in cognition/level of consciousness
Fluctuation in psychomotor activity [tremors, body movement]
Increased agitation/restlessness
Misperceptions [inappropriate responses]

Information in brackets added by the authors to clarify and enhance the use of nursing diagnoses.

 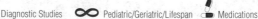

Lack of motivation to initiate/follow-through with purposeful behavior

Lack of motivation to initiate/follow-through with goal-directed behavior

Desired Outcomes/Evaluation Criteria—Client Will:

- Regain/maintain usual reality orientation and level of consciousness.
- Verbalize understanding of causative factors when known.
- Initiate lifestyle/behavior changes to prevent or minimize recurrence of problem.

Actions/Interventions

NURSING PRIORITY NO. 1. To assess causative/contributing factors:

- Identify factors present such as recent surgery, acute illness, trauma/fall, use of large numbers of medications (polypharmacy), intoxication, substance use/abuse, history/current seizures, episodes of fever/pain, presence of acute infection (especially urinary tract infection in elderly client), exposure to toxic substances, exposure to traumatic events, person with dementia experiencing sudden change in environment/unfamiliar surroundings or people. **Acute confusion is a symptom associated with numerous causes (e.g., hypoxia, abnormal metabolic conditions, ingestion of toxins or medications, electrolyte abnormalities, sepsis/systemic infections, nutritional deficiencies, endocrine disorders, CNS infections/other neurologic pathology, acute psychiatric disorders).**
- Investigate possibility of alcohol/other drug withdrawal.
- Evaluate vital signs **for indicators of poor tissue perfusion (i.e., hypotension, tachycardia, tachypnea), stress response (tachycardia/tachypnea).**
- Determine current medications/drug use—especially anti-anxiety agents, barbiturates, lithium, methyldopa, disulfiram, cocaine, alcohol, amphetamines, hallucinogens, opiates (**associated with high risk of confusion**)—and schedule of use, such as cimetidine + antacid or digoxin + diuretics (**combinations can increase risk of adverse reactions/interactions**).
- Assess diet/nutritional status **to identify possible deficiencies of essential nutrients and vitamins (e.g., thiamine) that could affect mental status.**
- Note presence of anxiety, agitation, fear.

Information in brackets added by the authors to clarify and enhance the use of nursing diagnoses.

  Cultural Collaborative Community/Home Care

- Evaluate for exacerbation of psychiatric conditions (e.g., mood or dissociative disorders, dementia).
- Monitor laboratory values (e.g., CBC, blood cultures, oxygen saturation, electrolytes, chemistries, ammonia levels, liver function studies, serum glucose, urinalysis, toxicology, and drug levels [including peak/trough, as appropriate]).
- Evaluate sleep/rest status, noting deprivation/oversleeping. (Refer to NDs Insomnia; Sleep Deprivation, as appropriate.)
- Review results of medical diagnostic studies (e.g., brain scans/imaging studies, EEG, cardiopulmonary tests, lumbar puncture/CSF studies).

NURSING PRIORITY NO. 2. To determine degree of impairment:

- Talk with SO(s) to determine historic baseline, observed changes, and onset/recurrence of changes **to understand and clarify current situation**.
- Evaluate mental status, noting extent of impairment in orientation, attention span, ability to follow directions, ability to send/receive communication, appropriateness of response.
- Note occurrence/timing of agitation, hallucinations, violent behaviors. (**"Sundown syndrome" may occur, with client oriented during daylight hours, but confused during nighttime.**)
- Determine threat to safety of client/others.

NURSING PRIORITY NO. 3. To maximize level of function, prevent further deterioration:

- Assist with treatment of underlying problem (e.g., drug intoxication/substance abuse, infectious process, hypoxemia, biochemical imbalances, nutritional deficits, pain management).
- Monitor/adjust medication regimen and note response. Determine medications that can be changed or eliminated **when polypharmacy, side effects, or adverse reactions are determined to be associated with current condition**.
- Orient client to surroundings, staff, necessary activities, as needed. Present reality concisely and briefly. Avoid challenging illogical thinking—**defensive reactions may result.**
- Encourage family/SO(s) to participate in reorientation as well as providing ongoing input (e.g., current news and family happenings).
- Maintain calm environment and eliminate extraneous noise/stimuli **to prevent overstimulation.** Provide normal levels of essential sensory/tactile stimulation—include personal items/pictures, and so forth.
- Encourage client to use vision/hearing aids when needed.

Information in brackets added by the authors to clarify and enhance the use of nursing diagnoses.

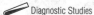

- Give simple directions. Allow sufficient time for client to respond, communicate, and make decisions.
- Provide for safety needs (e.g., supervision, seizure precautions, placing call bell within reach, positioning needed items within reach/clearing traffic paths, ambulating with devices).
- Note behavior that may be indicative of potential for violence and take appropriate actions.
- Assist with treatment of alcohol/drug intoxication and/or withdrawal, as indicated. Administer psychotropics cautiously **to control restlessness, agitation, hallucinations.**
- Avoid/limit use of restraints—**may worsen situation, increase likelihood of untoward complications.**
- Provide undisturbed rest periods.
- Administer short-acting, nonbenzodiazepine sleeping medication (e.g., Benadryl) at bedtime.
- Refer to NDs impaired Memory; disturbed Thought Processes; impaired verbal Communication, for additional interventions.

NURSING PRIORITY NO. 4. To promote wellness (Teaching/Discharge Considerations):

- Explain reason(s) for confusion, if known. **Although acute confusion usually subsides over time as client recovers from underlying cause and/or adjusts to situation, it can initially be frightening to client/SO. Therefore, information as to the cause and appropriate treatment to improve condition may be helpful in managing sense of fear and powerlessness.**
- Discuss need for ongoing medical review of client's medications **to limit possibility of misuse and/or potential for dangerous side effects/interactions.**
- Assist in identifying ongoing treatment needs and emphasize necessity of periodic evaluation **to support early intervention**.
- Stress importance of keeping vision/hearing aids in good repair **to improve client's interpretation of environmental stimuli and communication.**
- Discuss situation with family and involve in planning **to meet identified needs.**
- Review ways to maximize sleep environment (e.g., prefered bedtime rituals, room temperature, bedding/pillows, elimination or reduction of extraneous noise/stimuli and interruptions.)
- Provide appropriate referrals (e.g., cognitive retraining, substance abuse treatment/support groups, medication monitoring program, Meals on Wheels, home health, and adult daycare).

Information in brackets added by the authors to clarify and enhance the use of nursing diagnoses.

  Cultural Collaborative 🏠 Community/Home Care

Documentation Focus

ASSESSMENT/REASSESSMENT

• Nature, duration, frequency of problem.
• Current and previous level of function, effect on independ-ence/lifestyle (including safety concerns).

PLANNING

• Plan of care and who is involved in planning.
• Teaching plan.

IMPLEMENTATION/EVALUATION

• Response to interventions and actions performed.
• Attainment/progress toward desired outcomes.
• Modifications to plan of care.

DISCHARGE PLANNING

• Long-term needs and who is responsible for actions to be taken.
• Available resources and specific referrals.

SAMPLE NURSING OUTCOMES & INTERVENTIONS CLASSIFICATIONS (NOC/NIC)

NOC—Cognitive Ability
NIC—Delirium Management

chronic Confusion

Taxonomy II: Perception/Cognition—Class 4 Cognition (00129)
[Diagnostic Division: Neurosensory]
Submitted 1994

Definition: Irreversible, long-standing, and/or progressive deterioration of intellect and personality characterized by decreased ability to interpret environmental stimuli; decreased capacity for intellectual thought processes, manifested by disturbances of memory, orientation, and behavior

Related Factors

Alzheimer's disease [dementia of the Alzheimer's type]
Korsakoff's psychosis
Multi-infarct dementia

Information in brackets added by the authors to clarify and enhance the use of nursing diagnoses.

 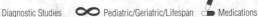

Cerebral vascular attack
Head injury

Defining Characteristics

OBJECTIVE

Clinical evidence of organic impairment
Altered interpretation
Altered response to stimuli
Progressive/long-standing cognitive impairment
No change in level of consciousness
Impaired socialization
Impaired short-term/long-term memory
Altered personality

Desired Outcome/Evaluation Criteria—Client Will:

• Remain safe and free from harm.

Family/SO Will:

• Verbalize understanding of disease process/prognosis and client's needs.
• Identify/participate in interventions to deal effectively with situation.
• Provide for maximal independence while meeting safety needs of client.

Actions/Interventions

NURSING PRIORITY NO. 1. To assess degree of impairment:

• Evaluate responses on diagnostic examinations (e.g., memory impairments, reality orientation, attention span, calculations). **A combination of tests (e.g., Confusion Assessment Method [CAM], Mini-Mental State Examination [MMSE], Alzheimer's Disease Assessment Scale [ADAS-cog], Brief Dementia Severity Rating Scale [BDSRS], Neuropsychiatric Inventory [NPI]) is often needed to complete an evaluation of the client's overall condition relating to a chronic/irreversible condition.**
• Test ability to receive and send effective communication. **Client may be nonverbal or require assistance with/interpretation of verbalizations.**

• Talk with SO(s) regarding baseline behaviors, length of time since onset/progression of problem, their perception of prognosis, and other pertinent information and concerns for

---

Information in brackets added by the authors to clarify and enhance the use of nursing diagnoses.

   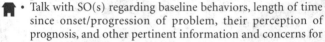 Cultural   Collaborative   Community/Home Care

client. **If the history reveals an insidious decline over months to years, and if abnormal perceptions, inattention, and memory problems are concurrent with confusion, a diagnosis of dementia is likely.**

- Ascertain interventions previously used/tried.
- Evaluate response to care providers and receptiveness to interventions **to determine areas of concern to be addressed.**
- Determine anxiety level in relation to situation and problem behaviors **that may be indicative of potential for violence.**

NURSING PRIORITY NO. 2. To limit effects of deterioration/maximize level of function:

- Assist in treating conditions (e.g., infections, malnutrition, electrolyte imbalances, and adverse medication reactions) **that may contribute to/exacerbate distress, discomfort, and agitation.**
- Provide calm environment, eliminate extraneous noise/stimuli **that may increase client's level of agitation/confusion.**
- Be open and honest in dicussing client's disease, abilities, and prognosis.
- Use touch judiciously. Tell client what is being done before initiating contact **to reduce sense of surprise/negative reaction.**
- Avoid challenging illogical thinking **because defensive reactions may result.**
- Use positive statements; offer guided choices between two options. Simplify client's tasks and routines **to reduce agitation associated with multiple options/demands.**
- Be supportive when client is attempting to communicate and be sensitive to increasing frustration, fears, and misperceived threats.
- Encourage family/SO(s) to provide ongoing orientation/input to include current news and family happenings.
- Maintain reality-oriented relationship/environment (e.g., clocks, calendars, personal items, seasonal decorations). Encourage participation in resocialization groups.
- Allow client to reminisce/exist in own reality, if not detrimental to well-being.
- Provide safety measures (e.g., close supervision, identification bracelet, medication lockup, lower temperature on hot water tank).
- Set limits on unsafe and/or inappropriate behavior, being alert to potential for violence.
- Avoid use of restraints as much as possible. Use vest (instead of wrist) restraints when required. **Although restraints may prevent falls, they can increase client's agitation and distress and are a safety risk.**

Information in brackets added by the authors to clarify and enhance the use of nursing diagnoses.

- Administer medications, as ordered (e.g., antidepressants, antipsychotics). Monitor for therapeutic action, as well as adverse reactions, side effects, and interactions. **Medications may be used judiciously to manage symptoms of psychosis, depression, or aggressive behavior**.
- Refer to NDs acute Confusion; impaired Memory; disturbed Thought Processes; impared verbal Communication, for additional interventions.

NURSING PRIORITY NO. 3. To assist SO(s) to develop coping strategies:

- Determine family resources, availability, and willingness to participate in meeting client's needs.
- Involve family/SO(s) in planning and care activities as needed/desired. Maintain frequent interactions with SO(s) **in order to relay information, change care strategies, obtain SO feedback, and offer support.**
- Discuss caregiver burden and signs of burnout, if appropriate.
- Provide educational materials, bibliographies, list of available local resources, help lines, websites, etc., as desired, **to assist SO(s) in dealing and coping with long-term care issues.**
- Identify appropriate community resources (e.g., Alzheimer's Disease and Related Disorders Association [ARDA], stroke or brain injury support group, senior support groups, clergy, social services, respite care) **to provide client/SO with support and assist with problem solving.**
- Refer to ND risk for Caregiver Role Strain.

NURSING PRIORITY NO. 4. To promote wellness (Teaching/ Discharge Considerations):

- Discuss nature of client's condition (e.g., chronic stable, progressive, or degenerative), treatment concerns, and follow-up needed **to maintain client at highest possible level of functioning.**
- Determine age-appropriate ongoing treatment and socialization needs and appropriate resources.
- Develop plan of care with family **to meet client's and SO's individual needs**.
- Provide appropriate referrals (e.g., Meals on Wheels, adult day care, home care agency, respite care).

Documentation Focus

ASSESSMENT/REASSESSMENT

- Individual findings, including current level of function and rate of anticipated changes.
- Safety issues.

Information in brackets added by the authors to clarify and enhance the use of nursing diagnoses.

  Cultural Collaborative 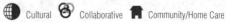 Community/Home Care

PLANNING

- Plan of care and who is involved in planning.

IMPLEMENTATION/EVALUATION

- Response to interventions and actions performed.
- Attainment/progress toward desired outcomes.
- Modifications to plan of care.

DISCHARGE PLANNING

- Long-term needs/referrals and who is responsible for actions to be taken.
- Available resources, specific referrals made.

SAMPLE NURSING OUTCOMES & INTERVENTIONS CLASSIFICATIONS (NOC/NIC)

NOC—Cognitive Ability
NIC—Dementia Management

risk for acute Confusion

Taxonomy II: Perception/Cognition—Class 4 Cognition (00173)
[Diagnostic Division: Neurosensory]
Submitted 2006

Definition: At risk for reversible disturbances of consciousness, attention, cognition, and perception that develop over a short period of time

Risk Factors

Alcohol use; substance abuse
Infection; urinary retention
Pain
Fluctuation in sleep-wake cycle
Medication/drugs: anesthesia, anticholinergics, diphenhydramine, opioids, psychoactive drugs, multiple medications
Metabolic abnormalities: decreased hemoglobin, electrolyte imbalances, dehydration, increased BUN/creatinine, azotemia, malnutrition
Decreased mobility; decreased restraints
History of stroke; impaired cognition; dementia; sensory deprivation
Over 50 years of age; male gender

Information in brackets added by the authors to clarify and enhance the use of nursing diagnoses.

 Diagnostic Studies   ∞ Pediatric/Geriatric/Lifespan   Medications   **191**

NOTE: A risk diagnosis is not evidenced by signs and symptoms, as the problem has not occurred and nursing interventions are directed at prevention.

Desired Outcomes/Evaluation Criteria—Client Will:

- Verbalize understanding of individual cause/risk factor(s).
- Identify interventions to prevent/reduce risk of confusion.

Actions/Interventions

NURSING PRIORITY NO. 1. To assess causative/contributing factors:

- Identify factors present such as recent trauma/fall; use of large numbers of medications/polypharmacy; substance use/abuse; history/current seizures; episodes of fever/pain; presence of acute infection; exposure to toxic substances; traumatic events in client's/SO's life; person with dementia experiencing sudden change in environment/unfamiliar surroundings or people. **Acute confusion is a symptom associated with numerous causes (e.g., hypoxia, abnormal metabolic conditions, ingestion of toxins or medications, electrolyte abnormalities, sepsis/systemic infections, nutritional deficiencies, endocrine disorders, CNS infections/other neurologic pathology, acute psychiatric disorders).**
- Investigate possibility of alcohol/other drug withdrawal, exacerbation of psychiatric conditions (e.g., mood disorder, dissociative disorders, dementia).
- Determine client's functional level, including ability to provide self-care and move about at will. **Conditions/situations that limit client's mobility and independence (e.g., acute or chronic physical/psychiatric illnesses and their therapies, trauma/extensive immobility, confinement in unfamiliar surroundings, sensory deprivation) potentiate prospect of acute confusional state.**
- Ascertain life events (e.g., death of spouse/other family member, absence of known care provider, move from lifelong home, catastrophic natural disaster) **that can affect client's perceptions, attention, and concentration.**
- Assess diet/nutritional status **to identify possible deficiencies of essential nutrients and vitamins that could affect mental status.**
- Evaluate sleep/rest status, noting deprivation/oversleeping. (Refer to NDs Insomnia; Sleep Deprivation, as appropriate.)

Information in brackets added by the authors to clarify and enhance the use of nursing diagnoses.

    Cultural   Collaborative   🏠 Community/Home Care

NURSING PRIORITY NO 2. To reduce/correct existing risk factors:

- Assist with treatment of underlying problem (e.g., drug intoxication/substance abuse, infectious processes, hypoxemia, biochemical imbalances, nutritional deficits, pain management).

- Monitor/adjust medication regimen and note response. **May identify medications that can be changed or eliminated in client who's prone to adverse or exaggerated responses (including confusion) to medications.**

- Administer medications, as appropriate (e.g., relieving pain in elderly client with hip fracture can improve cognitive responses).
- Orient client to surroundings, staff, necessary activities.
- Encourage family/SO(s) to participate in orientation by providing ongoing input (e.g., current news and family happenings).
- Maintain calm environment and eliminate extraneous noise/stimuli **to prevent overstimulation.** Provide normal levels of essential sensory/tactile stimulation—include personal items/pictures, desired music, activities, contacts, and so on.
- Encourage client to use vision/hearing aids/other adaptive equipment, as needed, **to assist client in interpretation of environment and communication.**
- Promote early ambulation activities **to enhance well-being and reduce effects of prolonged bedrest/inactivity.**
- Provide for safety needs (e.g., supervision; seizure precautions; placing needed items, such as a call bell, within reach; clearing traffic paths; ambulating with assistance; providing clear directions and instructions).

NURSING PRIORITY NO. 3. To promote wellness (Teaching/Discharge Considerations):

- Assist with treatment of underlying medical conditions and/or management of risk factors **to reduce/limit complications.**

- Stress importance of ongoing monitoring of medication regimen **for potential adverse actions/reactions.**
- Provide undisturbed rest periods.

- Review ways to maximize sleep environment (e.g., preferred bedtime rituals, room temperature, bedding/pillows, elimination or reduction of extraneous noise/stimuli and interruptions.)

- Provide appropriate referrals (e.g., medical/psychiatric specialists, medication monitoring program, nutritionist, substance abuse treatment, support groups, home health care, and adult day care).

Information in brackets added by the authors to clarify and enhance the use of nursing diagnoses.

 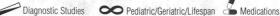

Documentation Focus

ASSESSMENT/REASSESSMENT

- Existing conditions/risk factors for individual.
- Current level of function, effect on independence and ability to meet own needs, including food/fluid intake and medication use.

PLANNING

- Plan of care and who is involved in planning.
- Teaching plan.

IMPLEMENTATION/EVALUATION

- Response to interventions and actions performed.
- Attainment/progress toward desired outcomes.
- Modifications to plan of care.

DISCHARGE PLANNING

- Long-term needs and who is responsible for actions to be taken.
- Available resources and specific referrals.

SAMPLE NURSING OUTCOMES & INTERVENTIONS CLASSIFICATIONS (NOC/NIC)

NOC—Cognitive Ability
NIC—Delirium Management

Constipation

Taxonomy II: Elimination—Class 2 Gastrointestinal System (00011)
[Diagnostic Division: Elimination]
Submitted 1975; Nursing Diagnosis Extension and Classification (NDEC) Revision 1998

Definition: Decrease in normal frequency of defecation accompanied by difficult or incomplete passage of stool and/or passage of excessively hard, dry stool

Related Factors

FUNCTIONAL

Irregular defecation habits; inadequate toileting (e.g., timeliness, positioning for defecation, privacy)

Information in brackets added by the authors to clarify and enhance the use of nursing diagnoses.

 Cultural Collaborative Community/Home Care

Insufficient physical activity; abdominal muscle weakness
Recent environmental changes
Habitual denial/ignoring of urge to defecate

PSYCHOLOGICAL

Emotional stress; depression; mental confusion

PHARMACOLOGICAL

Antilipemic agents; laxative overdose; calcium carbonate; aluminum-containing antacids; nonsteroidal anti-inflammatory agents; opiates; anticholinergics; diuretics; iron salts; phenothiazides; sedatives; sympathomimetics; bismuth salts; antidepressants; calcium channel blockers; anticonvulsants

MECHANICAL

Hemorrhoids; pregnancy; obesity
Rectal abscess/ulcer/prolapse; rectal anal fissures/strictures; rectocele
Prostate enlargement; postsurgical obstruction
Neurological impairment; Hirschsprung's disease; tumors
Electrolyte imbalance

PHYSIOLOGICAL

Poor eating habits; change in usual foods/eating patterns; insufficient fiber/fluid intake; dehydration
Inadequate dentition/oral hygiene
Decreased motility of gastrointestinal tract

Defining Characteristics

SUBJECTIVE

Change in bowel pattern; unable to pass stool; decreased frequency, decreased volume of stool
Increased abdominal pressure; feeling of rectal fullness/pressure
Abdominal pain; pain with defecation; nausea; vomiting; headache; indigestion; generalized fatigue

OBJECTIVE

Hard, formed stool
Straining with defecation
Hypoactive/hyperactive bowel sounds; borborygmi
Distended abdomen; abdominal tenderness with/without palpable muscle resistance; palpable abdominal/rectal mass
Percussed abdominal dullness

Information in brackets added by the authors to clarify and enhance the use of nursing diagnoses.

 Diagnostic Studies 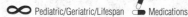 Pediatric/Geriatric/Lifespan Medications **195**

Presence of soft pastelike stool in rectum; oozing liquid stool; bright red blood with stool

Severe flatus; anorexia

Atypical presentations in older adults (e.g., change in mental status, urinary incontinence, unexplained falls, elevated body temperature)

Desired Outcomes/Evaluation Criteria—Client Will:

* Establish/regain normal pattern of bowel functioning.
* Verbalize understanding of etiology and appropriate interventions/solutions for individual situation.
* Demonstrate behaviors or lifestyle changes to prevent recurrence of problem.
* Participate in bowel program as indicated.

Actions/Interventions

NURSING PRIORITY NO. 1. To identify causative/contributing factors:

* Review medical/surgical/social history for conditions often associated with constipation (e.g., altered cognition; metabolic, endocrine, or neurological disorders; surgery; bowel disorders [e.g., irritable bowel syndrome, intestinal obstructions or tumors]; pregnancy; advanced age; immobility).
* Review daily dietary regimen, noting if diet is deficient in fiber.
* Note general oral/dental health **that can impact dietary intake.**
* Determine fluid intake **to evaluate client's hydration status.**
* Evaluate client's medication/drug regimen (e.g., opioids, pain relievers, antidepressants, anticonvulsants, aluminum-containing antacids, chemotherapy, iron, contrast media, steroids) **which could cause/exacerbate constipation.**
* Note energy/activity level and exercise pattern. **Sedentary lifestyle may affect elimination patterns.**
* Identify areas of stress (e.g., personal relationships, occupational factors, financial problems). **Individuals may fail to allow time for good bowel habits and/or suffer gastrointestinal effects from stress/tension.**
* Determine access to bathroom, privacy, and ability to perform self-care activities.
* Investigate reports of pain with defecation. Inspect perianal area for hemorrhoids, fissures, skin breakdown, or other abnormal findings.

Information in brackets added by the authors to clarify and enhance the use of nursing diagnoses.

  Cultural Collaborative Community/Home Care

- Determine laxative/enema use. Note signs/reports overuse of stimulant laxatives.
- Palpate abdomen **for presence of distention, masses.**
- Check rectum for presence of fecal impaction, as indicated.
- Assist with medical work-up (e.g., x-rays, abdominal imaging, proctosigmoidoscopy, colonic transit studies, stool sample tests) **for identification of other possible causative factors.**

NURSING PRIORITY NO. 2. To determine usual pattern of elimination:

- Discuss usual elimination habits (e.g., normal urge time) and problems (e.g., client unable to elimimate unless in own home, passing hard stool after prolonged effort, anal pain).
- Identify elements that usually stimulate bowel activity (e.g., caffeine, walking, laxative use) and any interfering factors (e.g., taking opioid pain medications, unable to ambulate to bathroom, pelvic surgery, etc.).

NURSING PRIORITY NO. 3. To assess current pattern of elimination:

- Note color, odor, consistency, amount, and frequency of stool. **Provides a baseline for comparison, promotes recognition of changes.**
- Ascertain duration of current problem and client's degree of concern (e.g., long-standing condition that client has "lived with" may not cause undue concern, whereas an acute post-surgical occurrence of constipation can cause great distress). **Client's response may/may not reflect severity of condition.**
- Auscultate abdomen for presence, location, and characteristics of bowel sounds **reflecting bowel activity.**
- Note treatments client has tried to relieve current situation (e.g., laxatives, suppositories, enemas) and document failure/lack of effectiveness.

NURSING PRIORITY NO. 4. To facilitate return to usual/acceptable pattern of elimination:

- Instruct in/encourage a diet of balanced fiber and bulk (e.g., fruits, vegetables, and whole grains) and fiber supplements (e.g., wheat bran, psyllium) **to improve consistency of stool and facilitate passage through colon.** Note: Improvement in elimination as a result of dietary changes takes time and is not a treatment for acute constipation.
- Promote adequate fluid intake, including high-fiber fruit juices; suggest drinking warm, stimulating fluids (e.g., coffee, hot water, tea) **to promote passage of soft stool.**
- Encourage activity/exercise within limits of individual ability **to stimulate contractions of the intestines.**

Information in brackets added by the authors to clarify and enhance the use of nursing diagnoses.

- Provide privacy and routinely scheduled time for defecation (bathroom or commode preferable to bedpan) **so that client can respond to urge.**
- Encourage/support treatment of underlying medical causes where appropriate **to improve organ function, including the bowel.**
- Administer stool softeners, mild stimulants, or bulk-forming agents, as ordered and/or routinely, when appropriate (e.g., for client receiving opiates, decreased level of activity/immobility).
- Apply lubricant/anesthetic ointment to anus, if needed.
- Administer enemas; digitally remove impacted stool.
- Provide sitz bath after stools **for soothing effect to rectal area.**
- Establish bowel program to include glycerin suppositories and digital stimulation, as appropriate, **when long-term or permanent bowel dysfunction is present.**
- Refer to primary care provider for medical therapies (e.g., added-emolient, saline, or hyperosmolar laxatives, enemas, or suppositories) **to best treat acute situation.**
- Discuss client's current medication regimen with physician **to determine if drugs contributing to constipation can be discontinued or changed.**

NURSING PRIORITY NO. 5. To promote wellness (Teaching/Discharge Considerations):

- Discuss client's particular physiology and acceptable variations in elimination.
- Provide information about relationship of diet, exercise, fluid, and appropriate use of laxatives, as indicated.
- Discuss rationale for and encourage continuation of successful interventions.
- Encourage client to maintain elimination diary, if appropriate, **to facilitate monitoring of long-term problem.**
- Identify specific actions to be taken if problem recurs **to promote timely intervention, enhancing client's independence.**

Documentation Focus

ASSESSMENT/REASSESSMENT

- Usual and current bowel pattern, duration of the problem, and individual contributing factors, including diet and exercise/activity level.
- Characteristics of stool.
- Underlying dynamics.

Information in brackets added by the authors to clarify and enhance the use of nursing diagnoses.

PLANNING

- Plan of care/interventions and changes in lifestyle that are necessary to correct individual situation, and who is involved in planning.
- Teaching plan.

IMPLEMENTATION/EVALUATION

- Responses to interventions/teaching and actions performed.
- Change in bowel pattern, character of stool.
- Attainment/progress toward desired outcomes.
- Modifications to plan of care.

DISCHARGE PLANNING

- Individual long-term needs, noting who is responsible for actions to be taken.
- Recommendations for follow-up care.
- Specific referrals made.

SAMPLE NURSING OUTCOMES & INTERVENTIONS CLASSIFICATIONS (NOC/NIC)

NOC—Bowel Elimination
NIC—Constipation/Impaction Management

perceived Constipation

Taxonomy II: Elimination—Class 2 Gastrointestinal System (00012)
[Diagnostic Division: Elimination]
Submitted 1988

Definition: Self-diagnosis of constipation and abuse of laxatives, enemas, and suppositories to ensure a daily bowel movement

Related Factors

Cultural/family health beliefs
Faulty appraisal [long-term expectations/habits]
Impaired thought processes

Defining Characteristics

SUBJECTIVE

Expectation of a daily bowel movement
Expected passage of stool at same time every day
Overuse of laxatives/enemas/suppositories

Information in brackets added by the authors to clarify and enhance the use of nursing diagnoses.

 Diagnostic Studies 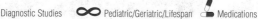 Pediatric/Geriatric/Lifespan Medications **199**

Desired Outcomes/Evaluation Criteria—Client Will:

- Verbalize understanding of physiology of bowel function.
- Identify acceptable interventions to promote adequate bowel function.
- Decrease reliance on laxatives/enemas.
- Establish individually appropriate pattern of elimination.

Actions/Interventions

NURSING PRIORITY NO. 1. To identify factors affecting individual beliefs:

- Determine client's understanding of a "normal" bowel pattern and cultural expectations.
- Compare with client's current bowel functioning.
- Identify interventions used by client to correct perceived problem **to identify strengths and areas of concern to be addressed.**

NURSING PRIORITY NO. 2. To promote wellness (Teaching/Discharge Considerations):

- Discuss physiology and acceptable variations in elimination.
- Identify detrimental effects of habitual laxative and/or enema use and discuss alternatives.
- Review relationship of diet, hydration, and exercise to bowel elimination.
- Provide support by active-listening and discussing client's concerns/fears.
- Encourage use of stress-reduction activities/refocusing of attention while client works to establish individually appropriate pattern.
- Offer educational materials/resources for client/SO **to peruse at home to assist them in making informed decisions regarding constipation and management options.**
- Refer to ND Constipation

Documentation Focus

ASSESSMENT/REASSESSMENT

- Assessment findings/client's perceptions of the problem.
- Current bowel pattern, stool characteristics.

PLANNING

- Plan of care/interventions and who is involved in the planning.
- Teaching plan.

Information in brackets added by the authors to clarify and enhance the use of nursing diagnoses.

 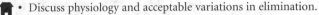 Cultural Collaborative Community/Home Care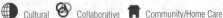

IMPLEMENTATION/EVALUATION

- Client's responses to interventions/teaching and actions performed.
- Changes in bowel pattern, character of stool.
- Attainment/progress toward desired outcome(s).
- Modifications to plan of care.

Discharge Planning

- Referral for follow-up care.

SAMPLE NURSING OUTCOMES & INTERVENTIONS CLASSIFICATIONS (NOC/NIC)

NOC—Health Beliefs
NIC—Bowel Management

risk for Constipation

Taxonomy II: Elimination—Class 2 Gastrointestinal
   System (00015)
[Diagnostic Division: Elimination]
Nursing Diagnosis Extension and Classification (NDEC)
   Submission 1998

Definition: At risk for a decrease in normal frequency of defecation accompanied by difficult or incomplete passage of stool and/or passage of excessively hard, dry stool

Risk Factors

FUNCTIONAL

Irregular defecation habits; inadequate toileting (e.g., timeliness, positioning for defecation, privacy)
Insufficient physical activity; abdominal muscle weakness
Recent environmental changes
Habitual denial/ignoring of urge to defecate

PSYCHOLOGICAL

Emotional stress; depression; mental confusion

PHYSIOLOGICAL

Change in usual foods/eating patterns; insufficient fiber/fluid intake, dehydration; poor eating habits

---

Information in brackets added by the authors to clarify and enhance the use of nursing diagnoses.

 Diagnostic Studies 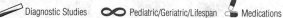 Pediatric/Geriatric/Lifespan   Medications **201**

Inadequate dentition or oral hygiene
Decreased motility of gastrointestinal tract

PHARMACOLOGICAL

Phenothiazides; nonsteroidal anti-inflammatory agents; sedatives; aluminum-containing antacids; laxative overuse; bismuth salts; iron salts; anticholinergics; antidepressants; anticonvulsants; antilipemic agents; calcium channel blockers; calcium carbonate; diuretics; sympathomimetics; opiates

MECHANICAL

Hemorrhoids; pregnancy; obesity
Rectal abscess/ulcer; rectal anal stricture/fissures; rectal prolapse; rectocele
Prostate enlargement; postsurgical obstruction
Neurological impairment; Hirschsprung's disease; tumors
Electrolyte imbalance

> NOTE: A risk diagnosis is not evidenced by signs and symptoms, as the problem has not occurred and nursing interventions are directed at prevention.

Desired Outcomes/Evaluation Criteria—Client Will:

- Maintain usual pattern of bowel functioning.
- Verbalize understanding of risk factors and appropriate interventions/solutions related to individual situation.
- Demonstrate behaviors or lifestyle changes to prevent developing problem.

Actions/Interventions

NURSING PRIORITY NO. **1.** To identify individual risk factors/needs:

- Review medical/surgical/social history (e.g., altered cognition; metabolic, endocrine, or neurological disorders; certain medications; surgery; bowel disorders [e.g., irritable bowel syndrome, intestinal obstructions or tumors, hemorrhoids/rectal bleeding]; pregnancy; advanced age; weakness/debilitation; conditions associated with immobility; recent travel; stressors/changes in lifestyle; depression) **to identify conditions commonly associated with constipation.**
- Auscultate abdomen for presence, location, and characteristics of bowel sounds **reflecting bowel activity.**

Information in brackets added by the authors to clarify and enhance the use of nursing diagnoses.

 Cultural Collaborative Community/Home Care

- Discuss usual elimination pattern and use of laxatives.
- Ascertain client's beliefs and practices about bowel elimination, such as "must have a bowel movement every day or I need an enema."
- Evaluate current dietary and fluid intake and implications for effect on bowel function.
- Review medications (new and chronic use) **for impact on/effects of changes in bowel function.**

NURSING PRIORITY NO. 2. To facilitate normal bowel function:

- Instruct in/encourage balanced fiber and bulk in diet (e.g., fruits, vegetables, and whole grains) and fiber supplements (e.g., wheat bran, psyllium) **to improve consistency of stool and facilitate passage through colon.**
- Promote adequate fluid intake, including water and high-fiber fruit juices; also suggest drinking warm fluids (e.g., coffee, hot water, tea) **to promote soft stool and stimulate bowel activity.**
- Encourage activity/exercise within limits of individual ability **to stimulate contractions of the intestines.**
- Provide privacy and routinely scheduled time for defecation (bathroom or commode preferable to bedpan) **so that client can respond to urge.**
- Administer routine stool softeners, mild stimulants, or bulk-forming agents prn and/or routinely, as appropriate (e.g., for client taking pain medications, especially opiates, or who is inactive, immobile, or unconscious).
- Ascertain frequency, color, consistency, amount of stools. **Provides a baseline for comparison, promotes recognition of changes.**

NURSING PRIORITY NO. 3. To promote wellness (Teaching/Discharge Considerations):

- Discuss physiology and acceptable variations in elimination. **May help reduce concerns/anxiety about situation.**
- Review individual risk factors/potential problems and specific interventions.
- Educate client/SO about safe and risky practices for managing constipation. **Information can help client to make beneficial choices when need arises.**
- Encourage client to maintain elimination diary, if appropriate, **to help monitor bowel pattern.**
- Review appropriate use of medications. Disscuss client's current medication regimen with physician **to determine if drugs contributing to constipation can be discontinued or changed.**

Information in brackets added by the authors to clarify and enhance the use of nursing diagnoses.

- Encourage/support treatment of underlying medical causes, where appropriate, **to improve organ function, including the bowel.**
- Refer to NDs Constipation; perceived Constipation.

Documentation Focus

ASSESSMENT/REASSESSMENT

- Current bowel pattern, characteristics of stool, medications/herbals used.
- Dietary intake.
- Exercise/activity level.

PLANNING

- Plan of care and who is involved in planning.
- Teaching plan.

IMPLEMENTATION/EVALUATION

- Responses to interventions/teaching and actions performed.
- Attainment/progress toward desired outcomes.
- Modifications to plan of care.

DISCHARGE PLANNING

- Individual long-term needs, noting who is responsible for actions to be taken.
- Specific referrals made.

SAMPLE NURSING OUTCOMES & INTERVENTIONS CLASSIFICATIONS (NOC/NIC)

NOC—Bowel Elimination
NIC—Constipation/Impaction Management

Contamination

Taxonomy II: Safety/Protection—Class 4 Environmental Hazards (00181)
[Diagnostic Division: Safety]
Submitted 2006

Definition: Exposure to environmental contaminants in doses sufficient to cause adverse health effects

---

Information in brackets added by the authors to clarify and enhance the use of nursing diagnoses.

  Cultural Collaborative Community/Home Care

Related Factors

EXTERNAL

Chemical contamination of food/water; presence of atmospheric pollutants

Inadequate municipal services (trash removal, sewage treatment facilities)

Geographic area (living in area where high level of contaminants exist)

Playing in outdoor areas where environmental contaminants are used

Personal/household hygiene practices

Living in poverty (increases potential for multiple exposure, lack of access to healthcare, and poor diet)

Use of environmental contaminants in the home (e.g., pesticides, chemicals, environmental tobacco smoke)

Lack of breakdown of contaminants once indoors (breakdown is inhibited without sun and rain exposure)

Flooring surface (carpeted surfaces hold contaminant residue more readily than hard floor surfaces)

Flaking, peeling paint/plaster in presence of young children

Paint, lacquer, etc., in poorly ventilated areas/without effective protection

Inappropriate use/lack of protective clothing

Unprotected contact with heavy metals or chemicals (e.g., arsenic, chromium, lead)

Exposure to radiation (occupation in radiography, employment in/living near nuclear industries and electrical generating plants)

Exposure to disaster (natural or man-made); exposure to bioterrorism

INTERNAL

Age (children less than age 5 years, older adults); gestational age during exposure; developmental characteristics of children

Female gender; pregnancy

Nutritional factors (e.g., obesity, vitamin and mineral deficiencies)

Preexisting disease states; smoking

Concomitant exposure; previous exposures

Defining Characteristics

(Defining characteristics are dependent on the causative agent. Agents cause a variety of individual organ responses as well as systemic responses.)

Information in brackets added by the authors to clarify and enhance the use of nursing diagnoses.

 Diagnostic Studies ∞ Pediatric/Geriatric/Lifespan 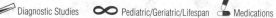 Medications

SUBJECTIVE/OBJECTIVE

Pesticides: (Major categories of pesticides: insecticides, herbicides, fungicides, antimicrobials, rodenticides; major pesticides: organophosphates, carbamates, organochlorines, pyrethrium, arsenic, glycophosphates, bipyridyis, chlorophenoxy)

Dermatological/gastrointestinal/neurological/pulmonary/renal effects of pesticide

Chemicals: (Major chemical agents: petroleum-based agents, anticholinesterases; Type I agents act on proximal tracheo-bronchial portion of the respiratory tract, Type II agents act on alveoli, Type III agents produce systemic effects)

Dermatological/gastrointestinal/immunologic/neurological/pulmonary/renal effects of chemical exposure

Biologics: Dermatological/gastrointestinal/neurological/pulmonary/renal effects of exposure to biologicals (toxins from living organisms—bacteria, viruses, fungi)

Pollution: (Major locations: air, water, soil; major agents: asbestos, radon, tobacco [smoke], heavy metal, lead, noise, exhaust)

Neurological/pulmonary effects of pollution exposure

Waste: (Categories of waste: trash, raw sewage, industrial waste)

Dermatological/gastrointestinal/hepatic/pulmonary effects of waste exposure

Radiation: (Categories: Internal—ingestion of radioactive material [e.g., food/water contamination]; External—exposure through direct contact with radioactive material)

Immunologic/genetic/neurological/oncologic effects of radiation exposure

Desired Outcomes/Evaluation Criteria—Client Will:

- Be free of injury.
- Verbalize understanding of individual factors that contributed to injury and plans for correcting situation(s) where possible.
- Modify environment, as indicated, to enhance safety.

Client/Community Will:

- Identify hazards that lead to exposure/contamination.
- Correct environmental hazards, as identified.
- Demonstrate necessary actions to promote community safety.

Information in brackets added by the authors to clarify and enhance the use of nursing diagnoses.

  Cultural Collaborative Community/Home Care

Actions/Interventions

In reviewing this ND, it is apparent there is overlap with other diagnoses. We have chosen to present generalized interventions. Although there are commonalities to Contamination situations, we suggest that the reader refer to other primary diagnoses as indicated, such as ineffective Airway Clearance, ineffective Breathing Pattern, impaired Gas Exchange, ineffective Home Maintenance, risk for Infection, risk for Injury, risk for Poisoning, impaired/risk for impaired Skin Integrity, Suffocation, ineffective Tissue Perfusion, Trauma.

NURSING PRIORITY NO. 1 To evaluate degree/source of exposure:

- Ascertain 1) type of contaminant(s) to which client has been exposed (e.g., chemical, biological, air pollutant), 2) manner of exposure (e.g., inhalation, ingestion, topical), 3) whether exposure was accidental or intentional, and 4) immediate/delayed reactions. **Determines course of action to be taken by all emergency/other care providers. Note: Intentional exposure to hazardous materials requires notification of law enforcement for further investigation and possible prosecution.**
- Note age and gender: **Children less than 5 years of age are at greater risk for adverse effects from exposure to contaminants because 1) smaller body size causes them to receive a more concentrated "dose" than adults; 2) they spend more time outside than most adults, increasing exposure to air and soil pollutants; 3) they spend more time on the floor, increasing exposure to toxins in carpets and low cupboards; 4) they consume more water and food per pound than adults, increasing their body weight to toxin ratio; and 5) fetus's/infant's and young children's developing organ systems can be disrupted. Older adults have a normal decline in function of immune, integumentary, cardiac, renal, hepatic, and pulmonary systems; an increase in adipose tissue mass; and a decline in lean body mass. Females, in general, have a greater proportion of body fat, increasing the chance of accumulating more lipid soluble toxins than males.**
- Ascertain geographic location (e.g., home/work) where exposure occurred. **Individual and/or community intervention may be needed to modify/correct problem.**
- Note socioeconomic status/availability and use of resources. **Living in poverty increases potential for multiple exposures, delayed/lack of access to healthcare, and poor general health, potentially increasing the severity of adverse effects of exposure.**

Information in brackets added by the authors to clarify and enhance the use of nursing diagnoses.

 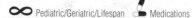

- Determine factors associated with particular contaminant:

  Pesticides: Determine if client has ingested contaminated foods (e.g., fruits, vegetables, commercially raised meats), or inhaled agent (e.g., aerosol bug sprays, in vicinity of crop spraying).

  Chemicals: Ascertain if client uses environmental contaminants in the home or at work (e.g., pesticides, chemicals, chlorine household cleaners), and fails to use/inappropriately uses protective clothing.

  Biologics: Determine if client may have been exposed to biological agents (bacteria, viruses, fungi) or bacterial toxins (e.g., botulinum, ricin). **Exposure occurring as a result of an act of terrorism would be rare; however, individuals may be exposed to bacterial agents or toxins through contaminated/poorly prepared foods.**

  Pollution air/water: Determine if client has been exposed/is sensitive to atmospheric pollutants (e.g., radon, benzene [from gasoline], carbon monoxide, automobile emissions [numerous chemicals], chlorofluorocarbons [refrigerants, solvents], ozone/smog particles [acids, organic chemicals; particles in smoke; commercial plants, such as pulp and paper mills]).

    Investigate possibility of home-based exposure to air pollution—carbon monoxide (e.g., poor ventilation, especially in the winter months [poor heating systems/use of charcoal grill indoors, leaves car running in garage]; cigarette/cigar smoke indoors; ozone [spending a lot of time outdoors, such as playing children, adults participating in moderate to strenuous work or recreational activities]).

  Waste: Determine if client lives in area where trash/garbage accumulates, is exposed to raw sewage or industrial wastes that **can contaminate soil and water.**

  Radiation: Ascertain if client/household member experienced accidental exposure (e.g., occupation in radiography, living near/working in nuclear industries or electrical generation plants).

- Observe for signs and symptoms of infective agent and sepsis such as fatigue, malaise, headache, fever, chills, diaphoresis, skin rash, altered level of consciousness. **Initial symptoms of some diseases may mimic influenza and be misdiagnosed if healthcare providers do not maintain an index of suspicion.**

- Note presence and degree of chemical burns and initial treatment provided.

Information in brackets added by the authors to clarify and enhance the use of nursing diagnoses.

  Cultural Collaborative 🏠 Community/Home Care

- Obtain/assist with diagnostic studies, as indicated. **Provides information about type and degree of exposure/organ involvement or damage.**
- Identify psychological response (e.g., anger, shock, acute anxiety, confusion, denial) to accidental or mass exposure incident. **Although these are normal responses, they may recycle repeatedly and result in post-trauma syndrome if not dealt with adequately.**
- Alert proper authorities to presence/exposure to contamination, as appropriate. **Depending on agent involved, there may be reporting requirements to local/state/national agencies, such as the local health department and Centers for Disease Control and Prevention (CDC).**

NURSING PRIORITY NO. 2. To assist in treating effects of exposure:

- Implement a coordinated decontamination plan (e.g., removal of clothing, showering with soap and water), when indicated, following consultation with medical toxicologist, hazardous materials team, and industrial hygiene and safety officer **to prevent further harm to client and to protect healthcare providers**.
- Insure availablity of/use of personal protective equipment (PPE) (e.g., high-efficiency particulate air [HEPA] filter masks, special garments, and barrier materials including gloves/face shield) **to protect from exposure to biological, chemical, and radioactive hazards.**
- Provide for isolation or group/cohort individuals with same diagnosis/exposure, as resources require. **Limited resources may dictate open ward-like environment; however, the need to control the spread of infection still exists. Only plague, smallpox, and viral hemorrhagic fevers require more than standard infection-control precautions.**
- Provide/assist with therapeutic interventions, as individually appropriate. **Specific needs of the client and the level of care available at a given time/location determine response.**
- Refer pregnant client for individually appropriate diagnostic procedures/screenings. **Helps to determine effects of teratogenic exposure on fetus, allowing for informed choices/preparations.**
- Screen breast milk in lactating client following radiation exposure. **Depending on type and amount of exposure, breastfeeding may need to be briefly interrupted or, occasionally, terminated.**

Information in brackets added by the authors to clarify and enhance the use of nursing diagnoses.

CONTAMINATION

Diagnostic Studies   Pediatric/Geriatric/Lifespan   Medications

209

- Cooperate with/refer to appropriate agencies (e.g., The Centers for Disease Control and Prevention [CDC]; U.S. Army Medical Research Institute of Infectious Diseases [USAMRIID]; Federal Emergency Management Agency [FEMA]; Department of Health and Human Services [DHHS]; Office of Emergency Preparedness [OEP]; Environmental Protection Agency [EPA]) **to prepare for/manage mass casualty incidents.**

NURSING PRIORITY NO. 3. To promote wellness (Teaching/Discharge Considerations):

CLIENT/CAREGIVER

- Identify individual safety needs and injury/illness prevention in home, community, and work setting.
- Install carbon monoxide monitors and a radon detector in home, as appropriate.
- Review individual nutritional needs, appropriate exercise program, and need for rest. **Essentials for well-being and recovery.**
- Repair/replace/correct unsafe household items/situations (e.g., storage of solvents in soda bottles, flaking/peeling paint or plaster, filtering unsafe tap water).
- Stress importance of supervising infant/child or individuals with cognitive limitations.
- Encourage removal of/cleaning of carpeted floors, especially for small children and persons with respiratory conditions. **Carpets hold up to 100 times as much fine particle material as a bare floor, and can contain metals and pesticides.**
- Identify commericial cleaning resources, if appropriate, **for safe cleaning of contaminated articles/surfaces.**
- Install dehumidifier in damp areas **to retard growth of molds.**
- Encourage timely cleaning/replacement of air filters on furnace and/or air conditioning unit. **Good ventilation cuts down on indoor air pollution from carpets, machines, paints, solvents, cleaning materials, and pesticides.**
- Discuss protective actions for specific "bad air" days (e.g., limiting /avoiding outdoor activities) **especially in sensitive groups (e.g., children who are active outdoors, adults involved in moderate or strenuous outdoor activities, persons with respiratory diseases).**
- Review effects of second-hand smoke and importance of refraining from smoking in home/car where others are likely to be exposed.

Information in brackets added by the authors to clarify and enhance the use of nursing diagnoses.

🏠 • Recommend periodic inspection of well water/tap water **to identify possible contaminants.**

🏠 • Encourage client/caregiver to develop a personal/family disaster plan, to gather needed supplies to provide for self/family during a community emergency, and to learn how specific public health threats might affect client and actions **to reduce the risk to health and safety.**

🏠 • Instruct client to always refer to local authorities and health experts for specific up-to-date information for the community and to follow their advice.

⊗ • Refer to counselor/support groups **for ongoing assistance in dealing with traumatic incident/after-effects of exposure.**

🏠 • Provide bibliotherapy/written resources and appropriate websites **for later review and self-paced learning.**

⊗ • Refer to smoking cessation program, as needed.

COMMUNITY

🏠 • Promote community education programs in different modalities/languages/cultures and educational levels geared to increasing awareness of safety measures and resources available to individuals/community.

🏠 • Review pertinent job-related health department/OSHA regulations.

🏠 • Refer to resources that provide information about air quality (e.g., pollen index, "bad air days").

🏠 • Encourage community members/groups to engage in problem-solving activities.

🏠 • Ascertain that there is a comprehensive disaster plan in place in the community to ensure an effective response to any emergency (e.g., flood, toxic spill, infectious disease outbreak, radiation release), including a chain of command, equipment, communication, training, decontamimation area(s), safety and security plans.

Documentation Focus

ASSESSMENT/REASSESSMENT

• Details of specific exposure including location and circumstances.
• Client's/caregiver's understanding of individual risks/safety concerns.

PLANNING

• Plan of care and who is involved in planning.
• Teaching plan.

Information in brackets added by the authors to clarify and enhance the use of nursing diagnoses.

IMPLEMENTATION/EVALUATION

- Individual responses to interventions/teaching and actions performed.
- Specific actions and changes that are made.
- Attainment/progress toward desired outcome(s).
- Modifications to plan of care.

DISCHARGE PLANNING

- Long-range plans for discharge needs, lifestyle and community changes, and who is responsible for actions to be taken.
- Specific referrals made.

SAMPLE NURSING OUTCOMES & INTERVENTIONS CLASSIFICATIONS (NOC/NIC)

NOC—Community Disaster Readiness
NIC—Environmental Risk Protection

risk for Contamination

Taxonomy II: Safety/Protection—Class 4 Environmental Hazards (00180)
[Diagnostic Division: Safety]
Submitted 2006

Definition: Accentuated risk of exposure to environmental contaminants in doses sufficient to cause adverse health effects

Risk Factors

EXTERNAL

Chemical contamination of food/water; presence of atmospheric pollutants

Inadequate municipal services (trash removal, sewage treatment facilities)

Geographic area (living in area where high level of contaminants exist)

Playing in outdoor areas where environmental contaminants are used

Personal/household hygiene practices

Living in poverty (increases potential for multiple exposure, lack of access to healthcare, and poor diet)

Use of environmental contaminants in the home (e.g., pesticides, chemicals, environmental tobacco smoke)

Information in brackets added by the authors to clarify and enhance the use of nursing diagnoses.

  Cultural Collaborative Community/Home Care

Lack of breakdown of contaminants once indoors (breakdown is inhibited without sun and rain exposure)

Flooring surface (carpeted surfaces hold contaminant residue more readily than hard floor surfaces)

Flaking, peeling paint/plaster in presence of young children

Paint, lacquer, etc., in poorly ventilated areas/without effective protection

Inappropriate use/lack of protective clothing

Unprotected contact with heavy metals or chemicals (e.g., arsenic, chromium, lead)

Exposure to radiation (occupation in radiography, employment in/living near nuclear industries and electrical generating plants)

Exposure to disaster (natural or man-made); exposure to bioterrorism

INTERNAL

Age (children less than age 5 years, older adults); gestational age during exposure; developmental characteristics of children

Female gender; pregnancy

Nutritional factors (e.g., obesity, vitamin and mineral deficiencies)

Preexisting disease states; smoking

Concomitant exposure; previous exposures

NOTE: A risk diagnosis is not evidenced by signs and symptoms, as the problem has not occurred and nursing interventions are directed at prevention.

Desired Outcomes/Evaluation Criteria—Client Will:

- Verbalize understanding of individual factors that contribute to possibility of injury and take steps to correct situation(s).
- Demonstrate behaviors/lifestyle changes to reduce risk factors and protect self from injury.
- Modify environment, as indicated, to enhance safety.
- Be free of injury.
- Support community activities for disaster preparedness.

Client/Community Will:

- Identify hazards that could lead to exposure/contamination.
- Correct environmental hazards, as identified.
- Demonstrate necessary actions to promote community safety/disaster preparedness.

Information in brackets added by the authors to clarify and enhance the use of nursing diagnoses.

 Diagnostic Studies 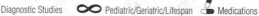 Pediatric/Geriatric/Lifespan Medications **213**

Actions/Interventions

NURSING PRIORITY NO. 1. To evaluate degree/source of risk inherent in the home/community/worksite:

- Ascertain type of contaminant(s) and exposure routes posing a potential hazard to client and/or community (e.g., air/soil/water pollutants, food source, chemical, biological, radiation) as listed in Risk Factors. **Determines course of action to be taken by client/community/care providers.**
- Note age and gender of client/community base (e.g., community health clinic serving primarily poor children or elderly; school near large industrial plant; family living in smog-prone area). **Young children, frail elderly, and females have been found to be at higher risk for effects of exposure to toxins.** (Refer to ND Contamination.)
- Ascertain client's geographic location at home/work (e.g., lives where crop spraying is routine; works in nuclear plant; contract worker/soldier returning from combat area). **Individual and/or community intervention may be needed to reduce risks of accidental/intentional exposures.**
- Note socioeconomic status/availability and use of resources. **Living in poverty increases the potential for multiple exposures, delayed/lack of access to healthcare, and poor general health.**
- Determine client's/SO's understanding of potential risk and appropriate protective measures.

NURSING PRIORITY NO. 2. To assist client to reduce or correct individual risk factors:

- Assist client to develop plan to address individual safety needs and injury/illness prevention in home, community, and work setting.
- Repair/replace/correct unsafe household items/situations (e.g., flaking/peeling paint or plaster, filtering unsafe tap water).
- Review effects of second-hand smoke and importance of refraining from smoking in home/car **where others are likely to be exposed**.
- Encourage removal of/cleaning of carpeted floors, especially for small children and persons with respiratory conditions. **Carpets hold up to 100 times as much fine particle material as a bare floor and can contain metals and pesticides.**
- Encourage timely cleaning/replacement of air filters on furnace and/or air conditioning unit. **Good ventilation cuts down on indoor air pollution from carpets, machines, paints, solvents, cleaning materials, and pesticides.**

Information in brackets added by the authors to clarify and enhance the use of nursing diagnoses.

 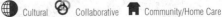

- Recommend periodic inspection of well water/tap water **to identify possible contaminants.**
- Encourage client to install carbon monoxide monitors and a radon detector in home, as appropriate.
- Recommend placing dehumidifier in damp areas **to retard growth of molds**.
- Review proper handling of household chemicals:

  Read chemical labels. Know primary hazards (especially in commonly used household cleaning/gardening products).

  Follow directions printed on product label (e.g., avoid use of certain chemicals on food preparation surfaces, refrain from spraying garden chemicals on windy days).

  Choose least hazardous products for the job, preferably multi-use products **to reduce number of different chemicals used/stored.** Use products labeled "non-toxic" wherever possible.

  Use form of chemical that most reduces risk of exposure (e.g., cream instead of liquid or aerosol).

  Wear protective clothing, gloves, and safety glasses when using chemicals. Avoid mixing chemicals at all times, and use in well-ventilated areas.

  Store chemicals in locked cabinets. Keep chemicals in original labeled containers and do not pour into other containers.

  Place safety stickers on chemicals **to warn children of harmful contents.**
- Review proper food handling/storage/cooking techniques.
- Stress importance of pregnant or lactating women following fish/wildlife consumption guidelines provided by state/U.S. territorial or Native American tribes. **Ingestion of noncommercial fish/wildlife can be a significant source of pollutants.**

NURSING PRIORITY NO. 3. To promote wellness (Teaching/Discharge Considerations):

HOME

- Discuss general safety concerns with client/SO.
- Stress importance of supervising infant/child or individuals with cognitive limitations.
- Stress importance of posting emergency and poison control numbers in a visible location.
- Encourage learning of CPR and first aid.
- Dissuss protective actions for specific "bad air" days (e.g., limiting /avoiding outdoor activities).
- Review pertinent job-related safety regulations. Stress necessity of wearing appropriate protective equipment.

Information in brackets added by the authors to clarify and enhance the use of nursing diagnoses.

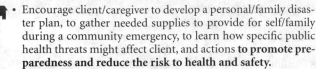

- Encourage client/caregiver to develop a personal/family disaster plan, to gather needed supplies to provide for self/family during a community emergency, to learn how specific public health threats might affect client, and actions **to promote preparedness and reduce the risk to health and safety.**
- Provide information/refer to appropriate resources about potential toxic hazards and protective measures. Provide bibliotherapy/written resources and appropriate websites **for client review and self-paced learning.**
- Refer to smoking cessation program as needed.

COMMUNITY

- Promote education programs **geared to increasing awareness of safety measures and resources available to individuals/community.**
- Review pertinent job-related health department/OSHA regulations **to safegaurd the workplace and the community.**
- Ascertain that there is a comprehensive plan in place in the community to ensure an effective response to any emergency (e.g., flood, toxic spill, infectious disease outbreak, radiation release), including a chain of command, protective equipment, communication, training, decontamination area(s), safety and security plans).
- Refer to appropriate agencies (e.g., The Centers for Disease Control and Prevention [CDC]; U.S. Army Medical Research Institute of Infectious Diseases [USAMRIID]; Federal Emergency Management Agency [FEMA]; Department of Health and Human Services [DHHS]; Office of Emergency Preparedness [OEP]; Environmental Protection Agency [EPA]) **to prepare for and manage mass casualty incidents.**

Documentation Focus

ASSESSMENT/REASSESSMENT

- Client's/caregiver's understanding of individual risks/safety concerns.

PLANNING

- Plan of care and who is involved in planning.
- Teaching plan.

IMPLEMENTATION/EVALUATION

- Individual responses to interventions/teaching and actions performed.

Information in brackets added by the authors to clarify and enhance the use of nursing diagnoses.

  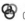 Cultural   Collaborative  Community/Home Care

- Specific actions and changes that are made.
- Attainment/progress toward desired outcome(s).
- Modifications to plan of care.

DISCHARGE PLANNING

- Long-range plans, lifestyle and community changes, and who is responsible for actions to be taken.
- Specific referrals made.

SAMPLE NURSING OUTCOMES & INTERVENTIONS CLASSIFICATIONS (NOC/NIC)

NOC—Community Disaster Readiness
NIC—Environmental Risk Protection

compromised family Coping

Taxonomy II: Coping/Stress Tolerance—Class 2 Coping Responses (00074)
[Diagnostic Division: Social Interaction]
Submitted 1980; Revised 1996

Definition: Usually supportive primary person (family member or close friend [SO]) provides insufficient, ineffective, or compromised support, comfort, assistance, or encouragement that may be needed by the client to manage or master adaptive tasks related to his/her health challenge

Related Factors

Coexisting situations affecting the significant person
Developmental/situational crises the significant person may be facing
Prolonged disease [or disability progression] that exhausts the supportive capacity of SO(s)
Exhaustion of supportive capacity of significant people
Inadequate/incorrect understanding of information by a primary person
Lack of reciprocal support; little support provided by client, in turn, for primary person; [unrealistic expectations of client/SO(s) or each other]
Temporary preoccupation by a significant person
Temporary family disorganization/role changes
[Lack of mutual decision-making skills]
[Diverse coalitions of family members]

Information in brackets added by the authors to clarify and enhance the use of nursing diagnoses.

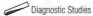 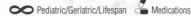

Defining Characteristics

SUBJECTIVE

Client expresses a complaint/concern about SO's response to health problem; SO expresses an inadequate knowledge base/understanding, which interferes with effective supportive behaviors

SO describes preoccupation with personal reaction (e.g., fear, anticipatory grief, guilt, anxiety) to client's need

OBJECTIVE

SO attempts assistive/supportive behaviors with less-than-satisfactory results

SO displays protective behavior disproportionate to the client's abilities/need for autonomy

SO enters into limited personal communication with client

SO withdraws from client

[SO displays sudden outbursts of emotions/emotional lability or interferes with necessary nursing/medical interventions]

Desired Outcomes/Evaluation Criteria—Family Will:

- Identify/verbalize resources within themselves to deal with the situation.
- Interact appropriately with the client, providing support and assistance as indicated.
- Provide opportunity for client to deal with situation in own way.
- Verbalize knowledge and understanding of illness/disability/disease.
- Express feelings honestly.
- Identify need for outside support and seek such.

Actions/Interventions

NURSING PRIORITY NO. 1. To assess causative/contributing factors:

- Identify underlying situation(s) that may contribute to the inability of family to provide needed assistance to the client. **Circumstances may have preceded the illness and now have a significant effect (e.g., client had a heart attack during sexual activity, mate is afraid any activity may cause repeat).**

 • Note cultural factors related to family relationships that may be involved in problems of caring for member who is ill.

- Note the length of illness, such as cancer, MS, and/or other long-term situations that may exist.

Information in brackets added by the authors to clarify and enhance the use of nursing diagnoses.

 Cultural Collaborative 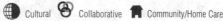 Community/Home Care

- Assess information available to and understood by the family/SO(s).
- Discuss family perceptions of situation. **Expectations of client and family members may/may not differ and/or be realistic.**
- Identify role of the client in family and how illness has changed the family organization.
- Note other factors besides the client's illness that are affecting abilities of family members **to provide needed support.**

NURSING PRIORITY NO. 2. To assist family to reactivate/develop skills to deal with current situation:

- Listen to client's/SO's comments, remarks, and expression of concern(s). Note nonverbal behaviors and/or responses and congruency.
- Encourage family members to verbalize feelings openly/clearly.
- Discuss underlying reasons for behaviors with family **to help them understand and accept/deal with client behaviors.**
- Assist the family and client to understand "who owns the problem" and who is responsible for resolution. Avoid placing blame or guilt.
- Encourage client and family to develop problem-solving skills **to deal with the situation.**

NURSING PRIORITY NO. 3. To promote wellness (Teaching/Discharge Considerations):

- Provide information for family/SO(s) about specific illness/condition.
- Involve client and family in planning care as often as possible. **Enhances commitment to plan.**
- Promote assistance of family in providing client care, as appropriate. **Identifies ways of demonstrating support while maintaining client's independence (e.g., providing favorite foods, engaging in diversional activities).**
- Refer to appropriate resources for assistance, as indicated (e.g., counseling, psychotherapy, financial, spiritual).
- Refer to NDs; Fear; Anxiety/death Anxiety; ineffective Coping; readiness for enhanced family Coping; disabled family Coping; anticipatory Grieving, as appropriate.

Documentation Focus

ASSESSMENT/REASSESSMENT

- Assessment findings, including current/past coping behaviors, emotional response to situation/stressors, support systems available.

Information in brackets added by the authors to clarify and enhance the use of nursing diagnoses.

PLANNING

- Plan of care, who is involved in planning and areas of responsibility.
- Teaching plan.

IMPLEMENTATION/EVALUATION

- Responses of family members/client to interventions/teaching and actions performed.
- Attainment/progress toward desired outcome(s).
- Modifications to plan of care.

DISCHARGE PLANNING

- Long-range plan and who is responsible for actions.
- Specific referrals made.

SAMPLE NURSING OUTCOMES & INTERVENTIONS CLASSIFICATIONS (NOC/NIC)

NOC—Family Coping
NIC—Family Involvement Promotion

defensive Coping

Taxonomy II: Coping/Stress Tolerance—Class 2 Coping
   Responses (00071)
[Diagnostic Division: Ego Integrity]
Submitted 1988

Definition: Repeated projection of falsely positive self-evaluation based on a self-protective pattern that defends against underlying perceived threats to positive self-regard

Related Factors

To be developed
[Refer to ND ineffective Coping]

Defining Characteristics

SUBJECTIVE

Denial of obvious problems/weaknesses
Projection of blame/responsibility
Hypersensitive to slight/criticism
Grandiosity

Information in brackets added by the authors to clarify and enhance the use of nursing diagnoses.

Rationalizes failures
[Refuses or rejects assistance]

OBJECTIVE

Superior attitude toward others
Difficulty establishing/maintaining relationships [avoidance of intimacy]
Hostile laughter; ridicule of others [aggressive behavior]
Difficulty in perception of reality/reality testing
Lack of follow-through in treatment/therapy
Lack of participation in treatment/therapy
[Attention-seeking behavior]

Desired Outcomes/Evaluation Criteria—Client Will:

- Verbalize understanding of own problems/stressors.
- Identify areas of concern/problems.
- Demonstrate acceptance of responsibility for own actions, successes, and failures.
- Participate in treatment program/therapy.
- Maintain involvement in relationships.

Actions/Interventions

- Refer to ND ineffective Coping for additional interventions.

NURSING PRIORITY NO. 1. To determine degree of impairment:

- Assess ability to comprehend current situation, developmental level of functioning.
- Determine level of anxiety and effectiveness of current coping mechanisms.
- Perform/review results of testing such as Taylor Manifest Anxiety Scale (B-MAS) and Marlowe–Crowne Social Desirability Scale (LMC), as indicated, to identify coping styles.
- Determine coping mechanisms used (e.g., projection, avoidance, rationalization) and purpose of coping strategy (e.g., may mask low self-esteem) **to note how these behaviors affect current situation.**
- Observe interactions with others **to note difficulties/ability to establish satisfactory relationships.**
- Note expressions of grandiosity in the face of contrary evidence (e.g., "I'm going to buy a new car" when the individual has no job or available finances).
- Assess physical condition. **Defensive coping style has been connected with a decline/alteration in physical well-being**

Information in brackets added by the authors to clarify and enhance the use of nursing diagnoses.

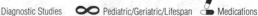

and illnesses, especially chronic health concerns (e.g., CHF, diabetes, chronic fatigue syndrome).

NURSING PRIORITY NO. 2. To assist client to deal with current situation:

- Develop therapeutic relationship to enable client **to test new behaviors in a safe environment.** Use positive, nonjudgmental approach and "I" language **to promote sense of self-esteem.**
- Assist client to identify/consider need to address problem differently.
- Use therapeutic communication skills such as active-listening to assist client to describe all aspects of the problem.
- Acknowledge individual strengths and incorporate awareness of personal assets/strengths in plan.
- Provide explanation of the rules of the treatment program and consequences of lack of cooperation.
- Set limits on manipulative behavior; be consistent in enforcing consequences when rules are broken and limits tested.
- Encourage control in all situations possible, include client in decisions and planning **to preserve autonomy.**
- Convey attitude of acceptance and respect (unconditional positive regard) **to avoid threatening client's self-concept, preserve existing self-esteem.**
- Encourage identification and expression of feelings.
- Provide healthy outlets for release of hostile feelings (e.g., punching bags, pounding boards). Involve client in outdoor recreation program/activities.
- Provide opportunities for client to interact with others in a positive manner, **promoting self-esteem.**
- Identify and discuss responses to situation, maladaptive coping skills. Suggest alternative responses to situation **to help client select more adaptive strategies for coping.**
- Use confrontation judiciously **to help client begin to identify defense mechanisms (e.g., denial/projection) that are hindering development of satisfying relationships.**
- Assist with treatments for physical illnesses, as appropriate.

NURSING PRIORITY NO. 3. To promote wellness (Teaching/Discharge Considerations):

- Use cognitive-behavioral therapy. **Helps change negative thinking patterns when rigidly held beliefs are used by client to defend against low self-esteem.**
- Encourage client to learn relaxation techniques, use of guided imagery, and positive affirmation of self **in order to incorporate and practice new behaviors.**

Information in brackets added by the authors to clarify and enhance the use of nursing diagnoses.

- Promote involvement in activities/classes where client can practice new skills and develop new relationships.
- Refer to additional resources (e.g., substance rehabilitation, family/marital therapy), as indicated.

Documentation Focus

ASSESSMENT/REASSESSMENT

- Assessment findings/presenting behaviors.
- Client perception of the present situation and usual coping methods/degree of impairment.
- Health concerns.

PLANNING

- Plan of care and interventions and who is involved in development of the plan.
- Teaching plan.

IMPLEMENTATION/EVALUATION

- Response to interventions/teaching and actions performed.
- Attainment/progress toward desired outcome(s).
- Modifications to plan of care.

DISCHARGE PLANNING

- Referrals and follow-up program.

SAMPLE NURSING OUTCOMES & INTERVENTIONS CLASSIFICATIONS (NOC/NIC)

NOC—Self-Esteem
NIC—Self-Awareness Enhancement

disabled family Coping

Taxonomy II: Coping/Stress Tolerance—Class 2 Coping Responses (00073)
[Diagnostic Division: Social Interaction]
Submitted 1980; Revised 1996

Definition: Behavior of significant person (family member or other primary person) that disables his/her capacities and the client's capacity to effectively address tasks essential to either person's adaptation to the health challenge

---

Information in brackets added by the authors to clarify and enhance the use of nursing diagnoses.

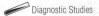 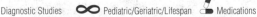

Related Factors

Significant person with chronically unexpressed feelings (e.g., guilt, anxiety, hostility, despair)

Dissonant coping styles for dealing with adaptive tasks by the significant person and client/among significant people

Highly ambivalent family relationships

Arbitrary handling of family's resistance to treatment [that tends to solidify defensiveness as it fails to deal adequately with underlying anxiety]

[High-risk family situations, such as single or adolescent parent, abusive relationship, substance abuse, acute/chronic disabilities, member with terminal illness]

Defining Characteristics

SUBJECTIVE

[Expresses despair regarding family reactions/lack of involvement]

OBJECTIVE

Psychosomaticism

Intolerance; rejection; abandonment; desertion; agitation; aggression; hostility; depression

Carrying on usual routines without regard for client's needs; disregarding client's needs

Neglectful care of the client in regard to basic human needs/ illness treatment

Neglectful relationships with other family members

Family behaviors that are detrimental to well-being

Distortion of reality regarding the client's health problem

Impaired restructuring of a meaningful life for self, impaired individualization, prolonged overconcern for client

Taking on illness signs of client

Client's development of dependence

Desired Outcomes/Evaluation Criteria—Family Will:

- Verbalize more realistic understanding and expectations of the client.
- Visit/contact client regularly.
- Participate positively in care of client, within limits of family's abilities and client's needs.
- Express feelings and expectations openly and honestly, as appropriate.

Information in brackets added by the authors to clarify and enhance the use of nursing diagnoses.

  Cultural Collaborative 🏠 Community/Home Care

Actions/Interventions

NURSING PRIORITY NO. 1. To assess causative/contributing factors:

- Ascertain pre-illness behaviors/interactions of the family. **Provides comparative baseline.**
- Identify current behaviors of the family members (e.g., withdrawal—not visiting, brief visits, and/or ignoring client when visiting; anger and hostility toward client and others; ways of touching between family members, expressions of guilt).
- Discuss family perceptions of situation. **Expectations of client and family members may/may not be realistic.**
- Note cultural factors related to family relationships that may be involved in problems of caring for member who is ill.
- Note other factors that may be stressful for the family (e.g., financial difficulties or lack of community support, as when illness occurs when out of town). **Provides opportunity for appropriate referrals.**
- Determine readiness of family members to be involved with care of the client.

NURSING PRIORITY NO. 2. To provide assistance to enable family to deal with the current situation:

- Establish rapport with family members who are available. **Promotes therapeutic relationship and support for problem-solving solutions.**
- Acknowledge difficulty of the situation for the family. **Reduces blaming/feelings of guilt.**
- Active-listen to concerns; note both overconcern/lack of concern, which may interfere with ability to resolve situation.
- Allow free expression of feelings, including frustration, anger, hostility, and hopelessness. Place limits on acting-out/inappropriate behaviors **to minimize risk of violent behavior.**
- Give accurate information to SO(s) from the beginning.
- Act as liaison between family and healthcare providers **to provide explanations and clarification of treatment plan.**
- Provide brief, simple explanations about use and alarms when equipment (such as a ventilator) is involved. Identify appropriate professional(s) **for continued support/problem solving.**
- Provide time for private interaction between client/family.
- Include SO(s) in the plan of care; provide instruction **to assist them to learn necessary skills to help client.**
- Accompany family when they visit **to be available for questions, concerns, and support.**
- Assist SO(s) to initiate therapeutic communication with client.

Information in brackets added by the authors to clarify and enhance the use of nursing diagnoses.

 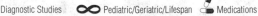

• Refer client to protective services as necessitated by risk of physical harm. **Removing client from home enhances individual safety and may reduce stress on family to allow opportunity for therapeutic intervention.**

NURSING PRIORITY NO. 3. To promote wellness (Teaching/Discharge Considerations):

 • Assist family to identify coping skills being used and how these skills are/are not helping them deal with current situation.

 • Answer family's questions patiently and honestly. Reinforce information provided by other healthcare providers.

 • Reframe negative expressions into positive, whenever possible. **(A positive frame contributes to supportive interactions and can lead to better outcomes.)**

 • Respect family needs for withdrawal and intervene judiciously. **Situation may be overwhelming and time away can be beneficial to continued participation.**

• Encourage family to deal with the situation in small increments rather than the whole picture at one time.

 • Assist the family to identify familiar items that would be helpful to the client (e.g., a family picture on the wall), especially when hospitalized for long period of time, **to reinforce/maintain orientation.**

 • Refer family to appropriate resources, as needed (e.g., family therapy, financial counseling, spiritual advisor).

• Refer to ND Grieving, as appropriate.

Documentation Focus

ASSESSMENT/REASSESSMENT

• Assessment findings, current/past behaviors, including family members who are directly involved and support systems available.
• Emotional response(s) to situation/stressors.
• Specific health/therapy challenges.

PLANNING

• Plan of care/interventions and who is involved in planning.
• Teaching plan.

IMPLEMENTATION/EVALUATION

• Responses of individuals to interventions/teaching and actions performed.
• Attainment/progress toward desired outcome(s).
• Modifications to plan of care.

Information in brackets added by the authors to clarify and enhance the use of nursing diagnoses.

DISCHARGE PLANNING

- Ongoing needs/resources/other follow-up recommendations and who is responsible for actions.
- Specific referrals made.

SAMPLE NURSING OUTCOMES & INTERVENTIONS CLASSIFICATIONS (NOC/NIC)

NOC—Family Normalization
NIC—Family Therapy

ineffective Coping

Taxonomy II: Coping/Stress Tolerance—Class 2 Coping Responses (00069)
[Diagnostic Division: Ego Integrity]
Submitted 1978; Nursing Diagnosis Extension and Classification (NDEC) Revision 1998

Definition: Inability to form a valid appraisal of the stressors, inadequate choices of practiced responses, and/or inability to use available resources

Related Factors

Situational/maturational crises
High degree of threat
Inadequate opportunity to prepare for stressor; disturbance in pattern of appraisal of threat
Inadequate level of confidence in ability to cope; inadequate level of perception of control; uncertainty
Inadequate resources available; inadequate social support created by characteristics of relationships
Disturbance in pattern of tension release
Inability to conserve adaptive energies
Gender differences in coping strategies
[Work overload, too many deadlines]
[Impairment of nervous system; cognitive/sensory/perceptual impairment, memory loss]
[Severe/chronic pain]

Defining Characteristics

SUBJECTIVE

Verbalization of inability to cope/ask for help
Sleep disturbance; fatigue

Information in brackets added by the authors to clarify and enhance the use of nursing diagnoses.

 Diagnostic Studies ∞ Pediatric/Geriatric/Lifespan 🔹 Medications **227**

Abuse of chemical agents
[Reports of muscular/emotional tension; lack of appetite]

OBJECTIVE

Lack of goal-directed behavior/resolution of problem, including inability to attend to and difficulty with organizing information [lack of assertive behavior]

Use of forms of coping that impede adaptive behavior [including inappropriate use of defense mechanisms, verbal manipulation]

Inadequate problem solving

Inability to meet role expectations/basic needs [including skipping meals, little or no exercise, no time for self/no vacations]

Decreased use of social support

Poor concentration

Change in usual communication patterns

High illness rate [including high blood pressure, ulcers, irritable bowel, frequent headaches/neckaches]

Risk taking

Destructive behavior toward self [including overeating, excessive smoking/drinking, overuse of prescribed/OTC medications, illicit drug use]

[Behavioral changes (e.g., impatience, frustration, irritability, discouragement)]

Desired Outcomes/Evaluation Criteria—Client Will:

- Assess the current situation accurately.
- Identify ineffective coping behaviors and consequences.
- Verbalize awareness of own coping abilities.
- Verbalize feelings congruent with behavior.
- Meet psychological needs as evidenced by appropriate expression of feelings, identification of options, and use of resources.

Actions/Interventions

NURSING PRIORITY NO. 1. To determine degree of impairment:

- Determine individual stressors (e.g., family, social, work environment, life changes, or nursing/healthcare management).
- Evaluate ability to understand events, provide realistic appraisal of situation.
- Identify developmental level of functioning. (**People tend to regress to a lower developmental stage during illness/crisis.**)

Information in brackets added by the authors to clarify and enhance the use of nursing diagnoses.

  Cultural Collaborative 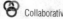 Community/Home Care

- Assess current functional capacity and note how it is affecting the individual's coping ability.
- Determine alcohol intake, drug use, smoking habits, sleeping and eating patterns. **These mechanisms are often used when individual is not coping effectively with stressors.**
- Ascertain impact of illness on sexual needs/relationship.
- Assess level of anxiety and coping on an ongoing basis.
- Note speech and communication patterns. Be aware of negative/catastrophizing thinking.
- Observe and describe behavior in objective terms. Validate observations.

NURSING PRIORITY NO. 2. To assess coping abilities and skills:

- Ascertain client's understanding of current situation and its impact on life and work.
- Active-listen and identify client's perceptions of what is happening.
- Evaluate client's decision-making ability.
- Determine previous methods of dealing with life problems **to identify successful techniques that can be used in current situation.**

NURSING PRIORITY NO. 3. To assist client to deal with current situation:

- Call client by name. Ascertain how client prefers to be addressed. **Using client's name enhances sense of self and promotes individuality/self-esteem.**
- Encourage communication with staff/SO(s).
- Use reality orientation (e.g., clocks, calendars, bulletin boards) and make frequent references to time, place, as indicated. Place needed/familiar objects within sight for visual cues.
- Provide for continuity of care with same personnel taking care of the client as often as possible.
- Explain disease process/procedures/events in a simple, concise manner. Devote time for listening. **May help client to express emotions, grasp situation, and feel more in control.**
- Provide for a quiet environment/position equipment out of view as much as possible **when anxiety is increased by noisy surroundings.**
- Schedule activities so periods of rest alternate with nursing care. Increase activity slowly.
- Assist client in use of diversion, recreation, relaxation techniques.
- Stress positive body responses to medical conditions, but do not negate the seriousness of the situation (e.g., stable blood

---

Information in brackets added by the authors to clarify and enhance the use of nursing diagnoses.

pressure during gastric bleed or improved body posture in depressed client).

 • Encourage client to try new coping behaviors and gradually master situation.

 • Confront client when behavior is inappropriate, pointing out difference between words and actions. **Provides external locus of control, enhancing safety.**

 • Assist in dealing with change in concept of body image, as appropriate. (Refer to ND disturbed Body Image.)

NURSING PRIORITY NO. 4. To provide for meeting psychological needs:

• Treat the client with courtesy and respect. Converse at client's level, providing meaningful conversation while performing care. (**Enhances therapeutic relationship.**)

 • Help client to learn how to substitute positive thoughts for negative ones (i.e., "I can do this; I am in charge of myself"). Take advantage of teachable moments.

• Allow client to react in own way without judgment by staff. Provide support and diversion, as indicated.

• Encourage verbalization of fears and anxieties and expression of feelings of denial, depression, and anger. Let the client know that these are normal reactions.

• Provide opportunity for expression of sexual concerns.

• Help client to set limits on acting-out behaviors and learn ways to express emotions in an acceptable manner. (**Promotes internal locus of control.**)

NURSING PRIORITY NO. 5. To promote wellness (Teaching/Discharge Considerations):

 • Give updated/additional information needed about events, cause (if known), and potential course of illness as soon as possible. **Knowledge helps reduce anxiety/fear, allows client to deal with reality.**

 • Provide and encourage an atmosphere of realistic hope.

 • Give information about purposes and side effects of medications/treatments.

 • Stress importance of follow-up care.

 • Encourage and support client in evaluating lifestyle, occupation, and leisure activities.

 • Discuss ways to deal with identified stressors (e.g., family, social, work environment, or nursing/healthcare management).

 • Provide for gradual implementation and continuation of necessary behavior/lifestyle changes. **Enhances commitment to plan.**

Information in brackets added by the authors to clarify and enhance the use of nursing diagnoses.

- ⌂ • Discuss/review anticipated procedures and client concerns, as well as postoperative expectations when surgery is recommended.
- ⊘ • Refer to outside resources and/or professional therapy, as indicated/ordered.
- ⌂ • Determine need/desire for religious representative/spiritual counselor and arrange for visit.
- ⌂ • Provide information, refer for consultation, as indicated, for
- ⊘   sexual concerns. Provide privacy when client is not in own home.
- • Refer to other NDs, as indicated (e.g., chronic Pain; Anxiety; impaired verbal Communication; risk for other-/self-directed Violence).

Documentation Focus

ASSESSMENT/REASSESSMENT

- Baseline findings, specific stressors, degree of impairment, and client's perceptions of situation.
- Coping abilities and previous ways of dealing with life problems.

PLANNING

- Plan of care/interventions and who is involved in planning.
- Teaching plan.

IMPLEMENTATION/EVALUATION

- Client's responses to interventions/teaching and actions performed.
- Medication dose, time, and client's response.
- Attainment/progress toward desired outcome(s).
- Modifications to plan of care.

DISCHARGE PLANNING

- Long-term needs and actions to be taken.
- Support systems available, specific referrals made, and who is responsible for actions to be taken.

SAMPLE NURSING OUTCOMES & INTERVENTIONS CLASSIFICATIONS (NOC/NIC)

NOC—Coping
NIC—Coping Enhancement

Information in brackets added by the authors to clarify and enhance the use of nursing diagnoses.

ineffective community Coping

Taxonomy II: Coping/Stress Tolerance—Class 2 Coping
  Responses (00077)
[Diagnostic Division: Social Interaction]
Submitted 1994; Nursing Diagnosis Extension and
  Classification (NDEC) Revision 1998

Definition: Pattern of community activities for
adaptation and problem solving that is unsatisfactory
for meeting the demands or needs of the community

Related Factors

Deficits in community social support services/resources
Inadequate resources for problem solving
Ineffective/nonexistent community systems (e.g., lack of
  emergency medical system, transportation system, or disas-
  ter planning systems)
Natural/man-made disasters

Defining Characteristics

SUBJECTIVE

Community does not meet its own expectations
Expressed vulnerability; community powerlessness
Stressors perceived as excessive

OBJECTIVE

Deficits of community participation
Excessive community conflicts
High illness rates
Increased social problems (e.g., homicides, vandalism, arson,
  terrorism, robbery, infanticide, abuse, divorce, unemploy-
  ment, poverty, militancy, mental illness)

Desired Outcomes/Evaluation
Criteria—Community Will:

- Recognize negative and positive factors affecting community's
  ability to meet its own demands or needs.
- Identify alternatives to inappropriate activities for adapta-
  tion/problem solving.
- Report a measurable increase in necessary/desired activities to
  improve community functioning.

Information in brackets added by the authors to clarify and enhance
the use of nursing diagnoses.

 Cultural Collaborative Community/Home Care

Actions/Interventions

NURSING PRIORITY NO. **1.** To identify causative or precipitating factors:

- Evaluate community activities **as related to meeting collective needs within the community itself and between the community and the larger society.**
- Note community reports of community functioning, (e.g., transportation, financial needs, emergency response) including areas of weakness or conflict.
- Identify effects of Related Factors on community activities.
- Determine availability and use of resources.
- Identify unmet demands or needs of the community.

NURSING PRIORITY NO. **2.** To assist the community to reactivate/develop skills to deal with needs:

- Determine community strengths.
- Identify and prioritize community goals.
- Encourage community members to join groups and engage in problem-solving activities.
- Develop a plan jointly with community **to deal with deficits in support to meet identified goals.**

NURSING PRIORITY NO. **3.** To promote wellness as related to community health:

- Create plans managing interactions within the community itself and between the community and the larger society **to meet collective needs.**
- Assist the community to form partnerships within the community and between the community and the larger society. **Promotes long-term development of the community to deal with current and future problems.**
- Promote community involvement in developing a comprehensive disaster plan to ensure an effective response to any emergency (e.g., flood, tornado, toxic spill, infectious disease outbreak). (Refer to ND Contamination for additional interventions.)
- Provide channels for dissemination of information to the community as a whole (e.g., print media; radio/television reports and community bulletin boards; speakers' bureau; reports to committees, councils, advisory boards), on file, and accessible to the public.
- Make information available in different modalities and geared to differing educational levels and cultural/ethnic populations of the community.

Information in brackets added by the authors to clarify and enhance the use of nursing diagnoses.

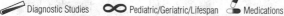

• Seek out and evaluate underserved populations, including the homeless.

Documentation Focus

ASSESSMENT/REASSESSMENT

• Assessment findings, including perception of community members regarding problems.
• Availability/use of resources.

PLANNING

• Plan of care and who is involved in planning.
• Teaching plan.

IMPLEMENTATION/EVALUATION

• Response of community entities to plan/interventions and actions performed.
• Attainment/progress toward desired outcome(s).
• Modifications to plan of care.

DISCHARGE PLANNING

• Long-range plans and who is responsible for actions to be taken.

SAMPLE NURSING OUTCOMES & INTERVENTIONS CLASSIFICATIONS (NOC/NIC)

NOC—Community Health Status
NIC—Community Health Development

readiness for enhanced Coping

Taxonomy II: Coping/Stress Tolerance—Class 2 Coping Responses (00158)
[Diagnostic Divisions: Ego Integrity]
Submitted 2002

Definition: A pattern of cognitive and behavioral efforts to manage demands that is sufficient for well-being and can be strengthened

Related Factors

To be developed

Information in brackets added by the authors to clarify and enhance the use of nursing diagnoses.

   Cultural Collaborative Community/Home Care

Defining Characteristics

SUBJECTIVE

Defines stressors as manageable
Seeks social support/knowledge of new strategies
Acknowledges power
Aware of possible environmental changes

OBJECTIVE

Uses a broad range of problem-/emotional-oriented strategies
Uses spiritual resources

Desired Outcomes/Evaluation Criteria—Client Will:

- Assess current situation accurately.
- Identify effective coping behaviors currently being used.
- Verbalize feelings congruent with behavior.
- Meet psychological needs as evidenced by appropriate expression of feelings, identification of options, and use of resources.

Actions/Interventions

NURSING PRIORITY NO. 1. To determine needs and desire for improvement:

- Evaluate ability to understand events, provide realistic appraisal of situation. **Provides information about client's perception, cognitive ability, and whether the client is aware of the facts of the situation. This is essential for planning care.**
- Determine stressors that are currently affecting client. **Accurate identification of situation that client is dealing with provides information for planning interventions to enhance coping abilities.**
- Ascertain motivation/expectations for change.
- Identify social supports available to client. **Available support systems, such as family and friends, can provide client with ability to handle current stressful events and often "talking it out" with an empathic listener will help client move forward to enhance coping skills.**
- Review coping strategies client is aware of and currently using. **The desire to improve one's coping ability is based on an awareness of the current status of the stressful situation.**
- Determine alcohol intake, other drug use, smoking habits, sleeping and eating patterns. **Use of these substances impairs**

Information in brackets added by the authors to clarify and enhance the use of nursing diagnoses.

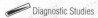

readiness for enhanced COPING

ability to deal with anxiety and affects ability to cope with life's stressors. **Identification of impaired sleeping and eating patterns provides clues to need for change.**

- Assess level of anxiety and coping on an ongoing basis. **Provides information for baseline to develop plan of care to improve coping abilities.**
- Note speech and communication patterns. **Assesses ability to understand and provides information necessary to help client make progress in desire to enhance coping abilities.**
- Evaluate client's decision-making ability. **Understanding client's ability provides a starting point for developing plan and determining what information client needs to develop more effective coping skills.**

NURSING PRIORITY NO. 2. To assist client to develop enhanced coping skills:

- Active-listen and clarify client's perceptions of current status. **Reflecting client's statements and thoughts can provide a forum for understanding perceptions in relation to reality for planning care and determining accuracy of interventions needed.**
- Review previous methods of dealing with life problems. **Enables client to identify successful techniques used in the past, promoting feelings of confidence in own ability.**
- Discuss desire to improve ability to manage stressors of life. **Understanding client's desire to seek new information to enhance life will help client determine what is needed to learn new skills of coping.**
- Discuss understanding of concept of knowing what can and cannot be changed. **Acceptance of reality that some things cannot be changed allows client to focus energies on dealing with things that can be changed.**
- Help client develop problem-solving skills. **Learning the process for problem solving will promote successful resolution of potentially stressful situations that arise.**

NURSING PRIORITY NO. 3. To promote optimum wellness:

- Discuss predisposing factors related to any individual's response to stress. **Understanding that genetic influences, past experiences, and existing conditions determine whether a person's response is adaptive or maladaptive will give client a base on which to continue to learn what is needed to improve life.**
- Encourage client to create a stress management program. **An individualized program of relaxation, meditation,**

Information in brackets added by the authors to clarify and enhance the use of nursing diagnoses.

 Cultural   Collaborative   Community/Home Care

involvement with caring for others/pets will enhance coping skills and strengthen client's ability to manage challenging situations.

- Recommend involvement in activities of interest, such as exercise/sports, music, and art. **Individuals must decide for themselves what coping strategies are adaptive for them. Most people find enjoyment and relaxation in these kinds of activities.**
- Discuss possibility of doing volunteer work in an area of the client's choosing. **Many people report satisfaction in helping others, and client may find pleasure in such involvement.**
- Refer to classes and/or reading material, as appropriate. **May be helpful to further learning and pursuing goal of enhanced coping ability.**

Documentation Focus

ASSESSMENT/REASSESSMENT

- Baseline information, client's perception of need to enhance abilities.
- Coping abilities and previous ways of dealing with life problems.
- Motivation and expectations for change.

PLANNING

- Plan of care/interventions and who is involved in planning.
- Teaching plan.

IMPLEMENTATION/EVALUATION

- Client's responses to interventions/teaching and actions performed.
- Attainment/progress toward desired outcome(s).
- Modifications to plan of care.

DISCHARGE PLANNING

- Long-term needs and actions to be taken.
- Support systems available, specific referrals made, and who is responsible for actions to be taken.

SAMPLE NURSING OUTCOMES & INTERVENTIONS CLASSIFICATIONS (NOC/NIC)

NOC—Coping
NIC—Coping Enhancement

Information in brackets added by the authors to clarify and enhance the use of nursing diagnoses.

readiness for enhanced community Coping

Taxonomy II: Coping/Stress Tolerance—Class 2 Coping Responses (00076)
[Diagnostic Division: Social Interaction]
Submitted 1994

Definition: Pattern of community activities for adaptation and problem solving that is satisfactory for meeting the demands or needs of the community but can be improved for management of current and future problems/stressors

Related Factors

Social supports available
Resources available for problem solving
Community has a sense of power to manage stressors

Defining Characteristics

One or more characteristics that indicate effective coping:

SUBJECTIVE

Agreement that community is responsible for stress management

OBJECTIVE

Active planning by community for predicted stressors
Active problem solving by community when faced with issues
Positive communication among community members
Positive communication between community/aggregates and larger community
Programs available for recreation/relaxation
Resources sufficient for managing stressors

Desired Outcomes/Evaluation Criteria—Community Will:

- Identify positive and negative factors affecting management of current and future problems/stressors.
- Have an established plan in place to deal with identified problems/stressors.
- Describe management of challenges in characteristics that indicate effective coping.
- Report a measurable increase in ability to deal with problems/stressors.

Information in brackets added by the authors to clarify and enhance the use of nursing diagnoses.

  Cultural Collaborative Community/Home Care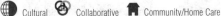

Actions/Interventions

NURSING PRIORITY NO. 1. To determine existence of and deficits or weaknesses in management of current and future problems/stressors:

 • Review community plan for dealing with problems/stressors.
 • Assess effects of Related Factors on management of problems/stressors.
 • Determine community's strengths and weaknesses.
 • Identify limitations in current pattern of community activities (such as transportation, water needs, roads) **that can be improved through adaptation and problem solving**.
 • Evaluate community activities as related to management of problems/stressors within the community itself and between the community and the larger society.

NURSING PRIORITY NO. 2. To assist the community in adaptation and problem solving for management of current and future needs/stressors:

 • Define and discuss current needs and anticipated or projected concerns. **Agreement on scope/parameters of needs is essential for effective planning.**
 • Prioritize goals **to facilitate accomplishment.**
• Identify available resources (e.g., persons, groups, financial, governmental, as well as other communities).
• Make a joint plan with the community to deal with adaptation and problem solving **for management of problems/stressors.**
 • Seek out and involve underserved/at-risk groups within the community. **Supports communication and commitment of community as a whole.**

NURSING PRIORITY NO. 3. To promote well-being of community:

• Assist the community to form partnerships within the community and between the community and the larger society **to promote long-term developmental growth of the community.**
 • Support development of plans for maintaining these interactions.
 • Establish mechanism for self-monitoring of community needs and evaluation of efforts. **Facilitates proactive rather than reactive responses by the community.**
 • Use multiple formats, such as TV, radio, print media, billboards and computer bulletin boards, speakers' bureau, reports to community leaders/groups on file and accessible to the public, **to keep community informed regarding plans, needs, outcomes.**

Information in brackets added by the authors to clarify and enhance the use of nursing diagnoses.

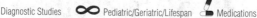

Documentation Focus

ASSESSMENT/REASSESSMENT

- Assessment findings and community's perception of situation.
- Identified areas of concern, community strengths/weaknesses.

PLANNING

- Plan of care and who is involved and responsible for each action.
- Teaching plan.

IMPLEMENTATION/EVALUATION

- Response of community entities to the actions performed.
- Attainment/progress toward desired outcomes.
- Modifications to plan of care.

DISCHARGE PLANNING

- Short-range and long-range plans to deal with current, anticipated, and potential needs and who is responsible for follow-through.
- Specific referrals made, coalitions formed.

SAMPLE NURSING OUTCOMES & INTERVENTIONS CLASSIFICATIONS (NOC/NIC)

NOC—Community Competence
NIC—Program Development

readiness for enhanced family Coping

Taxonomy II: Coping/Stress Tolerance—Class 2 Coping Responses (00075)
[Diagnostic Division: Social Interaction]
Submitted 1980

Definition: Effective managing of adaptive tasks by family member involved with the client's health challenge, who now exhibits desire and readiness for enhanced health and growth in regard to self and in relation to the client

Related Factors

Needs sufficiently gratified to enable goals of self-actualization to surface

---

Information in brackets added by the authors to clarify and enhance the use of nursing diagnoses.

240   Cultural   Collaborative 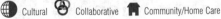 Community/Home Care

Adaptive tasks effectively addressed to enable goals of self-actualization to surface
[Developmental stage, situational crises/supports]

Defining Characteristics

SUBJECTIVE

Family member attempts to describe growth impact of crisis [on his or her own values, priorities, goals, or relationships]
Individual expresses interest in making contact with others who have experienced a similar situation

OBJECTIVE

Family member moves in direction of health-promotion/enriching lifestyle
Chooses experiences that optimize wellness

Desired Outcomes/Evaluation Criteria—Family Member Will:

- Express willingness to look at own role in the family's growth.
- Verbalize desire to undertake tasks leading to change.
- Report feelings of self-confidence and satisfaction with progress being made.

Actions/Interventions

NURSING PRIORITY NO. 1. To assess situation and adaptive skills being used by the family members:

- Determine individual situation and stage of growth family is experiencing/demonstrating. **Changes that are occurring may help family adapt and grow and thrive when faced with these transitional events.**
- Ascertain motivation/expectations for change.
- Note expressions, such as "Life has more meaning for me since this has occurred," **to identify changes in values.**
- Observe communication patterns of family. Listen to family's expressions of hope, planning, effect on relationships/life.
- Identify cultural/religious health beliefs and expectations. **For example: Navajo parents may define family as nuclear, extended, or a clan and it is important to identify who are the primary child-rearing persons.**

Information in brackets added by the authors to clarify and enhance the use of nursing diagnoses.

Diagnostic Studies   ∞ Pediatric/Geriatric/Lifespan   Medications   **241**

NURSING PRIORITY NO. 2. To assist family member to develop/ strengthen potential for growth:

 • Provide time to talk with family **to discuss their view of the situation.**

 • Establish a relationship with family/client **to foster trust/growth.**

 • Provide a role model with which the family member may identify.

 • Discuss importance of open communication and of not having secrets.

 • Demonstrate techniques, such as active-listening, I-messages, and problem-solving, **to facilitate effective communication.**

• Establish social goals of achieving and maintaining harmony with oneself, family, and community.

NURSING PRIORITY NO. 3. To promote wellness (Teaching/Discharge Considerations):

 • Assist family member to support the client in meeting own needs within ability and/or constraints of the illness/situation.

 • Provide experiences for the family **to help them learn ways of assisting/supporting client.**

• Identify other individuals/groups with similar conditions (e.g., Reach for Recovery, CanSurmount, Al-Anon, MS Society) and assist client/family member to make contact. **Provides ongoing support for sharing common experiences, problem solving, and learning new behaviors.**

 • Assist family member to learn new, effective ways of dealing with feelings/reactions.

 • Encourage family member to pursue personal interests/ hobbies/leisure activities **to promote individual well-being and strengthen coping abilities.**

Documentation Focus

ASSESSMENT/REASSESSMENT

• Adaptive skills being used, stage of growth.
• Family communication patterns.
• Motivation and expectations for change.

PLANNING

• Plan of care/interventions and who is involved in planning.
• Teaching plan.

IMPLEMENTATION/EVALUATION

• Client's/family's responses to interventions/teaching and actions performed.

Information in brackets added by the authors to clarify and enhance the use of nursing diagnoses.

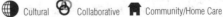 Cultural Collaborative Community/Home Care

- Attainment/progress toward desired outcome(s).
- Modifications to plan of care.

DISCHARGE PLANNING

- Identified needs/referrals for follow-up care, support systems.
- Specific referrals made.

SAMPLE NURSING OUTCOMES & INTERVENTIONS CLASSIFICATIONS (NOC/NIC)

NOC—Family Participation in Professional Care
NIC—Normalization Promotion

---

risk for sudden infant Death Syndrome

Taxonomy II: Safety/Protection—Class 2 Physical Injury (00156)
[Diagnostic Division: Safety]
Submitted 2002

Definition: Presence of risk factors for sudden death of an infant under 1 year of age

---

[Sudden Infant Death Syndrome (SIDS) is the sudden death of an infant under 1 year of age, which remains unexplained after a thorough case investigation, including performance of a complete autopsy, examination of the death scene, and review of the clinical history. SIDS is a subset of Sudden Unexpected Death in Infancy (SUDI) that is the sudden and unexpected death of an infant due to natural or unnatural causes.]

Risk Factors

MODIFIABLE

Delayed/lack of prenatal care
Infants placed to sleep in the prone/side-lying position
Soft underlayment (loose articles in the sleep environment)
Infant overheating/overwrapping
Prenatal/postnatal infant smoke exposure

POTENTIALLY MODIFIABLE

Young maternal age
Low birth weight; prematurity

NONMODIFIABLE

Male gender

Information in brackets added by the authors to clarify and enhance the use of nursing diagnoses.

 Diagnostic Studies   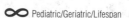 Pediatric/Geriatric/Lifespan   Medications   **243**

Ethnicity (e.g., African American or Native American)
Seasonality of SIDS deaths (higher in winter and fall months)
Infant age of 2 to 4 months

> NOTE: A risk diagnosis is not evidenced by signs and symptoms as the problem has not occurred; rather, nursing interventions are directed at prevention.

Desired Outcomes/Evaluation Criteria—Client Will:

- Verbalize understanding of modifiable factors.
- Make changes in environment to reduce risk of death occurring from other factors.
- Follow medically recommended prenatal and postnatal care.

Actions/Interventions

NURSING PRIORITY NO. 1. To assess causative/contributing factors:

 • Identify individual risk factors pertaining to situation. **Determines modifiable or potentially modifiable factors that can be addressed and treated. SIDS is the most common cause of unexplained death between 2 weeks and 1 year of age, with peak incidence occurring between the 2nd and 4th month.**

- Determine ethnicity, cultural background of family. **Although distribution is worldwide, African American infants are twice as likely to die of SIDS and Native American infants are nearly three times more likely to die than other infants.**

- Note whether mother smoked during pregnancy or is currently smoking. **Smoking is known to negatively affect the fetus prenatally as well as after birth. Some reports indicate an increased risk of SIDS in babies of smoking mothers.**

- Assess extent of prenatal care and extent to which mother followed recommended care measures. **Prenatal care is important for all pregnancies to afford the optimal opportunity for all infants to have a healthy start to life.**

- Note use of alcohol or other drugs/medications during and after pregnancy **that may have a negative impact on the developing fetus. Enables management to minimize any damaging effects.**

NURSING PRIORITY NO. 2. To promote use of activities to minimize risk of SIDS:

- Recommend that **infant** be placed on his or her back to sleep, both at nighttime and naptime. **Research comfirms that**

Information in brackets added by the authors to clarify and enhance the use of nursing diagnoses.

fewer infants die of SIDS when they sleep on their backs and that a side-lying position is not to be used.

- Advise all caregivers of the infant regarding the importance of maintaining correct sleep position. **Anyone who will have responsibility for the care of the child during sleep needs to be reminded of the importance of the back sleep position.**

- Encourage parents to schedule "tummy time" only while infant is awake. **This activity promotes strengthening of back and neck muscles while parents are close and baby is not sleeping.**

- Encourage early and medically recommended prenatal care and continue with well-baby checkups and immunizations after birth. Include information about signs of premature labor and actions to be taken to avoid problems if possible. **Prematurity presents many problems for the newborn and keeping babies healthy prevents problems that could put the infant at risk for SIDS. Immunizing infants prevents many illnesses that can also be life threatening.**

- Encourage breastfeeding, if possible. Recommend sitting up in chair when nursing at night. **Breastfeeding has many advantages, immunological, nutritional, and psychosocial, promoting a healthy infant. Although this does not preclude the occurrence of SIDS, healthy babies are less prone to many illnesses/problems. The risk of the mother falling asleep while feeding infant in bed with resultant accidental suffocation has been shown to be of concern.**

- Discuss issues of bedsharing and the concerns regarding sudden and unexpected infant deaths from accidental entrapment under a sleeping adult or suffocation by becoming wedged in a couch or cushioned chair. **Bedsharing or putting infant to sleep in an unsafe situation results in dangerous sleep environments that place infants at substantial risk for SUDI or SIDS.**

- Note cultural beliefs about bedsharing. **Bedsharing is more common among breastfed infants and mothers who are young, unmarried, low income, or from a minority group. (Additional study is needed to better understand bedsharing practices and its associated risks and benefits.)**

NURSING PRIORITY NO. 3. To promote wellness (Teaching/Discharge Considerations):

- Discuss known facts about SIDS with parents. **Corrects misconceptions and helps reduce level of anxiety.**

- Avoid overdressing or overheating infants during sleep. **Infants dressed in two or more layers of clothes as they slept had six times the risk of SIDS as those dressed in fewer layers.**

Information in brackets added by the authors to clarify and enhance the use of nursing diagnoses.

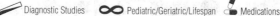

• Place the baby on a firm mattress in an approved crib. **Avoiding soft mattresses, sofas, cushions, waterbeds, other soft surfaces, while not known to prevent SIDS, will minimize chance of suffocation/SUDI.**

 • Remove fluffy and loose bedding from sleep area, making sure baby's head and face are not covered during sleep. **Minimizes possibility of suffocation.**

 • Discuss the use of apnea monitors. **Apnea monitors are not recommended to prevent SIDS, but may be used to monitor other medical problems.**

• Recommend public health nurse/or similar resource visit new mothers at least once or twice following discharge. **Researchers found that Native American infants whose mothers received such visits were 80% less likely to die from SIDS than those who were never visited.**

• Ascertain that day care center/provider(s) are trained in observation and modifying risk factors (e.g., sleeping position) **to reduce risk of death while infant is in their care.**

• Refer parents to local SIDS programs/other resources for learning (e.g., National SIDS/Infant Death Resource Center and similar websites) and encourage consultation with healthcare provider if baby shows any signs of illness or behaviors that concern them. **Can provide information and support for risk reduction and correction of treatable problems.**

Documentation Focus

ASSESSMENT/REASSESSMENT

• Baseline findings, degree of parental anxiety/concern.
• Individual risk factors.

PLANNING

• Plan of care/interventions and who is involved in planning.
• Teaching plan.

IMPLEMENTATION/EVALUATION

• Parent's responses to interventions/teaching and actions performed.
• Attainment/progress toward desired outcome(s).
• Modifications to plan of care.

DISCHARGE PLANNING

• Long-term needs and actions to be taken.
• Support systems available, specific referrals made, and who is responsible for actions to be taken.

Information in brackets added by the authors to clarify and enhance the use of nursing diagnoses.

  Cultural Collaborative Community/Home Care

NOC—Risk Detection
NIC—Risk Identification

readiness for enhanced Decision Making

Taxonomy II: Perception/Cognition—Class 4 Cognition
and Life Principles—Class 3 Value/Belief/Action
Congruence (00184)
[Diagnostic Division: Ego Integrity]
Submitted 2006

Definition: A pattern of choosing courses of action that
is sufficient for meeting short- and long-term health-
related goals and can be strengthened

Related Factors

To be developed

Defining Characteristics

SUBJECTIVE

Expresses desire to enhance decision making, congruency of
decisions with personal/sociocultural values and goals, use of
reliable evidence for decisions, risk-benefit analysis of decisions, understanding of choices for decision making, understanding of the meaning of choices

Desired Outcomes/Evaluation
Criteria—Client Will:

- Explain possible choices for decision making.
- Identify risks and benefit of decisions.
- Express beliefs about the meaning of choices.
- Make decisions that are congruent with personal and socio-
  cultural values/goals.
- Use reliable evidence in making decisions.

Actions/Interventions

NURSING PRIORITY NO. 1. To assess causative/contributing factors:

- Determine usual ability to manage own affairs. **Provides baseline for understanding client's decision-making process and
  measures growth.**

Information in brackets added by the authors to clarify and enhance
the use of nursing diagnoses.

- Note expressions of decision, dependability, and availability of support persons.
- Active-listen/identify reason(s) client would like to improve decision-making abilities and expectations of change. **As client articulates/clarifies reasons for improvement, direction is provided for change.**
- Note presence of physical signs of excitement. **Enhances energy for quest for improvement and personal growth.**
- Discuss meaning of life/reasons for living, belief in God or higher power, and how these relate to current desire for improvement.

NURSING PRIORITY NO. 2. To assist client to improve/effectively use problem-solving skills:

- Promote safe and hopeful environment. **Provides opportunity for client to discuss concerns/thoughts freely.**
- 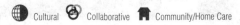 Provide opportunities for client to recognize own inner control in decision-making process. **Individuals with an internal locus of control believe they have some degree of control in outcomes and that their own actions/choices help determine what happens in their lives.**
- Encourage verbalization of ideas, concerns, particular decisions that need to be made.
- Clarify and prioritize individual's goals, noting possible conflicts or challenges that may be encountered.
- Identify positive aspects of this experience, encouraging client to view it as a learning opportunity.
- Assist client in learning how to find factual information (e.g., use of the library, reliable Internet websites).
- Review the process of problem solving and how to do risk-benefit analysis of decisions.
- Encourage children to make age-appropriate decisions. **Learning problem solving at an early age will enhance sense of self-worth and ability to exercise coping skills.**
- Discuss/clarify spiritual beliefs, accepting client's values in a nonjudgmental manner.

NURSING PRIORITY NO. 3. To promote optimum wellness:

- Identify opportunities for using conflict resolution skills, emphasizing each step as they are used.
- Provide positive feedback for efforts. **Enhances use of skills and learning efforts.**
- Encourage involvement of family/SO(s), as desired/appropriate, in decision-making process **to help all family members improve conflict-resolution skills**.
- Suggest participation in stress management or assertiveness classes, as appropriate.

Information in brackets added by the authors to clarify and enhance the use of nursing diagnoses.

Cultural Collaborative Community/Home Care

• Refer to other resources, as necessary (e.g., clergy, psychiatric clinical nurse specialist/psychiatrist, family/marital therapist).

Documentation Focus

ASSESSMENT/REASSESSMENT

• Assessment findings/behavioral responses.
• Motivation/expectations for change.
• Individuals involved in improving conflict skills.
• Personal values/beliefs.

PLANNING

• Plan of care/intervention and who is involved in the planning.
• Teaching plan.

IMPLEMENTATION/EVALUATION

• Clients and involved individual's responses to interventions/ teaching and actions performed.
• Ability to express feelings, identify options, use resources.
• Attainment/progress toward desired outcome(s).
• Modifications to plan of care.

DISCHARGE PLANNING

• Long-term needs, noting who is responsible for actions to be taken.
• Specific referrals made.

SAMPLE NURSING OUTCOMES & INTERVENTIONS CLASSIFICATIONS (NOC/NIC)

NOC—Decision Making
NIC— Decision-Making Support

ineffective Denial

Taxonomy II: Coping/Stress Tolerance—Class 2 Coping Responses (00072)
[Diagnostic Division: Ego Integrity]
Submitted 1988; Revised 2006

Definition: Conscious or unconscious attempt to disavow the knowledge or meaning of an event to reduce anxiety/fear, but leading to the detriment of health

---

Information in brackets added by the authors to clarify and enhance the use of nursing diagnoses.

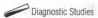 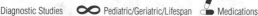

Related Factors

Anxiety; threat of inadequacy in dealing with strong emotions

Lack of control of life situation; fear of loss of autonomy

Overwhelming stress; lack of competency in using effective coping mechanisms

Threat of unpleasant reality

Fear of separation/death, loss of autonomy

Lack of emotional support from others

Defining Characteristics

SUBJECTIVE

Minimizes symptoms; displaces source of symptoms to other organs

Unable to admit impact of disease on life pattern

Displaces fear of impact of the condition

Does not admit fear of death/invalidism

OBJECTIVE

Delays seeking/refuses healthcare attention to the detriment of health

Does not perceive personal relevance of symptoms

Unable to admit impact of disease on life pattern; does not perceive personal relevance of danger

Makes dismissive gestures/comments when speaking of distressing events

Displays inappropriate affect

Uses self-treatment

Desired Outcomes/Evaluation Criteria—Client Will:

• Acknowledge reality of situation/illness.
• Express realistic concern/feelings about symptoms/illness.
• Seek appropriate assistance for presenting problem.
• Display appropriate affect.

Actions/Interventions

NURSING PRIORITY NO. 1. To assess causative/contributing factors:

• Identify situational crisis/problem and client's perception of the situation.
• Determine stage and degree of denial.
• Compare client's description of symptoms/conditions to reality of clinical picture.

Information in brackets added by the authors to clarify and enhance the use of nursing diagnoses.

  Cultural Collaborative Community/Home Care

- Note client's comments about impact of illness/problem on lifestyle.

NURSING PRIORITY NO. 2. To assist client to deal appropriately with situation:

- Use therapeutic communication skills of active-listening and I-messages **to develop trusting nurse-client relationship.**
- Provide safe, nonthreatening environment. **Encourages client to talk freely without fear of judgment.**
- Encourage expressions of feelings, accepting client's view of the situation without confrontation. Set limits on maladaptive behavior **to promote safety.**
- Present accurate information, as appropriate, without insisting that the client accept what has been presented. **Avoids confrontation, which may further entrench client in denial.**
- Discuss client's behaviors in relation to illness (e.g., diabetes, hypertension, alcoholism) and point out the results of these behaviors.
- Encourage client to talk with SO(s)/friends. **May clarify concerns and reduce isolation and withdrawal.**
- Involve client in group sessions **so client can hear other views of reality and test own perceptions.**
- Avoid agreeing with inaccurate statements/perceptions **to prevent perpetuating false reality.**
- Provide positive feedback for constructive moves toward independence **to promote repetition of behavior.**

NURSING PRIORITY NO. 3. To promote wellness (Teaching/Discharge Considerations):

- Provide written information about illness/situation **for client and family to refer to as they consider options.**
- Involve family members/SO(s) in long-range planning for meeting individual needs.
- Refer to appropriate community resources (e.g., Diabetes Association, Multiple Sclerosis Society, Alcoholics Anonymous) **to help client with long-term adjustment.**
- Refer to ND ineffective Coping.

Documentation Focus

ASSESSMENT/REASSESSMENT

- Assessment findings, degree of personal vulnerability/denial.
- Impact of illness/problem on lifestyle.

Information in brackets added by the authors to clarify and enhance the use of nursing diagnoses.

 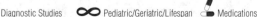

PLANNING

- Plan of care and who is involved in the planning.
- Teaching plan.

IMPLEMENTATION/EVALUATION

- Client's response to interventions/teaching and actions performed.
- Use of resources.
- Attainment/progress toward desired outcome(s).
- Modifications to plan of care.

DISCHARGE PLANNING

- Long-term needs and who is responsible for actions taken.
- Specific referrals made.

SAMPLE NURSING OUTCOMES & INTERVENTIONS CLASSIFICATIONS (NOC/NIC)

NOC—Acceptance: Health Status
NIC—Anxiety Reduction

impaired Dentition

Taxonomy II: Safety/Protection—Class 2 Physical Injury (00048)
[Diagnostic Division: Food/Fluid]
Nursing Diagnosis Extension and Classification (NDEC) Submission 1998

Definition: Disruption in tooth development/eruption patterns or structural integrity of individual teeth

Related Factors

Dietary habits; nutritional deficits
Selected prescription medications; chronic use of tobacco/coffee/tea/red wine
Ineffective oral hygiene, sensitivity to heat/cold; chronic vomiting
Deficient knowledge regarding dental health; excessive intake of fluorides/use of abrasive cleaning agents
Barriers to self-care; lack of access/economic barriers to professional care
Genetic predisposition; bruxism
[Traumatic injury/surgical intervention]

Information in brackets added by the authors to clarify and enhance the use of nursing diagnoses.

  Cultural Collaborative Community/Home Care

Defining Characteristics

SUBJECTIVE

Toothache

OBJECTIVE

Halitosis

Tooth enamel discoloration; erosion of enamel; excessive plaque

Worn down/abraded teeth; crown/root caries; tooth fracture(s); loose teeth; missing teeth; absence of teeth

Premature loss of primary teeth; incomplete eruption for age (may be primary or permanent teeth)

Excessive calculus

Malocclusion; tooth misalignment; asymmetrical facial expression

Desired Outcomes/Evaluation Criteria—Client Will:

- Display healthy gums, mucous membranes, and teeth in good repair.
- Report adequate nutritional/fluid intake.
- Verbalize and demonstrate effective dental hygiene skills.
- Follow-through on referrals for appropriate dental care.

Action/Interventions

NURSING PRIORITY NO. 1. To assess causative/contributing factors:

- Inspect oral cavity. Note presence/absence of teeth and/or dentures and ascertain its significance in terms of nutritional needs and aesthetics.
- Evaluate current status of dental hygiene and oral health **to determine need for instruction/coaching, assistive devices, and/or referral to dental care providers.**
- Document presence of factors affecting dentition (e.g., chronic use of tobacco, coffee, tea; bulimia/chronic vomiting; abscesses, tumors, braces, bruxism/chronic grinding of teeth) **to determine possible interventions and/or treatment needs.**
- Note current factors impacting dental health (e.g., presence of ET intubation, facial fractures, chemotherapy) **that require special mouth care.**
- Document (photo) facial injuries before treatment **to provide "pictorial baseline" for future comparison/evaluation.**

Information in brackets added by the authors to clarify and enhance the use of nursing diagnoses.

NURSING PRIORITY NO. 2. To treat/manage dental care needs:

- Ascertain client's usual method of oral care **to provide continuity of care or to build on client's existing knowledge base and current practices in developing plan of care.**
- Assist with/provide oral care, as indicated:

  Tap water or saline rinses, diluted alcohol-free mouthwashes.

  Gentle gum massage and tongue brushing with soft toothbrush, using fluoride toothpaste to manage tartar buildup, if appropriate.

  Brushing and flossing **when client is unable to do self-care.**

  Use of electric or battery-powered mouth care devices (e.g., toothbrush, plaque remover, water pic), as indicated.

  Denture care, when indicated (e.g., remove and clean after meals and at bedtime).
- Provide appropriate diet for optimal nutrition, limiting between-meal, sugary foods and bedtime snacks, as **food left on teeth at night is more likely to cause cavities.**
- Increase fluids, as needed, **to enhance hydration and general well-being of oral mucous membranes.**
- Reposition ET tubes and airway adjuncts routinely, carefully padding/protecting teeth/prosthetics. Suction with care, when indicated.
- Avoid thermal stimuli when teeth are sensitive. Recommend use of specific toothpastes **designed to reduce sensitivity of teeth.**
- Maintain good jaw/facial alignment when fractures are present.
- Administer antibiotics, as needed, **to treat oral/gum infections.**
- Recommend use of analgesics and topical analgesics, as needed, **when dental pain is present.**
- Administer antibiotic therapy prior to dental procedures in susceptible individuals (e.g., prosthetic heart valve clients) and/or ascertain that bleeding disorders or coagulation deficits are not present **to prevent excess bleeding.**
- Refer to appropriate care providers (e.g., dental hygienists, dentists, periodontists, oral surgeons).

NURSING PRIORITY NO. 3. To promote wellness (Teaching/Discharge Considerations):

- Instruct client/caregiver in home-care interventions **to treat condition and/or prevent further complications.**
- Review resources that are needed for the client to perform adequate dental hygiene care (e.g., toothbrush/paste, clean water, dental floss, personal care assistant).

Information in brackets added by the authors to clarify and enhance the use of nursing diagnoses.

  Cultural Collaborative 🏠 Community/Home Care

- Recommend that client (of any age) limit sugary/high carbo-hydrate foods in diet and snacks **to reduce buildup of plaque and risk of cavities caused by acids associated with break-down of sugar and starch.**
- Instruct older client and caregiver(s) concerning special needs and importance of regular dental care.
- Advise mother regarding age-appropriate concerns (e.g., refrain from letting baby fall asleep with milk or juice in bot-tle; use water and pacifier during night; avoid sharing eating utensils among family members; teach children to brush teeth while young; provide child with safety devices such as hel-met/face mask/mouth guard to prevent facial injuries).
- Discuss with pregnant women special needs and regular den-tal care **to maintain maternal dental health and promote strong teeth and bones in fetal development.**
- Encourage cessation of tobacco, especially smokeless, and enrollment in smoking-cessation classes **to reduce incidence of gum disorders, oral cancer, and other health problems.**
- Discuss advisability of dental checkup/care prior to initiating chemotherapy or radiation treatments **to minimize oral/dental tissue damage.**
- Refer to resources to maintain dental hygiene (e.g., dental care providers, financial assistance programs).

Documentation Focus

ASSESSMENT/REASSESSMENT

- Individual findings, including individual factors influencing dentition problems.
- Baseline photos/description of oral cavity/structures.

PLANNING

- Plan of care and who is involved in planning.
- Teaching plan.

IMPLEMENTATION/EVALUATION

- Responses to interventions/teaching and actions performed.
- Attainment/progress toward desired outcome(s).
- Modifications to plan of care.

DISCHARGE PLANNING

- Individual long-term needs, noting who is responsible for actions to be taken.
- Specific referrals made.

Information in brackets added by the authors to clarify and enhance the use of nursing diagnoses.

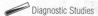

SAMPLE NURSING OUTCOMES & INTERVENTIONS CLASSIFICATIONS (NOC/NIC)

NOC—Oral Health
NIC—Oral Health Maintenance

risk for delayed Development

Taxonomy II: Growth/Development—Class 2
  Development (00112)
[Diagnostic Division: Teaching/Learning]
Nursing Diagnosis Extension and Classification (NDEC)
  Submission 1998

Definition: At risk for delay of 25% or more in one or more of the areas of social or self-regulatory behavior, or cognitive, language, gross or fine motor skills

Risk Factors

PRENATAL

Maternal age <15 or >35 years
Unplanned/unwanted pregnancy; lack of/late/poor prenatal
  care
Inadequate nutrition; poverty
Illiteracy
Genetic/endocrine disorders; infections; substance abuse

INDIVIDUAL

Prematurity; congenital/genetic disorders
Vision/hearing impairment; frequent otitis media
Inadequate nutrition; failure to thrive
Chronic illness; chemotherapy; radiation therapy
Brain damage (e.g., hemorrhage in postnatal period, shaken
  baby, abuse, accident); seizures
Positive drug screening(s); substance abuse; lead poisoning
Foster/adopted child
Behavior disorders
Technology dependent
Natural disaster

ENVIRONMENTAL

Poverty
Violence

Information in brackets added by the authors to clarify and enhance the use of nursing diagnoses.

 Cultural Collaborative Community/Home Care

CAREGIVER

Mental retardation; severe learning disability
Abuse
Mental illness

> NOTE: A risk diagnosis is not evidenced by signs and symptoms, as the problem has not occurred and nursing interventions are directed at prevention.

Desired Outcomes/Evaluation Criteria—Client Will:

- Perform motor, social, self-regulatory behavior, cognitive and language skills appropriate for age within scope of present capabilities.

Caregiver Will:

- Verbalize understanding of age-appropriate development/ expectations.
- Identify individual risk factors for developmental delay/ deviation.
- Formulate plan(s) for prevention of developmental deviation.
- Intiate interventions/lifestyle changes promoting appropriate development.

Actions/Interventions

NURSING PRIORITY NO. 1. To assess causative/contributing factors:

- Identify condition(s) that could contribute to developmental deviations; for example, genetic condition (e.g., Down syndrome, cerebral palsy) or complications of high-risk pregancy (e.g., prematurity, extremes of maternal age, maternal substance abuse, brain injury/damage), chronic severe illness, infections, mental illness, poverty, shaken baby syndrome/abuse, violence, failure to thrive, inadequate nutrition, and/or others as listed in Risk Factors.
 - Collaborate in multidisciplinary evaluation to assess client's development in following areas: gross motor, fine motor, cognitive, social/emotional, adaptive and communicative development **to determine area(s) of need/possible intervention.**
- Identify cultural beliefs, norms, and values **as they may impact parent/caregiver view of situation.**

Information in brackets added by the authors to clarify and enhance the use of nursing diagnoses.

 Diagnostic Studies Pediatric/Geriatric/Lifespan Medications

- Ascertain nature of caregiver-required activities and abilities to perform needed activities.
- Note severity/pervasiveness of situation (e.g., potential for long-term stress leading to abuse/neglect versus situational disruption during period of crisis or transition).
- Evaluate environment in which long-standing care will be provided **to determine ongoing services/other needs of child and care provider(s).**

NURSING PRIORITY NO. 2. To assist in preventing and/or limiting developmental delays:

- Avoid blame when discussing contributing factors. **Blame engenders negative feelings and does nothing to contribute to solution of the situation.**
- Note chronological age and review expectations for "normal" development at this age **to help determine developmental expectations.**
- Review expected skills/activities using authoritative text (e.g., Gesell, Musen/Congor) or assessment tools (e.g., Draw-a-Person, Denver Developmental Screening Test, Bender's Visual Motor Gestalt Test). **Provides guide for comparative measurement as child/individual progresses.**
- Consult professional resources (e.g., physical/occupational/rehabilitation/speech therapists; home health care agencies; social services; nutritionist; special-education teacher; family therapists; technological and adaptive equipment sources; vocational counselor) **to formulate plan and address specific individual needs/eligibility for intervention home- and/or community-based services.**
- Encourage setting of short-term realistic goals for achieving developmental potential. **Small incremental steps are often easier to deal with.**
- Identify equipment needs (e.g., adaptive/growth-stimulating computer programs, communication devices).

NURSING PRIORITY NO. 3. To promote wellness (Teaching/Discharge Considerations):

- Provide information regarding normal development, as appropriate, including pertinent reference materials.
- Encourage attendance at appropriate educational programs (e.g., parenting classes, infant stimulation sessions, seminars on life stresses, aging process).
- Identify available community resources, as appropriate (e.g., early-intervention programs, seniors' activity/support groups, gifted and talented programs, sheltered workshop, crippled

---

Information in brackets added by the authors to clarify and enhance the use of nursing diagnoses.

Cultural   Collaborative   Community/Home Care

children's services, medical equipment/supplier). **Provides additional assistance to support family efforts in treatment program.**

Documentation Focus

ASSESSMENT/REASSESSMENT

• Assessment findings/individual needs including developmental level and potential for improvement.
• Caregiver's understanding of situation and individual role.

PLANNING

• Plan of care and who is involved in the planning.
• Teaching plan.

IMPLEMENTATION/EVALUATION

• Client's response to interventions/teaching and actions performed.
• Caregiver response to teaching.
• Attainment/progress toward desired outcome(s).
• Modifications to plan of care.

DISCHARGE PLANNING

• Identified long-range needs and who is responsible for actions to be taken.
• Specific referrals made, sources for assistive devices, educational tools.

SAMPLE NURSING OUTCOMES & INTERVENTIONS CLASSIFICATIONS (NOC/NIC)

NOC—Child Development: [specify age]
NIC—Developmental Enhancement: Child [or] Adolescent

Diarrhea

Taxonomy II: Elimination—Class 2 Gastrointestinal System (0013)
[Diagnostic Division: Elimination]
Submitted 1975; Nursing Diagnosis Extension and Classification (NDEC) Revision 1998

Definition: Passage of loose, unformed stools

Information in brackets added by the authors to clarify and enhance the use of nursing diagnoses.

Related Factors

PSYCHOLOGICAL

High stress levels; anxiety

SITUATIONAL

Laxative/alcohol abuse; toxins; contaminants
Adverse effects of medications; radiation
Tube feedings
Travel

PHYSIOLOGICAL

Inflammation; irritation
Infectious processes; parasites
Malabsorption

Defining Characteristics

SUBJECTIVE

Abdominal pain
Urgency, cramping

OBJECTIVE

Hyperactive bowel sounds
At least three loose liquid stools per day

Desired Outcomes/Evaluation Criteria—Client Will:

• Reestablish and maintain normal pattern of bowel functioning.
• Verbalize understanding of causative factors and rationale for treatment regimen.
• Demonstrate appropriate behavior to assist with resolution of causative factors (e.g., proper food preparation or avoidance of irritating foods).

Actions/Interventions

NURSING PRIORITY NO. 1. To assess causative factors/etiology:

• Ascertain onset and pattern of diarrhea, noting whether acute or chronic. **Acute diarrhea (caused by viral/bacterial/parasitic infections [e.g. Norwalk, Rotovirus/Salmonella, Shigella/ Giardia, Amebiasis, respectively]; bacterial food-borne toxins [e.g., *Staphylococcus aureus, Escherichia coli*]; medications [e.g., antibiotics, chemotherapy agents, cholchicine,**

Information in brackets added by the authors to clarify and enhance the use of nursing diagnoses.

  Cultural Collaborative Community/Home Care

laxatives]; and enteral tube feedings) lasts a few days up to a week. Chronic diarrhea (caused by irritable bowel syndrome, infectious diseases affecting colon [e.g., inflammatory bowel disease], colon cancer and treatments, severe constipation, malabsorption disorders, laxative abuse, certain endocrine disorders [e.g., hyperthyroidism, Addison's disease]) almost always lasts more than three weeks.

- Obtain history/observe stools for volume, frequency (e.g., more than normal number of stools/day), characteristics (e.g., slightly soft to watery stools), and precipitating factors (e.g., travel, recent antibiotic use, day care center attendance) related to occurrence of diarrhea.
- Note client's age. **Diarrhea in infant/young child and older or debilitated client can cause complications of dehydration and electrolyte imbalances.**
- Determine if incontinence is present. (Refer to ND Bowel Incontinence.)
- Note reports of abdomimal or rectal pain associated with episodes.
- Auscultate abdomen **for presence, location, and characteristics of bowel sounds.**
- Observe for presence of associated factors, such as fever/chills, abdominal pain/cramping, bloody stools, emotional upset, physical exertion, and so forth.
- Evaluate diet history and note nutritional/fluid and electrolyte status.
- Determine recent exposure to different/foreign environments, change in drinking water/food intake, similar illness of others **that may help identify causative environmental factors.**
- Note history of recent gastrointestinal surgery; concurrent/chronic illnesses/treatment; food/drug allergies; lactose intolerance.
- Review results of laboratory testing (**e.g., parasites, cultures for bacteria, toxins, fat, blood) for acute diarrhea. Chronic diarrhea testing may include upper and lower gastrointestinal studies; stool examination for parasites; colonoscopy with biopsies, etc.**

NURSING PRIORITY NO. 2. To eliminate causative factors:

- Restrict solid food intake, as indicated, **to allow for bowel rest/reduced intestinal workload.**
- Provide for changes in dietary intake **to avoid foods/substances that precipitate diarrhea.**
- Limit caffeine and high-fiber foods; avoid milk and fruits, as appropriate.

Information in brackets added by the authors to clarify and enhance the use of nursing diagnoses.

DIARRHEA

- Adjust strength/rate of enteral tube feedings; change formula, as indicated, **when diarrhea is associated with tube feedings.**
- Assess for/remove fecal impaction, especially in an elderly client **where impaction may be accompanied by diarrhea.** (Refer to NDs Constipation; Bowel Incontinence.)
- Recommend change in drug therapy, as appropriate (e.g., choice of antibiotic).
- Assist in treatment of underlying conditions (e.g., infections, malabsorption syndrome, cancer) and complications of diarrhea. **Therapies can include treatment of fever, pain, and infectious/toxic agents; rehydration; oral refeeding, etc.**
- Promote use of relaxation techniques (e.g., progressive relaxation exercise, visualization techniques) **to decrease stress/anxiety.**

NURSING PRIORITY NO. 3. To maintain hydration/electrolyte balance:

- Assess for presence of postural hypotension, tachycardia, skin hydration/turgor, and condition of mucous membranes **indicating dehydration.**
- Weigh infant's diapers **to determine amount of output and fluid replacement needs.**
- Review laboratory studies for abnormalities.
- Administer antidiarrheal medications, as indicated, **to decrease gastrointestinal motility and minimize fluid losses.**
- Encourage oral intake of fluids containing electrolytes, such as juices, bouillon, or commercial preparations, as appropriate.
- Administer enteral and IV fluids, as indicated.

NURSING PRIORITY NO. 4. To maintain skin integrity:

- Assist, as needed, with pericare after each bowel movement.
- Provide prompt diaper change and gentle cleansing, **because skin breakdown can occur quickly when diarrhea is present.**
- Apply lotion/ointment as skin barrier, as needed.
- Provide dry linen, as necessary.
- Expose perineum/buttocks to air; use heat lamp with caution, if needed to keep area dry.
- Refer to ND impaired Skin Integrity.

NURSING PRIORITY NO. 5. To promote return to normal bowel functioning:

- Increase oral fluid intake and return to normal diet, as tolerated.
- Encourage intake of nonirritating liquids.

Information in brackets added by the authors to clarify and enhance the use of nursing diagnoses.

🌐 Cultural 🔗 Collaborative 🏠 Community/Home Care

- Discuss possible change in infant formula. **Diarrhea may be result of/aggravated by intolerance to specific formula.**
- Recommend products such as natural fiber, plain natural yogurt, Lactinex, **to restore normal bowel flora.**
- Administer medications, as ordered, **to treat infectious process, decrease motility, and/or absorb water.**
- Provide privacy during defecation and psychological support, as necessary.

NURSING PRIORITY NO. 6. To promote wellness (Teaching/Discharge Considerations):

- Review causative factors and appropriate interventions **to prevent recurrence.**
- Evaluate/identify individual stress factors and coping behaviors.
- Review food preparation, emphasizing adequate cooking time and proper refrigeration/storage **to prevent bacterial growth/contamination.**
- Emphasize importance of handwashing **to prevent spread of infectious causes of diarrhea** such as *Clostridium difficile* (*C. difficile*) or *S. aureus.*
- Discuss possibility of dehydration and the importance of proper fluid replacement.
- Discuss use of incontinence pads **to protect bedding/furniture, depending on the severity of the problem.**

Documentation Focus

ASSESSMENT/REASSESSMENT

- Assessment findings, including characteristics/pattern of elimination.
- Causative/aggravating factors.
- Methods used to treat problem.

PLANNING

- Plan of care and who is involved in planning.
- Teaching plan.

IMPLEMENTATION/EVALUATION

- Client's response to treatment/teaching and actions performed.
- Attainment/progress toward desired outcome(s).
- Modifications to plan of care.

DISCHARGE PLANNING

- Recommendations for follow-up care.

Information in brackets added by the authors to clarify and enhance the use of nursing diagnoses.

SAMPLE NURSING OUTCOMES & INTERVENTIONS CLASSIFICATIONS (NOC/NIC)

NOC—Bowel Elimination
NIC—Diarrhea Management

risk for compromised human Dignity

Taxonomy II: Self-Perception—Class 1 Self-Concept (00174)
[Diagnostic Division: Ego Integrity]
Submitted 2006

Definition: At risk for perceived loss of respect and honor

Risk Factors

Loss of control of body functions; exposure of the body
Perceived humiliation/invasion of privacy
Disclosure of confidential information; stigmatizing label; use of undefined medical terms
Perceived dehumanizing treatment/intrusion by clinicians
Inadequate participation in decision making
Cultural incongruity

Desired Outcomes/Evaluation Criteria—Client Will:

- Verbalize awareness of specific problem.
- Identify positive ways to deal with situation.
- Demonstrate problem-solving skills.
- Express sense of dignity in situation.

Actions/Interventions

NURSING PRIORITY NO. 1. To evaluate source/degree of risk:

- Determine client's perceptions and specific factors that could lead to sense of loss of dignity. **Human dignity is a totality of the individual's uniqueness—mind, body, and spirit.**
- Note labels/terms used by staff, friends/family that stigmatize the client. **Human dignity is threatened by insensitive, as well as inadequate, healthcare and lack of client participation in care decisions.**

 • Ascertain cultural beliefs/values and degree of importance to client. **Some individuals cling to their basic culture,**

Information in brackets added by the authors to clarify and enhance the use of nursing diagnoses.

 Cultural Collaborative Community/Home Care
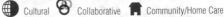

especially during times of stress, which may result in conflict with current circumstances.

- Identify healthcare goals/expectations.
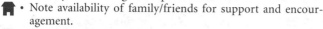 • Note availability of family/friends for support and encouragement.
- Ascertain response of family/SO(s) to client's situation.

NURSING PRIORITY NO. 2. To assist client/caregiver to reduce or correct individual risk factors:

- Ask client by what name he or she would like to be called. **A person's name is important to his or her identity and recognizes one's individuality. Many older people prefer to be addressed in a formal manner (e.g., Mr. or Mrs.).**
- Active-listen feelings and be available for support and assistance, as desired, **so client's concerns can be addressed.**
- Provide for privacy when discussing sensitive/personal issues.
- Encourage family/SO(s) to treat client with respect and understanding, especially when the client is older and may be irritable and difficult to deal with. **Everyone should be treated with respect and dignity regardless of individual ability/frailty.**
- Use understandable terms when talking to client/family about the medical condition/procedures/treatments. **Most lay people do not understand medical terms and may be hesitant to ask what is meant.**
- Respect the client's needs and wishes for quiet, privacy, talking, or silence.
- Include client and family in decision making, especially regarding end-of-life issues. **Helps the individuals feel respected/valued and that they are participants in the care process.**
- Protect client's privacy when providing personal care/during procedures. Assure client is covered adequately when care is being given **to prevent unnecessary exposure/embarrassment.**
- Cleanse client immediately when vomiting, bleeding, or incontinence occurs. Speak in a gentle voice and assure client that these things cannot be helped and nurses are glad to take care of the problem.
- Involve facility/local ethics committee, as appropriate, **to facilitate mediation/resolution of issues.**

NURSING PRIORITY NO. 3. To promote wellness (Teaching/Discharge Considerations):

- Discuss client's rights as an individual. **While hospitals and other care settings have a Patient's Bill of Rights, a broader view of human dignity is stated in the U.S. Constitution.**

Information in brackets added by the authors to clarify and enhance the use of nursing diagnoses.

risk for compromised human DIGNITY

 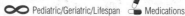

• Discuss/assist with planning for the future, taking into account client's desires and rights.

 • Incorporate identified familial, religious, and cultural factors that have meaning for client.

 • Refer to other resources (e.g., pastoral care, counseling, organized support groups, classes), as appropriate.

Documentation Focus

ASSESSMENT/REASSESSMENT

• Assessment findings, including individual risk factors, client's perceptions, and concerns about involvement in care.
• Individual cultural/religious beliefs, values, healthcare goals.
• Responses/involvement of family/SO(s).

PLANNING

• Plan of care and who is involved in planning.
• Teaching plan.

IMPLEMENTATION/EVALUATION

• Client's response to interventions/teaching and actions performed.
• Attainment/progress toward desired outcome(s).
• Modifications to plan of care.

DISCHARGE PLANNING

• Long-term needs and who is responsible for actions to be taken.
• Specific referrals made.

SAMPLE NURSING OUTCOMES & INTERVENTIONS CLASSIFICATIONS (NOC/NIC)

NOC—Client Satisfaction: Protection of Rights
NIC—Emotional Support

moral Distress

Taxonomy II: Life Principles—Class 3 Value/Belief/Action Congruence (00175)
[Diagnostic Division: Ego Integrity]
Submitted 2006

Definition: Response to the inability to carry out one's chosen ethical/moral decision/action

---

Information in brackets added by the authors to clarify and enhance the use of nursing diagnoses.

Related Factors

Conflict among decision makers [e.g., family, healthcare providers, insurance payers]

Conflicting information guiding moral/ethical decision making; cultural conflicts

Treatment decisions; end-of-life decisions; loss of autonomy

Time constraints for decision making; physical distance of decision maker

Defining Characteristics

OBJECTIVE

Expresses anguish (e.g., powerlessness, guilt, frustration, anxiety, self-doubt, fear) over difficulty acting on one's moral choice

Desired Outcomes/Evaluation Criteria — Client Will:

- Verbalize understanding of causes for conflict in own situation.
- Be aware of own moral values conflicting with desired/required course of action.
- Identify positive ways/actions necessary to deal with situation.
- Express sense of satisfaction with/acceptance of resolution.

Actions/Interventions

NURSING PRIORITY NO. 1. To identify cause/situation in which moral distress is occurring:

- Determine client's perceptions and specific factors resulting in a sense of distress and all parties involved in situation. **Moral conflict centers around lessening the amount of harm suffered, with the involved individuals usually struggling with decisions about what "can be done" to prevent, improve, or cure a medical condition or what "ought to be done" in a specific situation, often within financial constraints or scarcity of resources.**
- Note use of sarcasm, avoidance, apathy, crying, or reports of depression/loss of meaning. **Individuals may not understand their feelings of uneasiness/distress or know that the emotional basis for moral distress is anger.**
- Ascertain response of family/SO(s) to client's situation/healthcare choices.
- Identify healthcare goals/expectations. **New treatment options/technology can prolong life or postpone death**

Information in brackets added by the authors to clarify and enhance the use of nursing diagnoses.

based on the individual's personal viewpoint, increasing the possibility of conflict with others, including healthcare providers.

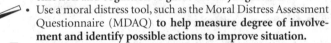

- Ascertain cultural beliefs/values and degree of importance to client. **Cultural diversity may lead to disparate views/expectations between clients, SO/family members, and healthcare providers. When tensions between conflicting values cannot be resolved, persons experience moral distress.**

- Note attitudes and expressions of dissatisfaction of caregivers/staff. **Client may feel pressure/disapproval if own views are not congruent with expectations of those perceived to be more knowledgeable or in "authority." Furthermore, healthcare providers may themselves feel moral distress in carrying out requested actions/interventions.**

- Determine degree of emotional and physical distress (e.g., fatigue, headaches, forgetfulness, anger, guilt, resentment) individual(s) are experiencing and impact on ability to function. **Moral distress can be very destructive, affecting one's ability to carry out daily tasks/care for self or others, and may lead to a crisis of faith.**

- Assess sleep habits of involved parties. **Evidence suggests that sleep-deprivation can harm a person's physical health and emotional well-being, hindering the ability to integrate emotion and cognition to guide moral judgments.**

- Use a moral distress tool, such as the Moral Distress Assessment Questionnaire (MDAQ) **to help measure degree of involvement and identify possible actions to improve situation.**

- Note availability of family/friends for support and encouragement.

NURSING PRIORITY NO. 2. To assist client/involved individuals to develop/effectively use problem-solving skills:

- Encourage involved individuals to recognize and name the experience resulting in moral sensitivity. **Brings concerns out in the open so they can be dealt with.**

- Use skills, such as active-listening, I-messages, and problem solving to assist individual(s) **to clarify feelings of anxiety and conflict.**

- Make time available for support and provide information as desired **to help individuals understand the ethical dilemma that led to moral distress.**

- Provide for privacy when discussing sensitive/personal issues.

- Ascertain coping behaviors client has used successfully in the past that may be helpful in dealing with current situation.

Information in brackets added by the authors to clarify and enhance the use of nursing diagnoses.

  Cultural Collaborative 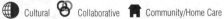 Community/Home Care

- Provide time for nonjudgmental discussion of philosophic issues/questions about impact of conflict leading to moral questioning of current situation.
- Identify role models (e.g., other individuals who have experienced similar problems in their lives). **Sharing of experiences, identifying options can be helpful to deal with current situation.**

 • Involve facility/local ethics committee or ethicist as appropriate **to educate, make recommendations, and facilitate mediation/resolution of issues.**

NURSING PRIORITY NO. 3. To promote wellness (Teaching/Discharge Considerations):

 • Engage all parties, as appropriate, in developing plan to address conflict. **Resolving one's moral distress requires making changes or compromises while preserving one's integrity and authenticity.**

 • Incorporate identified familial, religious, and cultural factors that have meaning for client.

 • Refer to appropriate resources for support/guidance (e.g., pastoral care, counseling, organized support groups, classes), as indicated.

 • Assist individuals to recognize that if they follow their moral decisions, they may clash with the legal system and refer to appropriate resource for legal opinion/options.

Documentation Focus

ASSESSMENT/REASSESSMENT

- Individual findings, including nature of moral conflict, individuals involved in conflict.
- Physical/emotional responses to conflict.
- Individual cultural/religious beliefs and values, healthcare goals.
- Responses/involvement of family/SOs.

PLANNING

- Plan of care and who is involved in planning.
- Teaching plan.

IMPLEMENTATION/EVALUATION

- Responses to interventions/teaching.
- Attainment/progress toward desired outcome(s).
- Modifications to plan of care.

Information in brackets added by the authors to clarify and enhance the use of nursing diagnoses.

Diagnostic Studies   ∞ Pediatric/Geriatric/Lifespan   Medications   **269**

DISCHARGE PLANNING

- Long-term needs and who is responsible for actions to be taken.
- Available resources.
- Specific referrals made.

SAMPLE NURSING OUTCOMES & INTERVENTIONS CLASSIFICATIONS (NOC/NIC)

NOC—Decision Making
NIC—Decision-Making Support

risk for Disuse Syndrome

Taxonomy II: Activity/Rest—Class 2 Activity/Exercise (00040)
[Diagnostic Division: Activity/Rest]
Submitted 1988

Definition: At risk for deterioration of body systems as the result of prescribed or unavoidable musculoskeletal inactivity

NOTE: Complications from immobility can include pressure ulcer, constipation, stasis of pulmonary secretions, thrombosis, urinary tract infection and/or retention, decreased strength or endurance, orthostatic hypotension, decreased range of joint motion, disorientation, body image disturbance, and powerlessness.

Risk Factors

Severe pain; [chronic pain]
Paralysis; [other neuromuscular impairment]
Mechanical/prescribed immobilization
Altered level of consciousness
[Chronic physical or mental illness]

NOTE: A risk diagnosis is not evidenced by signs and symptoms, as the problem has not occurred and nursing interventions are directed at prevention.

Desired Outcomes/Evaluation Criteria—Client Will:

- Display intact skin/tissues or achieve timely wound healing.
- Maintain/reestablish effective elimination patterns.

Information in brackets added by the authors to clarify and enhance the use of nursing diagnoses.

  Cultural Collaborative Community/Home Care

- Be free of signs/symptoms of infectious processes.
- Demonstrate absence of pulmonary congestion with breath sounds clear.
- Demonstrate adequate peripheral perfusion with stable vital signs, skin warm and dry, palpable peripheral pulses.
- Maintain usual reality orientation.
- Maintain/regain optimal level of cognitive, neurosensory, and musculoskeletal functioning.
- Express sense of control over the present situation and potential outcome.
- Recognize and incorporate change into self-concept in accurate manner without negative self-esteem.

Actions/Interventions

NURSING PRIORITY NO. 1. To evaluate probability of developing complications:

- Identify underlying conditions/pathology (e.g., cancer; trauma; fractures with casting; immobilization devices; surgery; chronic disease conditions; malnutrition; neurological conditions [e.g., stroke/other brain injury, post-polio syndrome, MS, spinal cord injury]; chronic pain conditions; use of predisposing medications [e.g., steroids]) **that cause/exacerbate problems associated with inactivity and immobility.**
- Note specific and potential concerns including client's age, cognition, mobility and exercise status, and whether current condition is acute/short-term or may be long-term/permanent. **Age-related physiological changes along with limitations imposed by illness/confinement predispose older adults to deconditioning and functional decline.**
- Assess/document client's ongoing functional status, including cognition, vision, and hearing; social support; psychological well-being; abilities in performance of ADLs **for comparative baseline; evaluate response to treatment and to identify preventative interventions or necessary services.**
- Evaluate client's risk for injury. **Risk is greater in client with cognitive difficulties, lack of safe or stimulating environment, inadequate/unsafe use of mobility aids, and/or sensory-perception problems.**
- Ascertain availability and use of support systems.
- Evaluate client's/family's understanding and ability to manage care for long period.

NURSING PRIORITY NO. 2. To identify individually appropriate preventive/corrective interventions:

Information in brackets added by the authors to clarify and enhance the use of nursing diagnoses.

🏠 SKIN

- Monitor skin over bony prominences.
- Reposition frequently as individually indicated **to relieve pressure.**
- Provide skin care daily and prn, drying well and using gentle massage and lotion **to stimulate circulation.**
- Use pressure-reducing devices (e.g., egg-crate/gel/water/air mattress or cushions).
- Review nutritional status and monitor nutritional intake.
- Provide/reinforce teaching regarding dietary needs, position changes, cleanliness.
- Refer to NDs impaired Skin Integrity; impaired Tissue Integrity.

🏠 ELIMINATION

- Encourage balanced diet, including fruits and vegetables high in fiber and with adequate fluids for optimal stool consistency and to facilitate passage through colon.
- Include 8 oz/day of cranberry juice cocktail to reduce risk of urinary infections.
- Maximize mobility at earliest opportunity

- Evaluate need for stool softeners, bulk-forming laxatives.
- Implement consistent bowel management/bladder training programs, as indicated.
- Monitor urinary output/characteristics. Observe for signs of infection.
- Refer to NDs Constipation; Diarrhea; Bowel Incontinence; impaired Urinary Elimination; Urinary Retention.

🏠 RESPIRATION

- Monitor breath sounds and characteristics of secretions for early detection of complications (e.g., pneumonia).
- Reposition, cough, deep-breathe on a regular schedule **to facilitate clearing of secretions/prevent atelectasis.**
- Suction, as indicated, **to clear airways.**
- Encourage use of incentive spirometry.
- Demonstrate techniques/assist with postural drainage.
- Assist with/instruct family and caregivers in quad coughing techniques/diaphragmatic weight training **to maximize ventilation in presence of spinal cord injury (SCI).**
- Discourage smoking. Involve in smoking-cessation program, as indicated.
- Refer to NDs ineffective Airway Clearance; ineffective Breathing Pattern.

Information in brackets added by the authors to clarify and enhance the use of nursing diagnoses.

  Cultural Collaborative Community/Home Care

🏠 VASCULAR (TISSUE PERFUSION)

- Monitor cognition and mental status. **Changes can reflect state of cardiac health, cerebral oxygenation impairment, or be indicative of mental/emotional state that could adversely affect safety and self-care.**
- Determine core and skin temperature. Investigate development of cyanosis, changes in mentation, **to identify changes in oxygenation status.**
- Routinely evaluate circulation/nerve function of affected body parts. Note changes in temperature, color, sensation, and movement.
- Institute peripheral vascular support measures (e.g., elastic hose, Ace wraps, sequential compression devices—SCDs) **to enhance venous return.**
- Encourage/provide adequate fluid **to prevent dehydration and circulatory stasis.**
- Monitor blood pressure before, during, and after activity—sitting, standing, and lying, if possible, **to ascertain response to/tolerance of activity.**
- Assist with position changes as needed. Raise head gradually. Institute use of tilt table where appropriate. **Injury may occur as a result of orthostatic hypotension.**
- Maintain proper body position; avoid use of constricting garments/restraints **to prevent vascular congestion.**
- Provide range-of-motion exercises for bed/chair. Ambulate as quickly and often as possible, using mobility aids and frequent rest stops **to assist client in continuing activity and prevent circulatory problems related to inactivity.**
- Refer to physical therapy **for strengthening and restoration of optimal range of motion and prevention of circulatory problems.**
- Refer to NDs ineffective Tissue Perfusion; risk for Peripheral Neurovascular Dysfunction.

🏠 MUSCULOSKELETAL (MOBILITY/RANGE OF MOTION, STRENGTH/ ENDURANCE)

- Perform range-of-motion (ROM) exercises and involve client in active exercises with physical/occupational therapy (e.g., muscle strengthening).
- Maximize involvement in self-care.
- Pace activities as possible to increase strength/endurance.
- Apply functional positioning splints as appropriate.
- Evaluate role of pain in mobility problem.
- Implement pain management program as individually indicated.

Information in brackets added by the authors to clarify and enhance the use of nursing diagnoses.

 Diagnostic Studies   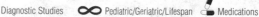 Pediatric/Geriatric/Lifespan   Medications   **273**

- Limit/monitor closely the use of restraints and immobilize client as little as possible. Remove restraints periodically and assist with ROM exercises.
- Refer to NDs Activity Intolerance; risk for Falls; impaired physical Mobility; acute or chronic Pain.

 SENSORY-PERCEPTION

- Orient client as necessary to time, place, person, and situation. Provide cues for orientation (e.g., clock, calendar).
- Provide appropriate level of environmental stimulation (e.g., music, TV/radio, personal possessions, visitors).
- Encourage participation in recreational/diversional activities and regular exercise program (as tolerated).
- Suggest use of sleep aids/usual presleep rituals to promote normal sleep/rest.
- Refer to NDs chronic Confusion; disturbed Sensory Perception; Insomnia; Social Isolation; deficient Diversional Activity.

 SELF-ESTEEM, POWERLESSNESS

- Explain/review all care procedures.
- Provide for/assist with mutual goal setting, involving SO(s). **Promotes sense of control and enhances commitment to goals.**
- Provide consistency in caregivers whenever possible.
- Ascertain that client can communicate needs adequately (e.g., call light, writing tablet, picture/letter board, interpreter).
- Encourage verbalization of feelings/questions.
- Refer to NDs Powerlessness; impaired verbal Communication; Self-Esteem [specify]; ineffective Role Performance.

BODY IMAGE

- Orient to body changes through verbal description, written information; encourage looking at and discussing changes **to promote acceptance**.
- Promote interactions with peers and normalization of activities within individual abilities.
- Refer to NDs disturbed Body Image; situational low Self-Esteem; Social Isolation; disturbed Personal Identity.

NURSING PRIORITY NO. 3. To promote wellness (Teaching/Discharge Considerations):

- Promote self-care and SO-supported activities **to gain/maintain independence.**

Information in brackets added by the authors to clarify and enhance the use of nursing diagnoses.

  Cultural   Collaborative   Community/Home Care

- Provide/review information about individual needs/areas of concerns (e.g., client's mental status, living environment, nutritional needs) **to enhance safety and prevent/limit effects of disuse.**
- Encourage involvement in regular exercise program, including isometric/isotonic activities, active or assistive ROM, to limit consequences of disuse and maximize level of function.
- Review signs/symptoms requiring medical evaluation/follow-up to promote timely interventions.
- Identify community support services (e.g., financial, counseling, home maintenance, respite care, transportation).
- Refer to appropriate rehabilitation/home-care resources.
- Note sources for assistive devices/necessary equipment.

Documentation Focus

ASSESSMENT/REASSESSMENT

- Assessment findings, noting individual areas of concern, functional level, degree of independence, support systems/available resources.

PLANNING

- Plan of care and who is involved in planning.
- Teaching plan.

IMPLEMENTATION/EVALUATION

- Client's response to interventions/teaching and actions performed.
- Changes in level of functioning.
- Attainment/progress toward desired outcome(s).
- Modifications to plan of care.

DISCHARGE PLANNING

- Long-term needs and who is responsible for actions to be taken.
- Specific referrals made, resources for specific equipment needs.

SAMPLE NURSING OUTCOMES & INTERVENTIONS CLASSIFICATIONS (NOC/NIC)

NOC—Immobility Consequences: Physiological
NIC—Energy Management

Information in brackets added by the authors to clarify and enhance the use of nursing diagnoses.

deficient Diversional Activity

Taxonomy II: Activity/Rest—Class 2 Activity/Exercise
(00097)
[Diagnostic Division: Activity/Rest]
Submitted 1980

Definition: Decreased stimulation from (or interest or engagement in) recreational or leisure activities [Note: Internal/external factors may or may not be beyond the individual's control.]

Related Factors

Environmental lack of diversional activity [e.g., long-term hospitalization; frequent, lengthy treatments; home-bound]
[Physical limitations; bedridden; fatigue; pain]
[Situational, developmental problem; lack of resources]
[Psychological condition, such as depression]

Defining Characteristics

SUBJECTIVE

Patient's statements regarding boredom (e.g., wish there were something to do, to read, etc.)
Usual hobbies cannot be undertaken in hospital [home or other care setting]
[Changes in abilities/physical limitations]

OBJECTIVE

[Flat effect; disinterest, inattentiveness]
[Restlessness; crying]
[Lethargy; withdrawal]
[Hostility]
[Overeating or lack of interest in eating; weight loss or gain]

Desired Outcomes/Evaluation Criteria—Client Will:

• Recognize own psychological response (e.g., hopelessness and helplessness, anger, depression) and initiate appropriate coping actions.
• Engage in satisfying activities within personal limitations.

Actions/Interventions

NURSING PRIORITY NO. 1. To assess precipitating/etiological factors:

Information in brackets added by the authors to clarify and enhance the use of nursing diagnoses.

  Cultural Collaborative 🏠 Community/Home Care

- Assess/review client's physical, cognitive, emotional, and environmental status. **Validates reality of environmental deprivation when it exists, or considers potential for loss of desired diversional activities in order to plan for prevention/early interventions.**
- Note impact of disability/illness on lifestyle (e.g., young child with leukemia, elderly person with fractured hip, individual with severe depression). **Provides comparative baseline for assessments and interventions.**
- Note age/developmental level, gender, cultural factors, and the importance of a given activity in client's life **in order to support client participation in something which promotes self-esteem and personal fulfillment.**
- Determine client's actual ability to participate/interest in available activities, noting attention span, physical limitations and tolerance, level of interest/desire, and safety needs. **Presence of acute illness, depression, problems of mobility, protective isolation, or sensory deprivation may interfere with desired activity.**

NURSING PRIORITY NO. 2. To motivate and stimulate client involvement in solutions:

- Institute/continue appropriate actions to deal with concomitant conditions such as anxiety, depression, grief, dementia, physical injury, isolation and immobility, malnutrition, acute or chronic pain. **These interfere with the individual's ability to engage in meaningful diversional activities.**
- Acknowledge reality of situation and feelings of the client **to establish therapeutic relationship and support hopeful emotions.**
- Review history of lifelong activities and hobbies client has enjoyed. Discuss reasons client is not doing these activities now and determine whether client can/would like to resume these activites.
- Encourage mix of desired activities/stimuli (e.g., music; news; educational presentations—TV/tapes; movies; computer/Internet access; books/other reading materials; visitors; games; arts and crafts; sensory enrichment [e.g., massage, aromatherapy]; grooming/beauty care; cooking; social outings; gardening; discussion groups, as appropriate). **Activities need to be personally meaningful and not physically/emotionally overwhelming for client to derive the most benefit.**
- Participate in decisions about timing and spacing of lengthy treatments to promote relaxation/reduce sense of boredom.

Information in brackets added by the authors to clarify and enhance the use of nursing diagnoses.

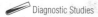 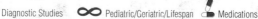

- Encourage client to assist in scheduling required and optional activity choices (e.g., if client's favorite TV show occurs at bathtime, reschedule bath for a later time), **enhancing client's sense of control.**
- Refrain from making changes in schedule without discussing with client. **It is important for staff to be responsible in making and following through on commitments to client.**
- Provide change of scenery (indoors and outdoors where possible) to **provide positive sensory stimulation, reduce sense of boredom, improve sense of normalcy and control.**
- Identify requirements for mobility (wheelchair/walker/van/volunteers and the like).
- Provide for periodic changes in the personal environment when the client is confined. Use the individual's input in creating the changes (e.g., seasonal bulletin boards, color changes, rearranging furniture, pictures).
- Suggest activities, such as bird feeders/baths for birdwatching, a garden in a window box/terrarium, or a fish bowl/aquarium **to stimulate observation as well as involvement and participation in activity, such as identification of birds, choice of seeds, and so forth.**
- Accept hostile expressions while limiting aggressive acting-out behavior. (**Permission to express feelings of anger, hopelessness allows for beginning resolution. However, destructive behavior is counterproductive to self-esteem and problem solving.**)
- Involve recreational/occupational/play/music/movement-therapist as appropriate **to help identify enjoyable activities for client; to procure assistive devices and/or modify activities for individual situation.**

NURSING PRIORITY NO. 3. To promote wellness (Teaching/Discharge Considerations):

- Explore options for useful activities using the person's strengths/abilities.
- Make appropriate referrals to available support groups, hobby clubs, service organizations.
- Refer to NDs Powerlessness; Social Isolation.

Documentation Focus

ASSESSMENT/REASSESSMENT

- Specific assessment findings, including blocks to desired activities.
- Individual choices for activities.

Information in brackets added by the authors to clarify and enhance the use of nursing diagnoses.

   Cultural Collaborative Community/Home Care

PLANNING

- Plan of care/interventions and who is involved in planning.

IMPLEMENTATION/EVALUATION

- Client's responses to interventions/teaching and actions performed.
- Attainment/progress toward desired outcome(s).
- Modifications to plan of care.

DISCHARGE PLANNING

- Long-term needs and who is responsible for actions to be taken.
- Referrals/community resources.

SAMPLE NURSING OUTCOMES & INTERVENTIONS CLASSIFICATIONS (NOC/NIC)

NOC—Leisure Participation
NIC—Recreation Therapy

disturbed Energy Field

Taxonomy II: Activity/Rest—Class 3 Energy Balance (00050)
[Diagnostic Division: Ego Integrity]
Submitted 1994, Revised 2004

Definition: Disruption of the flow of energy [aura] surrounding a person's being that results in a disharmony of the body, mind, and/or spirit

Related Factors

Slowing or blocking of energy flows secondary to:
  Pathophysological factors—Illness, pregnancy, injury
  Treatment-related factors—Immobility, labor and delivery, perioperative experience, chemotherapy
  Situational factors—Pain, fear, anxiety, grieving
  Maturational factors—Age-related developmental difficulties/ crisis

Defining Characteristics

OBJECTIVE

Perception of changes in patterns of energy flow, such as:
  Movement (wave, spike, tingling, dense, flowing)
  Sounds (tone, words)

Information in brackets added by the authors to clarify and enhance the use of nursing diagnoses.

 Diagnostic Studies   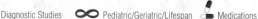 Pediatric/Geriatric/Lifespan   Medications   **279**

Temperature change (warmth, coolness)
Visual changes (image, color)
Disruption of the field (deficient, hole, spike, bulge, obstruction, congestion, diminished flow in energy field)

Desired Outcomes/Evaluation Criteria—Client Will:

• Acknowledge feelings of anxiety and distress.
• Verbalize sense of relaxation/well-being.
• Display reduction in severity/frequency of symptoms.

Actions/Interventions

NURSING PRIORITY NO. 1. To determine causative/contributing factors:

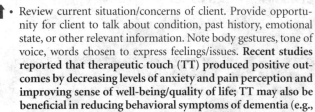

• Review current situation/concerns of client. Provide opportunity for client to talk about condition, past history, emotional state, or other relevant information. Note body gestures, tone of voice, words chosen to express feelings/issues. **Recent studies reported that therapeutic touch (TT) produced positive outcomes by decreasing levels of anxiety and pain perception and improving sense of well-being/quality of life; TT may also be beneficial in reducing behavioral symptoms of dementia (e.g., manual manipulation/restlessness, vocalization, pacing).**

• Determine client's motivation/desire for treatment. **Although attitude can affect success of therapy, TT is often successful even when the client is skeptical.**

• Note use of medications, other drug use (e.g., alcohol). **TT may be helpful in reducing anxiety level in individuals undergoing alcohol withdrawal.**

• Perform/review results of testing, as indicated, such as the State-Trait Anxiety Inventory (STAI) or the Affect Balance Scale, **to provide measures of the client's anxiety**.

NURSING PRIORITY NO. 2. To evaluate energy field:

• Develop therapeutic nurse-client relationship, initially accepting role of healer/guide as client desires.

• Place client in sitting or supine position with legs/arms uncrossed. Place pillows or other supports to enhance comfort and relaxation.

• Center self physically and psychologically **to quiet mind and turn attention to the healing intent.**

• Move hands slowly over the client at level of 2 to 6 inches above skin to assess state of energy field and flow of energy within the system.

Information in brackets added by the authors to clarify and enhance the use of nursing diagnoses.

 Cultural Collaborative Community/Home Care

- Identify areas of imbalance or obstruction in the field (i.e., areas of asymmetry; feelings of heat/cold, tingling, congestion, or pressure).

NURSING PRIORITY NO. **3.** To provide therapeutic intervention:

- Explain the process of TT and answer questions, as indicated, **to prevent unrealistic expectation. Fundamental focus of TT is on healing and wholeness, not curing signs/symptoms of disease.**
- Discuss findings of evaluation with client.
- Assist client with exercises to promote "centering" and increase potential to self-heal, enhance comfort, reduce anxiety.
- Perform unruffling process, keeping hands 2 to 6 inches from client's body **to dissipate impediments to free flow of energy within the system and between nurse and client**.
- Focus on areas of disturbance identified, holding hands over or on skin, and/or place one hand in back of body with other hand in front. **Allows client's body to pull/repattern energy as needed.** At the same time, concentrate on the intent to help the client heal.
- Shorten duration of treatment to 2 to 3 minutes, as appropriate. **Children, elderly individuals, those with head injuries, and others who are severely debilitated are generally more sensitive to overloading energy fields.**
- Make coaching suggestions (e.g., pleasant images/other visualizations, deep breathing) in a soft voice **for enhancing feelings of relaxation.**
- Use hands-on massage/apply pressure to acupressure points, as appropriate, during process.
- Note changes in energy sensations as session progresses. Stop when the energy field is symmetric and there is a change to feelings of peaceful calm.
- Hold client's feet for a few minutes at end of session **to assist in "grounding" the body energy.**
- Provide client time following procedure **for a period of peaceful rest.**

NURSING PRIORITY NO. **4.** To promote wellness (Teaching/Discharge Considerations):

- Allow period of client dependency, as appropriate, **for client to strengthen own inner resources.**
- Encourage ongoing practice of the therapeutic process.
- Instruct in use of stress-reduction activities (e.g., centering/meditation, relaxation exercises) **to promote harmony between mind-body-spirit.**

Information in brackets added by the authors to clarify and enhance the use of nursing diagnoses.

• Discuss importance of integrating techniques into daily activity plan **for sustaining/enhancing sense of well-being.**

 • Have client practice each step and demonstrate the complete TT process following the session as client displays readiness to assume responsibilities for self-healing.

 • Promote attendance at a support group **where members can help each other practice and learn the techniques of TT.**

 • Reinforce that TT is a complementary intervention and stress importance of seeking timely evaluation/continuing other prescribed treatment modalities, as appropriate.

 • Refer to other resources, as identified (e.g., psychotherapy, clergy, medical treatment of disease processes, hospice), **for the individual to address total well-being/facilitate peaceful death.**

Documentation Focus

ASSESSMENT/REASSESSMENT

• Assessment findings, including characteristics and differences in the energy field.
• Client's perception of problem/need for treatment.

PLANNING

• Plan of care and who is involved in planning.
• Teaching plan.

IMPLEMENTATION/EVALUATION

• Changes in energy field.
• Client's response to interventions/teaching and actions performed.
• Attainment/progress toward desired outcomes.
• Modifications to plan of care.

DISCHARGE PLANNING

• Long-term needs and who is responsible for actions to be taken.
• Specific referrals made.

SAMPLE NURSING OUTCOMES & INTERVENTIONS CLASSIFICATIONS (NOC/NIC)

NOC—Well-Being
NIC—Therapeutic Touch

Information in brackets added by the authors to clarify and enhance the use of nursing diagnoses.

  Cultural Collaborative Community/Home Care

impaired Environmental Interpretation Syndrome

Taxonomy II: Perception/Cognition—Class 2 Orientation (00127)
[Diagnostic Division: Safety]
Submitted 1994

Definition: Consistent lack of orientation to person, place, time, or circumstances over more than 3 to 6 months, necessitating a protective environment

Related Factors

Dementia [Alzheimer's disease, multi-infarct dementia, Pick's disease, AIDS dementia]
Huntington's disease
Depression

Defining Characteristics

OBJECTIVE

Consistent disorientation
Chronic confusional states
Inability to follow simple directions
Inability to reason/concentrate; slow in responding to questions
Loss of occupation/social functioning

Desired Outcomes/Evaluation Criteria—Client Will:

• Be free of harm.

Caregiver Will:

• Identify individual client safety concerns/needs.
• Modify activities/environment to provide for safety.

Actions/Interventions

NURSING PRIORITY NO. 1. To assess causative/precipitating factors:

Refer to NDs acute Confusion; chronic Confusion; impaired Memory; disturbed Thought Processes for additional relevant assessment and interventions.

Information in brackets added by the authors to clarify and enhance the use of nursing diagnoses.

 Diagnostic Studies   ∞ Pediatric/Geriatric/Lifespan   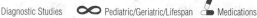 Medications   **283**

- Determine presence of medical conditions and/or behaviors leading to client's current situation **to identify potentially useful interventions and therapies.**
- **Note presence/reports of client's misinterpretation of environmental information** (e.g., sensory, cognitive, or social cues).
- **Discuss history and progression of condition, length of time since onset, future expectations, and incidents of injury/accidents.**
- Review client's behavioral changes with SO(s) **to note differences in viewpoint, as well as to identify additional impairments (e.g., decreased agility, reduced ROM of joints, loss of balance, decline in visual acuity, failure to eat, loss of interest in personal grooming, and forgetfulness resulting in unsafe actions).**
- Identify actual and/or potential environmental dangers and client's level of awareness (if any) of threat.
- Test ability to receive and send effective communication. **Client may be nonverbal or require assistance with/interpretation of verbalizations.**
- Review with client/SO(s) previous/usual habits for activities, such as sleeping, eating, self-care, **to include in plan of care.**
- Determine anxiety level in relation to situation. Note behavior **that may be indicative of potential for violence.**

- Evaluate responses on diagnostic examinations (e.g., memory impairments, reality orientation, attention span, calculations). **A combination of tests (e.g., Confusion Assessment Method [CAM], Mini-Mental State Examination [MMSE], Alzheimer's Disease Assessment Scale [ADAS-cog], Brief Dementia Severity Rating Scale [BDSRS], and Neuro Psychiatric Inventory [NPI]) is often needed to determine client's overall condition relating to chronic/irreversible condition.**

NURSING PRIORITY NO. 2. To promote safe environment:

- Collaborate in management of treatable conditions (e.g., infections, malnutrition, electrolyte imbalances, and adverse medication reactions) **that may contribute to/exacerbate confusion**.
- Provide calm environment; eliminate extraneous noise/stimuli **that may increase client's level of agitation/confusion**.
- Keep communication/questions simple. Use concrete terms and words that client can recognize. (Refer to ND impaired verbal Communication for additional interventions.)
- Use family/other interpreter, as needed, to comprehend client's communications.
- Provide/promote use of glasses, hearing aids, and adequate lighting **to optimize sensory input.**

Information in brackets added by the authors to clarify and enhance the use of nursing diagnoses.

 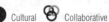 Cultural Collaborative Community/Home Care

- Use touch judiciously. Tell client what is being done before touching **to reduce sense of surprise/negative reaction.**
- Maintain reality-oriented environment (e.g., clocks, calendars, personal items, seasonal decorations, social events).
- Explain environmental cues to client (ongoing) **to protect safety/attempt to diminish fears.**
- Provide consistent caregivers and family-centered care as much as possible **for consistency/to decrease confusion.**
- Incorporate previous/usual patterns for activites (e.g., sleeping, eating, hygiene, desired clothing, leisure/play, or rituals) to the extent possible **to keep environment predictable and prevent client from feeling overwhelmed.**
- Limit number of visitors client interacts with at one time, if needed, **to prevent overstimulation.**
- Implement complementary therapies, as indicated/desired (e.g., music/movement therapy, massage, Therapeutic Touch, aromatherapy, bright-light treatment). **May help client relax, refocus attention, and stimulate memories.**
- Set limits on unsafe and/or inappropriate behavior, being alert to potential for violence.
- Provide for safety/protection against hazards, such as locking doors to unprotected areas/stairwells, prohibiting/supervising smoking, and monitoring ADLs (e.g., choice of clothing in relation to environment/season).
- Use identity tags in clothes/belongings, bracelet/necklace **to provide identification if client wanders away/gets lost.**
- Avoid use of restraints as much as possible. Use vest (instead of wrist) restraints, when required. **Although restraints can prevent falls, they can increase client's agitation and distress.**
- Administer medications, as ordered (e.g., antidepressants, antipsychotics). Monitor for expected and/or adverse reactions and side effects and interactions. **May be used to manage symptoms of psychosis, depression, or aggressive behavior.**

NURSING PRIORITY NO. 3. To assist caregiver to deal with situation:

- Determine family dynamics, cultural values, resources, and availability and willingness to participate in meeting client's needs.
- Involve family/SO(s) in planning and care activities, as needed/desired. Maintain frequent interactions with SO(s) **in order to relay information, change care strategies, obtain feedback, and offer support.**
- Evaluate SO's attention to own needs, including health status, grieving process, and respite. **Caregivers often feel guilty**

Information in brackets added by the authors to clarify and enhance the use of nursing diagnoses.

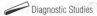 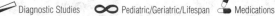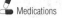

when taking time for themselves. **Without adequate support and respite, the caregiver cannot meet the needs of the client.**

 • Discuss caregiver burden, if appropriate. (Refer to NDs Caregiver Role Strain; risk for Caregiver Role Strain for additional interventions.)

• Provide educational materials and list of available resources, help lines, websites, etc., as desired, **to assist SO(s) in coping with long-term care issues.**

• Identify appropriate community resources (e.g., Alzheimer's Disease and Related Disorders Association [ARDA]; stroke or brain injury support group; senior support groups; clergy; social services; or respite care) **to provide client/SO with support and assist with problem solving.**

NURSING PRIORITY NO. **4.** To promote wellness (Teaching/Discharge Considerations):

 • Provide specific information about disease process/prognosis and client's particular needs. **Individuals with conditions requiring ongoing monitoring of their environment usually need more social and behavioral support than medical management, although medical concerns will occur occasionally.**

• Review age-appropriate ongoing treatment and social needs and appropriate resources for client and family.

 • Develop plan of care with family **to meet client's and SO's individual needs.**

 • Reinforce that caregiver cannot physically watch client at all times.

 • Perform home assessment/identify safety issues, such as locking up medications/poisonous substances and locking exterior doors **to prevent client from wandering off while SO is engaged in other household activities,** or removing matches/smoking material and knobs from the stove **to prevent client from turning on burner and leaving it unattended.**

• Refer to appropriate outside resources, such as adult day care, homemaker services, or support groups. **Provides assistance and promotes problem solving.**

Documentation Focus

ASSESSMENT/REASSESSMENT

• Assessment findings, including degree of impairment.
• Involvement/availability of family members to provide care.

PLANNING

• Plan of care and who is involved in planning.
• Teaching plan.

Information in brackets added by the authors to clarify and enhance the use of nursing diagnoses.

  Cultural Collaborative Community/Home Care

IMPLEMENTATION/EVALUATION

- Response to treatment plan/interventions and actions performed.
- Attainment/progress toward desired outcomes.
- Modifications to plan of care.

DISCHARGE PLANNING

- Long-range needs, who is responsible for actions to be taken.
- Specific referrals made.

SAMPLE NURSING OUTCOMES & INTERVENTIONS CLASSIFICATIONS (NOC/NIC)

NOC—Cognitive Ability
NIC—Reality Orientation

adult Failure to Thrive

Taxonomy II: Growth/Development—Class 1 Growth (00101)
[Diagnostic Division: Food/Fluid]
Submitted 1998

Definition: Progressive functional deterioration of a physical and cognitive nature. The individual's ability to live with multisystem diseases, cope with ensuing problems, and manage his/her care are remarkably diminished

Related Factors

Depression
[Major disease/degenerative condition]
[Aging process]

Defining Characteristics

SUBJECTIVE

Expresses loss of interest in pleasurable outlets
Altered mood state
Verbalizes desire for death

OBJECTIVE

Inadequate nutritional intake; consumption of minimal to no food at most meals (i.e., consumes less than 75% of normal requirements); anorexia

---

Information in brackets added by the authors to clarify and enhance the use of nursing diagnoses.

 Diagnostic Studies 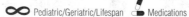 Pediatric/Geriatric/Lifespan Medications

Unintentional weight loss (e.g., 5% in 1 month, 10% in 6 months)

Physical decline (e.g., fatigue, dehydration, incontinence of bowel and bladder)

Cognitive decline: problems with responding to environmental stimuli; demonstrated difficulty in reasoning, decision making, judgment, memory, concentration; decreased perception

Apathy

Decreased participation in activities of daily living; self-care deficit; neglect of home environment/financial responsibilities

Decreased social skills; social withdrawal

Frequent exacerbations of chronic health problems

Desired Outcomes/Evaluation Criteria—Client Will:

- Acknowledge presence of factors affecting well-being.
- Identify corrective/adaptive measures for individual situation.
- Demonstrate behaviors/lifestyle changes necessary to enhance functional status.

Actions/Interventions

Refer to NDs Activity Intolerance; risk-prone health Behaviors; chronic Confusion; ineffective Coping; impaired Dentition; risk for Falls; complicated Grieving; risk for Loneliness; imbalanced Nutrition: less than body requirements; Relocation Stress Syndrome; chronic low Self-Esteem; Self-Care Deficit (specify); risk for Spiritual Distress; impaired Swallowing as appropriate, for additional relevant interventions.

NURSING PRIORITY NO. 1. To identify causative/contributing factors:

- Assess client's/SO's perception of factors leading to present condition, noting onset, duration, presence/absence of physical complaints, social withdrawal, **to provide comparative baseline**.
- Review with client previous and current life situations, including role changes and losses (e.g., death of loved ones; change in living arrangements, finances, independence), **to identify stressors affecting current situation.**
- Identify cultural beliefs/expectations regarding condition/situation, presence of conflicts.
- Determine presence of malnutrition and factors contributing to failure to eat (e.g., chronic nausea, loss of appetite, no access to food or cooking, poorly fitting dentures, no one with which to share meals, depression, financial problems).

Information in brackets added by the authors to clarify and enhance the use of nursing diagnoses.

  Cultural Collaborative Community/Home Care

- Determine client's medical, cognitive, emotional, and perceptual status and effect on self-care ability.
- Evaluate level of adaptive behavior, knowledge, and skills about health maintenance, environment, and safety.
- Ascertain safety and effectiveness of home environment, persons providing care, and potential for/presence of neglectful/abusive situations.

NURSING PRIORITY NO. 2. To assess degree of impairment:

- Collaborate in comprehensive assessment (e.g., physical, nutritional, self-care, and psychosocial) status **to determine the extent of limitations affecting ability to thrive and potential for positive intervention.**
- Obtain current weight **to provide comparative baseline and evaluate response to interventions.**
- Active-listen to client's/caregiver's perception of problem(s).
- Discuss individual concerns about feelings of loss/loneliness and relationship between these feelings and current decline in well-being. Note desire/willingness to change situation. **Motivation can impede—or facilitate—achieving desired outcomes.**
- Survey past and present availability/use of support systems.

NURSING PRIORITY NO. 3. To assist client to achieve/maintain general well-being:

- Assist with treatment of underlying medical/psychiatric conditions **that could positively influence current situation (e.g., resolution of infection, addressing depression).**
- Coordinate session with client/SO(s) and nutritionist **to identify specific dietary needs and creative ways to stimulate intake (e.g., offering client's favorite foods, family style meals, participation in social events such as ice cream social, happy hour).**
- Develop plan of action with client/caregiver **to meet immediate needs for nutrition, safety, and self-care and facilitate implementation of actions.**
- Explore strengths/successful coping behaviors the individual has used previously. **Incorporating these into problem solving builds on past successes.** Refine/develop new strategies as appropriate.
- Assist client to develop goals for dealing with life/illness situation. Involve SO/family in long-range planning. **Promotes commitment to goals and plan, maximizing outcomes.**

NURSING PRIORITY NO. 4. To promote wellness (Teaching/Discharge Considerations):

Information in brackets added by the authors to clarify and enhance the use of nursing diagnoses.

adult FAILURE TO THRIVE

- Assist client/SO(s) to identify useful community resources (e.g., support groups, Meals-on-Wheels, social worker, home care/assistive care, placement services). **Enhances coping, assists with problem solving, and may reduce risks to client and caregiver.**
- Encourge client to talk about positive aspects of life and to keep as physically active as possible **to reduce effects of dispiritedness (e.g., "feeling low," sense of being unimportant, disconnected).**
- Introduce concept of mindfulness (living in the moment). **Promotes feeling of capability and belief that this moment can be dealt with.**
- Offer opportunities to discuss life goals and support client/SO in setting/attaining new goals for this time of life to **enhance hopefulness for future**.
- Promote socialization within individual limitations. **Provides additional stimulation, reduces sense of isolation.**
- Assist client/SO/family to understand that failure to thrive commonly occurs near the end of life, and cannot always be reversed.
- Help client explore reasons for living, or begin to deal with end-of-life issues and provide support for grieving. **Enhances hope and sense of control.**
- Refer to pastoral care, counseling/psychotherapy **for grief work.**
- Discuss appropriateness of/refer to palliative services or hospice care as indicated.

Documentation Focus

ASSESSMENT/REASSESSMENT

- Individual findings, including current weight, dietary pattern, perceptions of self, food and eating.
- Perception of losses/life changes.
- Ability to perform ADLs/participate in care, meet own needs.
- Motivation for change, support/feedback from SO(s).

PLANNING

- Plan of care/interventions and who is involved in planning.
- Teaching plan.

IMPLEMENTATION/EVALUATION

- Responses to interventions and actions performed, general well-being, weekly weight.

Information in brackets added by the authors to clarify and enhance the use of nursing diagnoses.

- Attainment/progress toward desired outcome(s).
- Modifications to plan of care.

DISCHARGE PLANNING

- Long-term needs and who is responsible for actions to be taken.
- Community resources/support groups.
- Specific referrals made.

SAMPLE NURSING OUTCOMES & INTERVENTIONS CLASSIFICATIONS (NOC/NIC)

NOC—Will to Live
NIC—Mood Management

risk for Falls

Taxonomy II: Safety/Protection—Class 2 Physical Injury (00155)
[Diagnostic Division: Safety]
Submitted 2000

Definition: Increased susceptibility to falling that may cause physical harm

Risk Factors

ADULTS

History of falls
Wheelchair use; use of assistive devices (e.g., walker, cane)
Age 65 or over; lives alone
Lower limb prosthesis

PHYSIOLOGICAL

Presence of acute illness; postoperative conditions
Visual/hearing difficulties
Arthritis
Orthostatic hypotension; faintness when turning/extending neck
Sleeplessness
Anemias; vascular disease
Neoplasms (i.e., fatigue/limited mobility)
Urgency; incontinence; diarrhea
Postprandial blood sugar changes
Impaired physical mobility; foot problems; decreased lower extremity strength

---

Information in brackets added by the authors to clarify and enhance the use of nursing diagnoses.

Impaired balance; difficulty with gait; proprioceptive deficits [e.g., unilateral neglect]
Neuropathy

COGNITIVE

Diminished mental status [e.g., confusion, delirium, dementia, impaired reality testing]

MEDICATIONS

Antihypertensive agents; ACE inhibitors; diuretics; tricyclic antidepressants; antianxiety agents; hypnotics; tranquilizers; narcotics
Alcohol use

ENVIRONMENT

Restraints
Weather conditions (e.g., wet floors/ice)
Cluttered environment; throw rugs; no antislip material in bath/shower
Unfamiliar/dimly lit room

CHILDREN

<2 years of age; male gender when <1 year of age
Lack of: gate on stairs, window guards, auto restraints
Unattended infant on elevated surface (e.g., bed/changing table); bed located near window
Lack of parental supervision

NOTE: A risk diagnosis is not evidenced by signs and symptoms, as the problem has not occurred and nursing interventions are directed at prevention.

Desired Outcomes/Evaluation Criteria—Client/Caregivers Will:

- Verbalize understanding of individual risk factors that contribute to possibility of falls.
- Demonstrate behaviors, lifestyle changes to reduce risk factors and protect self from injury.
- Modify environment as indicated to enhance safety.
- Be free of injury.

Actions/Interventio

NURSING PRIORITY NO. 1. 1 .valuate source/degree of risk:

——————— *To evaluate*

Information in brackets added by the authors to clarify and enhance the use of nursing diagnoses.

 Cultural Collaborative Community/Home Care

- Observe individual's general health status, **noticing factors that might affect safety, such as chronic or debilitating conditions, use of multiple medications, recent trauma.**
- Note factors associated with age, gender, and developmental level. **Infants, young children (e.g., climbing on objects), young adults (e.g., sports activities), and elderly are at greatest risk because of developmental issues and impaired/lack of ability to self-protect.**
- Assess muscle strength, gross and fine motor coordination. Review history of past or current physical injuries (e.g., musculoskeletal injuries; orthopedic surgery) **altering coordination, gait, and balance.**
- Review history of prior falls associated with immobility, weakness, prolonged bedrest, sedentary lifestyle (changes in body due to disuse); unsafe environment **to predict current risk for falls.**
- Evaluate use/misuse/failure to use assistive aids, when indicated. **Client may have assistive device, but is at high risk for falls while adjusting to altered body state and use of unfamiliar device; or might refuse to use devices for various reasons (e.g., waiting for help; perception of weakness)**
- Evaluate client's cognitive status (e.g., brain injury, neurological disorders; depression). **Affects ability to perceive own limitations or recognize danger.**
- Assess mood, coping abilities, personality styles. **Individual's temperament, typical behavior, stressors, and level of self-esteem can affect attitude toward safety issues, resulting in carelessness or increased risk-taking without consideration of consequences.**
- Ascertain client's/SO's level of knowledge about/attendance to safety needs. **May reveal lack of understanding/resources or simple disregard for personal safety (e.g., "I can't watch him every minute; we can't hire a home assistant; it's not manly...").**
- Consider environmental hazards in the care setting and/or home/other environment. **Identifying needs/deficits provides opportunities for intervention and/or instruction (e.g., concerning clearing of hazards, intensifying client supervision, obtaining safety equipment, referring for vision evaluation).**
- Review results of various fall risk assessment tools (e.g., Functional Ambulation Profile [FAP]; the Johns Hopkins Hospital Fall Risk Assessment Tool; Tinetti Balance and Gait Assessment [not a comprehensive listing]).

Information in brackets added by the authors to clarify and enhance the use of nursing diagnoses.

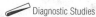 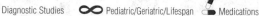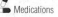

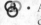

risk for FALLS

- Note socioeconomic status/availability and use of resources in other circumstances. **Can affect current coping abilities.**

NURSING PRIORITY NO. 2. To assist client/caregiver to reduce or correct individual risk factors:

- Assist in treatments and provide information regarding client's disease/condition(s) **that may result in increased risk of falls**.
- Discuss consequences of previously determined risk factors (e.g., falls caused by failure to make provisions for previously identified impairments/safety needs) **for follow-up instruction/interventions**.
- Review medication regimen and how it affects client. Instruct in monitoring of effects/side effects. **Use of certain medications (e.g., narcotics/optiates, psychotropics, antihypertensives, diuretics) can contribute to weakness, confusion, balance and gait disturbances).**
- Stress importance of monitoring conditions/risks that may contribute to occurrence of falls (e.g., client fatigue; acute illness; depression; objects that block traffic patterns in home; insufficient lighting; unfamiliar surroundings; client attempting tasks that are too difficult for present level of functioning; unable to contact someone when help is needed).
- Practice client safety. **Demonstrates behaviors for client/caregiver(s) to emulate.**
- Determine caregiver's expectations of children, cognitively impaired, and/or elderly family members and compare with actual abilities. **Reality of client's abilities and needs may be different than perception or desires of caregivers.**
- Discuss need for and sources of supervision (e.g., babysitters, before- and after-school programs, elderly day care, personal companions).
- Plan for home visit when appropriate. Determine that home safety issues are addressed, including supervision, access to emergency assistance, and client's ability to manage self-care in the home. **May be needed to adequately determine client's needs and available resources.**
- Refer to rehabilitation team, physical or occupational therapist, as appropriate, **to improve client's balance, strength, or mobility; to improve/relearn ambulation; to identify and obtain appropriate assistive devices for mobility, environmental safety, or home modification.**

NURSING PRIORITY NO. 3. To promote wellness (Teaching/Discharge Considerations):

- Refer to other resources as indicated. **Client/caregivers may need financial assistance, home modifications, referrals for**

Information in brackets added by the authors to clarify and enhance the use of nursing diagnoses.

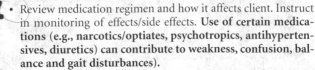 Cultural Collaborative Community/Home Care

counseling, home care, sources for safety equipment, or placement in extended care facility.

🏠 • Provide educational resources (e.g., home safety checklist; equipment directions for proper use, appropriate websites) **for later review/reinforcement of learning.**

🏠 • Promote community awareness about the problems of design of buildings, equipment, transportation, and workplace accidents that contribute to falls.

🏠 • Connect client/family with community resources, neighbors, friends **to assist elderly/handicapped individuals in providing such things as structural maintenance, clearing of snow, gravel, or ice from walks and steps, and so on.**

Documentation Focus

ASSESSMENT/REASSESSMENT

• Individual risk factors noting current physical findings (e.g., signs of injury—bruises, cuts; anemia, fatigue; use of alcohol, drugs, and prescription medications).
• Client's/caregiver's understanding of individual risks/safety concerns.

PLANNING

• Plan of care and who is involved in planning.
• Teaching plan.

IMPLEMENTATION/EVALUATION

• Individual responses to interventions/teaching and actions performed.
• Specific actions and changes that are made.
• Attainment/progress toward desired outcomes.
• Modifications to plan of care.

DISCHARGE PLANNING

• Long-range plans for discharge needs, lifestyle, home setting and community changes, and who is responsible for actions to be taken.
• Specific referrals made.

SAMPLE NURSING OUTCOMES & INTERVENTIONS CLASSIFICATIONS (NOC/NIC)

NOC—Safety Behavior: Fall Prevention
NIC—Fall Prevention

Information in brackets added by the authors to clarify and enhance the use of nursing diagnoses.

dysfunctional Family Processes: alcoholism / [substance abuse]

Taxonomy II: Role Relationships—Class 2 Family
   Relationships (00063)
[Diagnostic Division: Social Interaction]
Submitted 1994

Definition: Psychosocial, spiritual, and physiological
functions of the family unit are chronically disorganized,
which leads to conflict, denial of problems, resistance to
change, ineffective problem solving, and a series of self-
perpetuating crises

Related Factors

Abuse of alcohol/[addictive substances]
Family history of alcoholism/resistance to treatment
Inadequate coping skills; addictive personality; lack of problem-
   solving skills
Biochemical influences; genetic predisposition

Defining Characteristics

SUBJECTIVE

Feelings
Anxiety/tension/distress; decreased self-esteem/worthlessness;
   lingering resentment
Anger/suppressed rage; frustration; shame/embarrassment;
   hurt; unhappiness; guilt
Emotional isolation/loneliness; powerlessness; insecurity; hope-
   lessness; rejection
Responsibility for alcoholic's behavior; vulnerability; mistrust
Depression; hostility; fear; confusion; dissatisfaction; loss
Being different from other people; misunderstood
Emotional control by others; being unloved; lack of identity
Abandonment; confused love and pity; moodiness; failure

Roles and Relationships
Family denial; deterioration in family relationships/disturbed
   family dynamics; ineffective spouse communication; marital
   problems; intimacy dysfunction
Altered role function; disrupted family roles; inconsistent parenting; low perception of parental support; chronic family problems
Lack of skills necessary for relationships; lack of cohesiveness;
   disrupted family rituals
Pattern of rejection; economic problems; neglected obligations

---

Information in brackets added by the authors to clarify and enhance
the use of nursing diagnoses.

 Cultural   Collaborative   Community/Home Care

OBJECTIVE

Feelings
Repressed emotions

Roles and Relationships
Closed communication systems

Triangulating family relationships; reduced ability of family members to relate to each other for mutual growth and maturation

Family does not demonstrate respect for individuality/autonomy of its members

Behavioral
Alcohol abuse; substance abuse other than alcohol; nicotine addiction

Enabling to maintain drinking [substance use]; inadequate understanding/deficient knowledge about alcoholism [substance abuse]

Family special occasions are alcohol-centered

Rationalization/denial of problems; refusal to get help; inability to accept/receive help appropriately

Inappropriate expression of anger; blaming; criticizing; verbal abuse of children/spouse/parent

Lying; broken promises; lack of reliability; manipulation; dependency

Inability to express/accept wide range of feelings; difficulty with intimate relationships; diminished physical contact

Harsh self-judgment; difficulty having fun; self-blaming; isolation; unresolved grief; seeking approval/affirmation

Impaired communication; contradictory/paradoxical communication; controlling communication; power struggles

Ineffective problem-solving skills; lack of dealing with conflict; orientation toward tension relief rather than achievement of goals; agitation; escalating conflict; chaos

Disturbances in concentration; disturbances in academic performance in children; failure to accomplish developmental tasks; difficulty with lifecycle transitions

Inability to meet emotional/security/spiritual needs of its members

Inability to adapt to change; immaturity; stress-related physical illnesses; inability to accept health; inability to deal constructively with traumatic experiences

Desired Outcomes/Evaluation Criteria—Family Will:
- Verbalize understanding of dynamics of codependence.
- Participate in individual/family treatment programs.

Information in brackets added by the authors to clarify and enhance the use of nursing diagnoses.

- Identify ineffective coping behaviors/consequences of choices/actions.
- Demonstrate/plan for necessary lifestyle changes.
- Take action to change self-destructive behaviors/alter behaviors that contribute to client's drinking/substance use.
- Demonstrate improvement in parenting skills.

Actions/Interventions

NURSING PRIORITY NO. 1. To assess contributing factors/underlying problem(s):

- Assess current level of functioning of family members.
- Ascertain family's understanding of current situation; note results of previous involvement in treatment.
- Review family history, explore roles of family members and circumstances involving substance use.
- Determine history of accidents/violent behaviors within family and safety issues.
- Discuss current/past methods of coping. **May be able to identify methods that would be useful in the current situation.**
- Determine extent and understanding of enabling behaviors being evidenced by family members.
- Identify sabotage behaviors of family members. **Issues of secondary gain (conscious or unconscious) may impede recovery.**
- Note presence/extent of behaviors of family, client, and self that might be "too helpful," such as frequent requests for help, excuses for not following through on agreed-on behaviors, feelings of anger/irritation with others. **Enabling behaviors can complicate acceptance and resolution of problem.**

NURSING PRIORITY NO. 2. To assist family to change destructive behaviors:

- Mutually agree on behaviors/responsibilities for nurse and client. **Maximizes understanding of what is expected of each individual.**
- Confront and examine denial and sabotage behaviors used by family members. **Helps individuals recognize and move beyond blocks to recovery.**
- Discuss use of anger, rationalization, and/or projection and ways in which these interfere with problem resolution.
- Encourage family to deal with anger **to prevent escalation to violence.** Problem solve concerns.
- Determine family strengths, areas for growth, individual/family successes.
- Remain nonjudgmental in approach to family members and to member who uses alcohol/drugs.

Information in brackets added by the authors to clarify and enhance the use of nursing diagnoses.

   Cultural   Collaborative   Community/Home Care

- Provide information regarding effects of addiction on mood/personality of the involved person. **Helps family members understand and cope with negative behaviors without being judgmental or reacting angrily.**
- Distinguish between destructive aspects of enabling behavior and genuine motivation to aid the user.
- Identify use of manipulative behaviors and discuss ways to avoid/prevent these situations. **Manipulation has the goal of controlling others and when family members accept self-responsibility and commit to stop using it, new healthy behaviors will ensue.**

NURSING PRIORITY NO. 3. To promote wellness (Teaching/Discharge Considerations):

- Provide factual information to client/family about the effects of addictive behaviors on the family and what to expect after discharge.
- Provide information about enabling behavior, addictive disease characteristics for both user and nonuser who is codependent.
- Discuss importance of restructuring life activities, work/leisure relationships. **Previous lifestyle/relationships supported substance use, requiring change to prevent relapse.**
- Encourage family to refocus celebrations excluding alcohol use **to reduce risk of relapse.**
- Provide support for family members; encourage participation in group work. **Involvement in a group provides information about how others are dealing with problems, provides role models, and gives individual an opportunity to practice new healthy skills.**
- Encourage involvement with/refer to self-help groups (e.g., Al-Anon, AlaTeen, Narcotics Anonymous, family therapy groups) **to provide ongoing support and assist with problem solving.**
- Provide bibliotherapy as appropriate.
- In addition, refer to NDs interrupted Family Processes; compromised/disabled family Coping, as appropriate.

Documentation Focus

ASSESSMENT/REASSESSMENT

- Assessment findings, including history of substance(s) that have been used and family risk factors/safety concerns.
- Family composition and involvement.
- Results of prior treatment involvement.

Information in brackets added by the authors to clarify and enhance the use of nursing diagnoses.

PLANNING

- Plan of care and who is involved in planning.
- Teaching plan.

IMPLEMENTATION/EVALUATION

- Responses of family members to treatment/teaching and actions performed.
- Attainment/progress toward desired outcome(s).
- Modifications to plan of care.

DISCHARGE PLANNING

- Long-term needs, who is responsible for actions to be taken.
- Specific referrals made.

SAMPLE NURSING OUTCOMES & INTERVENTIONS CLASSIFICATIONS (NOC/NIC)

NOC—Family Environment: Internal
NIC—Substance Use Treatment

interrupted Family Processes

Taxonomy II: Role Relationships—Class 2 Family
  Relationships (00060)
[Diagnostic Division: Social Interactions]
Submitted 1982; Nursing Diagnosis Extension and
  Classification (NDEC) Revision 1998

Definition: Change in family relationships and/or
functioning

Related Factors

Situational transition/crises [e.g., economic, change in roles, illness, trauma, disabling/expensive treatments]
Developmental transition/crises [e.g., loss or gain of a family member, adolescence, leaving home for college]
Shift in health status of a family member
Family roles shift; power shift of family members
Modification in family finances/status
Interaction with community

Defining Characteristics

SUBJECTIVE

Changes in: power alliances; satisfaction with family; expressions of conflict within family; effectiveness in completing

Information in brackets added by the authors to clarify and enhance the use of nursing diagnoses.

assigned tasks; stress-reduction behaviors; expressions of conflict with/isolation from community resources; somatic complaints

[Family expresses confusion about what to do; verbalizes they are having difficulty responding to change]

OBJECTIVE

Changes in: assigned tasks; participation in problem solving/ decision making; communication patterns; mutual support; availability for emotional support/effective responsiveness; patterns; rituals; intimacy

Desired Outcomes/Evaluation Criteria—Family Will:

- Express feelings freely and appropriately.
- Demonstrate individual involvement in problem-solving processes directed at appropriate solutions for the situation/crisis.
- Direct energies in a purposeful manner to plan for resolution of the crisis.
- Verbalize understanding of illness/trauma, treatment regimen, and prognosis.
- Encourage and allow member who is ill to handle situation in own way, progressing toward independence.

Actions/Interventions

NURSING PRIORITY NO. 1. To assess individual situation for causative/contributing factors:

- Determine pathophysiology, illness/trauma, developmental crisis present.
- Identify family developmental stage (e.g., marriage, birth of a child, children leaving home). **Provides baseline for establishing plan of care.**
- Note components of family: parent(s), children, male/female, extended family available.
- Observe patterns of communication in family. Are feelings expressed? Freely? Who talks to whom? Who makes decisions? For whom? Who visits? When? What is the interaction between family members? **Identifies weakness/areas of concern to be addressed as well as strengths that can be used for resolution of problem.**
- Assess boundaries of family members. Do members share family identity and have little sense of individuality? Do they seem emotionally distant, not connected with one another?

Information in brackets added by the authors to clarify and enhance the use of nursing diagnoses.

Diagnostic Studies   ∞ Pediatric/Geriatric/Lifespan   Medications

Answers to these questions help identify specific problems needing to be addressed.

• Ascertain role expectations of family members. Who is the ill member (e.g., nurturer, provider)? How does the illness affect the roles of others?

• Identify "family rules." For example, how adult concerns (finances, illness, etc.) are kept from the children.

• Determine effectiveness of parenting skills and parents' expectations.

• Note energy direction. Are efforts at resolution/problem solving purposeful or scattered?

• Listen for expressions of despair/helplessness (e.g., "I don't know what to do") **to note degree of distress and inability to handle what is happening.**

• Note cultural and/or religious factors **that may affect perceptions/expectations of family members.**

• Assess availability/use of support systems outside of the family.

NURSING PRIORITY NO. 2. To assist family to deal with situation/crisis:

• Deal with family members in warm, caring, respectful way.

• Acknowledge difficulties and realities of the situation. **Reinforces that some degree of conflict is to be expected and can be used to promote growth.**

• Encourage expressions of anger. Avoid taking comments personally as the client is usually only angry at the situation over which he or she has little or no control. **Maintains boundaries between nurse and family.**

• Stress importance of continuous, open dialogue between family members **to facilitate ongoing problem solving.**

• Provide information, as necessary, in verbal and written formats. Reinforce, as necessary.

• Assist family to identify and encourage their use of previously successful coping behaviors.

• Recommend contact by family members on a regular, frequent basis.

• Arrange for/encourage family participation in multidisciplinary team conference/group therapy, as appropriate.

• Involve family in social support and community activities of their interest and choice.

NURSING PRIORITY NO. 3. To promote wellness (Teaching/Discharge Considerations):

• Encourage use of stress-management techniques (e.g., appropriate expression of feelings, relaxation exercises).

Information in brackets added by the authors to clarify and enhance the use of nursing diagnoses.

    Cultural   Collaborative   Community/Home Care

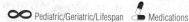

- Provide educational materials and information **to assist family members in resolution of current crisis.**
- Refer to classes (e.g., parent effectiveness, specific disease/disability support groups, self-help groups, clergy, psychological counseling/family therapy), as indicated.
- Assist family to identify situations that may lead to fear/anxiety. (Refer to NDs Fear; Anxiety.)
- Involve family in planning for future and mutual goal setting. **Promotes commitment to goals/continuation of plan.**
- Identify community agencies (e.g., Meals on Wheels, visiting nurse, trauma support group, American Cancer Society, Veterans Administration) for both immediate and long-term support.

Documentation Focus

ASSESSMENT/REASSESSMENT

- Assessment findings, including family composition, developmental stage of family, and role expectations.
- Family communication patterns.

PLANNING

- Plan of care/interventions and who is involved in planning.
- Teaching plan.

IMPLEMENTATION/EVALUATION

- Each individual's response to interventions/teaching and actions performed.
- Attainment/progress toward desired outcome(s).
- Modifications to plan of care.

DISCHARGE PLANNING

- Long-range needs, noting who is responsible for actions to be taken.
- Specific referrals made.

SAMPLE NURSING OUTCOMES & INTERVENTIONS CLASSIFICATIONS (NOC/NIC)

NOC—Family Functioning
NIC—Family Process Maintenance

Information in brackets added by the authors to clarify and enhance the use of nursing diagnoses.

readiness for enhanced Family Processes

Taxonomy II: Role Relationships—Class 2 Family Relationships (00159)
[Diagnostic Division: Social Interaction]
Submitted 2002

Definition: A pattern of family functioning that is sufficient to support the well-being of family members and can be strengthened

Defining Characteristics

SUBJECTIVE

Expresses willingness to enhance family dynamics
Communication is adequate
Relationships are generally positive; interdependent with community; family tasks are accomplished
Energy level of family supports activities of daily living
Family adapts to change

OBJECTIVE

Family functioning meets needs of family members
Activities support the safety/growth of family members
Family roles are appropriate/flexible for developmental stages
Family resilience is evident
Respect for family members is evident
Boundaries of family members are maintained
Balance exists between autonomy and cohesiveness

Desired Outcomes/Evaluation Criteria—Client Will:

- Express feelings freely and appropriately.
- Verbalize understanding of desire for enhanced family dynamics.
- Demonstrate individual involvement in problem solving to improve family communications.
- Acknowledge awareness of and respect for boundaries of family members.

Actions/Interventions

NURSING PRIORITY NO. 1. To determine status of family:

 • Determine family composition: parent(s), children, male/female, extended family. **Many family forms exist in society**

Information in brackets added by the authors to clarify and enhance the use of nursing diagnoses.

 Cultural Collaborative 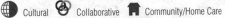 Community/Home Care

today, such as biological, nuclear, single-parent, step-family, communal, and same-sex couple or family. A better way to determine a family may be to determine the attribute of affection, strong emotional ties, a sense of belonging, and durability of membership.

- Identify participating members of family and how they define family. **Establishes members of family who need to be directly involved/taken into consideration when developing plan of care to improve family functioning.**

- Note stage of family development (e.g., single, young adult, newly married, family with young children, family with adolescents, grown children, later in life).

- Ascertain motivation/expectations for change.

- Observe patterns of communication in the family. Are feelings expressed? Freely? Who talks to whom? Who makes decisions? For whom? Who visits? When? What is the interaction between family members? **Identifies possible weaknesses to be addressed, as well as strengths that can be used for improving family communication.**

- Assess boundaries of family members. Do members share family identity and have little sense of individuality? Do they seem emotionally connected with one another? **Individuals need to respect one another and boundaries need to be clear so family members are free to be responsible for themselves.**

- Identify "family rules" that are accepted in the family. **Families interact in certain ways over time and develop patterns of behavior that are accepted as the way "we behave" in this family. "Functional family" rules are constructive and promote the needs of all family members.**

- Note energy direction. **Efforts at problem solving and resolution of different opinions may be purposeful or may be scattered and ineffective.**

- Determine cultural and/or religious factors influencing family interactions. **Expectations related to socioeconomic beliefs may be different in various cultures. For instance, traditional views of marriage and family life may be strongly influenced by Roman Catholicism in Italian-American and Latino-American families. In some cultures, the father is considered the authority figure and the mother is the homemaker. These beliefs may change with stressors/circumstances (e.g., financial, loss/gain of a family member, personal growth).**

- Note health of married individuals. **Recent reports have determined that marriage increases life expectancy by as much as five years.**

Information in brackets added by the authors to clarify and enhance the use of nursing diagnoses.

NURSING PRIORITY NO. 2. To assist the family to improve interactions:

• Establish nurse-family relationship. **Promotes a warm, caring atmosphere in which family members can share thoughts, ideas, and feelings openly and nonjudgmentally.**

• Acknowledge realities, and possible difficulties, of individual situation. **Reinforces that some degree of conflict is to be expected in family interactions that can be used to promote growth.**

 • Stress importance of continuous, open dialogue between family members. **Facilitates ongoing expression of open, honest feelings and opinions and effective problem solving.**

 • Assist family to identify and encourage use of previously successful coping behaviors. **Promotes recognition of previous successes and confidence in own abilities to learn and improve family interactions.**

 • Acknowledge differences among family members with open dialogue about how these differences have occurred. **Conveys an acceptance of these differences among individuals and helps to look at how they can be used to strengthen the family.**

 • Identify effective parenting skills already being used and additional ways of handling difficult behaviors. **Allows individual family members to realize that some of what has been done already has been helpful and encourages them to learn new skills to manage family interactions in a more effective manner.**

NURSING PRIORITY NO. 3. To promote optimum well-being:

 • Discuss and encourage use and participation in stress-management techniques. **Relaxation exercises, visualization, and similar skills can be useful for promoting reduction of anxiety and ability to manage stress that occurs in their lives.**

 • Encourage participation in learning role-reversal activities. **Helps individuals to gain insight and understanding of other person's feelings and perspective/point of view.**

 • Involve family members in setting goals and planning for the future. **When individuals are involved in the decision making, they are more committed to carrying out a plan to enhance family interactions as life goes on.**

 • Provide educational materials and information. **Enhances learning to assist in developing positive relationships among family members.**

 • Assist family members to identify situations that may create problems and lead to stress/anxiety. **Thinking ahead can help individuals anticipate helpful actions to handle/prevent conflict and untoward consequences.**

Information in brackets added by the authors to clarify and enhance the use of nursing diagnoses.

      Cultural   Collaborative   Community/Home Care

• Refer to classes/support groups, as appropriate. **Family effectiveness, self-help, psychology, and religious affiliations can
provide role models and new information to enhance family interactions.**

Documentation Focus

ASSESSMENT/REASSESSMENT

• Assessment findings, including family composition, develop-
mental stage of family, and role expectations.
• Cultural/religious values and beliefs regarding family and
family functioning.
• Family communication patterns.
• Motivation and expectations for change.

PLANNING

• Plan of care/interventions and who is involved in planning.
• Educational plan.

IMPLEMENTATION/EVALUATION

• Each individual's response to interventions/teaching and
actions performed.
• Attainment/progress toward desired outcome(s).
• Modifications to lifestyle/treatment plan.

DISCHARGE PLANNING

• Long-range needs, noting who is responsible for actions to be
taken.
• Specific referrals made.

SAMPLE NURSING OUTCOMES & INTERVENTIONS CLASSIFICATIONS (NOC/NIC)

NOC—Family Social Climate
NIC—Family Support

Fatigue

Taxonomy II: Activity/Rest—Class 3 Energy Balance
(00093)
[Diagnostic Division: Activity/Rest]
Submitted 1988; Nursing Diagnosis Extension and
Classification (NDEC) Revision 1998

Definition: An overwhelming sustained sense of
exhaustion and decreased capacity for physical and
mental work at usual level

Information in brackets added by the authors to clarify and enhance
the use of nursing diagnoses.

Related Factors

PSYCHOLOGICAL

Stress; anxiety; boring lifestyle; depression

ENVIRONMENTAL

Noise; lights; humidity; temperature

SITUATIONAL

Occupation; negative life events

PHYSIOLOGICAL

Increased physical exertion; sleep deprivation
Pregnancy; disease states; malnutrition; anemia
Poor physical condition
[Altered body chemistry (e.g., medications, drug withdrawal, chemotherapy)]

Defining Characteristics

SUBJECTIVE

Verbalization of an unremitting/overwhelming lack of energy; inability to maintain usual routines/level of physical activity
Perceived need for additional energy to accomplish routine tasks; increase in rest requirements
Tired; inability to restore energy even after sleep
Feelings of guilt for not keeping up with responsibilities
Compromised libido
Increase in physical complaints

OBJECTIVE

Lethargic; listless; drowsy; lack of energy
Compromised concentration
Disinterest in surroundings; introspection
Decreased performance [accident-prone]

Desired Outcomes/Evaluation
Criteria—Client Will:

- Report improved sense of energy.
- Identify basis of fatigue and individual areas of control.
- Perform ADLs and participate in desired activities at level of ability.
- Participate in recommended treatment program.

Information in brackets added by the authors to clarify and enhance the use of nursing diagnoses.

  Cultural Collaborative Community/Home Care

Actions/Interventions

NURSING PRIORITY NO. **1.** To assess causative/contributing factors:

- Identify presence of physical and/or psychological conditions (e.g., pregnancy; infectious processes; blood loss/anemia; connective tissue disorders [e.g., multiple sclerosis, lupus]; trauma/chronic pain syndromes [e.g., arthritis]; cardiopulmonary disorders; cancer and cancer treatments; hepatitis; AIDS; major depressive disorder; anxiety states; substance use/abuse).
- Note age, gender, and developmental stage. **Although some studies show a prevalence of fatigue in adolescent girls, the condition may be present in any person at any age.**
- Review medication regimen/use. **Certain medications, including prescription (especially beta-adrenergic blockers, chemotherapy), over-the-counter, herbal supplements, and combinations of drugs and/or substances, are known to cause and/or exacerbate fatigue.**
- Ascertain client's belief about what is causing the fatigue.
- Assess vital signs **to evaluate fluid status and cardiopulmonary response to activity.**
- Determine presence/degree of sleep disturbances. **Fatigue can be a consequence of, and/or exacerbated by, sleep deprivation.**
- Note recent lifestyle changes, including conflicts (e.g., expanded responsibilities/demands of others, job-related conflicts); maturational issues (e.g., adolescent with eating disorder); and developmental issues (e.g., new parenthood, loss of spouse/SO).
- Assess psychological and personality factors that may affect reports of fatigue level.
- Evaluate aspect of "learned helplessness" that may be manifested by giving up. **Can perpetuate a cycle of fatigue, impaired functioning, and increased anxiety and fatigue.**

NURSING PRIORITY NO. **2.** To determine degree of fatigue/impact on life:

- Obtain client/SO descriptions of fatigue (i.e., lacking energy or strength, tiredness, weakness lasting over length of time). Note presence of additional concerns (e.g., irritability, lack of concentration, difficulty making decisions, problems with leisure, relationship difficulties) **to assist in evaluating impact on client's life**.
- Ask client to rate fatigue (1–10 scale) and its effects on ability to participate in desired activities.

Information in brackets added by the authors to clarify and enhance the use of nursing diagnoses.

 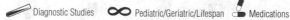

- Discuss lifestyle changes/limitations imposed by fatigue state.
- Interview parent/caregiver regarding specific changes observed in child/elder. **These individuals may not be able to verbalize feelings or relate meaningful information.**
- Note daily energy patterns (i.e., peaks/valleys). **Helpful in determining pattern/timing of activity.**

 Measure physiological response to activity (e.g., changes in blood pressure or heart/respiratory rate).

 Evaluate need for individual assistance/assistive devices.

 Review availability and current use of support systems/resources.

- Perform/review results of testing, such as the Multidimensional Assessment of Fatigue (MAF); Piper Fatigue Scale; Global Fatigue Index, as appropriate. **Can help determine manifestation, intensity, duration, and emotional meaning of fatigue.**

NURSING PRIORITY NO. 3. To assist client to cope with fatigue and manage within individual limits of ability:

 Accept reality of client reports of fatigue and do not underestimate effect on client's quality of life. **For example, clients with MS are prone to more frequent/severe fatigue following minimal energy expenditure and require a longer recovery period than is usual; post-polio clients often display a cumulative effect if they fail to pace themselves and rest when early signs of fatigue develop.**

 Establish realistic activity goals with client and encourage forward movement. **Enhances commitment to promoting optimal outcomes.**

 Plan interventions to allow individually adequate rest periods. Schedule activities for periods when client has the most energy **to maximize participation.**

 Involve client/SO(s) in schedule planning.

 Encourage client to do whatever possible (e.g., self-care, sit up in chair, go for walk, interact with family, play game). Increase activity level, as tolerated.

 Instruct in methods to conserve energy:
   Sit instead of stand during daily care/other activities.
   Carry several small loads instead of one large load.
   Combine and simplify activities.
   Take frequent short rest breaks during activities.
   Delegate tasks.
   Ask for/accept assistance.
   Say "no" or "later."
   Plan steps of activity before beginning so that all needed materials are at hand.

Information in brackets added by the authors to clarify and enhance the use of nursing diagnoses.

  Cultural Collaborative Community/Home Care

- Encourage use of assistive devices (e.g., wheeled walker, handicap parking spot, elevator, backpack for carrying objects), as needed, **to extend active time/conserve energy for other tasks**.
- Assist with self-care needs; keep bed in low position and travelways clear of furniture; assist with ambulation, as indicated.
- Avoid/limit exposure to temperature and humidity extremes, **which can negatively impact energy level.**
- Provide diversional activities. Avoid overstimulation/understimulation (cognitive and sensory). **Participating in pleasurable activities can refocus energy and diminish feelings of unhappiness, sluggishness, and worthlessness that can accompany fatigue.**
- Discuss routines to promote restful sleep. (Refer to ND Insomnia)
- Encourage nutritionally dense, easy to prepare/consume foods and to avoid caffeine and high sugar foods/drinks **to promote energy.**
- Instruct in/implement stress-management skills of visualization, relaxation, and biofeedback, when appropriate.
- Refer to comprehensive rehabilitation program, physical/occupational therapy for programmed daily exercises and activities **to improve stamina, strength, and muscle tone and to enhance sense of well-being.**

NURSING PRIORITY NO. 4. To promote wellness (Teaching/Discharge Considerations):

- Discuss therapy regimen relating to individual causative factors (e.g., physical and/or psychological illnesses) and help client/SO(s) to understand relationship of fatigue to illness.
- Assist client/SO(s) to develop plan for activity and exercise within individual ability. Stress necessity of allowing sufficient time to finish activities.
- Instruct client in ways to monitor responses to activity and significant signs/symptoms **that indicate the need to alter activity level.**
- Promote overall health measures (e.g., nutrition, adequate fluid intake, appropriate vitamin/iron supplementation).
- Provide supplemental oxygen, as indicated. **Presence of anemia/hypoxemia reduces oxygen available for cellular uptake and contributes to fatigue.**
- Encourage client to develop assertiveness skills, to prioritize goals/activities, to learn to delegate duties/tasks, or to say "No." Discuss burnout syndrome, when appropriate, and actions client can take to change individual situation.

Information in brackets added by the authors to clarify and enhance the use of nursing diagnoses.

Diagnostic Studies   Pediatric/Geriatric/Lifespan   Medications   **311**

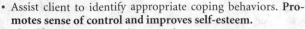

- Assist client to identify appropriate coping behaviors. **Promotes sense of control and improves self-esteem.**
- Identify support groups/community resources.
- Refer to counseling/psychotherapy, as indicated.
- Identify resources to assist with routine needs (e.g., Meals on Wheels, homemaker/housekeeper services, yard care).

Documentation Focus

ASSESSMENT/REASSESSMENT

- Manifestations of fatigue and other assessment findings.
- Degree of impairment/effect on lifestyle.
- Expectations of client/SO(s) relative to individual abilities/specific condition.

PLANNING

- Plan of care/interventions and who is involved in the planning.
- Teaching plan.

IMPLEMENTATION/EVALUATION

- Client's response to interventions/teaching and actions performed.
- Attainment/progress toward desired outcome(s).
- Modifications to plan of care.

DISCHARGE PLANNING

- Discharge needs/plan, actions to be taken, and who is responsible.
- Specific referrals made.

SAMPLE NURSING OUTCOMES & INTERVENTIONS CLASSIFICATIONS (NOC/NIC)

NOC—Endurance
NIC—Energy Management

Fear
[Specify Focus]

Taxonomy II: Coping/Stress Tolerance—Class 2 Coping
  Responses (00148)
[Diagnostic Division: Ego Integrity]
Submitted 1980; Revised 2000

Definition: Response to perceived threat [real or imagined] that is consciously recognized as a danger

Information in brackets added by the authors to clarify and enhance the use of nursing diagnoses.

 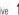

Related Factors

Innate origin (e.g., sudden noise, height, pain, loss of physical support); innate releasers (neurotransmitters); phobic stimulus

Learned response (e.g., conditioning, modeling from or identification with others)

Unfamiliarity with environmental experience(s)

Separation from support system in potentially stressful situation (e.g., hospitalization, hospital procedures [/treatments])

Language barrier; sensory impairment

Defining Characteristics

SUBJECTIVE

Report of apprehension; excitement; being scared; alarm; panic; terror; dread; decreased self-assurance; increased tension; jitteriness

Cognitive: Identifies object of fear; stimulus believed to be a threat

Physiological: Anorexia; nausea; fatigue; dry mouth; [palpitations]

OBJECTIVE

Cognitive: Diminished productivity/learning ability/problem solving

Behaviors: Increased alertness; avoidance[/flight]; attack behaviors; impulsiveness; narrowed focus on the source of the fear)

Physiological: Increased pulse; vomiting; diarrhea; muscle tightness; increased respiratory rate; dyspnea; increased systolic blood pressure; pallor; increased perspiration; pupil dilation

Desired Outcomes/Evaluation
Criteria—Client Will:

• Acknowledge and discuss fears, recognizing healthy versus unhealthy fears.

• Verbalize accurate knowledge of/sense of safety related to current situation.

• Demonstrate understanding through use of effective coping behaviors (e.g., problem solving) and resources.

• Display appropriate range of feelings and lessened fear.

Actions/Interventions

NURSING PRIORITY NO. 1. To assess degree of fear and reality of threat perceived by the client:

Information in brackets added by the authors to clarify and enhance the use of nursing diagnoses.

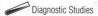 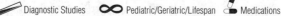

FEAR

- Ascertain client's/SO's perception of what is occurring and how this affects life. **Fear is a defensive mechanism in protecting oneself but, if left unchecked, can become disabling to the client's life.**

- Determine client's age/developmental level. **Helps in understanding usual/typical fears experienced by individuals (e.g., toddler often has different fears than adolescent or older person suffering with dementia).**

- Note degree of incapacitation (e.g., "frozen with fear," inability to engage in necessary activities).

- Compare verbal/nonverbal responses **to note congruencies or misperceptions of situation.**

- Be alert to signs of denial/depression.

- Identify sensory deficits that may be present, such as vision/hearing impairment. **Affects sensory reception and interpretation of environment.**

- Note degree of concentration, focus of attention.

- Investigate client's reports of subjective experiences, which could be indicative of delusions/hallucinations, **to help determine client's interpretation of surroundings and/or stimuli.**

- Be alert to and evaluate potential for violence.

- Measure vital signs/physiological responses to situation.

- Assess family dynamics. Refer to other NDs, such as interrupted Family Processes; readiness for enhanced family Coping; compromised/disabled family Coping; Anxiety.

NURSING PRIORITY NO. 2. To assist client/SO(s) in dealing with fear/situation:

- Stay with the client or make arrangements to have someone else be there. **Providing client with usual/desired support persons can diminish feelings of fear.**

- Discuss client's perceptions/fearful feelings. Listen/active-listen to client's concerns. **Promotes atmosphere of caring and permits explanation/correction of misperceptions.**

- Provide information in verbal and written form. Speak in simple sentences and concrete terms. **Facilitates understanding and retention of information.**

- Acknowledge normalcy of fear, pain, despair, and give "permission" to express feelings appropriately/freely. **Promotes attitude of caring, opens door for discussion about feelings and/or addressing reality of situation.**

- Provide opportunity for questions and answer honestly. **Enhances sense of trust and nurse-client relationship.**

- Provide presence/physical contact (e.g., hugging, refocusing attention, rocking a child), as appropriate, when painful procedures are anticipated **to soothe fears and provide assurance.**

Information in brackets added by the authors to clarify and enhance the use of nursing diagnoses.

 Cultural Collaborative   Community/Home Care

∞ • Modify procedures, if possible (e.g., substitute oral for intra-muscular medications, combine blood draws/use fingerstick method), **to limit degree of stress, avoid overwhelming a fearful individual.**

∞ • Manage environmental factors, such as loud noises, harsh lighting, changing person's location without knowledge of family/SO(s), strangers in care area/unfamiliar people, high traffic flow, **which can cause/exacerbate stress, especially to very young or to older individuals.**

🏠 • Present objective information, when available, and allow client to use it freely. Avoid arguing about client's perceptions of the situation. **Limits conflicts when fear response may impair rational thinking.**

🏠 • Promote client control, where possible, and help client identify and accept those things over which control is not possible. **Strengthens internal locus of control.**

🏠 • Encourage contact with a peer who has successfully dealt with a similarly fearful situation. **Provides a role model and client is more likely to believe others who have had similar experience(s).**

NURSING PRIORITY NO. 3. To assist client in learning to use own responses for problem solving:

🏠 • Acknowledge usefulness of fear for taking care of self.

🏠 • Identify client's responsibility for the solutions while reinforcing that the nurse will be available for help if desired/needed. **Enhances sense of control.**

🏠 • Determine internal/external resources for assistance (e.g., awareness/use of effective coping skills in the past; SOs who are available for support).

🏠 • Explain procedures within level of client's ability to understand and handle. (Be aware of how much information client wants **to prevent confusion/overload.**)

🏠 • Explain relationship between disease and symptoms, if appropriate.

💊 • Review use of antianxiety medications and reinforce use as prescribed.

NURSING PRIORITY NO. 4. To promote wellness (Teaching/Discharge Considerations):

🏠 • Support planning for dealing with reality. **Assists in identifying areas in which control can be exercised and those in which control is not possible, thus enabling client to handle fearful situations/feelings.**

🏠 • Instruct in use of relaxation/visualization and guided imagery skills.

Information in brackets added by the authors to clarify and enhance the use of nursing diagnoses.

- Encourage regular physical activity. Assist client/refer to physical therapist to develop exercise program (within limits of ability). **Provides a healthy outlet for energy generated by fearful feelings and promotes relaxation.**
- Provide for/deal with sensory deficits in appropriate manner (e.g., speak clearly and distinctly, use touch carefully, as indicated by situation).
- Refer to support groups, community agencies/organizations, as indicated. **Provides ongoing assistance for individual needs.**

Documentation Focus

ASSESSMENT/REASSESSMENT

- Assessment findings, noting individual factors contributing to current situation, source of fear.
- Manifestations of fear.

PLANNING

- Plan of care and who is involved in the planning.
- Teaching plan.

IMPLEMENTATION/EVALUATION

- Client's responses to treatment plan/interventions and actions performed.
- Attainment/progress toward desired outcome(s).
- Modifications to plan of care.

DISCHARGE PLANNING

- Long-term needs and who is responsible for actions to be taken.
- Specific referrals made.

SAMPLE NURSING OUTCOMES & INTERVENTIONS CLASSIFICATIONS (NOC/NIC)

NOC—Fear Self-Control
NIC—Anxiety Reduction

---

readiness for enhanced Fluid Balance

Taxonomy II: Nutrition—Class 5 Hydration (00160)
[Diagnostic Division: Food/Fluid]
Submitted 2002

Definition: A pattern of equilibrium between fluid volume and chemical composition of body fluids that is sufficient for meeting physical needs and can be strengthened

---

Information in brackets added by the authors to clarify and enhance the use of nursing diagnoses.

Related Factors

To be developed

Defining Characteristics

SUBJECTIVE

Expresses willingness to enhance fluid balance
No excessive thirst

OBJECTIVE

Stable weight; no evidence of edema
Moist mucous membranes
Intake adequate for daily needs
Straw-colored urine; specific gravity within normal limits; urine output appropriate for intake
Good tissue turgor; [no signs of] dehydration

Desired Outcomes/Evaluation Criteria—Client Will:

- Maintain fluid volume at a functional level as indicated by adequate urinary output, stable vital signs, moist mucous membranes, good skin turgor.
- Demonstrate behaviors to monitor fluid balance.
- Be free of thirst.
- Be free of evidence of fluid overload (e.g., absence of edema and adventitious lung sounds).

Actions/Interventions

NURSING PRIORITY NO. 1. To determine potential for fluid imbalance and ways that client is managing:

- Note presence of factors with potential for fluid imbalance: 1) diagnoses/disease processes (e.g., hyperglycemia, ulcerative colitis, COPD, burns, cirrhosis of the liver, vomiting, diarrhea, hemorrhage), or situations (e.g., diuretic therapy, hot/humid climate, prolonged exercise, getting overheated/fever, diuretic effect of caffeine/alcohol) that may lead to deficits; or 2) conditions/situations potentiating fluid excess (e.g., renal failure, cardiac failure, stroke, cerebral lesions, renal/adrenal insufficiency, psychogenic polydipsia, acute stress, surgical/anesthetic procedures, excessive or rapid infusion of IV fluids). **Body fluid balance is regulated by intake (food and fluid), output (kidney, gastrointestinal tract, skin, and lungs), and regulatory hormonal mechanisms. Balance is maintained**

Information in brackets added by the authors to clarify and enhance the use of nursing diagnoses.

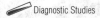 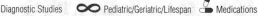

readiness for enhanced FLUID BALANCE

within a relatively narrow margin and can be easily disrupted by multiple factors.

- Determine potential effects of age and developmental stage. **Elderly individuals have less body water than younger adults, decreased thirst response, and reduced effectiveness of compensatory mechanisms (e.g., kidneys are less efficient in conserving sodium and water). Infants and children have a relatively higher percentage of total body water and metabolic rate and are often less able than adults to control their fluid intake.**

 • Evaluate environmental factors that could impact fluid balance. **Persons with impaired mobility, diminished vision, or confined to bed cannot as easily meet their own needs and may be reluctant to ask for assistance. Persons whose work environment is restrictive or outside may also have greater challenges in meeting fluid needs.**

- Assess vital signs (e.g., temperature, blood pressure, heart rate), skin/mucous membrane moisture, and urine output. Weigh, as indicated. **Predictors of fluid balance that should be in client's usual range in a healthy state.**

NURSING PRIORITY NO. 2. To prevent occurrence of imbalance:

- Monitor I/O (e.g., frequency of voids/diaper changes), as appropriate, being aware of insensible losses (e.g., diaphoresis in hot environment, use of oxygen/permanent tracheostomy), and "hidden sources" of intake (e.g., foods high in water content) **to ensure accurate picture of fluid status.**

- Weigh client and compare with recent weight history. **Provides baseline for future monitoring.**

 • Establish and review with client individual fluid needs/ replacement schedule. **Active participation in planning for own needs enhances likelihood of adhering to plan.**

 • Encourage regular oral intake (e.g., fluids between meals, additional fluids during hot weather or when exercising) **to maximize intake and maintain fluid balance.**

 • Distribute fluids over 24-hour period in presence of fluid restriction. **Prevents peaks/valleys in fluid level and associated thirst.**

- Administer/discuss judicious use of medications, as indicated (e.g., antiemetics, antidiarrheals, antipyretics, and diuretics). **Medications may be indicated to prevent fluid imbalance if individual becomes sick.**

NURSING PRIORITY NO. 3. To promote optimum wellness:

 • Discuss client's individual conditions/factors that could cause occurrence of fluid imbalance, as individually appropriate

---

Information in brackets added by the authors to clarify and enhance the use of nursing diagnoses.

(such as prevention of hyperglycemic episodes) **so that client/SO can take corrective action.**

🏠 • Identify and instruct in ways to meet specific fluid needs (e.g., client could carry water bottle when going to sports events or measure specific 24-hour fluid portions if restrictions apply) **to manage fluid intake over time.**

🏠 • Recommend restriction of caffeine, alcohol, as indicated. **Prevents untoward diuretic effect and possible dehydration.**

🏠 • Instruct client/SO(s) in how to measure and record I/O, if needed for home management. **Provides means of monitoring status and adjusting therapy to meet changing needs.**

🏠 • Establish regular schedule for weighing **to help monitor changes in fluid status.**

🏠 • Identify actions (if any) client may take to correct imbalance. **Encourages responsibility for self-care.**

🏠 • Review any dietary needs/restrictions and safe substitutes for salt, as appropriate. **Helps prevent fluid retention/edema formation.**

💊 • Review/instruct in medication regimen and administration and discuss potential for interactions/side effects that could disrupt fluid balance.

🔎 • Instruct in signs and symptoms indicating need for immediate/further evaluation and follow-up care **to prevent complications and/or allow for early intervention.**

Documentation Focus

ASSESSMENT/REASSESSMENT

• Individual findings, including factors affecting ability to manage (regulate) body fluids.
• I/O, fluid balance, changes in weight, and vital signs.

PLANNING

• Plan of care and who is involved in the planning.
• Teaching plan.

IMPLEMENTATION/EVALUATION

• Client's responses to treatment/teaching and actions performed.
• Attainment/progress toward desired outcome(s).
• Modifications to plan of care.

DISCHARGE PLANNING

• Long-term needs, noting who is responsible for actions to be taken.
• Specific referrals made.

Information in brackets added by the authors to clarify and enhance the use of nursing diagnoses.

SAMPLE NURSING OUTCOMES & INTERVENTIONS CLASSIFICATIONS (NOC/NIC)

NOC—Fluid Balance
NIC—Fluid Monitoring

[deficient Fluid Volume: hyper/hypotonic]

NOTE: NANDA has restricted Fluid Volume, deficient, to address only isotonic dehydration. For client needs related to dehydration associated with alterations in sodium, the authors have provided this second diagnostic category.

[Diagnostic Division: Food/Fluid]

Definition: [Decreased intravascular, interstitial, and/or intracellular fluid. This refers to dehydration with changes in sodium.]

Related Factors

[Hypertonic dehydration: uncontrolled diabetes mellitus/ insipidus, HHNC, increased intake of hypertonic fluids/IV therapy, inability to respond to thirst reflex/inadequate free water supplementation (high-osmolarity enteral feeding formulas), renal insufficiency/failure]

[Hypotonic dehydration: chronic illness/malnutrition, excessive use of hypotonic IV solutions (e.g., D5W), renal insufficiency]

Defining Characteristics

SUBJECTIVE

[Reports of fatigue, nervousness, exhaustion]
[Thirst]

OBJECTIVE

[Increased urine output, dilute urine (initially) and/or decreased output/oliguria]
[Weight loss]
[Decreased venous filling]; [hypotension (postural)]
[Increased pulse rate; decreased pulse volume and pressure]
[Decreased skin turgor]; [dry skin/mucous membranes]
[Increased body temperature]
[Change in mental status (e.g., confusion)]
[Hemoconcentration; altered serum sodium]

Information in brackets added by the authors to clarify and enhance the use of nursing diagnoses.

 Cultural   Collaborative   Community/Home Care

Desired Outcomes/Evaluation Criteria—Client Will:

- Maintain fluid volume at a functional level as evidenced by individually adequate urinary output, stable vital signs, moist mucous membranes, good skin turgor.
- Verbalize understanding of causative factors and purpose of individual therapeutic interventions and medications.
- Demonstrate behaviors to monitor and correct deficit, as indicated, when condition is chronic.

Actions/Interventions

NURSING PRIORITY NO. 1. To assess causative/precipitating factors:

- Note possible conditions/processes that may lead to deficits: 1) fluid loss (e.g., diarrhea/vomiting, excessive sweating; heat stroke; diabetic ketoacidosis; burns, other draining wounds; gastrointestinal obstruction; salt-wasting diuretics; rapid breathing/mechanical ventilation; surgical drains); 2) limited intake (e.g., sore throat or mouth; client dependent on others for eating/drinking; NPO status); 3) fluid shifts (e.g., ascites, effusions, burns, sepsis); and 4) environmental factors (e.g., isolation, restraints, malfunctioning air conditioning, exposure to extreme heat).

 - Determine effects of age. **Very young and extremely elderly individuals are quickly affected by fluid volume deficit, and are least able to express need. For example, elderly people often have a decreased thirst reflex and/or may not be aware of water needs. Infants/young children and other nonverbal persons cannot describe thirst.**

- Evaluate nutritional status, noting current intake, weight changes, problems with oral intake, use of supplements/tube feedings. Measure subcutaneous fat/muscle mass.

NURSING PRIORITY NO. 2. To evaluate degree of fluid deficit:

- Assess vital signs, including temperature (often elevated), pulse (may be elevated), and respirations. Note strength of peripheral pulses.
- Measure blood pressure (may be low) with the client lying/sitting/standing, when possible, and monitor invasive hemodynamic parameters, as indicated (e.g., CVP, PAP/PCWP).
- Note presence of physical signs (e.g., dry mucous membranes, poor skin turgor, delayed capillary refill).
- Note change in usual mentation/behavior/functional abilities (e.g., confusion, falling, loss of ability to carry out usual

---

Information in brackets added by the authors to clarify and enhance the use of nursing diagnoses.

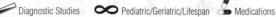

activities, lethargy, dizziness). **These signs indicate sufficient dehydration to cause poor cerebral perfusion and/or electrolyte imbalance.**

- Observe urinary output, color, and measure amount and specific gravity. Measure or estimate other fluid losses (e.g., gastric, respiratory, wound losses) **to more accurately determine replacement needs.**
- Review laboratory data (e.g., Hb/Hct; electrolytes [sodium, potassium, chloride, bicarbonate]; blood urea nitrogen [BUN]; creatinine; total protein/albumin).

NURSING PRIORITY NO. 3. To correct/replace fluid losses to reverse pathophysiological mechanisms:

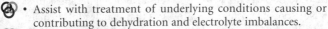

- Assist with treatment of underlying conditions causing or contributing to dehydration and electrolyte imbalances.
- Administer fluids and electrolytes, as indicated. **Fluids used for replacement depend on 1) the type of dehydration present (e.g., hypertonic/hypotonic), and 2) the degree of deficit determined by age, weight, and type of condition causing the deficit.**
- Establish 24-hour replacement needs and routes to be used (e.g., IV/PO, enteral feedings). **Steady rehydration over time prevents peaks/valleys in fluid level.**
- Note client preferences, and provide beverages and foods with high fluid content.
- Limit intake of alcohol/caffeinated beverages **that tend to exert a diuretic effect.**
- Provide nutritious diet via appropriate route; give adequate free water with enteral feedings.
- Maintain accurate intake and output (I/O), calculate 24-hour fluid balance, and weigh daily.

NURSING PRIORITY NO. 4. To promote comfort and safety:

- Bathe less frequently using mild cleanser/soap, and provide optimal skin care with suitable emollients **to maintain skin integrity and prevent excessive dryness.**
- Provide frequent oral and eye care **to prevent injury from dryness.**
- Change position frequently.
- Provide for safety measures when client is confused.
- Replace electrolytes, as ordered.
- Administer or discontinue medications, as indicated, **when disease process or medications are contributing to dehydration.**

Information in brackets added by the authors to clarify and enhance the use of nursing diagnoses.

   Cultural   Collaborative   Community/Home Care

NURSING PRIORITY NO. 5. To promote wellness (Teaching/Discharge Considerations):

- Discuss factors related to occurrence of deficit, as individually appropriate. **Early identification of risk factors can decrease occurrence and severity of complications associated with hypovolemia.**
- Identify and instruct in ways to meet specific nutritional needs.
- Instruct client/SO(s) in how to measure and record I/O, monitor fluid status.
- Identify actions (if any) client may take to correct deficiencies.
- Review/instruct in medication regimen and administration and interactions/side effects.
- Instruct in signs and symptoms indicating need for immediate/further evaluation and follow-up care.

Documentation Focus

ASSESSMENT/REASSESSMENT

- Individual findings, including factors affecting ability to manage (regulate) body fluids and degree of deficit.
- I/O, fluid balance, changes in weight, urine specific gravity, and vital signs.
- Results of diagnostic testing/laboratory studies.

PLANNING

- Plan of care and who is involved in the planning.
- Teaching plan.

IMPLEMENTATION/EVALUATION

- Client's responses to treatment/teaching and actions performed.
- Attainment/progress toward desired outcome(s).
- Modifications to plan of care.

DISCHARGE PLANNING

- Long-term needs, noting who is responsible for actions to be taken.
- Specific referrals made.

SAMPLE NURSING OUTCOMES & INTERVENTIONS CLASSIFICATIONS (NOC/NIC)

NOC—Fluid Balance
NIC—Fluid/Electrolyte Management

Information in brackets added by the authors to clarify and enhance the use of nursing diagnoses.

 Diagnostic Studies 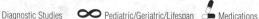 Pediatric/Geriatric/Lifespan Medications

deficient Fluid Volume
[Isotonic]

NOTE: This diagnosis has been structured to address isotonic dehydration (hypovolemia) excluding states in which changes in sodium occur. For client needs related to dehydration associated with alterations in sodium, refer to [deficient Fluid Volume: hyper/hypotonic].

Taxonomy II: Nutrition—Class 5 Hydration (00027)
[Diagnostic Division: Food/Fluid]
Submitted 1978; Revised 1996

Definition: Decreased intravascular, interstitial, and/or intracellular fluid. This refers to dehydration, water loss alone without change in sodium

Related Factors

Active fluid volume loss [e.g., hemorrhage, gastric intubation, acute/prolonged diarrhea, wounds, abdominal cancer; burns, fistulas, ascites (third spacing), use of hyperosmotic radiopaque contrast agents]
Failure of regulatory mechanisms [e.g., fever/thermoregulatory response, renal tubule damage]

Defining Characteristics

SUBJECTIVE

Thirst
Weakness

OBJECTIVE

Decreased urine output; increased urine concentration
Decreased venous filling; decreased pulse volume/pressure
Sudden weight loss (except in third spacing)
Decreased BP; increased pulse rate/body temperature
Decreased skin/tongue turgor; dry skin/mucous membranes
Change in mental state
Elevated Hct

Desired Outcomes/Evaluation
Criteria—Client Will:

• Maintain fluid volume at a functional level as evidenced by individually adequate urinary output with normal specific gravity, stable vital signs, moist mucous membranes, good skin turgor and prompt capillary refill, resolution of edema (e.g., ascites).

Information in brackets added by the authors to clarify and enhance the use of nursing diagnoses.

  Cultural Collaborative Community/Home Care

- Verbalize understanding of causative factors and purpose of individual therapeutic interventions and medications.
- Demonstrate behaviors to monitor and correct deficit, as indicated.

Actions/Interventions

NURSING PRIORITY NO. 1. To assess causative/precipitating factors:

- Note possible diagnoses that may create a fluid volume deficit (e.g., diarrhea, ulcerative colitis, burns, cirrhosis of the liver, abdominal cancer) and other factors (e.g., bleeding/drainage from wounds/fistulas or suction devices; hemorrhage; water deprivation/fluid restrictions; vomiting; dialysis; decreased level of consciousness; prolonged exercise; increased metabolic rate secondary to fever; hot/humid climate; overuse of diuretics/caffeine/alcohol.)
- Determine effects of age. **Elderly individuals are at higher risk because of decreasing response/effectiveness of compensatory mechanisms (e.g., kidneys are less efficient in conserving sodium and water). Infants and children have a relatively high percentage of total body water, are sensitive to loss, and are less able to control their fluid intake.**

NURSING PRIORITY NO. 2. To evaluate degree of fluid deficit:

- Estimate traumatic/procedural fluid losses and note possible routes of insensible fluid losses.
- Assess vital signs, noting low blood pressure/severe hypotension, rapid heart beat, and thready peripheral pulses.
- Note complaints and physical signs associated with dehydration (e.g., scanty/concentrated urine, lack of tears when crying [infant/child], dry/sticky mucous membranes, lack of sweating, delayed capillary refill, poor skin turgor, confusion, sleepiness/lethargy, muscle weakness, dizziness/lightheadedness, headache).
- Compare usual and current weight.
- Measure abdominal girth when ascites or third spacing of fluid occurs. Assess for peripheral edema formation.
- Review laboratory data (e.g., Hb/Hct, electrolytes, total protein/albumin, BUN/Cr).

NURSING PRIORITY NO. 3. To correct/replace losses to reverse pathophysiological mechanisms:

- Stop blood loss (e.g., gastric lavage with room temperature or cool saline solution, drug administration) and prepare for surgical intervention.

Information in brackets added by the authors to clarify and enhance the use of nursing diagnoses.

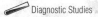

- Establish 24-hour fluid replacement needs and routes to be used. **Prevents peaks/valleys in fluid level.**
- Note client preferences regarding fluids and foods with high fluid content.
- Keep fluids within client's reach and encourage frequent intake, as appropriate.
 • Administer IV fluids, as indicated. Replace blood products/ plasma expanders, as ordered.
- Control humidity and ambient air temperature, as appropriate, especially when major burns are present; or increase/ decrease in presence of fever. Reduce bedding/clothes; provide tepid sponge bath. Assist with hypothermia, when ordered, **to reduce high fever and elevated metabolic rate.** (Refer to ND Hyperthermia.)
- Maintain accurate I/O and weigh daily. Monitor urine specific gravity.
- Monitor vital signs (lying/sitting/standing) and invasive hemodynamic parameters, as indicated (e.g., CVP, PAP/ PCWP).

NURSING PRIORITY NO. 4. To promote comfort and safety:
- Change position frequently.
- Bathe every other day, provide optimal skin care with emollients.
- Provide frequent oral as well as eye care **to prevent injury from dryness.**
- Change dressings frequently/use adjunct appliances, as indicated, for draining wounds **to protect skin and monitor losses.**
- Provide for safety measures when client is confused.
- Administer medications (**e.g., antiemetics or antidiarrheals to limit gastric/intestinal losses; antipyretics to reduce fever**).
- Refer to ND Diarrhea.

NURSING PRIORITY NO. 5. To promote wellness (Teaching/ Discharge Considerations):
- Discuss factors related to occurrence/ways client/SO(s) can prevent dehydration, as indicated.
- Assist client/SO(s) to learn to measure own I/O.
- Recommend restriction of caffeine, alcohol, as indicated.
- Review medications and interactions/side effects.
- Note signs/symptoms indicating need for emergent/further evaluation and follow-up care.

Information in brackets added by the authors to clarify and enhance the use of nursing diagnoses.

Documentation Focus

ASSESSMENT/REASSESSMENT

- Assessment findings, including degree of deficit and current sources of fluid intake.
- I/O, fluid balance, changes in weight/edema, urine specific gravity, and vital signs.
- Results of diagnostic studies.

PLANNING

- Plan of care and who is involved in planning.
- Teaching plan.

IMPLEMENTATION/EVALUATION

- Client's responses to interventions/teaching and actions performed.
- Attainment/progress toward desired outcome(s).
- Modifications to plan of care.

DISCHARGE PLANNING

- Long-term needs, plan for correction, and who is responsible for actions to be taken.
- Specific referrals made.

SAMPLE NURSING OUTCOMES & INTERVENTIONS CLASSIFICATIONS (NOC/NIC)

NOC—Hydration
NIC—Hypovolemia Management

excess Fluid Volume

Taxonomy II: Nutrition—Class 5 Hydration (00026)
[Diagnostic Division: Food/Fluid]
Submitted 1982; Revised 1996

Definition: Increased isotonic fluid retention

Related Factors

Compromised regulatory mechanism [e.g., syndrome of inappropriate antidiuretic hormone—SIADH—or decreased plasma proteins as found in conditions such as malnutrition, draining fistulas, burns, organ failure]

Information in brackets added by the authors to clarify and enhance the use of nursing diagnoses.

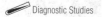 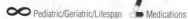

Excess fluid intake
Excess sodium intake
[Drug therapies, such as chlorpropamide, tolbutamide, vincristine, triptylines, carbamazepine]

Defining Characteristics

SUBJECTIVE

Orthopnea [difficulty breathing]
Anxiety

OBJECTIVE

Edema; anasarca; weight gain over short period of time
Intake exceeds output; oliguria
Adventitious breath sounds [rales or crackles]; changes in respiratory pattern; dyspnea
Increased central venous pressure; jugular vein distention; positive hepatojugular reflex
S3 heart sound
Pulmonary congestion, pleural effusion, pulmonary artery pressure changes; blood pressure changes
Change in mental status; restlessness
Specific gravity changes
Decreased Hb/Hct, azotemia, altered electrolytes

Desired Outcomes/Evaluation Criteria—Client Will:

- Stabilize fluid volume as evidenced by balanced I/O, vital signs within client's normal limits, stable weight, and free of signs of edema.
- Verbalize understanding of individual dietary/fluid restrictions.
- Demonstrate behaviors to monitor fluid status and reduce recurrence of fluid excess.
- List signs that require further evaluation.

Actions/Interventions

NURSING PRIORITY NO. 1. To assess causative/precipitating factors:

- Note presence of medical conditions/situations that potentiate fluid excess (e.g., cardiac failure, cerebral lesions, renal/adrenal insufficiency, psychogenic polydipsia, acute stress, surgical/anesthetic procedures, excessive or rapid infusion of IV fluids, decrease or loss of serum proteins).

Information in brackets added by the authors to clarify and enhance the use of nursing diagnoses.

🌐 Cultural   Collaborative 🏠 Community/Home Care

- Note amount/rate of fluid intake from all sources: PO, IV, ventilator, and so forth.
- Review intake of sodium (dietary, drug, IV) and protein.

NURSING PRIORITY NO. 2. To evaluate degree of excess:

- Compare current weight with admission and/or previously stated weight.
- Measure vital signs and invasive hemodynamic parameters (e.g., CVP, PAP/PCWP), if available.
- Auscultate breath sounds **for presence of crackles/congestion.**
- Record occurrence of dyspnea (exertional, nocturnal, and so forth).
- Auscultate heart tones for S_3, **ventricular gallop.**
- Assess for presence of neck vein distention/hepatojugular reflux.
- Note presence of edema (puffy eyelids, dependent swelling of ankles/feet if ambulatory or up in chair; sacrum and posterior thighs when recumbent), anasarca.
- Measure abdominal girth **for changes that may indicate increasing fluid retention/edema.**
- Note patterns and amount of urination (e.g., nocturia, oliguria).
- Evaluate mentation **for confusion, personality changes.**
- Assess neuromuscular reflexes **to evaluate for presence of electrolyte imbalances such as hypernatremia.**
- Assess appetite; note presence of nausea/vomiting.
- Observe skin and mucous membranes **for presence of decubitus/ulceration.**
- Note fever. **Client could be at increased risk of infection.**
 - Review laboratory data (e.g., BUN/Cr, Hb/Hct, serum albumin, proteins, and electrolytes; urine specific gravity/osmolality/sodium excretion) and chest x-ray **to evaluate degree of fluid and electrolyte imbalance and response to therapies.**

NURSING PRIORITY NO. 3. To promote mobilization/elimination of excess fluid:

- Restrict sodium and fluid intake, as indicated.
- Record I/O accurately; calculate 24-hour fluid balance (plus/minus).
- Set an appropriate rate of fluid intake/infusion throughout 24-hour period **to prevent peaks/valleys in fluid level and thirst.**
- Weigh daily or on a regular schedule, as indicated. **Provides a comparative baseline and evaluates the effectiveness of diuretic therapy when used (i.e., if I/O is 1 liter negative, weight loss of 2.2 pounds should be noted).**

Information in brackets added by the authors to clarify and enhance the use of nursing diagnoses.

- Administer medications (e.g., diuretics, cardiotonics, steroid replacement, plasma or albumin volume expanders).
- Elevate edematous extremities, change position frequently **to reduce tissue pressure and risk of skin breakdown.**
- Place in semi-Fowler's position, as appropriate, **to facilitate movement of diaphragm, thus improving respiratory effort.**
- Promote early ambulation.
- Provide quiet environment, limiting external stimuli.
- Use safety precautions if confused/debilitated.
- Assist with procedures, as indicated (e.g., dialysis).

NURSING PRIORITY NO. 4. To maintain integrity of skin and oral mucous membranes:

- Refer to NDs impaired/risk for impaired Skin Integrity; impaired Oral Mucous Membrane.

NURSING PRIORITY NO. 5. To promote wellness (Teaching/ Discharge Considerations):

- Review dietary restrictions and safe substitutes for salt (e.g., lemon juice or spices such as oregano).
- Discuss importance of fluid restrictions and "hidden sources" of intake (such as foods high in water content).
- Instruct client/family in use of voiding record, I/O.
- Consult dietitian, as needed.
- Suggest interventions, such as frequent oral care, chewing gum/hard candy, use of lip balm, **to reduce discomfort of fluid restrictions.**
- Review drug regimen (and side effects) used to increase urine output and/or manage hypertension, kidney disease, or heart failure.
- Stress need for mobility and/or frequent position changes **to prevent stasis and reduce risk of tissue injury.**
- Identify "danger" signs requiring notification of healthcare provider **to ensure timely evaluation/intervention.**

Documentation Focus

ASSESSMENT/REASSESSMENT

- Assessment findings, noting existing conditions contributing to and degree of fluid retention (vital signs; amount, presence, and location of edema; and weight changes).
- I/O, fluid balance.
- Results of laboratory tests/diagnostic studies.

Information in brackets added by the authors to clarify and enhance the use of nursing diagnoses.

 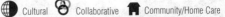

PLANNING

- Plan of care and who is involved in the planning.
- Teaching plan.

IMPLEMENTATION/EVALUATION

- Response to interventions/teaching and actions performed.
- Attainment/progress toward desired outcome(s).
- Modifications to plan of care.

DISCHARGE PLANNING

- Long-range needs, noting who is responsible for actions to be taken.

SAMPLE NURSING OUTCOMES & INTERVENTIONS CLASSIFICATIONS (NOC/NIC)

NOC—Fluid Balance
NIC—Hypervolemia Management

risk for deficient Fluid Volume

Taxonomy II: Nutrition—Class 5 Hydration (00028)
[Diagnostic Division: Food/Fluid]
Submitted 1978

Definition: At risk for experiencing vascular, cellular, or intracellular dehydration

Risk Factors

Extremes of age/weight
Loss of fluid through abnormal routes (e.g., indwelling tubes)
Knowledge deficiency
Factors influencing fluid needs (e.g., hypermetabolic state)
Medication (e.g., diuretics)
Excessive losses through normal routes (e.g., diarrhea)
Deviations affecting access/intake/absorption of fluids

> NOTE: A risk diagnosis is not evidenced by signs and symptoms as the problem has not occurred; rather, nursing interventions are directed at prevention.

Desired Outcomes/Evaluation Criteria—Client Will:

- Identify individual risk factors and appropriate interventions.

Information in brackets added by the authors to clarify and enhance the use of nursing diagnoses.

 Diagnostic Studies   ∞ Pediatric/Geriatric/Lifespan   Medications   **331**

- Demonstrate behaviors or lifestyle changes to prevent development of fluid volume deficit.

Actions/Interventions

NURSING PRIORITY NO. 1. To assess causative/contributing factors:

- Note possible conditions/processes that may lead to deficits: 1) fluid loss (e.g., fever, diarrhea/vomiting, excessive sweating; heat stroke; diabetic ketoacidosis; burns, other draining wounds; gastrointestinal obstruction; salt-wasting diruetics; rapid breathing/mechanical ventilation; surgical drains); 2) limited intake (e.g., sore throat or mouth; client dependent on others for eating and drinking; NPO status); 3) fluid shifts (e.g., ascites, effusions, burns, sepsis); and 4) environmental factors (e.g., isolation, restraints, malfunctioning air conditioning, exposure to extreme heat).
- Determine effects of age. **Very young and extremely elderly individuals are quickly affected by fluid volume deficit, and are least able to express need. For example, elderly people often have a decreased thirst reflex and/or may not be aware of water needs. Infants/young children and other nonverbal persons cannot describe thirst.**
- Note client's level of consciousness/mentation **to evaluate ability to express needs**.
- Evaluate nutritional status, noting current intake, type of diet (e.g., client is NPO or is on a restricted diet). Note problems (e.g., impaired mentation, nausea, fever, facial injuries, immobility, insufficient time for intake) **that can negatively affect fluid intake.**
- Review laboratory data (e.g., Hb/Hct, electrolytes, BUN/Cr).

NURSING PRIORITY NO. 2. To prevent occurrence of deficit:

- Monitor I/O balance, being aware of altered intake or output **to ensure accurate picture of fluid status.**
- Weigh client and compare with recent weight history. Perform serial weights **to determine trends.**
- Assess skin turgor/oral mucous membranes.
- Monitor vital signs for changes (e.g., orthostatic hypotension, tachycardia, fever).
- Establish individual fluid needs/replacement schedule. Distribute fluids over 24-hour period.
- Encourage oral intake:
  Provide water and other fluid needs to a minimum amount daily (up to 2.5 L/day or amount determined by healthcare provider for client's age, weight, and condition).

Information in brackets added by the authors to clarify and enhance the use of nursing diagnoses.

  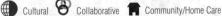 Cultural Collaborative Community/Home Care

Offer fluids between meals and regularly throughout the day.

Provide fluids in manageable cup, bottle, or with drinking straw.

Allow for adequate time for eating and drinking at meals.

Ensure that immobile/restrained client is assisted.

Encourage a variety of fluids in small frequent offerings, attempting to incorporate client's preferred beverages and temperature (e.g., iced or hot).

Limit fluids that tend to exert a diuretic effect (e.g., caffeine, alcohol).

Promote intake of high-water content foods (e.g., popsicles, gelatin, soup, eggnog, watermelon) and/or electrolyte replacement drinks (e.g., Smartwater, Gatorade, Pedialyte), as appropriate.

- Provide supplemental fluids (e.g., enteral, parenteral), as indicated. **Fluids may be given in this manner if client is unable to take oral fluid, is NPO for procedures, or when rapid fluid resuscitation is required.**

- Administer medications as indicated (e.g., antiemetics, antidiarrheals, antipyretics).

NURSING PRIORITY NO. 3. To promote wellness (Teaching/Discharge Considerations):

- Discuss individual risk factors/potential problems and specific interventions (e.g., proper clothing/bedding for infants and elderly during hot weather, use of room cooler/fan for comfortable ambient environment, fluid replacement options/schedule).

- Encourage client to increase fluid intake when exercising or during hot weather.

- Review appropriate use of medications **that have potential for causing/exacerbating dehydration**.

- Encourage client to maintain diary of food/fluid intake; number and amount of voidings and stools; and so forth.

- Refer to NDs [deficient Fluid Volume: hyper/hypotonic] or [isotonic].

Documentation Focus

ASSESSMENT/REASSESSMENT

- Individual findings, including individual factors influencing fluid needs/requirements.
- Baseline weight, vital signs.
- Results of laboratory tests.
- Specific client preferences for fluids.

Information in brackets added by the authors to clarify and enhance the use of nursing diagnoses.

 Diagnostic Studies   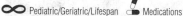 Pediatric/Geriatric/Lifespan   Medications   **333**

PLANNING

- Plan of care and who is involved in planning.
- Teaching plan.

IMPLEMENTATION/EVALUATION

- Responses to interventions/teaching and actions performed.
- Attainment/progress toward desired outcome(s).
- Modifications to plan of care.

DISCHARGE PLANNING

- Individual long-term needs, noting who is responsible for actions to be taken.
- Specific referrals made.

SAMPLE NURSING OUTCOMES & INTERVENTIONS CLASSIFICATIONS (NOC/NIC)

NOC—Fluid Balance
NIC—Fluid Monitoring

risk for imbalanced Fluid Volume

Taxonomy II: Nutrition—Class 5 Hydration (00025)
[Diagnostic Division: Food/Fluid]
Submitted 1998

Definition: At risk for a decrease, increase, or rapid shift from one to the other of intravascular, interstitial, and/or intracellular fluid. This refers to body fluid loss, gain, or both.

Risk Factors

Scheduled for major invasive procedures
[Rapid/sustained loss (e.g., hemorrhage, burns, fistulas)]
[Rapid fluid replacement]

> NOTE: A risk diagnosis is not evidenced by signs and symptoms, as the problem has not occurred and nursing interventions are directed at prevention.

Desired Outcomes/Evaluation Criteria—Client Will:

- Demonstrate adequate fluid balance as evidenced by stable vital signs; palpable pulses/good quality; normal skin turgor;

Information in brackets added by the authors to clarify and enhance the use of nursing diagnoses.

  Cultural Collaborative Community/Home Care

moist mucous membranes; individual appropriate urinary output; lack of excessive weight fluctuation (loss/gain); and no edema present.

Actions/Interventions

NURSING PRIORITY NO. 1. To determine risk/contributing factors:

- Note potential sources of fluid loss/intake (e.g., presence of conditions, such as diabetes insipidus, hyperosmolar nonketotic syndrome, bowel obstruction, heart/kidney/liver failure); major invasive procedures [e.g., surgery]; use of anesthesia; preoperative vomiting and dehydration; draining wounds; use/overuse of certain medications [e.g., diuretics, laxatives, anitcoagulants]; use of IV fluids and delivery device; administration of total parenteral nutrition [TPN]).
- Note client's age, current level of hydration, and mentation. **Provides information regarding ability to tolerate fluctuations in fluid level and risk for creating or failing to respond to problem (e.g., confused client may have inadequate intake, disconnect tubings, or readjust IV flow rate).**
- Review laboratory data, chest x-ray **to determine changes indicative of electrolyte and/or fluid status.**

NURSING PRIORITY NO. 2. To prevent fluctuations/imbalances in fluid levels:

- Measure and record intake:
  Include all sources (e.g., PO, IV, antibiotic additives, liquids with medications).
- Measure and record output:
  Monitor urine output (hourly or as needed). Report urine output <30 mL/hr or 0.5 mL/kg/hr **because it may indicate deficient fluid volume or cardiac or kidney failure.**
  Observe color of all excretions **to evaluate for bleeding.**
  Measure/estimate amount of liquid stool; weigh diapers/continence pads, when indicated.
  Measure emesis and output from drainage devices (e.g., gastric, wound, chest).
  Estimate/calculate insensible fluid losses **to include in replacement calculations.**
  Calculate 24-hour fluid balance (intake>output or output> intake).
- Weigh daily, or as indicated, and evaluate changes **as they relate to fluid status.**
- Auscultate BP, calculate pulse pressure. (**Pulse pressure widens before systolic BP drops in response to fluid loss.**)

Information in brackets added by the authors to clarify and enhance the use of nursing diagnoses.

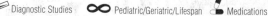

- Monitor vital sign responses to activities. **BP and heart/respiratory rate often increase initially when either fluid deficit or excess is present**.
- Assess for clinical signs of dehydration (e.g., hypotension, dry skin/mucous membranes, delayed capillary refill) or fluid excess (e.g., peripheral/dependent edema, adventitious breath sounds, distended neck veins).
- Note increased lethargy, hypotension, muscle cramping. **Electrolyte imbalances may be present**.
- Establish fluid oral intake, incorporating beverage preferences when possible.
- Maintain fluid/sodium restrictions, when needed.
- Administer IV fluids, as prescribed, using infusion pumps **to deliver fluids accurately and at desired rates to prevent either underinfusion/overinfusion**.
- Tape tubing connections longitudinally **to reduce risk of disconnection and loss of fluids**.
- Administer diuretics, antiemetics, antidiarrheals, as prescribed.
- Assist with rotating tourniquets (if used while awaiting response to pharmacologic therapies); dialysis; or ultrafiltration **to correct fluid overload situation**.

NURSING PRIORITY NO. 3. To promote wellness (Teaching/Discharge Considerations):

- Discuss individual risk factors/potential problems and specific interventions **to prevent/limit occurrence of fluid deficit/excess**.
- Instruct client/SO(s) in how to measure and record I/O, if indicated.
- Review/instruct in medication or nutritional regimen (e.g., enteral/parenteral feedings) **to alert to potential complications and appropriate management**.
- Identify signs and symptoms indicating need for prompt evaluation/follow-up care.
- Refer to NDs [deficient Fluid Volume: hyper/hypotonic] or [isotonic]; excess Fluid Volume; risk for deficient Fluid Volume for additional interventions.

Documentation Focus

ASSESSMENT/REASSESSMENT

- Individual findings, including individual factors influencing fluid needs/requirements.
- Baseline weight, vital signs.

Information in brackets added by the authors to clarify and enhance the use of nursing diagnoses.

  Cultural Collaborative Community/Home Care

- Results of laboratory test/diagnostic studies.
- Specific client preferences for fluids.

PLANNING

- Plan of care and who is involved in planning.
- Teaching plan.

IMPLEMENTATION/EVALUATION

- Responses to interventions/teaching and actions performed.
- Attainment/progress toward desired outcome(s).
- Modifications to plan of care.

DISCHARGE PLANNING

- Individual long-term needs, noting who is responsible for actions to be taken.
- Specific referrals made.

SAMPLE NURSING OUTCOMES & INTERVENTIONS CLASSIFICATIONS (NOC/NIC)

NOC—Fluid Balance
NIC—Fluid Monitoring

impaired Gas Exchange

Taxonomy II: Elimination—Class 4 Pulmonary System (00030)
[Diagnostic Division: Respiration]
Submitted 1980; Revised 1996, 1998 by Nursing Diagnosis Extension and Classification (NDEC)

Definition: Excess or deficit in oxygenation and/or carbon dioxide elimination at the alveoli-capillary membrane [This may be an entity of its own, but also may be an end result of other pathology with an interrelatedness between airway clearance and/or breathing pattern problems.]

Related Factors

Ventilation perfusion imbalance [as in: altered blood flow (e.g., pulmonary embolus, increased vascular resistance), vasospasm, heart failure, hypovolemic shock]
Alveolar-capillary membrane changes [e.g., acute respiratory distress syndrome; chronic conditions, such as restrictive/

Information in brackets added by the authors to clarify and enhance the use of nursing diagnoses.

 Diagnostic Studies   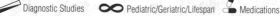 Pediatric/Geriatric/Lifespan   Medications   **337**

obstructive lung disease, pneumoconiosis, asbestosis/silicosis]
[Altered oxygen supply (e.g., altitude sickness)]
[Altered oxygen-carrying capacity of blood (e.g., sickle cell/other anemia, carbon monoxide poisoning)]

Defining Characteristics

SUBJECTIVE

Dyspnea
Visual disturbances
Headache upon awakening
[Sense of impending doom]

OBJECTIVE

Confusion [decreased mental acuity]
Restlessness; irritability; [agitation]
Somnolence; [lethargy]
Abnormal ABGs/arterial pH; hypoxia/hypoxemia; hypercapnia; hypercarbia; decreased carbon dioxide
Cyanosis (in neonates only); abnormal skin color (e.g., pale, dusky)
Abnormal breathing (e.g., rate, rhythm, depth); nasal flaring
Tachycardia; [development of dysrhythmias]
Diaphoresis
[Polycythemia]

Desired Outcomes/Evaluation Criteria—Client Will:

- Demonstrate improved ventilation and adequate oxygenation of tissues by ABGs within client's normal limits and absence of symptoms of respiratory distress (as noted in Defining Characteristics).
- Verbalize understanding of causative factors and appropriate interventions.
- Participate in treatment regimen (e.g., breathing exercises, effective coughing, use of oxygen) within level of ability/situation.

Actions/Interventions

NURSING PRIORITY NO. 1. To assess causative/contributing factors:
- Note presence of factors listed in Related Factors. Refer to NDs ineffective Airway Clearance; ineffective Breathing Pattern, as appropriate.

Information in brackets added by the authors to clarify and enhance the use of nursing diagnoses.

  Cultural Collaborative Community/Home Care

NURSING PRIORITY NO. 2. To evaluate degree of compromise:

- Note respiratory rate, depth, use of accessory muscles, pursed-lip breathing; and areas of pallor/cyanosis; for example, peripheral (nailbeds) versus central (circumoral) or general duskiness.
- Auscultate breath sounds, note areas of decreased/adventitious breath sounds as well as fremitus.
- Note character and effectiveness of cough mechanism (e.g, ability to clear airways of secretions).
- Assess level of consciousness and mentation changes. Note somnolence, restlessness, reports of headache on arising.
- Monitor vital signs and cardiac rhythm.
- Evaluate pulse oximetry to determine oxygenation; evaluate lung volumes and forced vital capacity **to assess for respiratory insufficiency.**
- Review other pertinent laboratory data (e.g., ABGs, CBC); chest x-rays.
- Assess energy level and activity tolerance.
- Note effect of illness on self-esteem/body image

NURSING PRIORITY NO. 3. To correct/improve existing deficiencies:

- Elevate head of bed/position client appropriately, provide airway adjuncts and suction, as indicated, **to maintain airway.**
- Encourage frequent position changes and deep-breathing/coughing exercises. Use incentive spirometer, chest physiotherapy, IPPB, and so forth, as indicated. **Promotes optimal chest expansion and drainage of secretions.**
- Provide supplemental oxygen at lowest concentration indicated by laboratory results and client symptoms/situation.
- Monitor for carbon dioxide narcosis (e.g., change in level of consciousness, changes in O_2 and CO_2 blood gas levels, flushing, decreased respiratory rate, headaches), **which may occur in client receiving long-term oxygen therapy.**
- Maintain adequate I/O **for mobilization of secretions,** but avoid fluid overload.
- Use sedation judiciously **to avoid depressant effects on respiratory functioning.**
- Ensure availability of proper emergency equipment, including ET/trach set and suction catheters appropriate for age and size of infant/child/adult.
- Avoid use of face mask in elderly emaciated client.
- Encourage adequate rest and limit activities to within client tolerance. Promote calm/restful environment. **Helps limit oxygen needs/consumption.**

Information in brackets added by the authors to clarify and enhance the use of nursing diagnoses.

 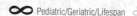

- Provide psychological support, active-listen questions/concerns **to reduce anxiety.**
- Administer medications, as indicated (e.g., inhaled and systemic glucocorticosteroids, antibiotics, bronchodilators, methylxanthines, expectorants), **to treat underlying conditions.**
- Monitor/instruct client in therapeutic and adverse effects as well as interactions of drug therapy.
- Minimize blood loss from procedures (e.g., tests, hemodialysis) **to limit adverse affects of anemia.**
- Assist with procedures as individually indicated (e.g., transfusion, phlebotomy, bronchoscopy) **to improve respiratory function/oxygen-carrying capacity.**
- Monitor/adjust ventilator settings (e.g., FIO_2, tidal volume, inspiratory/expiratory ratio, sigh, positive end-expiratory pressure [PEEP]), as indicated, when mechanical support is being used.
- Keep environment allergen/pollutant free **to reduce irritant effect of dust and chemicals on airways.**

NURSING PRIORITY NO. 4. To promote wellness (Teaching/Discharge Considerations):

- Review risk factors, particularly environmental/employment-related, **to promote prevention/management of risk.**
- Discuss implications of smoking related to the illness/condition.
- Encourage client and SO(s) to stop smoking, attend cessation programs, as necessary, **to reduce health risks and/or prevent further decline in lung function.**
- Discuss reasons for allergy testing when indicated. Review individual drug regimen and ways of dealing with side effects.
- Instruct in the use of relaxation, stress-reduction techniques, as appropriate.
- Reinforce need for adequate rest, while encouraging activity and exercise (e.g., upper and lower extremity endurance/strength training and flexibility) **to decrease dyspnea and improve quality of life.**
- Emphasize the importance of nutrition **in improving stamina and reducing the work of breathing.**
- Review oxygen-conserving techniques (e.g., sitting instead of standing to perform tasks; eating small meals; performing slower, purposeful movements).
- Review job description/work activities **to identify need for job modifications/vocational rehabilitation.**
- Discuss home oxygen therapy and safety measures, as indicated, when home oxygen implemented.

Information in brackets added by the authors to clarify and enhance the use of nursing diagnoses.

Cultural Collaborative Community/Home Care

• Identify specific supplier for supplemental oxygen/necessary respiratory devices, as well as other individually appropriate resources, such as home care agencies, Meals on Wheels, and so on, **to facilitate independence.**

Documentation Focus

ASSESSMENT/REASSESSMENT

• Assessment findings, including respiratory rate, character of breath sounds; frequency, amount, and appearance of secretions; presence of cyanosis; laboratory findings; and mentation level.
• Conditions that may interfere with oxygen supply.

PLANNING

• Plan of care/interventions and who is involved in the planning.
• Ventilator settings, liters of supplemental oxygen.
• Teaching plan.

IMPLEMENTATION/EVALUATION

• Client's responses to treatment/teaching and actions performed.
• Attainment/progress toward desired outcome(s).
• Modifications to plan of care.

DISCHARGE PLANNING

• Long-range needs, identifying who is responsible for actions to be taken.
• Community resources for equipment/supplies post-discharge.
• Specific referrals made.

SAMPLE NURSING OUTCOMES & INTERVENTIONS CLASSIFICATIONS (NOC/NIC)

NOC—Respiratory Status: Gas Exchange
NIC—Respiratory Monitoring

risk for unstable blood Glucose

Taxonomy II: Nutrition—Class 4 Metabolism (00179)
[Diagnostic Division: Food/Fluid]
Submitted 2006

Definition: Risk for variation of blood glucose/sugar levels from the normal range

---

Information in brackets added by the authors to clarify and enhance the use of nursing diagnoses.

 Diagnostic Studies ∞ Pediatric/Geriatric/Lifespan   Medications **341**

Risk Factors

Lack of acceptance of diagnosis; deficient knowledge of diabetes management (e.g., action plan)

Lack of diabetes management/adherence to diabetes management (e.g., action plan); inadequate blood glucose monitoring; medication management

Dietary intake; weight gain/loss; rapid growth periods; pregnancy

Physical health status/activity level

Stress; mental health status

Developmental level

NOTE: A risk diagnosis is not evidenced by signs and symptoms, as the problem has not occurred and nursing interventions are directed at prevention.

Desired Outcomes/Evaluation Criteria—Client/Caregivers Will:

• Acknowledge factors that may lead to unstable glucose.
• Verbalize understanding of body and energy needs.
• Verbalize plan for modifying factors to prevent/minimize shifts in glucose level.
• Maintain glucose in satisfactory range.

Actions/Interventions

NURSING PRIORITY NO. 1. To assess risk/contributing factors:

• Determine individual factors that may contribute to unstable glucose as listed in risk factors. **Client or family history of diabetes; known diabetic with poor glucose control; eating disorders (e.g., morbid obesity); poor exercise habits; failure to recognize changes in glucose needs/control due to adolescent growth spurts/pregnancy all can result in problems with glucose stability.**

• Ascertain client's/SO's knowledge/understanding of condition and treatment needs.

• Identify individual perceptions and expectations of treatment regimen.

 • Note influence of cultural/religious factors impacting dietary practices, taking responsibility for own care, expectations of outcomes.

• Determine client's awareness/ability to be responsible for dealing with situation. Age, maturity, current health status, and developmental stage affect client's ability to provide for own safety.

Information in brackets added by the authors to clarify and enhance the use of nursing diagnoses.

  Cultural Collaborative 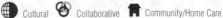 Community/Home Care

- Assess family/SO(s) support of client. Client may need assistance with lifestyle changes (e.g., food preparation/consumption, timing of intake and/or exercise, administration of medications).
- Note availability/use of resources.

NURSING PRIORITY NO. 2. To assist client to develop preventative strategies to avoid glucose instability:

- Ascertain whether client/SOs are adept at operating client's home glucose monitoring device. **All available machines will provide satisfactory readings if properly used and maintained and routinely calibrated.**
- Provide information on balancing food intake, antidiabetic agents, and energy expenditure.
- Review medical necessity for regularly scheduled lab screening tests for diabetes. Tests, including fasting and daily glucose and HgbA1c, help identify acute and long-term glucose control.
- Discuss home glucose monitoring according to individual parameters (e.g., 6 × day for normal day and more frequently during times of stress) **to identify and manage glucose variations.**
- Review client's common situations that contribute to glucose instability on daily, occasional, or crisis basis. **Multiple factors can play a role at any time, such as missing meals, adolescent growth spurt, or infection/other illness.**
- Review client's diet, especially carbohydrate intake. **Glucose balance is determined by the amount of carbohydrates consumed, which should be determined in needed grams/day.**
- Encourage client to read labels and choose foods described as having a low glycemic index (GI), higher fiber, and low-fat content. **These foods produce a slower rise in blood glucose.**
- Discuss how client's antidiabetic medication(s) work. **Drugs and combinations of drugs work in varying ways with different blood glucose control and side effects. Understanding drug actions can help client avoid/reduce risk of potential for hypoglycemic reactions.**

FOR CLIENT ON INSULIN

- Emphasize importance of checking expiration dates of medication, inspecting insulin for cloudiness if it is normally clear, and monitoring proper storage and preparation (when mixing required). **Affects insulin absorbability.**
- Review type(s) of insulin used (e.g., rapid, short, intermediate, long-acting, premixed) and delivery method (e.g., subcutaneous, intramuscular injection; inhaled, pump). Note time

---

Information in brackets added by the authors to clarify and enhance the use of nursing diagnoses.

when short-acting and long-acting insulins are administered. Remind client that only short-acting insulin is used in pump. **Affects timing of effects and provides clues to potential timing of glucose instability.**

• Check injection sites periodically. **Insulin absorption can vary from day to day in healthy sites and is less absorbable in lypohypertrophic (lumpy) tissues.**

∞ • Ascertain that all injections are being given. **Children, adolescents, and elderly clients may forget injections or be unable to self-inject and may need reminders and supervision.**

NURSING PRIORITY NO. 3. To promote wellness (Teaching/Discharge Considerations):

• Review individual risk factors and provide information to assist client in efforts to avoid complications, such as those caused by chronic hyperglycemia and acute hypoglycemia. **Note: Hyperglycemia is most commonly caused by alterations in nutrition needs, inactivity, and/or inadequate use of antidiabetic medications. Hypoglycemia is the most common complication of antidiabetic therapy, stress, and exercise.**

• Emphasize consequences of actions/choices—both immediate and long-term.

• Engage client/family/caregiver in formulating plan to manage blood glucose level incorporating lifestyle, age/developmental level, physical/psychological ability to manage condition.

• Consult with dietitian about specific dietary needs based on individual situation (e.g., growth spurt, pregnancy, change in activity level following injury).

• Encourage client to develop a system for self-monitoring to provide a sense of control and enable client to follow own progress and assist with making choices.

• Refer to appropriate community resources, diabetic educator, and/or support groups, as needed, **for lifestyle modification, medical management, referral for insulin pump or glucose monitor, financial assistance for supplies, etc.**

Documentation Focus

ASSESSMENT/REASSESSMENT

• Findings related to individual situation, risk factors, current caloric intake/dietary pattern; prescription medication use; monitoring of condition.
• Client's/caregiver's understanding of individual risks/potential complications.
• Results of laboratory tests/fingerstick testing.

Information in brackets added by the authors to clarify and enhance the use of nursing diagnoses.

 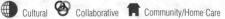

PLANNING

- Plan of care and who is involved in planning.
- Teaching plan.

IMPLEMENTATION/EVALUATION

- Individual responses to interventions/teaching and actions performed.
- Specific actions and changes that are made.
- Attainment/progress toward desired outcomes.
- Modifications to plan of care.

DISCHARGE PLANNING

- Long-range plans for ongoing needs, monitoring and management of condition, and who is responsible for actions to be taken.
- Sources for equipment/supplies.
- Specific referrals made.

SAMPLE NURSING OUTCOMES & INTERVENTIONS CLASSIFICATIONS (NOC/NIC)

NOC—Blood Glucose Level
NIC—Hyperglycemia Management

Grieving

Taxonomy II: Coping/Stress Tolerance—Class 2 Coping Responses (00136)
[Diagnostic Division: Ego Integrity]
Submitted 1980; Revised 1996, 2006

Definition: A normal complex process that includes emotional, physical, spiritual, social, and intellectual responses and behaviors by which individuals, families, and communities incorporate an actual, anticipated, or perceived loss into their daily lives

Related Factors

Anticipatory loss/loss of significant object (e.g., possessions, job, status, home, parts and processes of body)
Anticipatory loss/death of a significant other

Defining Characteristics

SUBJECTIVE

Anger; pain; suffering; despair; blame
Alteration in: activity level, sleep/dream patterns

Information in brackets added by the authors to clarify and enhance the use of nursing diagnoses.

 Diagnostic Studies 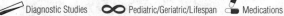 Pediatric/Geriatric/Lifespan Medications **345**

Making meaning of the loss; personal growth
Experiencing relief

OBJECTIVE

Detachment; disorganization; psychological distress; panic behavior
Maintaining the connection to the deceased
Alterations in immune/neuroendocrine function

Desired Outcomes/Evaluation Criteria—Client Will:

- Identify and express feelings (e.g., sadness, guilt, fear) freely/effectively.
- Acknowledge impact/effect of the grieving process (e.g., physical problems of eating, sleeping) and seek appropriate help.
- Look toward/plan for future, one day at a time.

Community Will:

- Recognize needs of citizens, including underserved population.
- Activate/develop plan to address identified needs.

Actions/Interventions

NURSING PRIORITY NO. 1. To identify causative/contributing factors:

- Determine circumstances of current situation (e.g., sudden death, prolonged fatal illness, loved one kept alive by extreme medical interventions). **Grief can be anticipatory (mourning the loss of loved one's former self before actual death), or actual. Both types of grief can provoke a wide range of intense and often conflicting feelings. Grief also follows losses other than death (e.g., traumatic loss of a limb, or loss of home by a tornado, loss of known self due to brain injury).**
- Evaluate client's perception of anticipated/actual loss and meaning to him or her: "What are your concerns?" "What are your fears?" "Your greatest fear?" "How do you see this affecting you/your lifestyle?"
 - Identify cultural/religious beliefs that may impact sense of loss.
 - Ascertain response of family/SO(s) to client's situation/concerns.
- Determine significance of loss to community (e.g., school bus accident with loss of life, major tornado damage to infrastructure, financial failure of major employer).

Information in brackets added by the authors to clarify and enhance the use of nursing diagnoses.

  Cultural 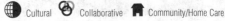 Collaborative 🏠 Community/Home Care

NURSING PRIORITY NO. 2. To determine current response:

🏠 • Note emotional responses, such as withdrawal, angry behavior, crying.

🏠 • Observe client's body language and check out meaning with the client. Note congruency with verbalizations.

🌐 • Note cultural/religious expectations that may dictate client's responses **to assess appropriateness of client's reaction to the situation.**

🏠 • Identify problems with eating, activity level, sexual desire, role performance (e.g., work, parenting). **Indicators of severity of feelings client is experiencing and need for specific interventions to address these issues.**

🏠 • Determine impact on general well-being (e.g., increased frequency of minor illnesses, exacerbation of chronic condition).

🏠 • Note family communication/interaction patterns.

🕸 • Determine use/availability of community resources/support groups.

• Note community plans in place to deal with major loss (e.g., team of crisis counselors stationed at a school to address the loss of classmates, vocational counselors/retraining programs, outreach of services from neighboring communities).

NURSING PRIORITY NO. 3. To assist client/community to deal with situation:

🏠 • Provide open environment and trusting relationship. **Promotes a free discussion of feelings and concerns.**

🏠 • Use therapeutic communication skills of active-listening, silence, acknowledgment. Respect client desire/request not to talk.

∞ • Inform children about death/anticipated loss in age-appropriate language. **Providing accurate information about impending loss or change in life situation will help child begin mourning process.**

∞ • Provide puppets or play therapy for toddlers/young children. **May help them more readily express grief and deal with loss.**

🏠 • Permit appropriate expressions of anger, fear. Note hostility toward/feelings of abandonment by spiritual power. (Refer to appropriate NDs, e.g., Spiritual Distress.)

🏠 • Provide information about normalcy of individual grief reaction.

• Be honest when answering questions, providing information. **Enhances sense of trust and nurse-client relationship.**

∞ • Provide assurance to child that cause for situation is not own doing, bearing in mind age and developmental level. **May lessen sense of guilt and affirm there is no need to assign blame to self or any family member.**

Information in brackets added by the authors to clarify and enhance the use of nursing diagnoses.

🏠 • Provide hope within parameters of specific situation. Refrain from giving false reassurance.

🏠 • Review past life experiences/previous loss(es), role changes, and coping skills, noting strengths/successes. **May be useful in dealing with current situation and problem solving existing needs.**

🏠 • Discuss control issues, such as what is in the power of the individual to change and what is beyond control. **Recognition of these factors helps client focus energy for maximal benefit/outcome.**

🏠 • Incorporate family/SO(s) in problem solving. **Encourages family to support/assist client to deal with situation while meeting needs of family members.**

🏠 • Determine client's status and role in family (e.g., parent, sibling, child) and address loss of family member role.

🏠 • Instruct in use of visualization and relaxation techniques.

💊 • Use sedatives/tranquilizers with caution. **May retard passage through the grief process, although short-term use may be beneficial to enhance sleep.**

• Encourage community members/groups to engage in talking about event/loss and verbalizing feelings. Seek out underserved populations to include in process.

• Encourage individuals to participate in activities to deal with loss/rebuild community.

🏠 NURSING PRIORITY NO. 4. To promote wellness (Teaching/Discharge Considerations):

🏠 • Give information that feelings are OK and are to be expressed appropriately. **Expression of feelings can facilitate the grieving process, but destructive behavior can be damaging.**

• Provide information that on birthdays, major holidays, at times of significant personal events, or anniversary of loss, client may experience/needs to be prepared for intense grief reactions. **If these reactions start to disrupt day-to-day functioning, client may need to seek help.** (Refer to NDs complicated Grieving; ineffective community Coping, as appropriate.)

🏠 • Encourage continuation of usual activities/schedule and involvement in appropriate exercise program.

🏠 • Identify/promote family and social support systems.

🏠 • Discuss and assist with planning for future/funeral, as appropriate.

🔯 • Refer to additional resources, such as pastoral care, counseling/psychotherapy, community/organized support groups, as indicated, for both client and family/SO(s), **to meet ongoing needs and facilitate grief work.**

Information in brackets added by the authors to clarify and enhance the use of nursing diagnoses.

  Cultural Collaborative 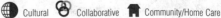 Community/Home Care

- Support community efforts to strengthen support/develop plan to foster recovery and growth.

Documentation Focus

ASSESSMENT/REASSESSMENT

- Assessment findings, including client's perception of anticipated loss and signs/symptoms that are being exhibited.
- Responses of family/SO(s) or community members, as indicated.
- Availability/use of resources.

PLANNING

- Plan of care and who is involved in planning.
- Teaching plan.

IMPLEMENTATION/EVALUATION

- Client's response to interventions/teaching and actions performed.
- Attainment/progress toward desired outcome(s).
- Modifications to plan of care.

DISCHARGE PLANNING

- Long-range needs and who is responsible for actions to be taken.
- Specific referrals made.

SAMPLE NURSING OUTCOMES & INTERVENTIONS CLASSIFICATIONS (NOC/NIC)

NOC—Grief Resolution
NIC—Grief Work Facilitation

complicated Grieving

Taxonomy II: Coping/Stress Tolerance—Class 2 Coping Responses (00135)
[Diagnostic Division: Ego Integrity]
Submitted 1980; Revised 1996, 2004, 2006

Definition: A disorder that occurs after the death of a significant other, in which the experience of distress accompanying bereavement fails to follow normative expectations and manifests in functional impairment

---

Information in brackets added by the authors to clarify and enhance the use of nursing diagnoses.

 Diagnostic Studies 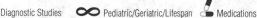 ∞ Pediatric/Geriatric/Lifespan 💊 Medications

Related Factors

GENERAL

Death/sudden death of a significant other
Emotional instability
Lack of social support
[Loss of significant object (e.g., possessions, job, status, home, parts and processes of body)]

Defining Characteristics

SUBJECTIVE

Verbalizes anxiety, lack of acceptance of the death, persistent painful memories, distressful feelings about the deceased, self-blame
Verbalizes feelings of anger, disbelief, detachment from others
Verbalizes feeling dazed, empty, stunned, in shock
Decreased sense of well-being, fatigue, low levels of intimacy, depression
Yearning

OBJECTIVE

Decreased functioning in life roles
Persistent emotional distress; separation/traumatic distress
Preoccupation with thoughts of the deceased, longing for the deceased, searching for the deceased, self-blame
Experiencing somatic symptoms of the deceased
Rumination
Grief avoidance

Desired Outcomes/Evaluation Criteria—Client Will:

• Acknowledge presence/impact of dysfunctional situation.
• Demonstrate progress in dealing with stages of grief at own pace.
• Participate in work and self-care/ADLs, as able.
• Verbalize a sense of progress toward grief resolution/hope for the future.

Actions/Interventions

NURSING PRIORITY NO. 1. To determine causative/contributing factors:

• Identify loss that is present. Note circumstances of death, such as sudden or traumatic (e.g., fatal accident, suicide, homicide),

---

Information in brackets added by the authors to clarify and enhance the use of nursing diagnoses.

related to socially sensitive issue (e.g., AIDS, suicide, murder), or associated with unfinished business (e.g., spouse died during time of crisis in marriage; son has not spoken to parent for years). **These situations can sometimes cause individual to become stuck in grief and unable to move forward with life.**

- Determine significance of the loss to client (e.g., presence of chronic condition leading to divorce/disruption of family unit and change in lifestyle/financial security).
- Identify cultural/religious beliefs and expectations that may impact or dictate client's response to loss.
- Ascertain response of family/SO(s) to client's situation (e.g., sympathetic or urging client to "just get over it").

NURSING PRIORITY NO. 2. To determine degree of impairment/dysfunction:

- Observe for cues of sadness (e.g., sighing; faraway look; unkempt appearance; inattention to conversation; somatic complaints, such as exhaustion, headaches).
- Listen to words/communications indicative of renewed/intense grief (e.g., constantly bringing up death/loss even in casual conversation long after event; outbursts of anger at relatively minor events; expressing desire to die), **indicating person is possibly unable to adjust/move on from feelings of severe grief.**
- Identify stage of grief being expressed: denial, isolation, anger, bargaining, depression, acceptance.
- Determine level of functioning, ability to care for self.
- Note availability/use of support systems and community resources.
- Be aware of avoidance behaviors (e.g., anger, withdrawal, long periods of sleeping, or refusing to interact with family; sudden or radical changes in lifestyle; inability to handle everyday responsiblities at home/work/school; conflict).
- Determine if client is engaging in reckless/self-destructive behaviors (e.g., substance abuse, heavy drinking, promiscuity, aggression) **to identify safety issues.**
- Identify cultural factors and ways individual has dealt with previous loss(es) **to put current behavior/responses in context.**
- Refer to mental health providers for specific diagnostic studies and intervention in issues associated with debilitating grief.
- Refer to ND Grieving for additional interventions, as appropriate.

Information in brackets added by the authors to clarify and enhance the use of nursing diagnoses.

 Diagnostic Studies ∞ Pediatric/Geriatric/Lifespan Medications **351**

NURSING PRIORITY NO. 3. To assist client to deal appropriately with loss:

- Encourage verbalization without confrontation about realities. **Helps to begin resolution and acceptance.**
- Encourage client to talk about what he or she chooses and refrain from forcing the client to "face the facts."
- Active-listen to feelings and be available for support/assistance. Speak in soft, caring tone.
- Encourage expression of anger/fear and anxiety. Refer to appropriate NDs.
- Permit verbalization of anger with acknowledgment of feelings and setting of limits regarding destructive behavior. **Enhances client safety and promotes resolution of grief process.**
- Acknowledge reality of feelings of guilt/blame, including hostility toward spiritual power. Do not minimize loss, avoid clichés and easy answers. (Refer to ND Spiritual Distress.) Assist client to take steps toward resolution.
- Respect the client's needs and wishes for quiet, privacy, talking, or silence.
- Give "permission" to be at this point when the client is depressed.
- Provide comfort and availability as well as caring for physical needs.
- Reinforce use of previously effective coping skills. Instruct in/encourage use of visualization and relaxation techniques.
- Assist SO(s) to cope with client's response and include age-specific interventions. **Family/SO(s) may not understand/be intolerant of client's distress and inadvertently hamper client's progress.**
- Include family/SO(s) in setting realistic goals for meeting needs of family members.
- Use sedatives/tranquilizers with caution **to avoid retarding resolution of grief process.**

NURSING PRIORITY NO. 4. To promote wellness (Teaching/Discharge Considerations):

- Discuss with client/SO(s) healthy ways of dealing with difficult situations.
- Have client identify familial, religious, and cultural factors that have meaning for him or her. **May help bring loss into perspective and promote grief resolution.**
- Encourage involvement in usual activities, exercise, and socialization within limits of physical ability and psychological state.
- Advocate planning for the future, as appropriate, to individual situation (e.g., staying in own home after death of spouse, returning to sporting activities following traumatic amputation,

---

Information in brackets added by the authors to clarify and enhance the use of nursing diagnoses.

  Cultural 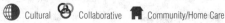 Collaborative 🏠 Community/Home Care

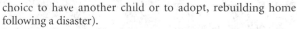

choice to have another child or to adopt, rebuilding home following a disaster).

- Refer to other resources (e.g., pastoral care, family counseling, psychotherapy, organized support groups). **Provides additional help, when needed, to resolve situation/continue grief work.**

Documentation Focus

ASSESSMENT/REASSESSMENT

- Assessment findings, including meaning of loss to the client, current stage of the grieving process, and responses of family/SO(s).
- Cultural/religious beliefs and expectations.
- Availability/use of resources.

PLANNING

- Plan of care and who is involved in the planning.
- Teaching plan.

IMPLEMENTATION/EVALUATION

- Client's response to interventions/teaching and actions performed.
- Attainment/progress toward desired outcome(s).
- Modifications to plan of care.

DISCHARGE PLANNING

- Long-term needs and who is responsible for actions to be taken.
- Specific referrals made.

SAMPLE NURSING OUTCOMES & INTERVENTIONS CLASSIFICATIONS (NOC/NIC)

NOC—Grief Resolution
NIC—Grief Work Facilitation

risk for complicated Grieving

Taxonomy II: Coping/Stress Tolerance – Class 2 Coping Responses (00172)
[Diagnostic Division: Ego Integrity]
Submitted 2004; Revised 2006

Definition: At risk for a disorder that occurs after the death of a significant other, in which the experience of distress accompanying bereavement fails to follow normative expectations and manifests in functional impairment

Information in brackets added by the authors to clarify and enhance the use of nursing diagnoses.

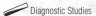 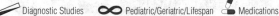

risk for complicated GRIEVING

Risk Factors

Death of a significant other
Emotional instability
Lack of social support
[Loss of significant object (e.g., possessions, job, status, home, parts and processes of body)]

> NOTE: A risk diagnosis is not evidenced by signs and symptoms, as the problem has not occurred and nursing interventions are directed at prevention.

Desired Outcomes/Evaluation Criteria—Client Will:

• Acknowledge awareness of individual factors affecting client in this situation. (See Risk Factors)
• Identify emotional responses and behaviors occurring after the death or loss.
• Participate in therapy to learn new ways of dealing with anxiety and feelings of inadequacy.
• Discuss meaning of loss to individual/family.
• Verbalize a sense of beginning to deal with grief process.

Actions/Interventions

NURSING PRIORITY NO. 1. To identify risk/contributing factors:

• Determine loss that has occurred and meaning to client. Note whether loss was sudden or expected.
• Ascertain gestational age of fetus at time of loss, or length of life of infant/child. **Death of child may be more difficult for parents/family to deal with based on individual values and sense of life unlived.**
• Note stage of grief client is experiencing. **Stages of grief may progress in a predictable manner or stages may be random/revisited.**
• Assess client's ability to manage activities of daily living and period of time since loss has occurred. **Periods of crying, feelings of overwhelming sadness, and loss of appetite and insomnia can occur with grieving; however, when they persist and interfere with normal activities, client may need additional assistance.**
• Note availability/use of support systems, community resources.
• Identify cultural/religious beliefs and expectations that may impact or dictate client's response to loss.

Information in brackets added by the authors to clarify and enhance the use of nursing diagnoses.

  Cultural Collaborative Community/Home Care

- Assess status of relationships/marital difficulties and adjustments to loss.

NURSING PRIORITY NO. 2. To assist client to deal appropriately with loss:

- Discuss meaning of loss to client, active-listen responses without judgment.
- Encourage expression of feelings, including anger/fear and anxiety. Let client know that all feelings are OK while setting limits on destructive behavior.
- Respect client's desire for quiet, privacy, talking, or silence.
- Acknowledge client's sense of relief/guilt at feeling relief when death follows a long and debilitating course. **Sadness and loss are still there, but the death may be a release; or, client may feel guilty about having a sense of relief.**
- Discuss the circumstances surrounding the death of a fetus/child. Was it sudden or expected? Have other children been lost (multiple miscarriages)? Was a congenital anomaly present? **Repeated losses increase sense of futility and compromise resolution of grieving process.**
- Meet with both members of the couple **to determine how they are dealing with the loss.**
- Encourage client/SOs to honor cultural practices through funerals, wakes, or sitting shiva, and so forth.
- Assist SO(s)/family to understand and be tolerant of client's feelings and behavior.

NURSING PRIORITY NO. 3. To promote wellness (Teaching/Discharge Considerations):

- Encourage client/SO(s) to identify healthy coping skills they have used in the past. **These can be used in current situation to facilitate dealing with grief.**
- Assist in setting goals for meeting needs of client and family members to move beyond the grieving process.
- Suggest resuming involvement in usual activities, exercise, and socialization within physical and psychological abilities.
- Discuss planning for the future, as appropriate to individual situation (e.g., staying in own home after death of spouse, returning to sporting activities following traumatic amputation, choice to have another child or to adopt, rebuilding home following a disaster).
- Refer to other resources, as needed, such as counseling, psychotherapy, religious references/pastor, grief support group. **Depending upon meaning of the loss, individual may require ongoing support to work through grief.**

Information in brackets added by the authors to clarify and enhance the use of nursing diagnoses.

Documentation Focus

ASSESSMENT/REASSESSMENT

- Assessment findings, including meaning of loss to the client, current stage of the grieving process, psychological status, and responses of family/SO(s).
- Availability/use of resources.

PLANNING

- Plan of care and who is involved in the planning.
- Teaching plan.

IMPLEMENTATION/EVALUATION

- Client's response to interventions/teaching and actions performed.
- Attainment/progress toward desired outcome(s).
- Modifications to plan of care.

DISCHARGE PLANNING

- Long-term needs and who is responsible for actions to be taken.
- Specific referrals made.

SAMPLE NURSING OUTCOMES & INTERVENTIONS CLASSIFICATIONS (NOC/NIC)

NOC—Grief Resolution
NIC—Grief Work Facilitation

risk for disproportionate Growth

Taxonomy II: Growth/Development—Class 1 Growth (00113)
[Diagnostic Division: Teaching/Learning]
Nursing Diagnosis Extension and Classification (NDEC) Submission 1998

Definition: At risk for growth above the 97th percentile or below the 3rd percentile for age, crossing two percentile channels

Risk Factors

PRENATAL

Maternal nutrition/infection; multiple gestation
Substance use/abuse; teratogen exposure

Information in brackets added by the authors to clarify and enhance the use of nursing diagnoses.

Congenital/genetic disorders [e.g., dysfunction of endocrine gland, tumors]

INDIVIDUAL

Prematurity

Malnutrition; caregiver/individual maladaptive feeding behaviors; insatiable appetite; anorexia [impaired metabolism, greater-than-normal energy requirements]

Infection; chronic illness [e.g., chronic inflammatory diseases]

Substance [use]/abuse [including anabolic steroids]

ENVIRONMENTAL

Deprivation; poverty

Violence; natural disasters

Teratogen; lead poisoning

CAREGIVER

Abuse

Mental illness/retardation, severe learning disability

NOTE: A risk diagnosis is not evidenced by signs and symptoms, as the problem has not occurred and nursing interventions are directed at prevention.

Desired Outcomes/Evaluation Criteria—Client Will:

- Receive appropriate nutrition as indicated by individual needs.
- Demonstrate weight/growth stabilizing or progress toward age-appropriate size.
- Participate in plan of care as appropriate for age/ability.

Caregiver Will:

- Verbalize understanding of potential for growth delay/deviation and plans for prevention.

Actions/Interventions

NURSING PRIORITY NO. 1. To assess causative/contributing factors:

- Determine factors/condition(s) existing that could contribute to growth deviation as listed in Risk Factors, including familial history of pituitary tumors, Marfan's syndrome, genetic anomalies, use of certain drugs/substances during pregnancy,

---

Information in brackets added by the authors to clarify and enhance the use of nursing diagnoses.

 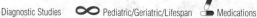

(side tab) **risk for disproportionate GROWTH**

maternal diabetes/other chronic illness, poverty/inability to attend to nutritional issues, eating disorders, etc.

 • Identify nature and effectiveness of parenting/caregiving activities (e.g., inadequate, inconsistent, unrealistic/insufficient expectations; lack of stimulation, limit setting, responsiveness).

 • Note severity/pervasiveness of situation (e.g., individual showing effects of long-term physical/emotional abuse/neglect versus individual experiencing recent-onset situational disruption or inadequate resources during period of crisis or transition).

 • Perform nutritional assessment. **Overfeeding or malnutrition (protein and other basic nutrients) on a constant basis prevents child from reaching healthy growth potential, even if no disorder/disease exists.** (Refer to ND imbalanced Nutrition: [specify].)

• Note results of laboratory tests.

• Determine cultural/familial/societal issues that may impact situation (e.g., childhood obesity now a risk for American children; parental concern for amount of food intake; expectations for "normal growth").

 • Assess significant stressful events, losses, separation, and environmental changes (e.g., abandonment, divorce, death of parent/sibling, aging, move).

 • Assess cognition, awareness, orientation, behavior (e.g., withdrawal/aggression), reaction to environment and stimuli.

• Active-listen concerns about body size, ability to perform competitively (e.g., sports, body building) **to ascertain the potential for use of anabolic steroids/other drugs.**

NURSING PRIORITY NO. 2. To prevent/limit deviation from growth norms:

 • Determine chronological age, familial factors (body build/stature) **to determine growth expectations.** Note reported losses/alterations in functional level. **Provides comparative baseline.**

 • Identify present growth age/stage. Review expectations for current height/weight percentiles and any degree of deviation.

• Investigate deviations from normal (e.g., height/weight, head/hand/feet size, facial features, etc.). **Deviations can be multifactorial and require varying interventions (e.g., weight deviation only [increased or decreased] may be remedied by changes in nutrition and exercise; other deviations may require in-depth evaluation and long-term treatment.)**

Information in brackets added by the authors to clarify and enhance the use of nursing diagnoses.

  Cultural Collaborative Community/Home Care

- Determine if child's growth is above 97th percentile (very tall and large) for age. **Suggests need for evaluation for endocrine/other disorders.**
- Determine if child's growth is below 3rd percentile (very short and small) for age. **May require evaluation for failure to thrive.**
- Note reports of changes in facial features, joint pain, lethargy, sexual dysfunction, and/or progressive increase in hat/glove/ring/shoe size in adults, especially after age 40. **Individual should be referred for further evaluation for hyperpituitarism/growth hormone imbalance/acromegaly.**
- Review results of x-rays/bone scans/MRIs **to determine bone age/extent of bone and soft-tissue overgrowth; presence of tumors;** note laboratory studies (e.g., growth hormone levels/other endocrine studies) **to identify pathology.**
- Assist with therapy to treat/correct underlying conditions (e.g., Crohn's disease, cardiac problems, renal disease); endocrine problems (e.g., hyperpituitarism, hypothyroidism, type 1 diabetes mellitus, growth hormone abnormalities); genetic/intrauterine growth retardation; infant feeding problems; nutritional deficits [specify].
- Include nutritionist and other specialists (e.g., physical/occupational therapist) in developing plan of care.
- Determine need for medications (e.g., appetite stimulants or antidepressants, growth hormones, etc.).
- Monitor growth periodically. **Aids in evaluating effectiveness of interventions/promotes early identification of need for additional actions.**

NURSING PRIORITY NO. 3. To promote wellness (Teaching/Discharge Considerations):

- Provide information regarding normal growth, as appropriate, including pertinent reference materials/credible websites.
- Address caregiver issues (e.g., parental abuse, learning deficiencies, environment of poverty) **that could impact client's ability to thrive.**
- Discuss appropriateness of appearance, grooming, touching, language, and other associated developmental issues. (Refer to NDs delayed Growth and Development; Self-Care Deficit [specify].)
- Recommend involvement in regular exercise/sports medicine program **to enhance muscle tone/strength and appropriate body building.**

Information in brackets added by the authors to clarify and enhance the use of nursing diagnoses.

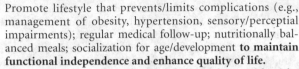

- Promote lifestyle that prevents/limits complications (e.g., management of obesity, hypertension, sensory/perceptual impairments); regular medical follow-up; nutritionally balanced meals; socialization for age/development **to maintain functional independence and enhance quality of life.**
- Discuss consequences of substance use/abuse with girls/women of childbearing age, and provide pregnant women with information regarding known teratogenic agents. **Education can influence mother to abstain from use of drugs/agents that may cause birth defects.**
- Refer for genetic screening, as appropriate.
- Identify available community resources, as appropriate (e.g., public health programs, such as WIC; medical equipment supplies; nutritionists; substance abuse programs; specialists in endocrine problems/genetics).

Documentation Focus

ASSESSMENT/REASSESSMENT

- Assessment findings/individual needs, including current growth status, and trends.
- Caregiver's understanding of situation and individual role.

PLANNING

- Plan of care and who is involved in the planning.
- Teaching plan.

IMPLEMENTATION/EVALUATION

- Client's responses to interventions/teaching and actions performed.
- Caregiver response to teaching.
- Attainment/progress toward desired outcome(s).
- Modifications to plan of care.

DISCHARGE PLANNING

- Identified long-range needs and who is responsible for actions to be taken.
- Specific referrals made, sources for assistive devices, educational tools.

SAMPLE NURSING OUTCOMES & INTERVENTIONS CLASSIFICATIONS (NOC/NIC)

NOC—Child Development: [specify age group]
NIC—Nutritional Monitoring

Information in brackets added by the authors to clarify and enhance the use of nursing diagnoses.

  Cultural Collaborative 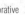 Community/Home Care

delayed Growth and Development

Taxonomy II: Growth/Development—Class 2
Development (00111)
[Diagnostic Division: Teaching/Learning]
Submitted 1986

Definition: Deviations from age-group norms

Related Factors

Inadequate caretaking; [physical/emotional neglect or abuse]
Indifference; inconsistent responsiveness; multiple caretakers
Separation from significant others
Environmental/stimulation deficiencies
Effects of physical disability [handicapping condition]
Prescribed dependence [insufficient expectations for self-care]
[Physical/emotional illness (chronic, traumatic) (e.g., chronic
inflammatory disease, pituitary tumors, impaired nutri-
tion/metabolism, greater-than-normal energy requirements,
prolonged/painful treatments, prolonged/repeated hospital-
izations)]
[Sexual abuse]
[Substance use/abuse]

Defining Characteristics

SUBJECTIVE

Inability to perform self-care/self-control activities appropriate
for age

OBJECTIVE

Delay/difficulty in performing skills typical of age group [loss of
previously acquired skills]
Altered physical growth
Flat effect; listlessness; decreased responses
[Sleep disturbances; negative mood/response]

Desired Outcomes/Evaluation
Criteria—Client Will:

• Perform motor, social, and/or expressive skills typical of age
  group within scope of present capabilities.
• Perform self-care and self-control activities appropriate for age.
• Demonstrate weight/growth stabilization or progress toward
  age-appropriate size.

Information in brackets added by the authors to clarify and enhance
the use of nursing diagnoses.

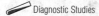 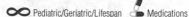

Parents/Caregivers Will:

- Verbalize understanding of growth/developmental delay or deviation and plan(s) for intervention.
- (Refer to ND risk for delayed Development for additonal actions/interventions.)

Actions/Interventions

NURSING PRIORITY NO. 1. To assess causative/contributing factors:

- Determine existing condition(s) contributing to growth/ developmental deviation, such as limited intellectual capacity, physical disabilities, chronic illness, genetic anomalies, substance use/abuse, multiple birth (e.g., twins)/minimal length of time between pregnancies.
- Determine nature of parenting/caretaking activities (e.g., inadequate, inconsistent, unrealistic/insufficient expectations; lack of stimulation, limit setting, responsiveness).
- Note severity/pervasiveness of situation (e.g., long-term physical/emotional abuse versus situational disruption or inadequate assistance during period of crisis or transition).
- Assess occurrence/frequency of significant stressful events, losses, separation, and environmental changes (e.g., abandonment; divorce; death of parent/sibling; aging; unemployment; new job; moves; new baby/sibling; marriage; new stepparent).
- Determine presence of environmental risk factors (e.g., child of parent(s) with active substance abuse issues, or who are abusive, neglectful, or mentally disabled).
- Active-listen to SO's concerns about client's body size, ability to communicate or perform desired/needed activites or participate competitively (e.g., sports, body building).
- Determine use of drugs, **which may affect body growth.**
- Evaluate home/day care/hospital/institutional environment **to determine adequacy of care provided, including nourishing meals, healthy sleep/rest time, stimulation, diversional or play activities.**

NURSING PRIORITY NO. 2. To determine degree of deviation from norms:

- Identify present growth age/stage. **Provides baseline for identification of needs and effectiveness of therapies.**
- Review expectations for current height/weight percentile. **Compares measurements to "standard" or normal range for children of same age and gender to determine degree of deviation.**

Information in brackets added by the authors to clarify and enhance the use of nursing diagnoses.

 Cultural Collaborative 🏠 Community/Home Care

- Note chronological age, familial factors (e.g., including body build/stature), and cultural concerns **to determine individual growth and developmental expectations.**
- Record height/weight over time **to determine trends.**
- Identify present developmental age/stage. Note reported deficits in functional level/evidence of precocious development. **Provides comparative baseline.**
- Review expected skills/activities, using authoritative text (e.g., Gesell, Musen/Congor) or assessment tools (e.g., Draw-a-Person, Denver Developmental Screening Test, Bender's Visual Motor Gestalt Test).
- Note degree of individual deviation, multiple skills affected (e.g., speech, motor activity, socialization), versus a single area of difficulty, such as toileting.
- Note whether difficulty is temporary or permanent (e.g., setback or delay versus irreversible condition, such as brain damage, stroke, dementia).
- Investigate sexual acting-out behaviors inappropriate for age. **May indicate sexual abuse.**
- Note findings of psychological evaluation of client and family **to determine factors that may impact development of client or impair psychological health of family.**

NURSING PRIORITY NO. 3. To correct/minimize growth deviations and associated complications:

- Participate in treatment of underlying medical/psychological conditions (e.g., malnourishment, kidney failure, congenital heart disease, cystic fibrosis, inflammatory bowel disease, bone/cartilage conditions, endocrine disorders, adverse effects of medications, mental illness, substance abuse), as appropriate.
- Review medication regimen given to stimulate/suppress growth, as appropriate, or possibly to shrink tumor when present.
- Stress necessity of not stopping medications without approval of healthcare provider.
- Discuss appropriateness and potential complications of bone-lengthening procedures.
- Review consequences of substance use/abuse.
- Include nutritionist and other specialists (e.g., physical/occupational therapists) in developing plan of care. Encourage "early intervention services" for children birth to 3 years of age with developmental delays. **Federally funded entitlement program for qualified child (e.g., Down syndrome or cerebral palsy; prematurity; deprived physical/social environment) aimed at maximizing child's development. Services include nursing,**

Information in brackets added by the authors to clarify and enhance the use of nursing diagnoses.

occupational/physical/speech therapy, service coordination, social work, and assistive technologies.

 • Monitor growth and development factors periodically. **Aids in evaluating effectiveness of interventions over time and promotes early identification of need for additional actions.**

NURSING PRIORITY NO. 4. To assist client (and/or caregivers) to prevent, minimize, or overcome delay/regressed development:

• Provide anticipatory guidance for parents/caregivers regarding expectations for client's development **to clarify misconceptions and assist them in dealing with reality of situation.**

• Consult appropriate professional resources (e.g., occupational/rehabilitation/speech therapists, special-education teacher, job counselor) **to address specific individual needs.**

 • Encourage recognition that deviation/behavior is appropriate for a specific age level (e.g., 14-year-old is functioning at level of 6-year-old or 16-year-old is not displaying pubertal changes). **Promotes acceptance of client, as presented, and helps shape expectations reflecting actual situation.**

 • Avoid blame when discussing contributing factors.

 • Maintain positive, hopeful attitude. Support self-actualizing nature of the individual and attempts to maintain or return to optimal level of self-control or self-care activities.

• Refer family/client for counseling/psychotherapy **to deal with issues of abuse/neglect.**

 • Encourage setting of short-term, realistic goals for achieving developmental potential.

 • Involve client in opportunities to practice new behaviors (e.g., role play, group activities). **Strengthens learning process.**

 • Identify equipment needs (e.g., adaptive/growth-stimulating computer programs, communication devices).

 • Evaluate progress on continual basis **to increase complexity of tasks/goals, as indicated.**

 • Provide positive feedback for efforts/successes and adaptation while minimizing failures. **Encourages continuation of efforts, thus improving outcome.**

 • Assist client/caregivers to accept and adjust to irreversible developmental deviations (e.g., Down syndrome).

 • Provide support for caregiver during transitional crises (e.g., residential schooling, institutionalization).

NURSING PRIORITY NO. 5. To promote wellness (Teaching/Discharge Considerations):

 • Provide information regarding normal growth and development process, as appropriate. Suggest genetic counseling for family/client dependent on causative factors.

Information in brackets added by the authors to clarify and enhance the use of nursing diagnoses.

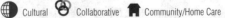
Cultural   Collaborative   Community/Home Care

- Determine reasonable expectations for individual without restricting potential (i.e., set realistic goals that, if met, can be advanced). **Provides hope for achievement and promotes continued personal growth.**
- Discuss appropriateness of appearance, grooming, touching, language, and other associated developmental issues. (Refer to ND Self-Care Deficit [specify].)
- Recommend involvement in regular exercise/sports medicine program **to enhance muscle tone/strength and appropriate body building.**
- Discuss actions to take to avoid preventable complications (e.g., periodic laboratory studies **to monitor hormone levels/nutritional status**).
- Recommend wearing medical alert bracelet when taking replacement hormones.
- Encourage attendance at appropriate educational programs (e.g., parenting and expectant parent classes; infant stimulation sessions; seminars on life stresses, aging process).
- Provide pertinent reference materials and pamphlets. **Enhances learning at own pace.**
- Discuss community responsibilities (e.g., services required to be provided to school-age child). Include social worker/special-education team in planning process **for meeting educational, physical, psychological, and monitoring needs of child.**
- Identify community resources, as appropriate: public health programs, such as Women, Infants, and Children (WIC); well-baby care provider; nutritionist; substance abuse programs; early-intervention programs; seniors' activity/support groups; gifted and talented programs; sheltered workshop; disabled children's services; medical equipment/supplier. **Provides additional assistance to support family efforts in treatment program.**
- Evaluate/refer to social services, as indicated, **to determine safety of client and consideration of placement in foster care.**
- Refer to the NDs impaired Parenting; interrupted Family Processes.

Documentation Focus

ASSESSMENT/REASSESSMENT

- Assessment findings/individual needs, including current growth status/trends and developmental level/evidence of regression.
- Caregiver's understanding of situation and individual role.
- Safety of individual/need for placement.

Information in brackets added by the authors to clarify and enhance the use of nursing diagnoses.

 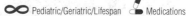

PLANNING

- Plan of care and who is involved in the planning.
- Teaching plan.

IMPLEMENTATION/EVALUATION

- Client's responses to interventions/teaching and actions performed.
- Caregiver response to teaching.
- Attainment/progress toward desired outcome(s).
- Modifications to plan of care.

DISCHARGE PLANNING

- Identified long-range needs and who is responsible for actions to be taken.
- Specific referrals made; sources for assistive devices, educational tools.

SAMPLE NURSING OUTCOMES & INTERVENTIONS CLASSIFICATIONS (NOC/NIC)

NOC—Child Development: [specify age group]
NIC—Developmental Enhancement: Child/Adolescent

ineffective Health Maintenance

Taxonomy II: Health Promotion—Class 2 Health Management (00099)
[Diagnostic Division: Safety]
Submitted 1982

Definition: Inability to identify, manage, and/or seek out help to maintain health

[This diagnosis contains components of other NDs. We recommend subsuming health maintenance interventions under the "basic" nursing diagnosis when a single causative factor is identified (e.g., deficient Knowledge [specify]; ineffective Therapeutic Regimen Management; chronic Confusion; impaired verbal Communication; disturbed Thought Processes; ineffective Coping; compromised family Coping; delayed Growth and Development).]

Related Factors

Deficient communication skills [written, verbal, and/or gestural]
Unachieved developmental tasks

Information in brackets added by the authors to clarify and enhance the use of nursing diagnoses.

  Cultural Collaborative  Community/Home Care

Inability to make appropriate judgments
Perceptual/cognitive impairment
Diminished/lack of gross/fine motor skills
Ineffective individual/family coping; complicated grieving; spiritual distress
Insufficient resources (e.g., equipment, finances); [lack of psychosocial supports]

Defining Characteristics

SUBJECTIVE

Lack of expressed interest in improving health behaviors
[Reported compulsive behaviors]

OBJECTIVE

Demonstrated lack of knowledge regarding basic health practices
Inability to take the responsibility for meeting basic health practices; history of lack of health-seeking behavior
Demonstrated lack of adaptive behaviors to environmental changes
Impairment of personal support system
[Observed compulsive behaviors]

Desired Outcomes/Evaluation Criteria—Client Will:

- Identify necessary health maintenance activities.
- Verbalize understanding of factors contributing to current situation.
- Assume responsibility for own healthcare needs within level of ability.
- Adopt lifestyle changes supporting individual healthcare goals.

SO/Caregiver Will:

- Verbalize ability to cope adequately with existing situation, provide support/monitoring as indicated.

Actions/Interventions

NURSING PRIORITY NO. 1. To assess causative/contributing factors:

- Identify risk factors in client's personal and family history. Note health values/religious/cultural beliefs and expectations regarding healthcare.
- Assess level of client's cognitive, emotional, physical functioning. Determine type/presence of developmental disabilities.

Information in brackets added by the authors to clarify and enhance the use of nursing diagnoses.

 Diagnostic Studies   Pediatric/Geriatric/Lifespan   Medications

• Determine whether impairment is an acute/sudden onset situation, a progressive illness/long-term health problem, or exacerbation or complication of chronic illness. **May require more intensive/long-lasting support.**

 • Note client's age (e.g., very young or elderly) and level of dependence/independence. **May range from complete dependence (dysfunctional) to partial or relative independence requiring support in a single area.**

• Evaluate for substance use/abuse (e.g., alcohol/other drugs). **Affects client's desire/ability to help self.**

• Ascertain recent changes in lifestyle (e.g., man whose wife dies and he has no skills for taking care of his own/family's health needs; loss of independence; changing support systems).

• Note setting where client lives (e.g., long-term care facility, homebound, homeless).

• Note desire/level of ability to meet health maintenance needs, as well as self-care ADLs.

• Determine level of adaptive behavior, knowledge, and skills about health maintenance, environment, and safety. **Determines beginning point for planning and interventions to assist client in addressing needs.**

• Assess client's ability and desire to learn. Determine barriers to learning (e.g., can't read, speaks/understands nondominant language, is overcome with grief or stress, has no interest in subject.)

• Assess communication skills/ability/need for interpreter. Identify support person requesting/willing to accept information.

• Note client's use of professional services and resources (e.g., appropriate or inappropriate/nonexistent).

NURSING PRIORITY NO. 2. To assist client/caregiver(s) to maintain and manage desired health practices:

• Discuss with client/SO(s) beliefs about health and reasons for not following prescribed plan of care. **Determines client's view about current situation and potential for change.**

• Evaluate environment **to note individual adaptation needs.**

• Develop plan with client/SO(s) for self-care. **Allows for incorporating existing disabilities with client's/SO's desires and ability to adapt and organize care activites.**

• Involve comprehensive specialty health teams when available/indicated (e.g., pulmonary, psychiatric, enterostomal, IV therapy, nutritional support, substance-abuse counselors).

• Provide anticipatory guidance **to maintain and manage effective health practices during periods of wellness and identify ways client can adapt when progressive illness/long-term health problems occur.**

Information in brackets added by the authors to clarify and enhance the use of nursing diagnoses.

Cultural   Collaborative   Community/Home Care

• Encourage socialization and personal involvement **to enhance support system, provide pleasant stimuli, and prevent permanent regression.**

• Provide for communication and coordination between the healthcare facility team and community healthcare providers **to provide continuation of care.**

• Monitor adherence to prescribed medical regimen **to problem solve difficulties in adherence and alter the plan of care, as needed.**

NURSING PRIORITY NO. 3. To promote wellness (Teaching/Discharge Considerations):

• Provide information about individual healthcare needs, using client's/SO's perferred learning style (e.g., pictures, words, video, Internet) **to assist client in understanding own situation and enhance interest/involvement in meeting own health needs.**

• Limit amount of information presented at one time, especially when dealing with elderly or cognitively/developmentally impaired client. Present new material through self-paced instruction when possible. **Allows client time to process and store new information.**

• Help client/SO(s) develop realistic healthcare goals. Provide a written copy to those involved in planning process **for future reference/revision, as appropriate.**

• Assist client/SO(s) to develop stress management skills.

• Identify ways to adapt things in current circumstances **to meet client's changing needs/abilities and environmental concerns.**

• Identify signs and symptoms requiring further screening, evaluation, and follow-up care.

• Make referral, as needed, for community support services (e.g., homemaker/home attendant, Meals on Wheels, skilled nursing care, well-baby clinic, senior citizen healthcare activities).

• Refer to social services, as indicated, **for assistance with financial, housing, or legal concerns (e.g., conservatorship).**

• Refer to support groups, as appropriate (e.g., senior citizens, Salvation Army/Red Cross Shelter, homeless clinic, Alcoholics/Narcotics Anonymous).

• Arrange for hospice service for client with terminal illness.

Documentation Focus

ASSESSMENT/REASSESSMENT

• Assessment findings, including individual abilities; family involvement; and support factors/availability of resources.
• Cultural/religious beliefs and healthcare values.

Information in brackets added by the authors to clarify and enhance the use of nursing diagnoses.

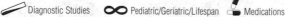

PLANNING

- Plan of care and who is involved in planning.
- Teaching plan.

IMPLEMENTATION/EVALUATION

- Responses of client/SO(s) to plan/interventions/teaching and actions performed.
- Attainment/progress toward desired outcome(s).
- Modifications to plan of care.

DISCHARGE PLANNING

- Long-range needs and who is responsible for actions to be taken.
- Specific referrals made.

SAMPLE NURSING OUTCOMES & INTERVENTIONS CLASSIFICATIONS (NOC/NIC)

NOC—Health Promoting Behavior
NIC—Health System Guidance

Health-Seeking Behaviors (specify)

Taxonomy II: Health Promotion—Class 2 Health
Management (00084)
[Diagnostic Division: Teaching/Learning]
Submitted 1988

Definition: Active seeking (by a person in stable health) of ways to alter personal health habits and/or the environment in order to move toward a higher level of health (Note: Stable health is defined as achievement of age-appropriate illness-prevention measures; client reports good or excellent health; and signs and symptoms of disease, if present, are controlled.)

Related Factors

To be developed
[Situational/maturational occurrence precipitating concern about current health status]

Defining Characteristics

SUBJECTIVE

Expressed desire to seek a higher level of wellness
Expressed desire for increased control of health practice

Information in brackets added by the authors to clarify and enhance the use of nursing diagnoses.

  Cultural Collaborative 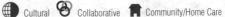 Community/Home Care

Expressed concern about current environmental conditions on health status

Stated unfamiliarity with wellness community resources

[Expressed desire to modify codependent behaviors]

OBJECTIVE

Observed unfamiliarity with wellness community resources

Demonstrated lack of knowledge in health promotion behaviors

Desired Outcomes/Evaluation Criteria—Client Will:

- Express desire to change specific habit/lifestyle patterns to achieve/maintain optimal health.
- Participate in planning for change.
- Seek community resources to assist with desired change.

Actions/Interventions

NURSING PRIORITY NO. 1. To assess specific concerns/habits/issues client desires to change:

- Determine client's current health status and perception of possible threats to health.
- Address barriers to healthcare (e.g., transportation, lack of insurance, costs of services, communication barriers, fear of/actual criticism from family/peers).
- Identify behaviors (e.g., tobacco use; behavior that results in injury and violence; alcohol and substance use; dietary and hygienic practices that cause disease; sedentary lifestyle; sexual behavior that causes unintended pregnancy and disease) **associated with health habits/poor health practices and proliferation of chronic health problems.**
- Note cultural/religious beliefs and practices that impact perceptions of health status and expectations for change.
- Active-listen/discuss concerns with client **to identify underlying issues (e.g., physical and/or emotional stressors and/or external factors, such as environmental pollutants or other hazards) that could impact client's ability to control own health.**
- Review knowledge base and note coping skills that have been used previously to change behavior/promote health.
- Use screening/testing, as indicated, and review results with client/SO(s) **to help with development of plan of action.**

Information in brackets added by the authors to clarify and enhance the use of nursing diagnoses.

HEALTH-SEEKING BEHAVIORS (specify)

NURSING PRIORITY NO. 2. To assist client to develop plan for improving health:

- Discuss with client his or her particular risk-taking behavior (e.g., smoking, drinking, self-medicating, lack of healthy food or exercise) **to provide information and encourage client to make healthy choices for future.**

 • Explore with client/SO(s) areas of health over which each individual has control and possible barriers (e.g., lack of time, access to convenient facilites or safe environment in which to exercise, etc.). Problem solve options for change. **Helps identify actions to be taken to achieve desired improvement.**

 • Provide information about conditions/health risk factors or concerns in written and audiovisual forms, Internet websites, as appropriate. **Use of multiple modalities enhances acquisition/retention of information.**

 • Discuss assertive behaviors and provide opportunity for client to practice new behaviors.

 • Use therapeutic communication skills **to provide support for desired changes.**

NURSING PRIORITY NO. 3. To promote wellness (Teaching/Discharge Considerations):

 • Acknowledge client's strengths in present health management and build on in planning for future.

 • Encourage use of relaxation skills, medication, visualization, and guided imagery **to assist in management of stress.**

• Instruct in individually appropriate wellness behaviors (e.g., breast/testicle self-examination, immunizations, smoking cessation, regular medical and dental examinations, healthy diet, exercise program, early intervention and treatment of risk factors [e.g., hypertension, obesity]).

• Identify and refer child/family member to health resources for immunizations, basic health services, and to learn health promotion/monitoring skills (e.g., monitoring hydration, measuring fever). **May facilitate long-term attention to health issues.**

• Refer to community resources (e.g., dietitian/weight control program, smoking cessation groups, Alcoholics Anonymous, codependency support groups, assertiveness training/parent effectiveness classes, driving safety, violence prevention, clinical nurse specialists/psychiatrists) **to address specific concerns.**

Documentation Focus

ASSESSMENT/REASSESSMENT

- Assessment findings, including individual concerns/risk factors.

Information in brackets added by the authors to clarify and enhance the use of nursing diagnoses.

  Cultural Collaborative Community/Home Care

- Pertinent cultural/religious beliefs and values.
- Client's request for change.

PLANNING

- Plan of care and who is involved in planning.
- Teaching plan.

IMPLEMENTATION/EVALUATION

- Responses to wellness plan, interventions/teaching, and actions performed.
- Attainment/progress toward desired outcome(s).
- Modifications to plan of care.

DISCHARGE PLANNING

- Long-range needs and who is responsible for actions to be taken.
- Specific referrals.

SAMPLE NURSING OUTCOMES & INTERVENTIONS CLASSIFICATIONS (NOC/NIC)

NOC—Health-Seeking Behavior
NIC—Self-Modification Assistance

impaired Home Maintenance

Taxonomy II: Health Promotion—Class 2 Health Management (00098)
[Diagnostic Division: Safety]
Submitted 1980

Definition: Inability to independently maintain a safe growth-promoting immediate environment

Related Factors

Disease; injury
Insufficient family organization/planning
Insufficient finances
Impaired functioning
Lack of role modeling
Unfamiliarity with neighborhood resources
Deficient knowledge
Inadequate support systems

Information in brackets added by the authors to clarify and enhance the use of nursing diagnoses.

 Diagnostic Studies 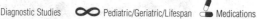 Pediatric/Geriatric/Lifespan   Medications

Defining Characteristics

SUBJECTIVE

Household members express difficulty in maintaining their home in a comfortable [safe] fashion

Household members request assistance with home maintenance

Household members describe outstanding debts/financial crises

OBJECTIVE

Disorderly/unclean surroundings; offensive odors

Inappropriate household temperature

Presence of vermin

Repeated unhygienic disorders/infections

Lack of necessary equipment; unavailable cooking equipment

Insufficient/lack of clothes/linen

Overtaxed family members

Desired Outcomes/Evaluation Criteria—Client/Caregiver Will:

- Identify individual factors related to difficulty in maintaining a safe environment.
- Verbalize plan to eliminate health and safety hazards.
- Adopt behaviors reflecting lifestyle changes to create and sustain a healthy/growth-promoting environment.
- Demonstrate appropriate, effective use of resources.

Actions/Interventions

NURSING PRIORITY NO. 1. To assess causative/contributing factors:

- Identify presence of/potential for physical/mental conditions (e.g., advanced age, chronic illnesses, brain/other traumatic injuries; severe depression/other mental illness; multiple persons in one home incapable of handling home tasks) **that compromise client's/SO's functional abilities in taking care of home.**
- Note presence of personal and/or environmental factors (e.g., family member with multiple care tasks; substance abuse; absence of family/support systems; lifestyle of self-neglect; client comfortable with home environment/has no desire for change).
- Determine problem in household and degree of discomfort/unsafe conditons noted by client/SO(s). **Safety problems may be obvious (e.g., lack of heat or water; unsanitary rooms) while other problems may be more subtle and difficult to manage (e.g., lack of finances for home repair, or lack of knowledge about food storage, rodent control).**

Information in brackets added by the authors to clarify and enhance the use of nursing diagnoses.

  Cultural Collaborative Community/Home Care

- Assess client/SO's level of cognitive/emotional/physical functioning **to ascertain needs and capabilities in handling tasks of home management.**
- Identify lack of knowledge/misinformation.
- Discuss home environment/perform home visit, as appropriate, **to determine ability to care for self and to identify potential health and safety hazards.**
- Identify support systems available to client/SO(s) **to determine needs and initiate referrals (e.g., companionship, daily care, household cleaning/homemaking, running errands).**
- Determine financial resources to meet needs of individual situation.

NURSING PRIORITY NO. 2. To help client/SO(s) create/maintain a safe, growth-promoting environment:

- Coordinate planning with multidisciplinary team, as appropriate.
- Assist client/SO(s) to develop plan for maintaining a clean, healthful environment (e.g., sharing of household tasks/repairs between family members, contract services, exterminators, trash removal).
- Assist client/SO(s) to identify and acquire necessary equipment (e.g., lifts, commode chair, safety grab bars, cleaning supplies, structural adaptations) **to meet individual needs.**
- Identify resources available for appropriate assistance (e.g., visiting nurse, budget counseling, homemaker, Meals on Wheels, physical/occupational therapy, social services).

NURSING PRIORITY NO. 3. To promote wellness (Teaching/Discharge Considerations):

- Discuss environmental hazards **that may negatively affect health or ability to perform desired activities.**
- Develop long-term plan for taking care of environmental needs (e.g., assistive personnel to clean house/do laundry; trash removal and pest control services).
- Identify ways to access/use community resources and support systems (e.g., extended family, neighbors).
- Refer to NDs deficient Knowledge (specify); Self-Care Deficit [specify]; ineffective Coping; compromised family Coping; Caregiver Role Strain; risk for Injury.

Documentation Focus

ASSESSMENT/REASSESSMENT

- Assessment findings include individual/environmental factors, presence and use of support systems.

Information in brackets added by the authors to clarify and enhance the use of nursing diagnoses.

 Diagnostic Studies ∞ Pediatric/Geriatric/Lifespan Medications

PLANNING

- Plan of care and who is involved in planning; support systems and community resources identified.
- Teaching plan.

IMPLEMENTATION/EVALUATION

- Client's/SO's responses to interventions/teaching and actions performed.
- Attainment/progress toward desired outcome(s).
- Modifications to plan of care.

DISCHARGE PLANNING

- Long-term needs and who is responsible for actions to be taken.
- Specific referrals made, equipment needs/resources.

SAMPLE NURSING OUTCOMES & INTERVENTIONS CLASSIFICATIONS (NOC/NIC)

NOC—Self-Care: Instrumental Activities of Daily Living (IADL)
NIC—Home Maintenance Assistance

readiness for enhanced Hope

Taxonomy II: Life Principles—Class 1 Values (00185)
   Class 2 Beliefs
[Diagnostic Division: Ego Integrity]
Submitted 2006

Definition: A pattern of expectations and desires that is sufficient for mobilizing energy on one's own behalf and can be strengthened

Related Factors

To be developed

Defining Characteristics

SUBJECTIVE

Expresses desire to enhance hope; belief in possibilities; congruency of expectations with desires; ability to set achievable goals; problem solving to meet goals
Expresses desire to enhance sense of meaning to life; interconnectedness with others; spirituality

---

Information in brackets added by the authors to clarify and enhance the use of nursing diagnoses.

  Cultural Collaborative Community/Home Care

Desired Outcomes/Evaluation Criteria—Client Will:

- Identify and verbalize feelings related to expectations and desires.
- Verbalize belief in possibilities for the future.
- Discuss current situation and desire to enhance hope.
- Set short-term goals that will lead to behavioral changes to meet desire for enhanced hope.

Actions/Interventions

NURSING PRIORITY NO. 1. To determine needs and desire for improvement:

- Review familial/social history to identify past situations (e.g., illness, emotional conflicts, alcoholism) that have led to decision to improve life.
- Determine current physical condition of client/SO(s). **Treatment regimen can influence ability to promote positive feelings of hope.**
- Ascertain client's perception of current state and expectations/goals for the future (e.g., general well-being, prosperity, independence).
- Identify spiritual beliefs/cultural values that influence sense of hope and connectedness and give meaning to life.
- Note degree of involvement in activities/relationships with others. **Superficial interactions with others can limit sense of connectedness and reduce enjoyment of relationships.**
- Determine level of commitment and expectations for change and congruency of expectations with desires.

NURSING PRIORITY NO. 2. To assist client to achieve goals and strengthen sense of hope:

- Establish a therapeutic relationship, showing positive regard and sense of hope for the client. **Enhances feelings of worth and comfort, inspiring client to continue pursuit of goals.**
- Help client recognize areas that are in his or her control versus those that are not. **To be most effective, client needs to expend energy in those areas where he or she has control/can make changes and let the others go.**
- Assist client to develop manageable short-term goals.
- Identify activities to achieve goals and facilitate contingency planning. **Helps client deal with situation in manageable steps, enhancing chances for success and sense of control.**
- Explore interrelatedness of unresolved emotions, anxieties, fears, and guilt. **Provides opportunity to address issues**

Information in brackets added by the authors to clarify and enhance the use of nursing diagnoses.

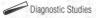 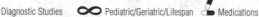

that may be limiting individual's ability to improve life situation.

- Assist client to acknowledge current coping behaviors and defense mechanisms that are not helping client move toward goals. **Allows client to focus on coping mechanisms that are more successful in problem solving.**

- Encourage client to concentrate on progress not perfection. **If client can accept that perfection is difficult and generally not the focus, rather achieving the desired goal is, then he or she may be able to view own accomplishments with pride.**

- Involve client in care and explain all procedures thoroughly, answering questions truthfully. **Enhances trust and relationship, promoting hope for a positive outcome.**

- Express hope to client and encourage SO(s) and other heath team members to do so. **Enhances client's sense of hope and belief in possibility of a positive outcome.**

 • Identify ways to strengthen sense of interconnectedness or harmony with others **to support sense of belonging and connection that promotes feelings of wholeness and hopefulness.**

NURSING PRIORITY NO. 3. To promote optimum wellness:

 • Demonstrate and encourage use of relaxation techniques, guided imagery, and meditation activities.

 • Provide positive feedback for actions taken to improve problem-solving skills and for setting achievable goals. **Acknowledges client's efforts and reinforces gains.**

 • Explore how beliefs give meaning and value to daily living. **As client's understanding of these issues improves, hope for the future is strengthened.**

 • Encourage life-review by client **to acknowledge own successes, identify opportunity for change, and clarify meaning in life.**

 • Identify ways for client to express/strengthen spirituality. **There are many options for enhancing spirituality through connectedness with self/others (e.g., volunteering, mentoring, involvement in religious activities).** (Refer to ND readiness for enhanced Spiritual Well-Being.)

 • Encourage client to join groups with similar or new interests. **Expanding knowledge and making friendships with new people will broaden horizons for the individual.**

 • Refer to community resources/support groups, spiritual advisor, as indicated.

Information in brackets added by the authors to clarify and enhance the use of nursing diagnoses.

🌐 Cultural   Collaborative   Community/Home Care

Documentation Focus

ASSESSMENT/REASSESSMENT

- Assessment findings, including client's perceptions of current situation, relationships, sense of desire for enhancing life.
- Motivation and expectations for improvement.

PLANNING

- Plan of care and who is involved in planning.
- Teaching plan.

IMPLEMENTATION/EVALUATION

- Responses to interventions/teaching and actions performed.
- Attainment/progress toward desired outcome(s).
- Modifications to plan of care.

DISCHARGE PLANNING

- Long-range needs/goals for change and who is responsible for actions to be taken.
- Specific referrals made.

SAMPLE NURSING OUTCOMES & INTERVENTIONS CLASSIFICATIONS (NOC/NIC)

NOC—Hope
NIC—Spiritual Growth Facilitation

Hopelessness

Taxonomy II: Self-Perception—Class 1 Self-Concept (00124)
[Diagnostic Division: Ego Integrity]
Submitted 1986

Definition: Subjective state in which an individual sees limited or no alternatives or personal choices available and is unable to mobilize energy on own behalf

Related Factors

Prolonged activity restriction creating isolation
Deteriorating physiological condition
Long-term stress; abandonment
Lost belief in spiritual power/transcendent values[/God]

Information in brackets added by the authors to clarify and enhance the use of nursing diagnoses.

 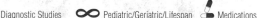

Defining Characteristics

SUBJECTIVE

Verbal cues (despondent content, "I can't," sighing) [believes things will not change/problems will always be there]

OBJECTIVE

Passivity; decreased verbalization
Decreased affect/appetite/response to stimuli
[Depressed cognitive functions; problems with decisions, thought processes; regression]
Lack of initiative/lack of involvement in care
Sleep pattern disturbance [increased/decreased sleep]
Turning away from speaker; shrugging in response to speaker; [withdrawal from environs; closing eyes]
[Lack of involvement/interest in SO(s) (children, spouse)]
[Angry outbursts]
[Substance abuse]

Desired Outcomes/Evaluation Criteria—Client Will:

- Recognize and verbalize feelings.
- Identify and use coping mechanisms to counteract feelings of hopelessness.
- Involve self in and control (within limits of the individual situation) own self-care and ADLs.
- Set progressive short-term goals that develop/foster/sustain behavioral changes/positive outlook.
- Participate in diversional activities of own choice.

Actions/Interventions

NURSING PRIORITY NO. 1. To identify causative/contributing factors:

- Review familial/social history and physiological history for problems, such as history of poor coping abilities, disorder of familial relating patterns, emotional problems, (**leading to feelings of isolation**), recent or long-term illness of client or family member, multiple social and/or physiological traumas to individual or family members.

- Note current familial/social/physical situation of client (e.g., newly diagnosed with chronic/terminal disease, lack of support system, recent job loss, loss of spiritual/religious faith, recent multiple traumas, alcoholism/substance abuse).

Information in brackets added by the authors to clarify and enhance the use of nursing diagnoses.

  Cultural Collaborative 🏠 Community/Home Care

- Identify cultural/spiritual values **that can impact beliefs in own ability to change situation.** Note language barriers.
- Determine coping behaviors and defense mechanisms displayed.
- Discuss problem of alcohol/drug abuse. **Client may feel hopeless about stopping behavior and believe that it is impossible.**
- Determine suicidal thoughts and if the client has a plan. **Hopelessness is a symptom of suicidal ideation.**

NURSING PRIORITY NO. 2. To assess level of hopelessness:

- Note behaviors indicative of hopelessness. (Refer to Defining Characteristics.)
- Determine coping behaviors previously used and client's perception of effectiveness then and now.
- Evaluate/discuss use of defense mechanisms (useful or not), such as increased sleeping, use of drugs (including alcohol), illness behaviors, eating disorders, denial, forgetfulness, daydreaming, ineffectual organizational efforts, exploiting own goal setting, regression.

NURSING PRIORITY NO. 3. To assist client to identify feelings and to begin to cope with problems as perceived by the client:

- Establish a therapeutic/facilitative relationship showing positive regard for the client. **Client may then feel safe to disclose feelings and feel understood and listened to.**
- Complete Beck's Depression Scale. Explain all tests/procedures thoroughly. Involve client in planning schedule for care. Answer questions truthfully. **Enhances trust and therapeutic relationship enabling client to talk freely about concerns.**
- Discuss initial signs of hopelessness (e.g., procrastination, increasing need for sleep, decreased physical activity, and withdrawal from social/familial activities).
- Encourage client to verbalize and explore feelings and perceptions (e.g., anger, helplessness, powerlessness, confusion, despondency, isolation, grief).
- Provide opportunity for children to "play out" feelings (e.g., puppets or art for preschooler, peer discussions for adolescents). **Provides insight into perceptions and may give direction for coping strategies.**
- Engage teens in discussions and arrange to do activities with them. **Parents can make a difference in their children's lives by being with them, discussing sensitive topics, and going different places with them.**

Information in brackets added by the authors to clarify and enhance the use of nursing diagnoses.

 Diagnostic Studies   ∞ Pediatric/Geriatric/Lifespan   Medications

HOPELESSNESS

- Express hope to client and encourage SO(s) and other health-team members to do so. **Client may not identify positives in own situation.**

- Assist client to identify short-term goals. Encourage activities to achieve goals, and facilitate contingency planning. **Promotes dealing with situation in manageable steps, enhancing chances for success and sense of control.**

- Discuss current options and list actions that may be taken to gain some control of situation. Correct misconceptions expressed by the client.

- Endeavor to prevent situations that might lead to feelings of isolation or lack of control in client's perception.

- Promote client control in establishing time, place, and frequency of therapy sessions. Involve family members in the therapy situation, as appropriate.

- Help client recognize areas in which he or she has control versus those that are not within his or her control.

- Encourage risk taking in situations in which the client can succeed.

- Help client begin to develop coping mechanisms that can be learned and used effectively **to counteract hopelessness.**

- Encourage structured/controlled increase in physical activity. **Enhances sense of well-being.**

- Demonstrate and encourage use of relaxation exercises, guided imagery.

- Discuss safe use of prescribed antidepressants.

NURSING PRIORITY NO. 4. To promote wellness (Teaching/Discharge Considerations):

- Provide positive feedback for actions taken to deal with and overcome feelings of hopelessness. **Encourages continuation of desired behaviors.**

- Assist client/family to become aware of factors/situations leading to feelings of hopelessness. **Provides opportunity to avoid/modify situation.**

- Facilitate client's incorporation of personal loss. **Enhances grief work and promotes resolution of feelings.**

- Encourage client/family to develop support systems in the immediate community.

- Help client to become aware of, nurture, and expand spiritual self. (Refer to ND Spiritual Distress.)

- Introduce the client into a support group before the individual therapy is terminated **for continuation of therapeutic process.**

- Stress need for continued monitoring of medication regimen by healthcare provider.

Information in brackets added by the authors to clarify and enhance the use of nursing diagnoses.

  Cultural Collaborative Community/Home Care

• Refer to other resources for assistance, as indicated (e.g., clinical nurse specialist, psychiatrist, social services, spiritual advisor, Alcoholics/Narcotics Anonymous, Al-Anon/Alateen).

Documentation Focus

ASSESSMENT/REASSESSMENT

• Assessment findings, including degree of impairment, use of coping skills, and support systems.

PLANNING

• Plan of care and who is involved in planning.
• Teaching plan.

IMPLEMENTATION/EVALUATION

• Responses to interventions/teaching and actions performed.
• Attainment/progress toward desired outcome(s).
• Modifications to plan of care.

DISCHARGE PLANNING

• Identified long-range needs/client's goals for change and who is responsible for actions to be taken.
• Specific referrals made.

SAMPLE NURSING OUTCOMES & INTERVENTIONS CLASSIFICATIONS (NOC/NIC)

NOC—Depression Control
NIC—Hope Instillation

Hyperthermia

Taxonomy II: Safety/Protection—Class 6
   Thermoregulation (00007)
[Diagnostic Division: Safety]
Submitted 1986

Definition: Body temperature elevated above normal range

Related Factors

Exposure to hot environment; inappropriate clothing
Vigorous activity; dehydration

Information in brackets added by the authors to clarify and enhance the use of nursing diagnoses.

 Diagnostic Studies   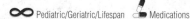 Pediatric/Geriatric/Lifespan   Medications   **383**

Decreased perspiration
Medications; anesthesia
Increased metabolic rate; illness; trauma

Defining Characteristics

SUBJECTIVE

[Headache]

OBJECTIVE

Increase in body temperature above normal range
Flushed skin; warm to touch
Tachypnea; tachycardia; [unstable BP]
Seizures; convulsions; [muscle rigidity/fasciculations]
[Confusion]

Desired Outcomes/Evaluation Criteria—Client Will:

- Maintain core temperature within normal range.
- Be free of complications such as irreversible brain/neurological damage, acute renal failure.
- Identify underlying cause/contributing factors and importance of treatment, as well as signs/symptoms requiring further evaluation or intervention.
- Demonstrate behaviors to monitor and promote normothermia.
- Be free of seizure activity.

Actions/Interventions

NURSING PRIORITY NO. 1. To assess causative/contributing factors:

- Identify underlying cause (e.g., excessive heat production, such as hyperthyroid state; malignant hyperpyrexia; impaired heat dissipation, such as heatstroke; dehydration; autonomic dysfunction as occurs with spinal cord transection; hypothalamic dysfunction, such as CNS infection; brain lesions; drug overdose; infection).

 • Note chronological and developmental age of client. **Children are more susceptible to heatstroke; elderly or impaired individuals may not be able to recognize and/or act on symptoms of hyperthermia.**

NURSING PRIORITY NO. 2. To evaluate effects/degree of hyperthermia:

- Monitor core temperature. Note: Rectal and tympanic temperatures most closely approximate core temperature; however,

---

Information in brackets added by the authors to clarify and enhance the use of nursing diagnoses.

abdominal temperature monitoring may be done in the premature neonate.

- Assess neurological response, noting level of consciousness and orientation, reaction to stimuli, reaction of pupils, presence of posturing or seizures.
- Monitor BP and invasive hemodynamic parameters if available (e.g., mean arterial pressure—MAP, CVP, PAP, PCWP). **Central hypertension or peripheral/postural hypotension can occur.**
- Monitor heart rate and rhythm. **Dysrhythmias and ECG changes are common due to electrolyte imbalance, dehydration, specific action of catecholamines, and direct effects of hyperthermia on blood and cardiac tissue.**
- Monitor respirations. **Hyperventilation may initially be present, but ventilatory effort may eventually be impaired by seizures, hypermetabolic state (shock and acidosis).**
- Auscultate breath sounds, noting adventitious sounds such as crackles (rales).
- Monitor/record all sources of fluid loss such as urine (**oliguria and/or renal failure may occur due to hypotension, dehydration, shock, and tissue necrosis**); vomiting and diarrhea; wounds/fistulas; and insensible losses (**potentiates fluid and electrolyte losses**).
- Note presence/absence of sweating as body attempts to increase heat loss by evaporation, conduction, and diffusion. **Evaporation is decreased by environmental factors of high humidity and high ambient temperature, as well as body factors producing loss of ability to sweat or sweat gland dysfunction (e.g., spinal cord transection, cystic fibrosis, dehydration, vasoconstriction).**
- Monitor laboratory studies, such as ABGs, electrolytes, cardiac and liver enzymes (**may reveal tissue degeneration**); glucose; urinalysis (**myoglobinuria, proteinuria, and hemoglobinuria can occur as products of tissue necrosis**); and coagulation profile (**for presence of disseminated intravascular coagulation—DIC**).

NURSING PRIORITY NO. 3. To assist with measures to reduce body temperature/restore normal body/organ function:

- Administer antipyretics, orally/rectally (e.g., aspirin, acetaminophen), as ordered. Refrain from use of aspirin products in children (**may cause Reye's syndrome**) or individuals with a clotting disorder or receiving anticoagulant therapy.
- Promote surface cooling by means of undressing (**heat loss by radiation and conduction**); cool environment and/or fans

---

Information in brackets added by the authors to clarify and enhance the use of nursing diagnoses.

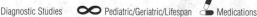

(heat loss by convection); cool/tepid sponge baths or immersion (heat loss by evaporation and conduction); local ice packs, especially in groin and axillae (areas of high blood flow). Note: In pediatric clients, tepid water is preferred. Alcohol sponge baths are contraindicated because they increase peripheral vascular constriction and CNS depression; cold-water sponges/immersion can increase shivering, producing heat.

- Monitor use of hypothermia blanket and wrap extremities with bath towels to minimize shivering. Turn off hypothermia blanket when core temperature is within 1 to 3 degrees of desired temperature to allow for downward drift.
- Administer medications (e.g., chlorpromazine or diazepam), as ordered, to control shivering and seizures.
- Assist with internal cooling methods to treat malignant hyperthermia to promote rapid core cooling.
- Promote client safety (e.g., maintain patent airway; padded siderails; skin protection from cold, such as when hypothermia blanket is used; observation of equipment safety measures).
- Provide supplemental oxygen to offset increased oxygen demands and consumption.
- Administer medications, as indicated, to treat underlying cause, such as antibiotics (for infection), dantrolene (for malignant hyperthermia), beta blockers (for thyroid storm).
- Administer replacement fluids and electrolytes to support circulating volume and tissue perfusion.
- Maintain bedrest to reduce metabolic demands/oxygen consumption.
- Provide high-calorie diet, tube feedings, or parenteral nutrition to meet increased metabolic demands.

NURSING PRIORITY NO. 4. To promote wellness (Teaching/Discharge Considerations):

- Review specific risk factor/cause, such as underlying conditions (hyperthyroidism, dehydration, neurologic diseases, nausea/vomiting, sepsis, use of certain medications [diruetics, blood pressure medications], alcohol/other drugs [cocaine/amphetamines]), environmental factors (exercise or labor in hot environment, lack of air conditioning, lack of acclimatization), reaction to anesthesia (malignant hyperthermia), other risk factors (salt or water depletion, elderly living alone).
- Identify those factors that client can control (if any), such as correction of underlying disease process (e.g., thyroid control medication), ways to protect oneself from excessive exposure to envi-

---

Information in brackets added by the authors to clarify and enhance the use of nursing diagnoses.

 Cultural 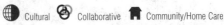 Collaborative   Community/Home Care ronmental heat (e.g., proper clothing, restriction of activity, scheduling outings during cooler part of day, use of fans/air-conditioning where possible), and understanding of family traits **(e.g., malignant hyperthermia reaction to anesthesia is often familial).**

- Instruct parents to avoid leaving young children in unattended car **to prevent heat injury/death.**
- Discuss importance of adequate fluid intake **to prevent dehydration.**
- Review signs/symptoms of hyperthermia (e.g., flushed skin, increased body temperature, increased respiratory/heart rate, fainting, loss of consciousness, seizures). **Indicates need for prompt intervention.**
- Recommend avoidance of hot tubs/saunas, as appropriate **(e.g., clients with MS, cardiac conditions, pregnancy that may affect fetal development or increase cardiac workload).**
- Identify community resources, especially for elderly clients, to address specific needs **(e.g., provision of fans for individual use, location of cooling rooms—usually in a community center—during heat waves, daily telephone contact to assess wellness).**

Documentation Focus

ASSESSMENT/REASSESSMENT

- Temperature and other assessment findings, including vital signs and state of mentation.

PLANNING

- Plan of care/interventions and who is involved in the planning.
- Teaching plan.

IMPLEMENTATION/EVALUATION

- Responses to interventions/teaching and actions performed.
- Attainment/progress toward desired outcome(s).
- Modifications to plan of care.

DISCHARGE PLANNING

- Referrals that are made, those responsible for actions to be taken.

SAMPLE NURSING OUTCOMES & INTERVENTIONS CLASSIFICATIONS (NOC/NIC)

NOC—Thermoregulation
NIC—Temperature Regulation

Information in brackets added by the authors to clarify and enhance the use of nursing diagnoses.

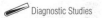 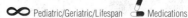

HYPOTHERMIA

Hypothermia

Taxonomy II: Safety/Protection—Class 6
   Thermoregulation (00006)
[Diagnostic Division: Safety]
Submitted 1986; Revised 1988

Definition: Body temperature below normal range

Related Factors

Exposure to cool environment [prolonged exposure, e.g., homeless, immersion in cold water/near-drowning, induced hypothermia/cardiopulmonary bypass]
Inadequate clothing
Evaporation from skin in cool environment
Decreased ability to shiver
Aging [or very young]
[Debilitating] illness; trauma; damage to hypothalamus
Malnutrition; decreased metabolic rate, inactivity
Consumption of alcohol; medications[/drug overdose]

Defining Characteristics

OBJECTIVE

Body temperature below normal range
Shivering; piloerection
Cool skin
Pallor; slow capillary refill; cyanotic nailbeds
Hypertension; tachycardia
[Core temperature 95°F/35°C: increased respirations, poor judgment, shivering]
[Core temperature 95°F to 93.2°F/35°C to 34°C: bradycardia or tachycardia, myocardial irritability/dysrhythmias, muscle rigidity, shivering, lethargic/confused, decreased coordination]
[Core temperature 93.2°F to 86°F/34°C to 30°C: hypoventilation, bradycardia, generalized rigidity, metabolic acidosis, coma]
[Core temperature below 86°F/30°C: no apparent vital signs, heart rate unresponsive to drug therapy, comatose, cyanotic, dilated pupils, apneic, areflexic, no shivering (appears dead)]

Desired Outcomes/Evaluation
Criteria—Client Will:

- Display core temperature within normal range.
- Be free of complications, such as cardiac failure, respiratory infection/failure, thromboembolic phenomena.

Information in brackets added by the authors to clarify and enhance the use of nursing diagnoses.

  Cultural Collaborative 🏠 Community/Home Care

- Identify underlying cause/contributing factors that are within client control.
- Verbalize understanding of specific interventions to prevent hypothermia.
- Demonstrate behaviors to monitor and promote normo-thermia.

Actions/Interventions

NURSING PRIORITY NO. 1. To assess causative/contributing factors:

- Note underlying cause (e.g., exposure to cold weather/winter outdoor activities; cold-water immersion; surgery; open wounds/exposed viscera; large burns; multiple rapid transfusions of banked blood; cooling therapy for hyperthermia).
- Note contributing factors: age of client (e.g., premature neonate, child, elderly person); concurrent/coexisting medical problems (e.g., brainstem injury, CNS trauma, near-drowning, sepsis, hypothyroidism); other factors (e.g., alcohol/other drug use/abuse; homelessness); living condition/relationship status (e.g., mentally impaired client alone).

NURSING PRIORITY NO. 2. To prevent further decrease in body temperature:

- Remove wet clothing. Wrap in warm blankets, extra clothing, as appropriate.
- Place knit cap on infant's head.
- Prevent pooling of antiseptic/irrigating solutions under client in operating room. Cover skin areas outside of operative field.
- Prevent drafts in room; raise ambient temperature.
- Place infant under radiant warmer/in isolet and monitor temperature closely.
- Avoid use of heat lamps or hot water bottles. (**Surface rewarming can result in rewarming shock due to surface vasodilation.**)
- Provide warm liquids if client can swallow.
- Warm IV solutions, as appropriate.

NURSING PRIORITY NO. 3. To evaluate effects of hypothermia:

- Measure core temperature with low register thermometer (measuring below 94°F/34°C).
- Assess respiratory effort (**rate and tidal volume are reduced when metabolic rate decreases and respiratory acidosis occurs**).
- Auscultate lungs, noting adventitious sounds (**pulmonary edema, respiratory infection, and pulmonary embolus are possible complications of hypothermia**).

Information in brackets added by the authors to clarify and enhance the use of nursing diagnoses.

 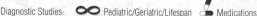

- Monitor heart rate and rhythm. **Cold stress reduces pacemaker function, and bradycardia (unresponsive to atropine), atrial fibrillation, atrioventricular blocks, and ventricular tachycardia can occur. Ventricular fibrillation occurs most frequently when core temperature is 82°F/28°C or below.**
- Monitor BP, noting hypotension. **Can occur due to vasoconstriction and shunting of fluids as a result of cold injury effect on capillary permeability.**
- Measure urine output. **Oliguria/renal failure can occur due to low flow state and/or following hypothermic osmotic diuresis.**
- Note CNS effects (e.g., mood changes, sluggish thinking, amnesia, complete obtundation) and peripheral CNS effects (e.g., paralysis—87.7°F/31°C, dilated pupils—below 86°F/30°C, flat EEG—68°F/20°C).
- Monitor laboratory studies, such as ABGs (**respiratory and metabolic acidosis**); electrolytes; CBC (**increased hematocrit, decreased white blood cell count**); cardiac enzymes (**myocardial infarct may occur owing to electrolyte imbalance, cold stress catecholamine release, hypoxia, or acidosis**); coagulation profile; glucose; pharmacological profile (**for possible cumulative drug effects**).

NURSING PRIORITY NO. 4. To restore normal body temperature/organ function:

- Assist with measures to normalize core temperature, such as warmed IV solutions and warm solution lavage of body cavities (gastric, peritoneal, bladder) or cardiopulmonary bypass, if indicated.
- Rewarm no faster than 1 to 2 degrees per hr **to avoid sudden vasodilation, increased metabolic demands on heart, and hypotension (rewarming shock).**
- Assist with surface warming by means of warmed blankets, warm environment/radiant heater, electronic warming devices. Cover head/neck and thorax, leaving extremities uncovered, as appropriate, **to maintain peripheral vasoconstriction.** Refrain from instituting surface rewarming prior to core rewarming in severe hypothermia (**causes after drop of temperature by shunting cold blood back to heart in addition to rewarming shock as a result of surface vasodilation).**
- Protect skin/tissues by repositioning, applying lotion/lubricants, and avoiding direct contact with heating appliance/blanket. **Impaired circulation can result in severe tissue damage.**

Information in brackets added by the authors to clarify and enhance the use of nursing diagnoses.

  Cultural Collaborative Community/Home Care

- Keep client quiet; handle gently **to reduce potential for fibrillation in cold heart.**
- Provide CPR, as necessary, with compressions initially at one-half normal heart rate (**severe hypothermia causes slowed conduction, and cold heart may be unresponsive to medications, pacing, and defibrillation**).
- Maintain patent airway. Assist with intubation, if indicated.
- Provide heated, humidified oxygen when used.
- Turn off warming blanket when temperature is within 1 to 3 degrees of desired temperature **to avoid hyperthermia situation.**
- Administer IV fluids with caution **to prevent overload as the vascular bed expands** (**cold heart is slow to compensate for increased volume**).
- Avoid vigorous drug therapy. (**as rewarming occurs, organ function returns, correcting endocrine abnormalities, and tissues become more receptive to the effects of drugs previously administered**).
- Immerse hands/feet in warm water/apply warm soaks once body temperature is stabilized. Place sterile cotton between digits and wrap hands/feet with a bulky gauze wrap.
- Perform range-of-motion exercises, provide support hose, reposition, encourage coughing/deep-breathing exercises, avoid restrictive clothing/restraints **to reduce circulatory stasis.**
- Provide well-balanced, high-calorie diet/feedings **to replenish glycogen stores and nutritional balance.**

NURSING PRIORITY NO. 5. To promote wellness (Teaching/Discharge Considerations):

- Review specific risk factors/causes of hypothermia. Note that hypothermia can be *accidental* (see Related Factors) or *intentional* (such as occurs when induced-hypothermia therapy is used after cardiac arrest or brain injury), requiring interventions to protect client from adverse effects.
- Discuss signs/symptoms of early hypothermia (e.g., changes in mentation, poor judgment, somnolence, impaired coordination, slurred speech) **to facilitate recognition of problem and timely intervention.**
- Identify factors that client can control (if any), such as protection from environment/adequate heat in home; layering clothing and blankets; minimize heat loss from head with hat/scarf; appropriate cold-weather clothing; avoidance of alcohol/other drugs if anticipating exposure to cold; potential risk for future hypersensitivity to cold, etc.

Information in brackets added by the authors to clarify and enhance the use of nursing diagnoses.

Documentation Focus

ASSESSMENT/REASSESSMENT

- Findings, noting degree of system involvement, respiratory rate, ECG pattern, capillary refill, and level of mentation.
- Graph temperature.

PLANNING

- Plan of care and who is involved in planning.
- Teaching plan.

IMPLEMENTATION/EVALUATION

- Responses to interventions/teaching, actions performed.
- Attainment/progress toward desired outcome(s).
- Modifications to plan of care.

DISCHARGE PLANNING

- Long-term needs, identifying who is responsible for each action.

SAMPLE NURSING OUTCOMES & INTERVENTIONS CLASSIFICATIONS (NOC/NIC)

NOC—Thermoregulation
NIC—Hypothermia Treatment

readiness for enhanced Immunizations

Taxonomy II: Health Promotion—Class 2 Health Management (00186)
Safety/Protection—Class 1 Infection
[Diagnostic Division: Safety]
Submitted 2006

Definition: A pattern of conforming to local, national, and/or international standards of immunization to prevent infectious disease(s) that is sufficient to protect a person, family, or community and can be strengthened

Related Factors

To be developed

Defining Characteristics

SUBJECTIVE

Expresses desire to enhance:
Knowledge of immunization standards

Information in brackets added by the authors to clarify and enhance the use of nursing diagnoses.

  Cultural Collaborative Community/Home Care

Immunization status
Identification of providers of immunizations
Recordkeeping of immunizations
Identification of possible problems associated with immu-
nizations
Behavior to prevent infectious diseases

Desired Outcomes/Evaluation Criteria—Client Will:

- Express understanding of immunization recommendations.
- Develop plan to obtain appropriate immunizations.
- Identify/adopt behaviors to reduce risk of infectious disease.
- Maintain and update immunization records.

Community Will:

- Provide information to community regarding immunization requirements/recommendations.
- Identify underserved populations requiring immunization support and ways to meet their needs.
- Develop plan to provide mass immunizations in time of major threat/disease outbreak.

Actions/Interventions

NURSING PRIORITY NO. 1. To determine current immunization status:

- Assess client's history of immunizations. Response may vary widely, depending on client's age (infant to adult); cultural influences; travel history; family beliefs about immunization; and medical conditions (**e.g., some vaccines should not be given to children with certain cancers, persons taking immunosuppressant drugs, or those with serious allergies to eggs**).
- Ascertain motivation/expectations for change.
- Determine if adult client works in/frequents high-risk areas (e.g., doctor's office, home care, homeless or immigrant shelters or clinics, correctional facility) **to review potential exposures and determine new vaccines or boosters client may need.**
- Address client's/SO's concerns (e.g., client may wonder if annual flu shots are truly beneficial, or whether adult boosters may be needed for particular immunizations received in childhood; parent may be concerned about safety of vaccine supply). **Helps to clarify plans and deal with misconceptions or myths.**

Information in brackets added by the authors to clarify and enhance the use of nursing diagnoses.

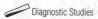 Diagnostic Studies   ∞ Pediatric/Geriatric/Lifespan   Medications   **393**

- Ascertain/discuss conditions that may preclude client receiving specific immunizations (e.g., history of prior adverse reaction, current fever/illness, pregnancy, undergoing cancer/other immunosuppressant treatments).
 • Review community plan for dealing with immunizations/disease outbreak. **Identifies strengths/limitations.**

NURSING PRIORITY NO. 2. To assist client/SO/community to develop/strengthen plan to meet identified needs:

 • Review parents' knowledge/information regarding immunizations recommended/required to enter school (e.g., hepatitis B, rotavirus, *Haemophilus influenza*, mumps/measles/rubella, varicella, and hepatitis A prior to kindergarten; tetanus/diphtheria/pertussis, human papillomavirus by junior high age; meningitis for college freshmen planning to live in dorm) **to document status, plan for boosters, and/or discuss appropriate intervals for follow-up.**

 • Examine/discuss protective benefit of each vaccine, route of administration, expected side effects, and potential adverse reactions **so that client/SO(s) can make informed decisions.**

∞ • Discuss appropriate time intervals for all recommended immunizations, as well as catch-up and booster options for children birth to 18 years.

 • Review requirements for client preparing for international travel **to ascertain potential for contracting vaccine-preventable disease in geographic area of client's travel, so that vaccines can be provided, if needed.**

 • Inform of exemptions when client/SO desires. **Some states permit medical, religious, personal, and philosophical exemptions when parent does not want child to participate in immunization programs.** Refer to appropriate care providers for further discussion/intervention.

 • Define and discuss current needs and anticipated or projected concerns of community health promotion programs. **Agreement on scope/parameters of needs is essential for effective planning.**

 • Prioritize goals **to facilitate accomplishment.**

 • Identify available community resources (**e.g., persons, groups, financial, governmental, as well as other communities**).

 • Seek out and involve underserved/at-risk groups within the community. **Supports communication and commitment of community as a whole.**

NURSING PRIORITY NO. 3. To promote optimum wellness:

 • Review reasons to continue immunization programs. **Viruses and bacteria that cause vaccine-preventable disease and death**

Information in brackets added by the authors to clarify and enhance the use of nursing diagnoses.

Cultural   Collaborative   Community/Home Care

still exist and can be passed on to people who are not protected, thus increasing medical, social, and economic costs.

- Provide reliable vaccine information in written form or Internet websites (**e.g., brochures/fact sheets from the CDC, American Academy of Pediatrics, National Network for Immunization Information, etc.**).
- Identify community resources for obtaining immunizations, such as Public Health Department, family physician.
- Discuss management of common side effects (e.g., muscle pain, rash, fever, site swelling).
- Support development of community plans for maintaining/enhancing efforts **to increase immunization level of population.**
- Establish mechanism for self-monitoring of community needs and evaluation of efforts.
- Use multiple formats; for example, TV, radio, print media, billboards and computer bulletin boards, speakers' bureau, reports to community leaders/groups on file and accessible to the public, **to keep community informed regarding immunization needs, disease prevention.**

Documentation Focus

ASSESSMENT/REASSESSMENT

- Assessment findings of immunization status, potential risks/disease exposure.
- Identified areas of concern, strengths/limitations.
- Understanding of immuniztion needs/safety, and disease prevention.
- Motivation and expectations for change.

PLANNING

- Action plan and who is involved in planning.
- Teaching plan.

IMPLEMENTATION/EVALUATION

- Individual/family responses to interventions/teaching and actions performed.
- Response of community entities to the actions performed.
- Attainment/progress toward desired outcome(s).
- Modifications to plan.

DISCHARGE PLANNING

- Identified needs/referrals for follow-up care, support systems.

Information in brackets added by the authors to clarify and enhance the use of nursing diagnoses.

- Short- and long-term plans to deal with current, anticipated, and potential community needs and who is responsible for follow-through.
- Specific referrals made, coalitions formed.

SAMPLE NURSING OUTCOMES & INTERVENTIONS CLASSIFICATIONS (NOC/NIC)

NOC—Immunization Behavior
NIC—Immunization/Vaccination Management

disorganized Infant Behavior

Taxonomy II: Coping/Stress Tolerance—Class 3
Neurobehavioral Stress (00116)
[Diagnostic Division: Neurosensory]
Submitted 1994; Nursing Diagnosis Extension and
Classification (NDEC) Revision 1998

Definition: Disintegrated physiological and neurobehavioral responses of infant to the environment

Related Factors

PRENATAL

Congenital/genetic disorders; teratogenic exposure; [exposure to drugs]

POSTNATAL

Prematurity; oral/motor problems; feeding intolerance; malnutrition
Invasive procedures; pain

INDIVIDUAL

Gestational/postconceptual age; immature neurological system
Illness; [infection]; [hypoxia/birth asphyxia]

ENVIRONMENTAL

Physical environment inappropriateness
Sensory inappropriateness/overstimulation/deprivation
Lack of containment/boundaries

CAREGIVER

Cue misreading; cue knowledge deficit
Environmental stimulation contribution

Information in brackets added by the authors to clarify and enhance the use of nursing diagnoses.

  Cultural Collaborative Community/Home Care

Defining Characteristics

OBJECTIVE

Regulatory Problems
Inability to inhibit startle; irritability

State-Organization System
Active-awake (fussy, worried gaze); quiet-awake (staring, gaze aversion)
Diffuse sleep, state-oscillation
Irritable crying

Attention-Interaction System
Abnormal response to sensory stimuli (e.g., difficult to soothe, inability to sustain alert status)

Motor System
Finger splaying, fisting; hands to face; hyperextension of extremities
Tremors, startles, twitches; jittery; uncoordinated movement
Changes to motor tone; altered primitive reflexes

Physiological
Bradycardia, tachycardia, arrhythmias
Skin color changes; desaturation
"Time-out signals" (e.g., gaze, grasp, hiccough, cough, sneeze, sigh, slack jaw, open mouth, tongue thrust)
Feeding intolerances

Desired Outcomes/Evaluation Criteria—Infant Will:

- Exhibit organized behaviors that allow the achievement of optimal potential for growth and development as evidenced by modulation of physiological, motor, state, and attentional-interactive functioning.

Parent/Caregiver Will:

- Recognize individual infant cues.
- Identify appropriate responses (including environmental modifications) to infant's cues.
- Verbalize readiness to assume caregiving independently.

Actions/Interventions

NURSING PRIORITY NO. 1. To assess causative/contributing factors:

- Determine infant's chronological and developmental age; note length of gestation.

Information in brackets added by the authors to clarify and enhance the use of nursing diagnoses.

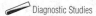 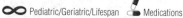

- Observe for cues suggesting presence of situations that may result in pain/discomfort.
- Determine adequacy of physiological support.
- Evaluate level/appropriateness of environmental stimuli.
- Ascertain parents' understanding of infant's needs/abilities.
- Listen to parents' concerns about their capabilities to meet infant's needs.

NURSING PRIORITY NO. 2. To assist parents in providing co-regulation to the infant:

- Provide a calm, nurturant physical and emotional environment.
- Encourage parents to hold infant, including skin-to-skin contact (kangaroo care [KC]), as appropriate. **Research suggests KC may have a positive effect on infant development by enhancing neurophysiological organization as well as an indirect effect by improving parental mood, perceptions, and interactive behavior.**
- Model gentle handling of baby and appropriate responses to infant behavior. **Provides cues to parent.**
- Support and encourage parents to be with infant and participate actively in all aspects of care. **Situation may be overwhelming, and support may enhance coping and strengthen attachment.**
- Provide positive feedback for progressive parental envolvement in caregiving process. **Transfer of care from staff to parents progresses along a continuum as parents' confidence level increases and they are able to take on more complex care activities.**
- Discuss infant growth/development, pointing out current status and progressive expectations, as appropriate. **Augments parents' knowledge of co-regulation.**
- Incorporate the parents' observations and suggestions into plan of care. **Demonstrates valuing of parents' input and encourages continued involvement.**

NURSING PRIORITY NO. 3. To deliver care within the infant's stress threshold:

- Provide a consistent caregiver. **Facilitates recognition of infant cues/changes in behavior.**
- Identify infant's individual self-regulatory behaviors, e.g., sucking, mouthing, grasp, hand-to-mouth, face behaviors, foot clasp, brace, limb flexion, trunk tuck, boundary seeking.
- Support hands to mouth and face; offer pacifier or non-nutritive sucking at the breast with gavage feedings. **Provides opportunities for infant to suck.**

Information in brackets added by the authors to clarify and enhance the use of nursing diagnoses.

 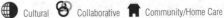 Cultural Collaborative Community/Home Care

- Avoid aversive oral stimulation, such as routine oral suction-ing; suction ET tube only when clinically indicated.
- Use oxy-hood large enough to cover the infant's chest so arms will be inside the hood. **Allows for hand-to-mouth activities during this therapy.**
- Provide opportunities for infant to grasp.
- Provide boundaries and/or containment during all activi-ties. Use swaddling, nesting, bunting, caregiver's hands as indicated.
- Allow adequate time/opportunities to hold infant. Handle infant very gently, move infant smoothly, slowly, and con-tained, avoiding sudden/abrupt movements.
- Maintain normal alignment, position infant with limbs softly flexed, shoulders and hips adducted slightly. Use appropriate-sized diapers.
- Evaluate chest for adequate expansion, placing rolls under trunk if prone position indicated.
- Avoid restraints, including at IV sites. If IV board is necessary, secure to limb positioned in normal alignment.
- Provide a sheepskin, egg-crate mattress, water bed, and/or gel pillow/mattress for infant who does not tolerate frequent position changes. **Minimizes tissue pressure, lessens risk of tissue injury.**
- Visually assess color, respirations, activity, invasive lines with-out disturbing infant. Assess with "hands on" every 4 hours as indicated and prn. **Allows for undisturbed rest/quiet periods.**
- Schedule daily activities, time for rest, and organization of sleep/wake states to maximize tolerance of infant. Defer rou-tine care when infant in quiet sleep.
- Provide care with baby in side-lying position. Begin by talking softly to the baby, then placing hands in containing hold on baby, **allows baby to prepare.** Proceed with least-invasive manipulations first.
- Respond promptly to infant's agitation or restlessness. Provide "time out" when infant shows early cues of overstimulation. Comfort and support the infant after stressful interventions.
- Remain at infant's bedside for several minutes after proce-dures/caregiving **to monitor infant's response and provide necessary support.**
- Administer analgesics as individually appropriate.

NURSING PRIORITY NO. 4. To modify the environment to provide appropriate stimulation:

- Introduce stimulation as a single mode and assess individual tolerance.

Information in brackets added by the authors to clarify and enhance the use of nursing diagnoses.

 Diagnostic Studies 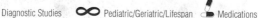 ∞ Pediatric/Geriatric/Lifespan Medications **399**

LIGHT/VISION

- Reduce lighting perceived by infant; introduce diurnal lighting (and activity) when infant achieves physiological stability. (Daylight levels of 20 to 30 candles and night light levels of less than 10 candles are suggested.) Change light levels gradually **to allow infant time to adjust.**
- Protect the infant's eyes from bright illumination during examinations/procedures, as well as from indirect sources, such as neighboring phototherapy treatments, **to prevent retinal damage.**
- Deliver phototherapy (when required) with Biliblanket devices if available **(alleviates need for eye patches).**
- Provide caregiver face (preferably parent's) as visual stimulus when infant shows readiness (awake, attentive).

SOUND

- Identify sources of noise in environment and eliminate or reduce (e.g., speak in a low voice; reduce volume on alarms/telephones to safe but not excessive volume; pad metal trash can lids; open paper packages, such as IV tubing and suction catheters, slowly and at a distance from bedside; conduct rounds/report away from bedside; place soft/thick fabric, such as blanket rolls and toys, near infant's head to absorb sound).
- Keep all incubator portholes closed, closing with two hands **to avoid loud snap with closure and associated startle response.**
- Refrain from playing musical toys or tape players inside incubator.
- Avoid placing items on top of incubator; if necessary to do so, pad surface well.
- Conduct regular decibel checks of interior noise level in incubator (recommended not to exceed 60 dB).
- Provide auditory stimulation **to console, support infant before and through handling or to reinforce restfulness.**

OLFACTORY

- Be cautious in exposing infant to strong odors (e.g., alcohol, Betadine, perfumes), **as olfactory capability of the infant is very sensitive.**
- Place a cloth or gauze pad scented with milk near the infant's face during gavage feeding. **Enhances association of milk with act of feeding/gastric fullness.**
- Invite parents to leave a handkerchief that they have scented by wearing close to their body near infant. **Strengthens infant recognition of parents.**

Information in brackets added by the authors to clarify and enhance the use of nursing diagnoses.

 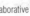

VESTIBULAR

- Move and handle the infant slowly and gently. Do not restrict spontaneous movement.
- Provide vestibular stimulation **to console, stabilize breathing/heart rate, or enhance growth.** Use a water bed (with or without oscillation), a motorized/moving bed or cradle, or rocking in the arms of a caregiver.

GUSTATORY

- Dip pacifier in milk and offer to infant during gavage feeding **for sucking and to stimulate tasting.**

TACTILE

- Maintain skin integrity and monitor closely. Limit frequency of invasive procedures.
- Minimize use of chemicals on skin (e.g., alcohol, Betadine, solvents) and remove afterward with warm water **because skin is very sensitive/fragile.**
- Limit use of tape and adhesives directly on skin. Use Duo-Derm under tape **to prevent dermal injury.**
- Touch infant with a firm containing touch, avoid light stroking. Provide a sheepskin, soft linen. **Note: Tactile experience is the primary sensory mode of the infant.**
- Encourage frequent parental holding of infant (including skin-to-skin). Supplement activity with extended family, staff, volunteers.

NURSING PRIORITY NO. 5. To promote wellness (Teaching/Discharge Considerations):

- Evaluate home environment **to identify appropriate modifications.**
- Identify community resources (e.g., early stimulation program, qualified childcare facilities/respite care, visiting nurse, home-care support, specialty organizations).
- Determine sources for equipment/therapy needs.
- Refer to support/therapy groups, as indicated, **to provide role models, facilitate adjustment to new roles/responsibilities, and enhance coping.**
- Provide contact number, as appropriate (e.g., primary nurse), **to support adjustment to home setting.**
- Refer to additional NDs, such as risk for impaired parent/child Attachment; compromised/disabled or readiness for enhanced family Coping; delayed Growth and Development; risk for Caregiver Role Strain.

Information in brackets added by the authors to clarify and enhance the use of nursing diagnoses.

Documentation Focus

ASSESSMENT/REASSESSMENT

- Findings, including infant's cues of stress, self-regulation, and readiness for stimulation; chronological/developmental age.
- Parents' concerns, level of knowledge.

PLANNING

- Plan of care and who is involved in the planning.
- Teaching plan.

IMPLEMENTATION/EVALUATION

- Infant's responses to interventions/actions performed.
- Parents' participation and response to interactions/teaching.
- Attainment/progress toward desired outcome(s).
- Modifications of plan of care.

DISCHARGE PLANNING

- Long-term needs and who is responsible for actions to be taken.
- Specific referrals made.

SAMPLE NURSING OUTCOMES & INTERVENTIONS CLASSIFICATIONS (NOC/NIC)

NOC—Neurological Status
NIC—Environmental Management

readiness for enhanced organized Infant Behavior

Taxonomy II: Coping/Stress Tolerance—Class 3 Neurobehavioral (00117)
[Diagnostic Division: Neurosensory]
Submitted 1994

Definition: A pattern of modulation of the physiological and behavioral systems of functioning (i.e., autonomic, motor, state-organizational, self-regulators, and attentional-interactional systems) in an infant that is satisfactory but that can be improved

Related Factors

Prematurity
Pain

Information in brackets added by the authors to clarify and enhance the use of nursing diagnoses.

 Cultural Collaborative Community/Home Care

Defining Characteristics

OBJECTIVE

Stable physiological measures
Definite sleep-wake states
Use of some self-regulatory behaviors
Response to stimuli (e.g., visual, auditory)

Desired Outcomes/Evaluation Criteria—Infant Will:

* Continue to modulate physiological and behavioral systems of functioning.
* Achieve higher levels of integration in response to environmental stimuli.

Parent/Caregiver Will:

* Identify cues reflecting infant's stress threshold and current status.
* Develop/modify responses (including environment) to promote infant adaptation and development.

Actions/Interventions

NURSING PRIORITY NO. 1. To assess infant status and parental skill level:

* Determine infant's chronological and developmental age; note length of gestation.
* Identify infant's individual self-regulatory behaviors: suck, mouth, grasp, hand-to-mouth, face behaviors, foot clasp, brace, limb flexion, trunk tuck, boundary seeking.
* Observe for cues suggesting presence of situations that may result in pain/discomfort.
* Evaluate level/appropriateness of environmental stimuli.
* Ascertain parents' understanding of infant's needs/abilities.
* Listen to parents' perceptions of their capabilities to promote infant's development.

NURSING PRIORITY NO. 2. To assist parents to enhance infant's integration:

* Review infant growth/development, pointing out current status and progressive expectations. Identify cues reflecting infant stress.
* Discuss possible modifications of environmental stimuli/activity schedule, sleep, and pain control needs.

Information in brackets added by the authors to clarify and enhance the use of nursing diagnoses.

 Diagnostic Studies   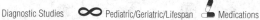 Pediatric/Geriatric/Lifespan   Medications   **403**

- Provide positive feedback for parental involvement in caregiving process. **Transfer of care from staff to parents progresses along a continuum as parents' confidence level increases and they are able to take on more responsibility.**
 - Discuss use of skin-to-skin contact (kangaroo care [KC]), as appropriate. **Research suggests KC may have a positive effect on infant development by enhancing neurophysiological organization as well as an indirect effect by improving parental mood, perceptions, and interactive behavior.**
 - Incorporate parents' observations and suggestions into plan of care. **Demonstrates value of and regard for parents' input and enhances sense of ability to deal with situation.**

NURSING PRIORITY NO. 3. To promote wellness (Teaching/Learning Considerations):

- Identify community resources (e.g., visiting nurse, home-care support, child care).
- Refer to support group/individual role model **to facilitate adjustment to new roles/responsibilities.**
- Refer to additional NDs; for example, readiness for enhanced family Coping.

Documentation Focus

ASSESSMENT/REASSESSMENT

- Findings, including infant's self-regulation and readiness for stimulation; chronological/developmental age.
- Parents' concerns, level of knowledge.

PLANNING

- Plan of care and who is involved in the planning.
- Teaching plan.

IMPLEMENTATION/EVALUATION

- Infant's responses to interventions/actions performed.
- Parents' participation and response to interactions/teaching.
- Attainment/progress toward desired outcome(s).
- Modifications of plan of care.

DISCHARGE PLANNING

- Long-term needs and who is responsible for actions to be taken.
- Specific referrals made.

Information in brackets added by the authors to clarify and enhance the use of nursing diagnoses.

 Cultural   Collaborative   Community/Home Care

NOC—Neurological Status
NIC—Developmental Care

risk for disorganized Infant Behavior

Taxonomy II: Coping/Stress Tolerance—Class 3
  Neurobehavioral Stress (00115)
[Diagnostic Division: Neurosensory]
Submitted 1994

Definition: Risk for alteration in integration and
modulation of the physiological and behavioral systems
of functioning (i.e., autonomic, motor, state,
organizational, self-regulatory, and attentional-
interactional systems).

Risk Factors

Pain; invasive/painful procedures
Oral/motor problems
Environmental overstimulation
Lack of containment within enviroment
Prematurity; [immaturity of the CNS; genetic problems that
  alter neurological and/or physiological functioning; condi-
  tions resulting in hypoxia and/or birth asphyxia]
[Malnutrition; infection; drug addiction]
[Environmental events or conditions, such as separation from
  parents, exposure to loud noise, excessive handling, bright
  lights]

> NOTE: A risk diagnosis is not evidenced by signs and symptoms, as
> the problem has not occurred and nursing interventions are
> directed at prevention.

Desired Outcomes/Evaluation
Criteria—Infant Will:

• Exhibit organized behaviors that allow the achievement of
  optimal potential for growth and development as evidenced
  by modulation of physiological, motor, state, and attentional-
  interactive functioning.

Information in brackets added by the authors to clarify and enhance
the use of nursing diagnoses.

 Diagnostic Studies 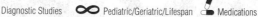 Pediatric/Geriatric/Lifespan Medications

risk for disorganized INFANT BEHAVIOR

Parent/Caregiver Will:

- Identify cues reflecting infant's stress threshold and current status.
- Develop/modify responses (including environment) to promote infant adaptation and development.
- Verbalize readiness to assume caregiving independently.

Refer to ND disorganized Infant Behavior for Actions/Interventions and Documentation Focus.

SAMPLE NURSING OUTCOMES & INTERVENTIONS CLASSIFICATIONS (NOC/NIC)

NOC—Neurological Status
NIC—Environmental Management

ineffective Infant Feeding Pattern

Taxonomy II: Nutrition—Class 1 Ingestion (00107)
[Diagnostic Division: Food/Fluid]
Submitted 1992; Revised 2006

Definition: Impaired ability of an infant to suck or coordinate the suck/swallow response resulting in inadequate oral nutrition for metabolic needs

Related Factors

Prematurity
Neurological impairment/delay
Oral hypersensitivity
Prolonged NPO
Anatomic abnormality

Defining Characteristics

SUBJECTIVE

[Caregiver reports infant is unable to initiate/sustain an effective suck]

OBJECTIVE

Inability to initiate/sustain an effective suck
Inability to coordinate sucking, swallowing, and breathing

Desired Outcomes/Evaluation Criteria—Client Will:

- Display adequate output as measured by sufficient number of wet diapers daily.

Information in brackets added by the authors to clarify and enhance the use of nursing diagnoses.

 Cultural Collaborative Community/Home Care

- Demonstrate appropriate weight gain.
- Be free of aspiration.

Actions/Interventions

NURSING PRIORITY NO. 1. To identify contributing factors/degree of impaired function:

- Assess infant's suck, swallow, and gag reflexes. **Provides comparative baseline and is useful in determining appropriate feeding method.**
- Note developmental age, structural abnormalities (e.g., cleft lip/palate), mechanical barriers (e.g., ET tube, ventilator).
- Determine level of consciousness, neurological impairment, seizure activity, presence of pain.
- Observe parent/infant interactions **to determine level of bonding/comfort that could impact stress level during feeding activity.**
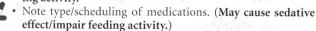
- Note type/scheduling of medications. (**May cause sedative effect/impair feeding activity.**)
- Compare birth and current weight/length measurements.
- Assess signs of stress when feeding (e.g., tachypnea, cyanosis, fatigue/lethargy).
- Note presence of behaviors indicating continued hunger after feeding.

NURSING PRIORITY NO. 2. To promote adequate infant intake:

- Determine appropriate method for feeding (e.g., special nipple/feeding device, gavage/enteral tube feeding) and choice of breast milk/formula to meet infant needs.
- Review early infant feeding cues (e.g., rooting, lip smacking, sucking fingers/hand) versus late cue of crying. **Early recognition of infant hunger promotes timely/more rewarding feeding experience for infant and mother.**
- Demonstrate techniques/procedures for feeding. Note proper positioning of infant, "latching-on" techniques, rate of delivery of feeding, frequency of burping. (Refer to ND ineffective Breastfeeding, as appropriate.)
- Limit duration of feeding to maximum of 30 minutes based on infant's response (e.g., signs of fatigue) **to balance energy expenditure with nutrient intake.**
- Monitor caregiver's efforts. Provide feedback and assistance, as indicated. **Enhances learning, encourages continuation of efforts.**
- Refer mother to lactation specialist for assistance and support in dealing with unresolved issues (e.g., teaching infant to suck).

Information in brackets added by the authors to clarify and enhance the use of nursing diagnoses.

 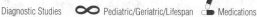

- Emphasize importance of calm/relaxed environment during feeding **to reduce detrimental stimuli and enhance mother's/ infant's focus on feeding activity.**
- Adjust frequency and amount of feeding according to infant's response. **Prevents stress associated with underfeeding/ overfeeding.**
- Advance diet, adding solids or thickening agent, as appropriate for age and infant needs.
- Alternate feeding techniques (e.g., nipple and gavage) according to infant's ability and level of fatigue.
- Alter medication/feeding schedules, as indicated, **to minimize sedative effects and have infant in alert state.**

NURSING PRIORITY NO. 3. To promote wellness (Teaching/ Discharge Considerations):

- Instruct caregiver in techniques to prevent/alleviate aspiration.
- Discuss anticipated growth and development goals for infant, corresponding caloric needs.
- Suggest monitoring infant's weight and nutrient intake periodically.
- Recommend participation in classes, as indicated (e.g., first aid, infant CPR).
- Refer to support groups (e.g., La Leche League, parenting support groups, stress reduction, or other community resources, as indicated).
- Provide bibliotherapy/appropriate websites for further information.

Documentation Focus

ASSESSMENT/REASSESSMENT

- Type and route of feeding, interferences to feeding and reactions.
- Infant's measurements.

PLANNING

- Plan of care/interventions and who is involved in planning.
- Teaching plan.

IMPLEMENTATION/EVALUATION

- Infant's response to interventions (e.g., amount of intake, weight gain, response to feeding) and actions performed.

Information in brackets added by the authors to clarify and enhance the use of nursing diagnoses.

  Cultural Collaborative 🏠 Community/Home Care

- Caregiver's involvement in infant care, participation in activities, response to teaching.
- Attainment of/progress toward desired outcome(s).
- Modifications to plan of care.

DISCHARGE PLANNING

- Long-term needs/referrals and who is responsible for follow-up actions.

SAMPLE NURSING OUTCOMES & INTERVENTIONS CLASSIFICATIONS (NOC/NIC)

NOC—Swallowing Status: Oral Phase
NIC—Nutritional Monitoring

risk for Infection

Taxonomy II: Safety/Protection—Class 1 Infection (00004)
[Diagnostic Division: Safety]
Submitted 1986

Definition: At increased risk for being invaded by pathogenic organisms

Risk Factors

Inadequate primary defenses (broken skin, traumatized tissue, decrease in ciliary action, stasis of body fluids, change in pH secretions, altered peristalsis)

Inadequate secondary defenses (e.g., decreased hemoglobin, leukopenia, suppressed inflammatory response)

Inadequate acquired immunity; immunosuppression

Tissue destruction; increased environmental exposure to pathogens; invasive procedures

Chronic disease; malnutrition; trauma

Pharmaceutical agents (e.g., immunosuppressants, [antibiotic therapy])

Rupture of amniotic membranes

Insufficient knowledge to avoid exposure to pathogens

> NOTE: A risk diagnosis is not evidenced by signs and symptoms, as the problem has not occurred and nursing interventions are directed at prevention.

Information in brackets added by the authors to clarify and enhance the use of nursing diagnoses.

 Diagnostic Studies   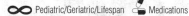 Pediatric/Geriatric/Lifespan   Medications   **409**

Desired Outcomes/Evaluation Criteria—Client Will:

- Verbalize understanding of individual causative/risk factor(s).
- Identify interventions to prevent/reduce risk of infection.
- Demonstrate techniques, lifestyle changes to promote safe environment.
- Achieve timely wound healing; be free of purulent drainage or erythema; be afebrile.

Actions/Interventions

NURSING PRIORITY NO. 1. To assess causative/contributing factors:

- Note risk factors for occurrence of infection (e.g., extremes of age; immunocompromised host; skin/tissue wounds; communities or persons sharing close quarters and/or equipment [e.g., college dorm, group home/long-term care facility, day care, correctional facility]; IV drug use; prolonged illness/hospitalization; multiple surgeries/invasive procedures; indwelling catheters; accidental or intentional environmental exposure [e.g., act of bioterrorism]).
- Observe for localized signs of infection at insertion sites of invasive lines, sutures, surgical incisions/wounds.
- Assess and document skin conditions around insertions of pins, wires, and tongs, noting inflammation and drainage.
- Note signs and symptoms of sepsis (systemic infection): fever, chills, diaphoresis, altered level of consciousness, positive blood cultures.
- Obtain appropriate tissue/fluid specimens for observation and culture/sensitivities testing.

NURSING PRIORITY NO. 2. To reduce/correct existing risk factors:

- Stress proper hand hygiene by all caregivers between therapies/clients. **A first-line defense against healthcare-associated infections (HAI).**
- Monitor client's visitors/caregivers for respiratory illnesses. Offer masks and tissues to client/visitors who are coughing/sneezing **to limit exposures, thus reduce cross-contamination.**
- Post visual alerts in healthcare settings instructing clients/SO(s) to inform healthcare providers if they have symptoms of respiratory infections/influenza-like symptoms.
- Encourage parents of sick children to keep them away from childcare settings and school until afebrile for 24 hours.

Information in brackets added by the authors to clarify and enhance the use of nursing diagnoses.

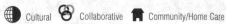 Cultural   Collaborative   Community/Home Care

- Provide for isolation, as indicated (e.g., wound/skin, respiratory, reverse). Educate staff in infection control procedures. **Reduces risk of cross-contamination.**
- Stress proper use of personal protective equipment (PPE) by staff/visitors, as dictated by agency policy.
- Perform/instruct in daily mouth care. Include use of antiseptic mouthwash for individuals in acute/long-term care settings **at high-risk for nosocomial/healthcare associated infections.**
- Recommend routine or preoperative body shower/scrubs, when indicated (e.g., orthopedic, plastic surgery) **to reduce bacterial colonization.**
- Maintain sterile technique for all invasive procedures (e.g., IV, urinary catheter, pulmonary suctioning).
- Fill bubbling humidifiers/nebulizers with *sterile* water, not distilled or tap water. Avoid use of room-air humidifiers unless unit is sterilized daily and filled with sterile water.
- Use heat and moisture exchangers (HME) instead of heated humidifier with mechanical ventilator.
- Assist with weaning from mechanical ventilator as soon as possible **to reduce risk of ventilator-associated pneumonia (VAP).**
- Choose proper vascular access device based on anticipated treatment duration and solution/medication to be infused and best available aseptic insertion techniques; cleanse incisions/insertion sites per facility protocol with appropriate solution **to reduce potential for catheter-related bloodstream infections.**
- Change surgical/other wound dressings, as indicated, using proper technique for changing/disposing of contaminated materials.
- Separate touching surfaces when skin is excoriated, such as in herpes zoster. Use gloves when caring for open lesions to minimize autoinoculation/transmission of viral diseases (e.g., herpes simplex virus, hepatitis, AIDS).
- Cover perineal/pelvic region dressings/casts with plastic when using bedpan **to prevent contamination.**
- Encourage early ambulation, deep breathing, coughing, position changes, and early removal of endotracheal and/or nasal/oral feeding tubes **for mobilization of respiratory secretions and prevention of aspiration/respiratory infections.**
- Monitor/assist with use of adjuncts (e.g., respiratory aids, such as incentive spirometry) **to prevent pneumonia.**

Information in brackets added by the authors to clarify and enhance the use of nursing diagnoses.

- Maintain adequate hydration, stand/sit to void, and catheterize, if necessary, **to avoid bladder distention/urinary stasis.**
- Provide regular urinary catheter/perineal care. **Reduces risk of ascending urinary tract infection.**
- Assist with medical procedures (e.g., wound/joint aspiration, incision and drainage of abscess, bronchoscopy), as indicated.
- Administer/monitor medication regimen (e.g., antimicrobials, drip infusion into osteomyelitis, subeschar clysis, topical antibiotics) and note client's response **to determine effectiveness of therapy/presence of side effects.**
- Administer prophylactic antibiotics and immunizations, as indicated.

NURSING PRIORITY NO. 3. To promote wellness (Teaching/Discharge Considerations):

- Review individual nutritional needs, appropriate exercise program, and need for rest.
- Instruct client/SO(s) in techniques to protect the integrity of skin, care for lesions, and prevention of spread of infection.
- Emphasize necessity of taking antivirals/antibiotics, as directed (e.g., dosage and length of therapy). **Premature discontinuation of treatment when client begins to feel well may result in return of infection and potentiate drug-resistant strains.**
- Discuss importance of not taking antibiotics/using "leftover" drugs unless specifically instructed by healthcare provider. **Inappropriate use can lead to development of drug-resistant strains/secondary infections.**
- Discuss the role of smoking in respiratory infections.
- Promote safer-sex practices and report sexual contacts of infected individuals **to prevent the spread of HIV/other sexually transmitted diseases.**
- Provide information/involve in appropriate community and national education programs **to increase awareness of and prevention of communicable diseases.**
- Discuss precautions with client engaged in international travel, and refer for immunizations **to reduce incidence/transmission of global infections.**
- Promote childhood immunization program. Encourage adults to obtain/update immunizations as appropriate.
- Include information in preoperative teaching about ways to reduce potential for postoperative infection (e.g., respiratory

---

Information in brackets added by the authors to clarify and enhance the use of nursing diagnoses.

measures to prevent pneumonia, wound/dressing care, avoidance of others with infection).

 • Review use of prophylactic antibiotics if appropriate (e.g., prior to dental work for clients with history of rheumatic fever/valvular heart disease).

 • Encourage contacting healthcare provider for prophylactic therapy, as indicated, following exposure to individuals with infectious disease (e.g., tuberculosis, hepatitis, influenza).

 • Identify resources available to the individual (e.g., substance abuse/rehabilitation or needle exchange program, as appropriate; available/free condoms, etc.).

• Refer to NDs readiness for enhanced Immunization; risk for Disuse Syndrome; impaired Home Maintenance; ineffective Health Maintenance.

Documentation Focus

ASSESSMENT/REASSESSMENT

• Individual risk factors that are present including recent/current antibiotic therapy.
• Wound and/or insertion sites, character of drainage/body secretions.
• Signs/symptoms of infectious process

PLANNING

• Plan of care/interventions and who is involved in planning.
• Teaching plan.

IMPLEMENTATION/EVALUATION

• Responses to interventions/teaching and actions performed.
• Attainment/progress toward desired outcome(s).
• Modifications to plan of care.

DISCHARGE PLANNING

• Discharge needs/referrals and who is responsible for actions to be taken.
• Specific referrals made.

SAMPLE NURSING OUTCOMES & INTERVENTIONS CLASSIFICATIONS (NOC/NIC)

NOC—Immune Status
NIC—Infection Protection

Information in brackets added by the authors to clarify and enhance the use of nursing diagnoses.

risk for INFECTION

risk for Injury

Taxonomy II: Safety/Protection—Class 2 Physical Injury
(00035)
[Diagnostic Division: Safety]
Submitted 1978

Definition: At risk of injury as a result of environmental
conditions interacting with the individual's adaptive and
defensive resources

Risk Factors

INTERNAL

Physical (e.g., broken skin, altered mobility); tissue hypoxia;
malnutrition

Abnormal blood profile (e.g., leukocytosis/leukopenia, altered
clotting factors, thrombocytopenia, sickle cell, thalassemia,
decreased hemoglobin)

Biochemical dysfunction; sensory dysfunction

Integrative/effector dysfunction; immune-autoimmune dysfunction

Psychological (affective, orientation); developmental age
(physiological, psychosocial)

EXTERNAL

Biological (e.g., immunization level of community, microor-
ganism)

Chemical (e.g., pollutants, poisons, drugs, pharmaceutical
agents, alcohol, nicotine, preservatives, cosmetics, dyes);
nutritional (e.g., vitamins, food types)

Physical (e.g., design, structure, and arrangement of community, building, and/or equipment), mode of transport

Human (e.g., nosocomial agents, staffing patterns; cognitive,
affective, psychomotor factors)

> NOTE: A risk diagnosis is not evidenced by signs and symptoms, as
> the problem has not occurred and nursing interventions are
> directed at prevention.

Desired Outcomes/Evaluation
Criteria—Client/Caregivers Will:

• Verbalize understanding of individual factors that contribute
to possibility of injury.

Information in brackets added by the authors to clarify and enhance
the use of nursing diagnoses.

 Cultural Collaborative 🏠 Community/Home Care

- Demonstrate behaviors, lifestyle changes to reduce risk factors and protect self from injury.
- Modify environment as indicated to enhance safety.
- Be free of injury.

Actions/Interventions

In reviewing this ND, it is apparent there is much overlap with other diagnoses. We have chosen to present generalized interventions. Although there are commonalities to injury situations, we suggest that the reader refer to other primary diagnoses as indicated, such as Activity Intolerance; risk for Aspiration; risk for imbalanced Body Temperature; decreased Cardiac Output; acute or chronic Confusion; risk for Contamination; risk for Falls; impaired Environmental Interpretation; impaired Gas Exchange; impaired Home Maintenance; impaired Mobility (specify); impaired/risk for impaired Parenting; imbalanced Nutrition [specify]; risk for Poisoning; disturbed Sensory Perception; impaired/risk for impaired Skin Integrity; Sleep Deprivation; risk for Suffocation; disturbed Thought Processes; ineffective Tissue Perfusion; risk for Infection; risk for Trauma; risk for other-directed/self-directed Violence; Wandering.

NURSING PRIORITY NO. 1. To evaluate degree/source of risk inherent in the individual situation:

- Perform thorough assessments regarding safety issues when planning for client care and/or preparing for discharge from care. **Failure to accurately assess and intervene or refer these issues can place the client at needless risk and creates negligence issues for the healthcare practitioner.**
- Ascertain knowledge of safety needs/injury prevention and motivation **to prevent injury in home, community, and work setting.**
- Note client's age, gender, developmental stage, decision-making ability, level of cognition/competence. **Affects client's ability to protect self and/or others, and influences choice of interventions and/or teaching.**
- Assess mood, coping abilities, personality styles (e.g., temperament, aggression, impulsive behavior, level of self-esteem) **that may result in carelessness/increased risk-taking without consideration of consequences.**
- Assess client's muscle strength, gross and fine motor coordination **to identify risk for falls.**
- Note socioeconomic status/availability and use of resources.

Information in brackets added by the authors to clarify and enhance the use of nursing diagnoses.

 Diagnostic Studies Pediatric/Geriatric/Lifespan Medications

• Evaluate individual's emotional and behavioral response to violence in environmental surroundings (e.g., home, neighborhood, peer group, media). **May affect client's veiw of and regard for own/others' safety.**

 • Determine potential for abusive behavior by family members/SO(s)/peers.

 • Observe for signs of injury and age (e.g., old/new bruises, history of fractures, frequent absences from school/work) **to determine need for evaluation of intentional injury/abuse in client relationship/living environment.**

NURSING PRIORITY NO. 2. To assist client/caregiver to reduce or correct individual risk factors:

• Provide healthcare within a culture of safety (e.g., adherence to nursing standards of care and facility safe-care policies) **to prevent errors resulting in client injury, promote client safety, and model safety behaviors for client/SO(s):**

Maintain bed/chair in lowest position with wheels locked

Ensure that pathway to bathroom is unobstructed and properly lighted

Place assistive devices (e.g., walker, cane, glasses, hearing aid) within reach

Instruct client/SO(s) to request assistance as needed; make sure call light is within reach and client knows how to operate

Monitor environment for potentially unsafe conditions and modify as needed

Administer medications and infusions using "5 rights" system (right patient, right medication, right route, right dose, right time)

Inform and educate client/SO(s) regarding all treatments and medications, etc.

Refer to NDs previously listed for additional interventions

 • Develop plan of care with family to meet client's and SO's individual needs.

 • Provide information regarding disease/condition(s) that may result in increased risk of injury (e.g., weakness, dementia, head injury, immunosuppression, use of multiple medications, use of alcohol/other drugs, exposure to environmental chemical/other hazards).

 • Identify interventions/safety devices **to promote safe physical environment and individual safety.** Refer to physical or occupational therapist, as appropriate.

 • Demonstrate/encourage use of techniques to reduce/manage stress and vent emotions, such as anger, hostility.

 • Review consequences of previously determined risk factors that client is reluctant to modify (e.g., oral cancer in teenager

Information in brackets added by the authors to clarify and enhance the use of nursing diagnoses.

 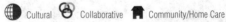

using smokeless tobacco, occurrence of spontaneous abortion, fetal alcohol syndrome/neonatal addiction in prenatal woman using drugs, fall related to failure to use assistive equipment, toddler getting into medicine cabinet, binge drinking while skiing, health/legal implications of illicit drug use, working too many hours for safe operation of machinery/vehicles, etc.).

- Discuss importance of self-monitoring of conditions/emotions **that can contribute to occurrence of injury (e.g., fatigue, anger, irritability).**

- Encourage participation in self-help programs, such as assertiveness training, positive self-image, to enhance self-esteem/sense of self-worth.

- Perform home assessment/identify safety issues, such as locking up medications/poisonous substances, locking exterior doors **to prevent client from wandering off while SO is engaged in other household activities,** or removing matches/smoking material and knobs from the stove **so confused client does not turn on burner and leave it unattended.**

- Review expectations caregivers have of children, cognitively impaired, and/or elderly family members.

- Discuss need for and sources of supervision (e.g., before- and after-school programs, elderly day care).

- Discuss concerns about childcare, discipline practices.

NURSING PRIORITY NO. 3. To promote wellness (Teaching/Discharge Considerations):

- Identify individual needs/resources **for safety education,** such as first aid/CPR classes, babysitter class, water or gun safety, smoking cessation, substance abuse program, weight and exercise management, industry and community safety courses.

- Provide telephone numbers and other contact numbers, as individually indicated (e.g., doctor, 911, poison control, police, lifeline, hazardous materials handler).

- Refer to other resources, as indicated (e.g., counseling/psychotherapy, budget counseling, parenting classes).

- Provide bibliotherapy/written resources **for later review and self-paced learning.**

- Promote community education programs geared to increasing awareness of safety measures and resources available to the individual (e.g., correct use of child safety seats, bicycle helmets, home hazard information, firearm safety, fall prevention, CPR/first aid, etc.).

- Promote community awareness about the problems of design of buildings, equipment, transportation, and workplace practices that contribute to accidents.

Information in brackets added by the authors to clarify and enhance the use of nursing diagnoses.

• Identify community resources/neighbors/friends to assist elderly/handicapped individuals in providing such things as structural maintenance, snow and ice removal from walks and steps, and so forth.

Documentation Focus

ASSESSMENT/REASSESSMENT

- Individual risk factors, noting current physical findings (e.g., bruises, cuts).
- Client's/caregiver's understanding of individual risks/safety concerns.
- Availability/use of resources.

PLANNING

- Plan of care and who is involved in planning.
- Teaching plan.

IMPLEMENTATION/EVALUATION

- Individual responses to interventions/teaching and actions performed.
- Specific actions and changes that are made.
- Attainment/progress toward desired outcome(s).
- Modifications to plan of care.

DISCHARGE PLANNING

- Long-range plans for discharge needs, lifestyle and community changes, and who is responsible for actions to be taken.
- Specific referrals made.

SAMPLE NURSING OUTCOMES & INTERVENTIONS CLASSIFICATIONS (NOC/NIC)

NOC—Safety Behavior: Personal
NIC—Surveillance: Safety

risk for perioperative positioning Injury

Taxonomy II: Safety/Protection—Class 2 Physical Injury (00087)
[Diagnostic Division: Safety]
Submitted 1994; Revised 2006

Definition: At risk for injury as a result of the environmental conditions found in the perioperative setting

---

Information in brackets added by the authors to clarify and enhance the use of nursing diagnoses.

Risk Factors

Disorientation; sensory/perceptual disturbances due to anesthesia

Immobilization, muscle weakness; [preexisting musculoskeletal conditions]

Obesity; emaciation; edema

[Elderly]

> NOTE: A risk diagnosis is not evidenced by signs and symptoms, as the problem has not occurred and nursing interventions are directed at prevention.

Desired Outcomes/Evaluation Criteria—Client Will:

- Be free of injury related to perioperative disorientation.
- Be free of untoward skin and tissue injury or changes lasting beyond 24 to 48 hours post-procedure.
- Report resolution of localized numbness, tingling, or changes in sensation related to positioning within 24 to 48 hours, as appropriate.

Actions/Interventions

NURSING PRIORITY NO. 1. To identify individual risk factors/needs:

- Review client's history, noting age, weight/height, nutritional status, physical limitations/preexisting conditions (e.g., elderly person with arthritis; extremes of weight; diabetes/other conditions affecting peripheral vascular health; nutrition/hydration impairments, etc.). **Affects choice of perioperative positioning and affects skin/tissue integrity during surgery.**
- Evaluate/document client's preoperative reports of neurologic, sensory, or motor deficits **for comparative baseline of perioperative/postoperative sensations.**
- Note anticipated length of procedure and customary position **to increase awareness of potential postoperative complications (e.g., supine position may cause low back pain and skin pressure at heels/elbows/sacrum; lateral chest position can cause shoulder and neck pain, or eye and ear injury on the client's downside).**
- Assess the individual's responses to preoperative sedation/medication, noting level of sedation and/or adverse effects (e.g., drop in BP) and report to surgeon, as indicated.

Information in brackets added by the authors to clarify and enhance the use of nursing diagnoses.

 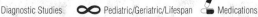

- Evaluate environmental conditions/safety issues surrounding the sedated client (e.g., client holding area, side rails up on bed/cart, someone with the client, etc.).

NURSING PRIORITY NO. 2. To position client to provide protection for anatomic structures and to prevent client injury:

- Lock cart/bed in place; support client's body and limbs; use adequate numbers of personnel during transfers **to prevent shear and friction injuries.**
- Place safety strap strategically to secure client for specific procedure **to prevent unintended movement.**
- Maintain body alignment as much as possible using pillows/padding/safety straps **to reduce potential for neurovascular complications associated with compression, overstretching, or ischemia of nerve(s).**
- Apply and reposition padding of pressure points/bony prominences (e.g., arms, elbows, sacrum, ankles, heels) and neurovascular pressure points (e.g., breasts, knees) **to maintain position of safety, especially when repositioning client and/or table attachments.**
- Check peripheral pulses and skin color/temperature periodically **to monitor circulation.**
- Protect body from contact with metal parts of the operating table, **which could produce burns/electric shock injury.**
- Reposition slowly at transfer and in bed (especially halothane-anesthetized client) **to prevent severe drop in BP, dizziness, or unsafe transfer.**
- Protect airway and facilitate respiratory effort following extubation.
- Determine specific position reflecting procedure guidelines (e.g., head of bed elevated following spinal anesthesia, turn to unoperated side following pneumonectomy).
- Identify potential hazards in the surgical suite and implement corrections, as appropriate.

NURSING PRIORITY NO. 3. To promote wellness (Teaching/Discharge Considerations):

- Provide perioperative teaching relative to client safety issues, including not crossing legs during procedures performed under local or light anesthesia, postoperative needs/limitations, and signs/symptoms requiring medical evaluation.
- Inform client and postoperative caregivers of expected/transient reactions (such as low backache, localized numbness, and reddening or skin indentations, all of which should disappear in 24 hours).

Information in brackets added by the authors to clarify and enhance the use of nursing diagnoses.

  Cultural Collaborative 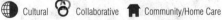 Community/Home Care

- Assist with therapies/nursing actions, including skin care measures, application of elastic stockings, early mobilization **to promote skin and tissue integrity.**
- Encourage/assist with frequent range-of-motion exercises, especially when joint stiffness occurs.
- Refer to appropriate resources, as needed.

Documentation Focus

ASSESSMENT/REASSESSMENT

- Findings, including individual risk factors for problems in the perioperative setting/need to modify routine activities or positions.
- Periodic evaluation of monitoring activities.

PLANNING

- Plan of care and who is involved in planning.
- Teaching plan.

IMPLEMENTATION/EVALUATION

- Response to interventions and actions performed.
- Attainment/progress toward desired outcome(s).
- Modifications to plan of care.

DISCHARGE PLANNING

- Long-term needs and who is responsible for actions to be taken.

SAMPLE NURSING OUTCOMES & INTERVENTIONS CLASSIFICATIONS (NOC/NIC)

NOC—Risk Control
NIC—Positioning: Intraoperative

Insomnia

Taxonomy II: Activity/Rest—Class 1 Sleep/Rest (00095)
[Diagnostic Division: Activity/Rest]
Submitted 2006 [Original submission 1980 as disturbed Sleep Pattern; Nursing Diagnosis Extension and Classification (NDEC) Revised 1998]

Definition: A sustained disruption in amount and quality of sleep that impairs functioning

---

Information in brackets added by the authors to clarify and enhance the use of nursing diagnoses.

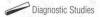 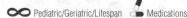

Related Factors

Intake of stimulants/alcohol; medications; gender-related hormonal shifts

Stress (e.g., ruminative pre-sleep pattern); depression, fear, anxiety, grief

Impairment of normal sleep pattern (e.g., travel, shift work, parental responsibilities, interruptions for interventions); inadequate sleep hygiene (current)

Activity pattern (e.g., timing, amount)

Physical discomfort (e.g., body temperature, pain, shortness of breath, cough, gastroesophageal reflux, nausea, incontinence/urgency)

Environmental factors (e.g., ambient noise, daylight/darkness exposure, ambient temperature/humidity, unfamiliar setting)

Defining Characteristics

SUBJECTIVE

Difficulty falling/staying asleep

Waking up too early

Dissatisfaction with sleep (current); nonrestorative sleep

Sleep disturbances that produce next-day consequences; lack of energy; difficulty concentrating; changes in mood

Decreased health status/quality of life

Increased accidents

OBJECTIVE

Observed lack of energy

Observed changes in affect

Increased work/school absenteeism

Desired Outcomes/Evaluation Criteria—Client Will:

* Verbalize understanding of sleep impairment.
* Identify individually appropriate interventions to promote sleep.
* Adjust lifestyle to accommodate chronobiological rhythms.
* Report improvement in sleep/rest pattern.
* Report increased sense of well-being and feeling rested.

Actions/Interventions

NURSING PRIORITY NO. 1. To identify causative/contributing factors:

* Identify presence of Related Factors **that can contribute to insomnia** (e.g., chronic pain, arthritis, dyspnea, movement

---

Information in brackets added by the authors to clarify and enhance the use of nursing diagnoses.

    Cultural   Collaborative   Community/Home Care

disorders, dementia, obesity, pregnancy, menopause, psychiatric disorders); metabolic diseases (such as hyperthyroidism and diabetes); prescribed/OTC drugs; alcohol, stimulant/other recreational drug use; circadian rhythm disorders (e.g., shift work, jet lag); environmental factors (e.g., noise, no control over thermostat, uncomfortable bed); major life stressors (e.g., grief, loss, finances).

- ∞ • Note age (**high percentage of elderly individuals are affected by sleep problems**).
- ∞ • Observe parent-infant interactions/provision of emotional support. Note mother's sleep-wake pattern. **Lack of knowledge of infant cues/problem relationships may create tension interfering with sleep. Structured sleep routines based on adult schedules may not meet child's needs.**
- • Ascertain presence/frequency of enuresis, incontinence, or need for frequent nighttime voidings, **interrupting sleep**.
- • Review psychological assessment, noting individual and personality characteristics **if anxiety disorders or depression could be affecting sleep**.
- • Determine recent traumatic events in client's life (e.g., death in family, loss of job).
- • Review client's medications, including prescription (e.g., beta-blockers, bronchodilators, weight-loss drugs, thyroid preparations, etc.); OTC products; herbals; **to determine if adjustments may be needed (such as change in dose or time medication is taken)**.
- • Evaluate use of caffeine and alcoholic beverages (**overindulgence interferes with REM sleep**).
- • Assist with diagnostic testing (e.g., EEG, full-night sleep studies) **to determine cause/type of sleep disturbance**.

NURSING PRIORITY NO. 2. To evaluate sleep pattern and dysfunction(s):

- • Observe and/or obtain feedback from client/SO(s) regarding client's sleep problems, usual bedtime, rituals/routines, number of hours of sleep, time of arising, and environmental needs **to determine usual sleep pattern and provide comparative baseline**.
- • Listen to subjective reports of sleep quality (e.g., client never feels rested, or feels sleepy during day).
- • Identify circumstances that interrupt sleep and the frequency at which they occur.
- • Determine client's/SO's expectations of adequate sleep. **Provides opportunity to address misconceptions/unrealistic expectations.**

Information in brackets added by the authors to clarify and enhance the use of nursing diagnoses.

• Investigate whether client snores and in what position(s) this occurs **to determine if further evaluation is needed to rule out obstructive sleep disorder.**

• Note alteration of habitual sleep time, such as change of work pattern/rotating shifts, change in normal bedtime (hospitalization).

• Observe physical signs of fatigue (e.g., restlessness, hand tremors, thick speech).

• Develop a chronological chart **to determine peak performance rhythm.**

• Graph "circadian" rhythms of individual's biological internal chemistry per protocol, as indicated. **Note: Studies have shown sleep cycles are affected by body temperature at onset of sleep.**

NURSING PRIORITY NO. 3. To assist client to establish optimal sleep/rest patterns:

• Arrange care to provide for uninterrupted periods for rest, especially allowing for longer periods of sleep at night when possible. Do as much care as possible without waking client.

• Explain necessity of disturbances for monitoring vital signs and/or other care when client is hospitalized.

• Provide quiet environment and comfort measures (e.g., back rub, washing hands/face, cleaning and straightening sheets) in preparation for sleep.

∞ • Discuss/implement effective age-appropriate bedtime rituals (e.g., going to bed at same time each night, drinking warm milk, rocking, story reading, cuddling, favorite blanket/toy) **to enhance client's ability to fall asleep, reinforce that bed is a place to sleep, and promote sense of security for child.**

• Recommend limiting intake of chocolate and caffeine/alcoholic beverages, especially prior to bedtime.

• Limit fluid intake in evening if nocturia is a problem **to reduce need for nighttime elimination.**

• Explore other sleep aids (e.g., warm bath, protein intake before bedtime).

• Administer pain medications (if required) 1 hour before sleep **to relieve discomfort and take maximum advantage of sedative effect.**

• Monitor effects of drug regimen—amphetamines or stimulants (e.g., methylphenidate—Ritalin used in narcolepsy).

• Use barbiturates and/or other sleeping medications sparingly. **Research indicates long-term use of these medications can actually induce sleep disturbances.**

Information in brackets added by the authors to clarify and enhance the use of nursing diagnoses.

  Cultural Collaborative 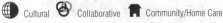 Community/Home Care

- Encourage routine use of continuous positive airway pressure (CPAP) therapy, when indicated, **to obtain optimal benefit of treatment for sleep apnea.**
- Develop behavioral program for insomnia, such as:
  Establishing routine bedtime and arising
  Thinking relaxing thoughts when in bed
  Not napping in the daytime
  Not reading or watching TV in bed
  Getting out of bed if not asleep in 15 minutes
  Limiting sleep to 7 hours a night
  Getting up the same time each day—even on weekends/ days off
  Getting adequate exposure to bright light during day
  Individually tailoring stress reduction program, music therapy, relaxation routine
- Collaborate in treatment of underlying medical problem (e.g., obstructive sleep apnea, pain, GERD, lower UTI/prostatic hypertrophy, depression, complicated grief).
- Refer to sleep specialist, as indicated/desired. **Follow-up evaluation/intervention may be needed when insomnia is seriously impacting client's quality of life, productivity, and safety (e.g., on the job, at home, on the road).**

NURSING PRIORITY NO. 4. To promote wellness (Teaching/ Discharge Considerations):

- Assure client that occasional sleeplessness should not threaten health. **Worrying about not sleeping can perpetuate the problem.**
- Assist client to develop individual program of relaxation. Demonstrate techniques (e.g., biofeedback, self-hypnosis, visualization, progressive muscle relaxation).
- Encourage participation in regular exercise program during day **to aid in stress control/release of energy. Exercise at bedtime may stimulate rather than relax client and actually interfere with sleep.**
- Recommend inclusion of bedtime snack (e.g., milk or mild juice, crackers, protein source such as cheese/peanut butter) in dietary program **to reduce sleep interference from hunger/hypoglycemia.**
- Suggest that bed/bedroom be used only for sleep, not for working, watching TV.
- Provide for child's (or impaired individual's) sleep time safety (e.g., infant placed on back, bed rails/bed in low position, nonplastic sheets).

Information in brackets added by the authors to clarify and enhance the use of nursing diagnoses.

• Investigate use of aids to block out light/noise, such as sleep mask, darkening shades/curtains, earplugs, monotonous sounds such as low-level background noise (white noise).

 • Participate in program to "reset" the body's sleep clock (chronotherapy) **when client has delayed sleep-onset insomnia.**

 • Assist individual to develop schedules that take advantage of peak performance times as identified in chronobiological chart.

 • Recommend midmorning nap if one is required. **Napping, especially in the afternoon, can disrupt normal sleep patterns.**

 • Assist client to deal with grieving process when loss has occurred. (Refer to ND Grieving.)

Documentation Focus

ASSESSMENT/REASSESSMENT

• Assessment findings, including specifics of sleep pattern (current and past) and effects on lifestyle/level of functioning.
• Medications/interventions, previous therapies.

PLANNING

• Plan of care and who is involved in planning.
• Teaching plan.

IMPLEMENTATION/EVALUATION

• Client's response to interventions/teaching and actions performed.
• Attainment/progress toward desired outcome(s).
• Modifications to plan of care.

DISCHARGE PLANNING

• Long-term needs and who is responsible for actions to be taken.
• Specific referrals made.

SAMPLE NURSING OUTCOMES & INTERVENTIONS CLASSIFICATIONS (NOC/NIC)

NOC—Sleep
NIC—Sleep Enhancement

Information in brackets added by the authors to clarify and enhance the use of nursing diagnoses.

    Cultural   Collaborative   Community/Home Care

decreased Intracranial Adaptive Capacity

Taxonomy II: Coping/Stress Tolerance—Class 3 Neurobe-
havioral Stress (00049)
[Diagnostic Division: Circulation]
Submitted 1994

Definition: Intracranial fluid dynamic mechanisms that
normally compensate for increases in intracranial
volume are compromised, resulting in repeated disproportionate increases in intracranial pressure (ICP) in
response to a variety of noxious and non-noxious stimuli

Related Factors

Brain injuries
Sustained increase in ICP = 10–15 mm Hg
Decreased cerebral perfusion pressure 50–60 mm Hg
Systemic hypotension with intracranial hypertension

Defining Characteristics

OBJECTIVE

Repeated increases of ICP >10 mm Hg for more than 5 minutes
    following a variety of external stimuli
Disproportionate increase in ICP following stimulus
Elevated P_2 ICP waveform
Volume pressure response test variation (volume-pressure ratio
    2, pressure-volume index <10)
Baseline ICP 10 mm Hg
Wide amplitude ICP waveform
[Altered level of consciousness—coma]
[Changes in vital signs, cardiac rhythm]

Desired Outcomes/Evaluation Criteria—Client Will:

• Demonstrate stable ICP as evidenced by normalization of
  pressure waveforms/response to stimuli.
• Display improved neurological signs.

Actions/Interventions

NURSING PRIORITY NO. 1. To assess causative/contributing factors:

• Determine factors related to individual situation (e.g., cause
  of loss of consciousness/coma; accompanying symptoms;
  early Glasgow Coma Scale).

Information in brackets added by the authors to clarify and enhance
the use of nursing diagnoses.

 Diagnostic Studies ∞ Pediatric/Geriatric/Lifespan 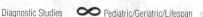 Medications **427**

decreased INTRACRANIAL ADAPTIVE CAPACITY

- Monitor/document changes in intracranial pressure (ICP); monitor waveform and corresponding event (e.g., suctioning, position change, monitor alarms, family visit) **to alter care appropriately.**

NURSING PRIORITY NO. 2. To note degree of impairment:

- Assess/document client's eye opening and position/movement, pupils (size, shape, equality, light reactivity), and consciousness/mental status (Glasgow Coma Scale) **to determine client's baseline neurological status and monitor changes over time.**
- Note purposeful and nonpurposeful motor response (posturing, etc.), comparing right/left sides.
- Test for presence/absence of reflexes (e.g., blink, cough, gag, Babinski's reflex), nuchal rigidity.
- Monitor vital signs and cardiac rhythm before/during/after activity.
- Review results of diagnostic imaging (e.g., CT scans) **to note location, type, and severity of tissue injury.**

NURSING PRIORITY NO. 3. To minimize/correct causative factors/ maximize perfusion:

- Elevate head of bed (HOB), as individually appropriate. **Although some researchers recommend head elevation up to 45 degrees, recent studies suggest a 30-degree head elevation for maximum benefit.**
- Maintain head/neck in neutral position, support with small towel rolls or pillows **to maximize venous return.** Avoid placing head on large pillow or causing hip flexion of 90 degrees or more.
- Decrease extraneous stimuli/provide comfort measures (e.g., quiet environment, soft voice, tapes of familiar voices played through earphones, back massage, gentle touch as tolerated) **to reduce CNS stimulation and promote relaxation.**
- Limit painful procedures (e.g., venipunctures, redundant neurological evaluations) to those that are absolutely necessary.
- Provide rest periods between care activities and limit duration of procedures. Lower lighting/noise level, schedule and limit activities **to provide restful environment and promote regular sleep patterns (i.e., day/night pattern).**
- Limit/prevent activities that increase intrathoracic/abdominal pressures (e.g., coughing, vomiting, straining at stool). Avoid/ limit use of restraints. **These factors markedly increase ICP.**
- Suction with caution—only when needed—to just beyond end of endo/tracheal tube without touching tracheal wall or

---

Information in brackets added by the authors to clarify and enhance the use of nursing diagnoses.

 Cultural Collaborative 🏠 Community/Home Care

carina. Administer lidocaine intratracheally (**reduces cough reflex**), hyperoxygenate before suctioning as appropriate **to minimize hypoxia.**

- Maintain patency of urinary drainage system **to reduce risk of hypertension, increased ICP, and associated dysreflexia when spinal cord injury is also present and spinal cord shock is past.** (Refer to ND Autonomic Dysreflexia.)
- Weigh, as indicated. Calculate fluid balance every shift/daily **to determine fluid needs/maintain hydration, prevent fluid overload.**
- Restrict fluid intake, as necessary, administer IV fluids via pump/control device **to prevent inadvertent fluid bolus or vascular overload.**
- Regulate environmental temperature; use cooling blanket as indicated **to decrease metabolic and O_2 needs when fever present or therapeutic hypothermia therapy is used.**
- Investigate increased restlessness **to determine causative factors and initiate corrective measures as early as possible.**
- Provide appropriate safety measures/initiate treatment for seizures **to prevent injury/increase of ICP/hypoxia.**
- Administer supplemental oxygen, as indicated, **to prevent cerebral ischemia**; hyperventilate (as indicated/per protocol) when on mechanical ventilation.**Therapeutic hyperventilation may be used (PaCO$_2$ of 30–35 mm) to reduce intracranial hypertension for a short period of time, while other methods of ICP control are initiated.**
- Administer medications (e.g., antihypertensives, diuretics, analgesics/sedatives, antipyretics, vasopressors, antiseizure drugs, neuromuscular blocking agents, and corticosteroids), as appropriate, **to maintain cerebral homeostasis and manage symptoms associated with neuological injury.**
- Prepare client for surgery, as indicated (e.g., evacuation of hematoma/space-occupying lesion), **to reduce ICP/enhance circulation.**

NURSING PRIORITY NO. 4. To promote wellness (Teaching/Discharge Considerations):

- Discuss with caregivers specific situations (e.g., if client choking or experiencing pain, needing to be repositioned, constipated, blocked urinary flow) and review appropriate interventions **to prevent/limit episodic increases in ICP.**
- Identify signs/symptoms suggesting increased ICP (in client at risk without an ICP monitor); for example, restlessness, deterioration in neurological responses. Review appropriate interventions.

Information in brackets added by the authors to clarify and enhance the use of nursing diagnoses.

decreased INTRACRANIAL ADAPTIVE CAPACITY

Documentation Focus

ASSESSMENT/REASSESSMENT

- Neurological findings noting right/left sides separately (such as pupils, motor response, reflexes, restlessness, nuchal rigidity); Glasgow Coma Scale.
- Response to activities/events (e.g., changes in pressure wave-forms/vital signs).
- Presence/characteristics of seizure activity.

PLANNING

- Plan of care and who is involved in planning.
- Teaching plan.

IMPLEMENTATION/EVALUATION

- Response to interventions and actions performed.
- Attainment/progress toward desired outcome(s).
- Modifications to plan of care.

DISCHARGE PLANNING

- Future needs, plan for meeting them, and determining who is responsible for actions.
- Referrals as identified.

SAMPLE NURSING OUTCOMES & INTERVENTIONS CLASSIFICATIONS (NOC/NIC)

NOC—Neurological Status
NIC—Cerebral Edema Management

disturbed personal Identity

Taxonomy II: Self-Perception—Class 1 Self-Concept (00121)
[Diagnostic Division: Ego Integrity]
Submitted 1978

Definition: Inability to distinguish between self and nonself

Related Factors

To be developed
[Organic brain syndrome; traumatic brain injury]
[Poor ego differentiation, as in schizophrenia]
[Panic/dissociative states]
[Biochemical body change, e.g., eating disorders]

Information in brackets added by the authors to clarify and enhance the use of nursing diagnoses.

 Cultural Collaborative Community/Home Care

[Illnesses/trauma affecting body image, e.g., multiple sclerosis, amputation]

Defining Characteristics

To be developed

SUBJECTIVE

[Confusion about sense of self, purpose or direction in life, sexual identity/preference]

[Questioning "Who am I?"; what does it take to be a person as opposed to a nonperson]

OBJECTIVE

[Difficulty in making decisions]
[Poorly differentiated ego boundaries]
[Problems with physical ability to move as desired]
[See ND Anxiety for additional characteristics]

Desired Outcomes/Evaluation Criteria—Client Will:

- Acknowledge threat to personal identity.
- Integrate threat in a healthy, positive manner (e.g., states anxiety is reduced, makes plans for the future).
- Verbalize acceptance of changes that have occurred.
- State ability to identify and accept self (long-term outcome).

Actions/Interventions

NURSING PRIORITY NO. 1. To assess causative/contributing factors:

- Ascertain client's perception of the extent of the threat to self and how client is handling the situation.
- Determine speed of occurrence of threat. **An event that has happened quickly may be more threatening (e.g., a traumatic event resulting in change in body image).**
- Have client define own body image. (**Body image is the basis of personal identity. Erikson's stages of psychosocial development describe an identity crisis during the teenage years as a struggle between feelings of identity versus role confusion.**)
- Be aware of physical signs of panic state. (Refer to ND Anxiety.)
- Note age of client. **An adolescent may struggle with the developmental task of personal/sexual identity, whereas an older person may have more difficulty accepting/dealing with a threat to identity, such as progressive loss of memory.**
- Assess availability and use of support systems. Note response of family/SO(s).

Information in brackets added by the authors to clarify and enhance the use of nursing diagnoses.

- Note withdrawn/automatic behavior, regression to earlier developmental stage, general behavioral disorganization, or display of self-mutilation behaviors in adolescent or adult; delayed development, preference for solitary play, display of self-stimulation in child.

• Determine presence of hallucinations/delusions, distortions of reality.

NURSING PRIORITY NO. 2. To assist client to manage/deal with threat:

- Make time to listen to client, encouraging appropriate expression of feelings, including anger and hostility.
- Provide calm environment. **Helps client to remain calm and able to discuss important issues related to the identity crisis.**
- Use crisis-intervention principles **to restore equilibrium when possible.**
- Discuss client's commitment to an identity. **Those who have made a strong commitment to an identity tend to be more comfortable with self and happier than those who have not.**
- Assist client to develop strategies to cope with threat to identity. **Helps reduce anxiety and promotes self-awareness and self-esteem.**
- Engage client in activities to help in identifying self as an individual (e.g., use of mirror for visual feedback, tactile stimulation).
- Provide for simple decisions, concrete tasks, calming activities.
- Allow client to deal with situation in small steps. **May be unable to cope with larger picture when in stress overload.**
- Encourage client to develop/participate in an individualized exercise program (walking is an excellent beginning).
- Provide concrete assistance, as needed (e.g., help with ADLs, providing food).
- Take advantage of opportunities to promote growth. Realize that client will have difficulty learning while in a dissociative state.
- Maintain reality orientation without confronting client's irrational beliefs. **Client may become defensive, blocking opportunity to look at other possibilities.**
- Use humor judiciously, when appropriate.
- Discuss options for dealing with issues of sexual gender (e.g., therapy/gender-change surgery when client is a transsexual).
- Refer to NDs disturbed Body Image; Self-Esteem [specify]; Spiritual Distress.

NURSING PRIORITY NO. 3. To promote wellness (Teaching/Discharge Considerations):

- Provide accurate information about threat to and potential consequences for individual. **Helps client to make positive decisions for future.**

Information in brackets added by the authors to clarify and enhance the use of nursing diagnoses.

    Cultural   Collaborative   Community/Home Care

- Assist client and SO(s) to acknowledge and integrate threat into future planning (e.g., wearing ID bracelet when prone to mental confusion; change of lifestyle to accommodate change of gender for transsexual client).

- Refer to appropriate support groups (e.g., day-care program, counseling/psychotherapy, gender identity).

Documentation Focus

ASSESSMENT/REASSESSMENT

- Findings, noting degree of impairment.
- Nature of and client's perception of the threat.
- Degree of commitment to own identity.

PLANNING

- Plan of care and who is involved in the planning.
- Teaching plan.

IMPLEMENTATION/EVALUATION

- Client's response to interventions/teaching and actions performed.
- Attainment/progress toward desired outcome(s).
- Modifications to plan of care.

DISCHARGE PLANNING

- Long-term needs and who is responsible for actions to be taken.
- Specific referrals made.

SAMPLE NURSING OUTCOMES & INTERVENTIONS CLASSIFICATIONS (NOC/NIC)

NOC—Identity
NIC—Self-Esteem Enhancement

deficient Knowledge
[Learning Need] (specify)

Taxonomy II: Perception/Cognition—Class 4 Cognition (00126)
[Diagnostic Division: Teaching/Learning]
Submitted 1980

Definition: Absence or deficiency of cognitive information related to specific topic [Lack of specific information necessary for clients/SO(s) to make informed choices regarding condition/treatment/lifestyle changes]

Information in brackets added by the authors to clarify and enhance the use of nursing diagnoses.

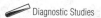 Diagnostic Studies 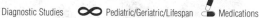 Pediatric/Geriatric/Lifespan Medications   **433**

Related Factors

Lack of exposure/recall
Information misinterpretation [inaccurate/incomplete information presented]
Unfamiliarity with information resources
Cognitive limitation
Lack of interest in learning [client's request for no information]

Defining Characteristics

SUBJECTIVE

Verbalization of the problem
[Request for information]
[Statements reflecting misconceptions]

OBJECTIVE

Inaccurate follow-through of instruction/performance of test
Inappropriate/exaggerated behaviors (e.g., hysterical, hostile, agitated, apathetic)
[Development of preventable complication]

Desired Outcomes/Evaluation Criteria—Client Will:

- Participate in learning process.
- Identify interferences to learning and specific action(s) to deal with them.
- Exhibit increased interest/assume responsibility for own learning by beginning to look for information and ask questions.
- Verbalize understanding of condition/disease process and treatment.
- Identify relationship of signs/symptoms to the disease process and correlate symptoms with causative factors.
- Perform necessary procedures correctly and explain reasons for the actions.
- Initiate necessary lifestyle changes and participate in treatment regimen.

Actions/Interventions

NURSING PRIORITY NO. 1. To assess readiness to learn and individual learning needs:

- Ascertain level of knowledge, including anticipatory needs.
- Determine client's ability/readiness and barriers to learning. **Individual may not be physically, emotionally, or mentally capable at this time.**

Information in brackets added by the authors to clarify and enhance the use of nursing diagnoses.

  Cultural Collaborative 🏠 Community/Home Care

- Be alert to signs of avoidance. **Client may need to suffer consequences of lack of knowledge before he or she is ready to accept information.**
- Identify support persons/SO(s) requiring information (e.g., parent, caregiver, spouse).

NURSING PRIORITY NO. 2. To determine other factors pertinent to the learning process:

- Note personal factors (e.g., age/developmental level, gender, social/cultural influences, religion, life experiences, level of education, emotional stability).
- Determine blocks to learning: language barriers (e.g., client can't read; speaks/understands a different language than healthcare provider); physical factors (e.g., cognitive impairment, aphasia, dyslexia); physical stability (e.g., acute illness, activity intolerance); difficulty of material to be learned.
- Assess the level of the client's capabilities and the possibilities of the situation. **May need to help SO(s) and/or caregivers to learn.**

NURSING PRIORITY NO. 3. To assess the client's/SO's motivation:

- Identify motivating factors for the individual (e.g., client needs to stop smoking because of advanced lung cancer, or client wants to lose weight because family member died of complications of obesity). **Motivation may be a negative stimulus (e.g., smoking caused lung cancer); or positive (e.g., client wants to promote health/prevent disease).**
- Provide information relevant only to the situation **to prevent overload.**
- Provide positive reinforcement. **Can encourage continuation of efforts.** Avoid use of negative reinforcers (e.g., criticism, threats).

NURSING PRIORITY NO. 4. To establish priorities in conjunction with client:

- Determine client's most urgent need from both client's and nurse's viewpoint **(which may differ and require adjustments in teaching plan).**
- Discuss client's perception of need. Relate information to client's personal desires/needs and values/beliefs **so that client feels competent and respected.**
- Differentiate "critical" content from "desirable" content. **Identifies information that can be addressed at a later time.**

NURSING PRIORITY NO. 5. To establish the content to be included:

- Identify information that needs to be remembered (cognitive).

Information in brackets added by the authors to clarify and enhance the use of nursing diagnoses.

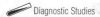

deficient KNOWLEDGE

- Identify information having to do with emotions, attitudes, and values (affective).
- Identify psychomotor skills that are necessary for learning.

NURSING PRIORITY NO. **6.** To develop learner's objectives:

- State objectives clearly in learner's terms **to meet learner's (not instructor's) needs.**
- Identify outcomes (results) to be achieved.
- Recognize level of achievement, time factors, and short-term and long-term goals.
- Include the affective goals (e.g., reduction of stress).

NURSING PRIORITY NO. **7.** To identify teaching methods to be used:

- Determine client's method of accessing information (visual, auditory, kinesthetic, gustatory/olfactory) and include in teaching plan **to facilitate learning/recall.**
- Involve the client/SO(s) by using age-appropriate materials tailored to client's literacy skills; questions/dialogue, audiovisual materials.
- Involve with others who have same problems/needs/concerns (e.g., group presentations, support groups). **Provides role model and sharing of information.**
- Provide mutual goal setting and learning contracts. **Clarifies expectations of teacher and learner.**
- Use team and group teaching as appropriate.

NURSING PRIORITY NO. **8.** To facilitate learning:

- Use short, simple sentences and concepts. Repeat and summarize as needed.
- Use gestures and facial expressions that help convey meaning of information.
- Discuss one topic at a time; avoid giving too much information in one session.
- Provide written information/guidelines and self-learning modules for client to refer to as necessary. **Reinforces learning process, allows client to proceed at own pace.**
- Pace and time learning sessions and learning activities to individual's needs. Evaluate effectiveness of leaning activities with client.
- Provide an environment that is conducive to learning.
- Be aware of factors related to teacher in the situation (e.g., vocabulary, dress, style, knowledge of the subject, and ability to impart information effectively).
- Begin with information the client already knows and move to what the client does not know, progressing from simple to

---

Information in brackets added by the authors to clarify and enhance the use of nursing diagnoses.

  Cultural Collaborative Community/Home Care

complex. **Can arouse interest/limit sense of being over-whelmed.**

- Deal with the client's anxiety/other strong emotions. Present information out of sequence, if necessary, dealing first with material that is most anxiety-producing **when the anxiety is interfering with the client's ability to learn.**
- Provide active role for client in learning process. **Promotes sense of control over situation and is means for determining that client is assimilating/using new information.**
- Provide for feedback (positive reinforcement) and evaluation of learning/acquisition of skills.
- Be aware of informal teaching and role modeling that takes place on an ongoing basis (e.g., answering specific questions/ reinforcing previous teaching during routine care).
- Assist client to use information in all applicable areas (e.g., situational, environmental, personal).

NURSING PRIORITY NO. 9. To promote wellness (Teaching/ Discharge Considerations):

- Provide access information for contact person **to answer questions/validate information post-discharge.**
- Identify available community resources/support groups.
- Provide information about additional learning resources (e.g., bibliography, websites, tapes). **May assist with further learning/promote learning at own pace.**

Documentation Focus

ASSESSMENT/REASSESSMENT

- Individual findings/learning style and identified needs, presence of learning blocks (e.g., hostility, inappropriate behavior).

PLANNING

- Plan for learning, methods to be used, and who is involved in the planning.
- Teaching plan.

IMPLEMENTATION/EVALUATION

- Responses of the client/SO(s) to the learning plan and actions performed. How the learning is demonstrated.
- Attainment/progress toward desired outcome(s).
- Modifications to plan of care.

DISCHARGE PLANNING

- Additional learning/referral needs.

Information in brackets added by the authors to clarify and enhance the use of nursing diagnoses.

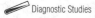 Diagnostic Studies ∞ Pediatric/Geriatric/Lifespan Medications **437**

SAMPLE NURSING OUTCOMES & INTERVENTIONS CLASSIFICATIONS (NOC/NIC)

NOC—Knowledge: [specify—25 choices]
NIC—Teaching: Individual

readiness for enhanced Knowledge (Specify)

Taxonomy II: Perception/Cognition—Class 4 Cognition (00161)
[Diagnostic Division: Teaching/Learning]
Submitted 2002

Definition: The presence or acquisition of cognitive information related to a specific topic is sufficient for meeting health-related goals and can be strengthened

Related Factors

To be developed

Defining Characteristics

SUBJECTIVE

Expresses an interest in learning
Explains knowledge of the topic; describes previous experiences pertaining to the topic

OBJECTIVE

Behaviors congruent with expressed knowledge

Desired Outcomes/Evaluation Criteria—Client Will:

- Exhibit responsibility for own learning by seeking answers to questions.
- Verify accuracy of informational resources.
- Verbalize understanding of information gained.
- Use information to develop individual plan to meet health-care needs/goals.

Actions/Interventions

NURSING PRIORITY NO. 1. To develop plan for learning:

 • Verify client's level of knowledge about specific topic. **Provides opportunity to assure accuracy and completeness of knowledge base for future learning.**

Information in brackets added by the authors to clarify and enhance the use of nursing diagnoses.

 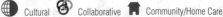 Cultural Collaborative Community/Home Care

- Determine motivation/expectations for learning. **Provides insight useful in developing goals and identifying information needs.**
- Assist client to identify learning goals. **Helps to frame or focus content to be learned and provides measure to evaluate learning process.**
- Ascertain preferred methods of learning (e.g., auditory, visual, interactive, or "hands-on"). **Identifies best approaches to facilitate learning process.**
- Note personal factors (e.g., age/developmental level, gender, social/cultural influences, religion, life experiences, level of education) **that may impact learning style, choice of informational resources.**
- Determine any challenges to learning: language barriers (e.g., client can't read, speaks/understands language other than that of care provider, dyslexia); physical factors (e.g., sensory deficits, such as vision/hearing deficits, aphasia); physical stability (e.g., acute illness, activity intolerance); difficulty of material to be learned. **Identifies special needs to be addressed if learning is to be successful.**

NURSING PRIORITY NO. **2.** To facilitate learning:

- Identify/provide information in varied formats appropriate to client's learning style (e.g., audiotapes, print materials, videos, classes/seminars, Internet). **Use of multiple formats increases learning and retention of material.**
- Provide information about additional/outside learning resources (e.g., bibliography, pertinent websites). **Promotes ongoing learning at own pace**.
- Discuss ways to verify accuracy of informational resources. **Encourages independent search for learning opportunities while reducing likelihood of acting on erroneous or unproven data that could be detrimental to client's well-being.**
- Identify available community resources/support groups. **Provides additional opportunities for role modeling, skill training, anticipatory problem solving, and so forth.**
- Be aware of informal teaching and role modeling that takes place on an ongoing basis (e.g., community/peer role models, support group feedback, print advertisements, popular music/videos). **Incongruencies may exist, creating questions/potentially undermining learning process.**

NURSING PRIORITY NO. **3.** To enhance optimum wellness:

- Assist client to identify ways to integrate and use information in all applicable areas (e.g., situational, environmental, personal).

Information in brackets added by the authors to clarify and enhance the use of nursing diagnoses.

readiness for enhanced KNOWLEDGE

Ability to apply/use information increases desire to learn and retention of information.

 • Encourage client to journal, keep a log, or graph as appropriate. **Provides opportunity for self-evaluation of effects of learning, such as better management of chronic condition, reduction of risk factors, acquisition of new skills.**

Documentation Focus

ASSESSMENT/REASSESSMENT

- Individual findings/learning style and identified needs, presence of challenges to learning.
- Motivation/expectations for learning.

PLANNING

- Plan for learning, methods to be used, and who is involved in the planning.
- Educational plan.

IMPLEMENTATION/EVALUATION

- Responses of the client/SO(s) to the learning plan and actions performed.
- How the learning is demonstrated.
- Attainment/progress toward desired outcome(s).
- Modifications to lifestyle/treatment plan.

DISCHARGE PLANNING

- Additional learning/referral needs.

SAMPLE NURSING OUTCOMES & INTERVENTIONS CLASSIFICATIONS (NOC/NIC)

NOC—Knowledge: [specify—25 choices]
NIC—Teaching: Individual

sedentary Lifestyle

Taxonomy II: Activity/Rest—Class 2 Activity/Exercise (00168)
[Diagnostic Division: Activity/Rest]
Submitted 2004

Definition: Reports a habit of life that is characterized by a low physical activity level

---

Information in brackets added by the authors to clarify and enhance the use of nursing diagnoses.

 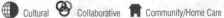

Related Factors

Lack of interest/motivation/resources (time, money, companionship, facilities)
Lack of training for accomplishment of physical exercise
Deficient knowledge of health benefits of physical exercise

Defining Characteristics

SUBJECTIVE

Verbalizes preference for activities low in physical activity

OBJECTIVE

Chooses a daily routine lacking physical exercise
Demonstrates physical deconditioning

Desired Outcomes/Evaluation Criteria—Client Will:

- Verbalize understanding of importance of regular exercise to general well-being.
- Identify necessary precautions/safety concerns and self-monitoring techniques.
- Formulate realistic exercise program with gradual increase in activity.

NURSING PRIORITY NO. 1. To assess precipitating/etiological factors:

- Identify conditions that may contribute to immobility or the onset and continuation of inactivity/sedentary lifestyle (e.g., obesity, depression, MS, arthritis, Parkinson's, surgery, hemiplegia/paraplegia, chronic pain, brain injury).
- Assess client's developmental level, motor skills, ease and capability of movement, posture, and gait.
- Note emotional/behavioral responses to problems associated with self- or condition-imposed sedentary lifestyle. **Feelings of frustration and powerlessness may impede attainment of goals.**
- Determine usual exercise and dietary habits, physical limitations, work environment, family dynamics, available resources.

NURSING PRIORITY NO. 2. To motivate and stimulate client involvement:

- Establish therapeutic relationship acknowledging reality of situation and client's feelings. **Changing a lifelong habit can be difficult, and client may be feeling discouragement with**

Information in brackets added by the authors to clarify and enhance the use of nursing diagnoses.

body and hopeless to turn situation around into a positive experience.

- Ascertain client's perception of current activity/exercise patterns, impact on life, and cultural expectations of client/others.
- Determine client's actual ability to participate in exercise/activities, noting attention span, physical limitations/tolerance, level of interest/desire, and safety needs. **Identifies barriers that need to be addressed.**
- Discuss motivation for change. **Concerns of SO(s) regarding threats to personal health/longevity, or acceptance by teen peers may be sufficient to cause client to initiate change; however, client must want to change for himself or herself in order to sustain change.**
- Review necessity for/benefits of regular exercise. **Research confirms that exercise has benefits for the whole body (e.g., can boost energy, enhance coordination, reduce muscle deterioration, improve circulation, lower blood pressure, produce healthier skin and a toned body, prolong youthful appearance. Exercise has also been found to boost cardiac fitness in both conditioned and out-of-shape individuals.**
- Involve client, SO, parent, or caregiver in developing exercise plan and goals to meet individual needs, desires, and available resources.
- Introduce activities at client's current level of functioning, progressing to more complex activities, as tolerated.
- Recommend mix of age/gender appropriate activities/stimuli (e.g., movement classes, walking/hiking, jazzercise, swimming, biking, skating, bowling, golf, weight training). **Activities need to be personally meaningful for client to derive the most enjoyment and to sustain motivation to continue with program.**
- Encourage change of scenery (indoors and out, where possible), and periodic changes in the personal environment when client is confined inside.

NURSING PRIORITY NO. 3. To promote optimal level of function and prevent exercise failure:

- Assist with treatment of underlying condition impacting participation in activities **to maximize function within limitations of situation.**
- Collaborate with physical medicine specialist or occupational/physical therapist in providing active or passive range-of-motion exercise, isotonic muscle contractions. **Techniques such as gait training, strength training, and exercise to**

Information in brackets added by the authors to clarify and enhance the use of nursing diagnoses.

  Cultural Collaborative  Community/Home Care

**improve balance and coordination can be helpful in reha-
bilitating client.**

 • Schedule ample time to perform exercise activities balanced with adequate rest periods.

 • Provide for safety measures as indicated by individual situation, including environmental management/fall prevention. (Refer to ND risk for Falls.)

 • Reevaluate ability/commitment periodically. **Changes in strength/endurance signal readiness for progression of activities or possibly to decrease exercise if overly fatigued. Wavering commitment may require change in types of activities, addition of a workout buddy to reenergize involvement.**

 • Discuss discrepancies in planned and performed activities with client aware and unaware of observation. Suggest methods for dealing with identified problems. **May be necessary when client is using avoidance or controlling behavior, or is not aware of own abilities due to anxiety/fear.**

 • Review importance of adequate intake of fluids, especially during hot weather/strenuous activity.

NURSING PRIORITY NO. 4. To promote wellness (Teaching/Discharge Considerations):

 • Review components of physical fitness: 1) muscle strength and endurance, 2) flexibility, 3) body composition (muscle mass, percentage of body fat), and 4) cardiovascular health. **Fitness routines need to include all elements to attain maximum benefits/prevent deconditioning.**

 • Instruct in safety measures as individually indicated (e.g., warm-up and cool down activities, taking pulse before/during/after activity, wearing reflective clothing when jogging/reflectors on bicycle, locking wheelchair before transfers, judicious use of medications, supervision as indicated).

 • Recommend keeping an activity/exercise log, including physical/psychological responses, changes in weight, endurance, body mass. **Provides visual evidence of progress/goal attainment and encouragement to continue with program.**

 • Encourage client to involve self in exercise as part of wellness management for the whole person; encourage parents to set a positive example for children by participating in exercise and an active lifestyle.

 • Identify community resources, charity activities, support groups. **Community walking/hiking trails, sports leagues, etc., provide free/low cost options. Activities such as 5K walks for charity, participation in Special Olympics, or**

_____

Information in brackets added by the authors to clarify and enhance the use of nursing diagnoses.

sedentary LIFESTYLE

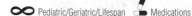

age-related competitive games provide goals to work toward. Note: Some individuals may prefer solitary activities; however, most individuals enjoy supportive companionship when exercising.

 • Discuss alternatives for exercise program in changing circumstances (e.g., walking the mall during inclement weather, using exercise facilities at hotel when traveling, water aerobics at local swimming pool, joining a gym).

 • Promote individual participation in community awareness of problem and discussion of solutions. **Physical inactivity (and associated diseases) is a major public health problem that affects huge numbers of people in all regions of the world. Recognizing the problem and future consequences may empower the global community to develop effective measures to promote physical activity and improve public health.**

 • Introduce/promote established goals for increasing physical activity, such as Sports, Play, and Active Recreation for Kids (SPARK) and Physician-Based Assessment and Counseling for Exercise (PACE) **to address national concerns about obesity and major barriers to physical activity, such as time constraints, lack of training in physical activity or behavioral change methods, and lack of standard protocols.**

Documentation Focus

ASSESSMENT/REASSESSMENT

• Individual findings, including level of function/ability to participate in specific/desired activities, motivation for change.

PLANNING

• Plan of care and who is involved in the planning.
• Teaching plan.

IMPLEMENTATION/EVALUATION

• Responses to interventions/teaching and actions performed.
• Attainment/progress toward desired outcome(s).
• Modifications to plan of care.

DISCHARGE PLANNING

• Discharge/long-range needs, noting who is responsible for each action to be taken.
• Specific referrals made.
• Sources of/maintenance for assistive devices.

Information in brackets added by the authors to clarify and enhance the use of nursing diagnoses.

Cultural   Collaborative   Community/Home Care

SAMPLE NURSING OUTCOMES & INTERVENTIONS CLASSIFICATIONS (NOC/NIC)

NOC—Knowledge: Prescribed Activity
NIC—Exercise Promotion

risk for impaired Liver Function

Taxonomy II: Nutrition—Class 4 Metabolism (0000178)
[Diagnostic Division: Food/Fluid]
Submitted 2006

Definition: At risk for liver dysfunction

Risk Factors

Viral infection (e.g., hepatitis A, hepatitis B, hepatitis C, Epstein-Barr)
HIV co-infection
Hepatotoxic medications (e.g., acetaminophen, statins)
Substance abuse (e.g., alcohol, cocaine)

> NOTE: A risk diagnosis is not evidenced by signs and symptoms, as the problem has not occurred and nursing interventions are directed at prevention.

Desired Outcomes/Evaluation Criteria—Client Will:

- Verbalize understanding of individual risk factors that contribute to possibility of liver damage/failure.
- Demonstrate behaviors, lifestyle changes to reduce risk factors and protect self from injury.
- Be free of signs of liver failure as evidenced by liver function studies within normal levels, and absence of jaundice, hepatic enlargement, or altered mental status.

Actions/Interventions

NURSING PRIORITY NO. 1. To identify individual risk factors/needs:

- Determine presence of condition(s) as listed in Risk Factors, noting whether problem is acute (e.g., viral hepatitis, acetaminophen overdose) or chronic (e.g., alcoholic cirrhosis). **Influences choice of interventions.**

Information in brackets added by the authors to clarify and enhance the use of nursing diagnoses.

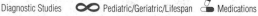

- Note if client works in high-risk occupation (e.g., performs tasks that involve contact with blood, blood-contaminated body fluids, other body fluids, or sharps/needles). **Carries high risk for exposure to hepatitis B and C.**
- Assess for exposure to contaminated food or poor sanitation practices by food service workers. **Poses risk for exposure to enteric viruses (hepatitis A and E).**

NURSING PRIORITY NO. 2. To assist client to reduce or correct individual risk factors:

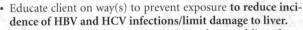

- Educate client on way(s) to prevent exposure **to reduce incidence of HBV and HCV infections/limit damage to liver.**
- Review results of laboratory tests (e.g., abnormal liver function studies, drug toxicity, HepB positive, etc.)/diagnostic studies **that indicate presence of hepatotoxic condition and need for medical treatment.**
- Assist with medical treatment of underlying condition **to support organ function and minimize liver damage.**
- Stress importance of responsible drinking or avoiding alcohol, when indicated, **to reduce incidence of cirrhosis/severity of liver damage/failure.**
- Encourage client with liver dysfunction to avoid fatty foods. Fat interferes with normal function of liver cells and can cause additional damage/permanent scarring to liver cells when they can no longer regenerate.
- Refer to nutritionist, as indicated, for dietary needs, including intake of proteins, vitamins, etc., to promote healing.
- Discuss safe use/concerns about client's medication regimen (e.g., acetaminophen; NSAIDs; herbal/vitamin supplements; phenobarbitol; cholesterol-lowering drugs, such as "statins;" certain antibiotics [e.g., sulfonamides, INH]; certain cardiovascular drugs [e.g., amiodarone, hydralazine]; antidepressants [e.g., tricyclics]) **known to cause hepatotoxicity, either alone or in combination, or in overdose situation.**
- Identify signs/symptoms that warrant prompt notification of healthcare provider (e.g., increased abdominal girth; rapid weight loss/gain; increased peripheral edema; dyspnea, fever; blood in stool or urine; excess bleeding of any kind; jaundice). **Indicators of severe liver dysfunction, possible organ failure.**
- Refer to specialist/liver treatment center, as indicated. **May be beneficial for person with chronic liver disease when decompensating, or client with hepatitis and other coexisting disease condition (e.g., HIV), or intolerance to treatment due to side effects.**

Information in brackets added by the authors to clarify and enhance the use of nursing diagnoses.

  Cultural Collaborative Community/Home Care

NURSING PRIORITY NO. 3. To promote wellness (Teaching/ Discharge Considerations):

- Encourage client routinely taking acetaminophen for pain management to read labels, determine strength of medication, note safe number of doses over 24 hours, become familiar with "hidden" sources of acetaminophen, limit alcohol intake (e.g., Nyquil, Vicodin) **to avoid/limit risk of liver damage.**

- Emphasize importance of hand hygiene and avoidance of fresh produce, use of bottled water and avoidance of raw meat/seafood (**if client is traveling to area where hepatitis A is endemic or food/waterborne illness is a risk**).

- Instruct in measures including protection from blood/other body fluids, sharps safety, safer sex practices, avoiding needle sharing, avoiding body tattoos/piercings **to prevent occupational and nonoccupational exposures to hepatitis.**

- Discuss need/refer for vaccination, as indicated (e.g., healthcare and public safety worker, children under 18, international traveler, recreational drug user, men who have sexual relationships with other men, client with clotting disorders or liver disease, anyone sharing household with an infected person), **to prevent exposure/transmission of blood/body fluid hepatitis/limit risk of liver injury.**

- Discuss appropriateness of prophylaxis immunizations. **Although the best way to protect against hepatitis B and C infections is to prevent exposure to viruses, post-exposure prophylaxis (PEP) should be initiated promptly to prevent/ limit severity of infection.**

- Provide information regarding availability of gamma globulin, ISG, H-BIG, HB vaccine (Recombivax HB, Engerix-B) through health department or family physician.

- Stress necessity of follow-up care (in client with chronic liver disease) and adherence to therapeutic regimen.

- Refer to community resources, drug/alcohol treatment program, as indicated.

Documentation Focus

ASSESSMENT/REASSESSMENT

- Assessment findings, including individual risk factors.
- Results of laboratory tests/diagnostic studies.

PLANNING

- Plan of care and who is involved in planning.
- Teaching plan.

Information in brackets added by the authors to clarify and enhance the use of nursing diagnoses.

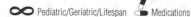

IMPLEMENTATION/EVALUATION

- Response to interventions/teaching and actions performed.
- Attainment/progress toward desired outcome(s).
- Modifications to plan of care.

DISCHARGE PLANNING

- Long-term needs, plan for follow-up, and who is responsible for actions to be taken.
- Specific referrals made.

SAMPLE NURSING OUTCOMES & INTERVENTIONS CLASSIFICATIONS (NOC/NIC)

NOC— Treatment Behavior: Illness or Injury
NIC—Substance Use Treatment

risk for Loneliness

Taxonomy II: Self-Perception—Class 1 Self-Concept (00054)
[Diagnostic Division: Social Interaction]
Submitted 1994

Definition: At risk for experiencing discomfort associated with a desire or need for more contact with others

Risk Factors

Affectional deprivation
Physical/social isolation
Cathectic deprivation
[Problems of attachment for infants or adolescents]
[Chaotic family relationships]

NOTE: A risk diagnosis is not evidenced by signs and symptoms, as the problem has not occurred and nursing interventions are directed at prevention.

Desired Outcomes/Evaluation Criteria—Client Will:

- Identify individual difficulties and ways to address them.
- Engage in social activities.
- Report involvement in interactions/relationship client views as meaningful.

Information in brackets added by the authors to clarify and enhance the use of nursing diagnoses.

 Cultural Collaborative Community/Home Care
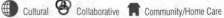

Parent/Caregiver Will:

- Provide infant with consistent and loving caregiving.
- Participate in programs for adolescents and families.

Actions/Interventions

NURSING PRIORITY NO. 1. To identify causative/precipitating factors:

- Differentiate between ordinary loneliness and a state or constant sense of dysphoria.
- Note client's age and duration of problem; that is, situational (such as leaving home for college) or chronic. **Adolescents may experience lonely feelings related to the changes that are happening as they become adults. Elderly individuals incur multiple losses associated with aging, loss of spouse, decline in physical health, and changes in roles intensifying feelings of loneliness.**
- Determine degree of distress, tension, anxiety, restlessness present. Note history of frequent illnesses, accidents, crises. **Most people feel lonely at some time in their lives related to situational occurrences that engender these feelings which are normal in the circumstances.**
- Note presence/proximity of family, SO(s), and whether they are helpful or not.
- Discuss with client whether there is a person or persons in his or her life who can be trustworthy and who will listen with empathy to the feelings that are expressed.
- Determine how individual perceives/deals with solitude. A person may feel alone in a crowd or may choose to be alone and enjoy the quiet.
- Review issues of separation from parents as a child, loss of SO(s)/spouse.
- Assess sleep/appetite disturbances, ability to concentrate. **Indicators of distress related to feelings of loneliness and low self-esteem.**
- Note expressions of "yearning" for an emotional partnership.

NURSING PRIORITY NO. 2. To assist client to identify feelings and situations in which he or she experiences loneliness:

- Establish nurse-client relationship. Client may feel free to talk about feelings in an empathetic relationship.
- Discuss individual concerns about feelings of loneliness and relationship between loneliness and lack of SO(s). Note desire/willingness to change situation. **Motivation can impede—or facilitate—achieving desired outcomes.**

Information in brackets added by the authors to clarify and enhance the use of nursing diagnoses.

• Support expression of negative perceptions of others and whether client agrees. **Provides opportunity for client to clarify reality of situation, recognize own denial.**

• Accept client's expressions of loneliness as a primary condition and not necessarily as a symptom of some underlying condition.

NURSING PRIORITY NO. 3. To assist client to become involved:

• Discuss reality versus perceptions of situation.

• Discuss importance of emotional bonding (attachment) between infants/young children, parents/caregivers as appropriate.

• Involve in classes, such as assertiveness, language/communication, social skills, **to address individual needs/enhance socialization.**

• Role play situations **to develop interpersonal skills.**

• Discuss positive health habits, including personal hygiene, exercise activity of client's choosing.

• Identify individual strengths, areas of interest **that provide opportunities for involvement with others.**

• Encourage attendance at support group activities to meet individual needs (e.g., therapy, separation/grief, religious).

• Help client establish plan for progressive involvement, beginning with a simple activity (e.g., call an old friend, speak to a neighbor) and leading to more complicated interactions/activities.

• Provide opportunities for interactions in a supportive environment (e.g., have client accompanied, as in a "buddy system") during initial attempts to socialize. **Helps reduce stress, provides positive reinforcement, and facilitates successful outcome.**

NURSING PRIORITY NO. 4. To promote wellness (Teaching/Discharge Considerations):

• Let client know that loneliness can be overcome. **It is up to the individual to build self-esteem and learn to feel good about self.**

• Encourage involvement in special-interest groups (e.g., computers, bird watchers); charitable services (e.g., serving in a soup kitchen, youth groups, animal shelter).

• Suggest volunteering for church committee or choir; attending community events with friends and family; becoming involved in political issues/campaigns; enrolling in classes at local college/continuing education programs.

• Refer to appropriate counselors for help with relationships and so on.

• Refer to NDs Hopelessness; Anxiety; Social Isolation.

Information in brackets added by the authors to clarify and enhance the use of nursing diagnoses.

  Cultural Collaborative Community/Home Care

Documentation Focus

ASSESSMENT/REASSESSMENT

- Assessment findings, including client's perception of problem, availability of resources/support systems.
- Client's desire/commitment to change.

PLANNING

- Plan of care and who is involved in planning.
- Teaching plan.

IMPLEMENTATION/EVALUATION

- Response to interventions/teaching and actions performed.
- Attainment/progress toward desired outcome(s).
- Modifications to plan of care.

DISCHARGE PLANNING

- Long-term needs, plan for follow-up, and who is responsible for actions to be taken.
- Specific referrals made.

SAMPLE NURSING OUTCOMES & INTERVENTIONS CLASSIFICATIONS (NOC/NIC)

NOC—Loneliness
NIC—Socialization Enhancement

---

impaired Memory

Taxonomy II: Perception/Cognition—Class 4 Cognition (00131)
[Diagnostic Division: Neurosensory]
Submitted 1994

Definition: Inability to remember or recall bits of information or behavioral skills [Impaired memory may be attributed to physiopathological or situational causes that are either temporary or permanent]

Related Factors

Hypoxia; anemia
Fluid and electrolyte imbalance; decreased cardiac output
Neurological disturbances [e.g., brain injury/concussion]
Excessive environmental disturbances; [manic state, fugue, traumatic event]

Information in brackets added by the authors to clarify and enhance the use of nursing diagnoses.

 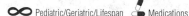

[Substance use/abuse; effects of medications]
[Age]

Defining Characteristics

SUBJECTIVE

[Reported] experience of forgetting
Inability to recall events/factual information [or familiar persons, places, items]

OBJECTIVE

[Observed] experience of forgetting
Inability to determine if a behavior was performed
Inability to learn/retain new skills/information
Inability to perform a previously learned skill
Forgets to perform a behavior at a scheduled time

Desired Outcomes/Evaluation Criteria—Client Will:

• Verbalize awareness of memory problems.
• Establish methods to help in remembering essential things when possible.
• Accept limitations of condition and use resources effectively.

Actions/Interventions

NURSING PRIORITY NO. 1. To assess causative factor(s)/degree of impairment:

• Determine physical/biochemical/environmental factors (e.g, systemic infections; brain injury; pulmonary disease with hypoxia; use of multiple medications; exposure to toxic substances; use/abuse of alcohol/other drugs; rape/trauma; removal from known environment; etc.) that may be associated with confusion and loss of memory.

 • Note client's age and potential for depression. **Depressive disorders affecting memory and concentration are particularly prevalent in older adults; however, impairments can occur in depressed persons of any age.**

 • Collaborate with medical and psychiatric provider in evaluating orientation, attention span, ability to follow directions, send/receive communication, appropriateness of response **to determine presence.**

 • Assist with/review results of cognitive testing (e.g., Blessed Information-Memory-Concentration [BIMC] test, Mini-Mental

---

Information in brackets added by the authors to clarify and enhance the use of nursing diagnoses.

  Cultural Collaborative Community/Home Care

State Examination [MMSE]), **to complete picture of client's overall condition and prognosis.**

- Evaluate skill proficiency levels, including self-care activities and driving ability.
- Ascertain how client/family view the problem (e.g., practical problems of forgetting and/or role and responsibility impairments related to loss of memory and concentration) **to determine significance/impact of problem.**

NURSING PRIORITY NO. 2. To maximize level of function:

- Assist with treatment of underlying conditions (e.g., electrolyte imbalances, reaction to medications, drug intoxication) **where treatment can improve memory processes.**
- Orient/reorient client as needed. Introduce self with each client contact **to meet client's safety and comfort needs.** (Refer to NDs acute/chronic Confusion, for additional interventions.)
- Implement appropriate memory retraining techniques (e.g., keeping calendars, writing lists, memory cue games, mnemonic devices, using computers).
- Assist in/instruct client and family in associate-learning tasks, such as practice sessions recalling personal information, reminiscing, locating a geographic location (Stimulation Therapy).
- Encourage ventilation of feelings of frustration, helplessness, etc. Refocus attention to areas of control and progress **to diminish feelings of powerlessness/hopelessness.**
- Provide for/emphasize importance of pacing learning activities and getting sufficient rest **to avoid fatigue that may further impair cognitive abilities.**
- Monitor client's behavior and assist in use of stress-management techniques (e.g., music therapy, reading, television, games, socialization) **to reduce frustration and enhance enjoyment of life.**
- Structure teaching methods and interventions to client's level of functioning and/or potential for improvement.
- Determine client's response to/effects of medications prescribed to improve attention, concentration, memory processes and to lift spirits/modify emotional responses. **Medication for cognitive enhancement can be effective, but benefits need to be weighed against whether quality of life is improved when considering side effects/cost of drugs.**

NURSING PRIORITY NO. 3. To promote wellness (Teaching/Discharge Considerations):

- Assist client/SO(s) to establish compensation strategies (e.g., menu planning with a shopping list, timely completion of

---

Information in brackets added by the authors to clarify and enhance the use of nursing diagnoses.

tasks on a daily planner, checklists at the front door to ascertain that lights and stove are off before leaving) **to improve functional lifestyle and safety.** (Refer to NDs acute/chronic Confusion for additional interventions.)

- Refer to/encourage follow-up with counselors, rehabilitation programs, job coaches, social/financial support systems **to help deal with persistent/difficult problems.**
- Assist client to deal with functional limitations (such as loss of driving privileges) and identify resources **to meet individual needs, maximizing independence.**

Documentation Focus

ASSESSMENT/REASSESSMENT

- Individual findings, testing results, and perceptions of significance of problem.
- Actual impact on lifestyle and independence.

PLANNING

- Plan of care and who is involved in planning process.
- Teaching plan.

IMPLEMENTATION/EVALUATION

- Responses to interventions/teaching and actions performed.
- Attainment/progress toward desired outcome(s).
- Modifications to plan of care.

DISCHARGE PLANNING

- Long-term needs and who is responsible for actions to be taken.
- Specific referrals made.

SAMPLE NURSING OUTCOMES & INTERVENTIONS CLASSIFICATIONS (NOC/NIC)

NOC—Memory
NIC—Memory Training

impaired bed Mobility

Taxonomy II: Activity/Rest—Class 2 Activity/Exercise (00091)
[Diagnostic Division: Safety]
Submitted 1998; Revised 2006

Definition: Limitation of independent movement from one bed position to another

---

Information in brackets added by the authors to clarify and enhance the use of nursing diagnoses.

 Cultural Collaborative Community/Home Care

Related Factors

Neuromuscular/musculoskeletal impairment

Insufficient muscle strength; deconditioning; obesity

Environmental contraints (i.e., bed size/type, treatment equipment, restraints)

Pain; sedating medications

Deficient knowledge

Cognitive impairment

Defining Characteristics

SUBJECTIVE

[Reported difficulty performing activities]

OBJECTIVE

Impaired ability to: turn side to side; move from supine to sitting/sitting to supine; "scoot" or reposition self in bed; move from supine to prone/prone to supine; move from supine to long-sitting/long-sitting to supine

Desired Outcomes/Evaluation Criteria—Client/Caregiver Will:

- Verbalize willingness to/and participate in repositioning program.
- Verbalize understanding of situation/risk factors, individual therapeutic regimen, and safety measures.
- Demonstrate techniques/behaviors that enable safe repositioning.
- Maintain position of function and skin integrity as evidenced by absence of contractures, footdrop, decubitus, and so forth.
- Maintain or increase strength and function of affected and/or compensatory body part.

Actions/Interventions

NURSING PRIORITY NO. 1. To identify causative/contributing factors:

- Determine diagnoses that contribute to immobility (e.g., MS, arthritis, Parkinson's, hemi/para/tetraplegia, fractures/multiple trauma, burns, head injury, depression, dementia).
- Note individual risk factors and current situation, such as surgery, casts, amputation, traction, pain, age, general weakness/debilitation.
- Determine degree of perceptual/cognitive impairment and/or ability to follow directions.

Information in brackets added by the authors to clarify and enhance the use of nursing diagnoses.

 Diagnostic Studies   Pediatric/Geriatric/Lifespan   Medications   **455**

NURSING PRIORITY NO. 2. To assess functional ability:

- Determine functional level classification 1 to 4 (1 = requires use of equipment or device, 2 = requires help from another person for assistance, 3 = requires help from another person and equipment device, 4 = dependent, does not participate in activity).
- Note cognitive/emotional/behavioral conditions/concerns impacting mobility.
- Note presence of complications related to immobility. (Refer to ND Disuse Syndrome.)

NURSING PRIORITY NO. 3. To promote optimal level of function and prevent complications:

- Ascertain that dependent client is placed in best bed for situation (e.g., correct size, support surface, and mobility functions) **to promote mobility and enhance environmental safety.**
- Turn dependent client frequently, utilizing bed and mattress positioning settings to assist movements; reposition in good body alignment, using appropriate supports.
- Instruct client and caregivers in methods of moving client relative to specific situations and mobility needs.
- Observe skin for reddened areas/shearing. Provide appropriate pressure relief/surface support mattress **to reduce friction, maintain safe skin/tissue pressures, and wick away moisture.** Provide regular skin care, as appropriate.
- Assist on/off bedpan and into sitting position (or use cardioposition bed or foot-egress bed) **to facilitate elimination.**
- Administer medication prior to activity as needed for pain relief **to permit maximal effort/involvement in activity.**
- Observe for change in strength to do more or less self-care **to adjust care as indicated.**
- Assist with activities of hygiene, toileting, feeding, as indicated.
- Provide diversional activities, as appropriate.
- Ensure telephone/call bell is within reach **to promote safety and timely response.**
- Provide individually appropriate methods to communicate adequately with client.
- Provide extremity protection (padding, exercises, etc.). (Refer to NDs impaired Skin Integrity; risk for Peripheral Neurovascular Dysfunction, for additional interventions.)
- Include physical/occupational therapists and rehabilitation providers in creating movement program and identifying assistive devices.

NURSING PRIORITY NO. 4. To promote wellness (Teaching/Discharge Considerations):

Information in brackets added by the authors to clarify and enhance the use of nursing diagnoses.

  Cultural Collaborative 🏠 Community/Home Care

- 🏠 • Involve client/SO(s) in determining activity schedule. **Promotes commitment to plan, maximizing outcomes.**
- 🏠 • Encourage continuation of exercises **to maintain/enhance gains in strength/muscle control.**
- 🏠 • Obtain/identify sources for assistive devices. Demonstrate safe use and proper maintenance.

Documentation Focus

ASSESSMENT/REASSESSMENT

- Individual findings, including level of function/ability to participate in specific/desired activities.

PLANNING

- Plan of care and who is involved in the planning.

IMPLEMENTATION/EVALUATION

- Responses to interventions/teaching and actions performed.
- Attainment/progress toward desired outcome(s).
- Modification to plan of care.

DISCHARGE PLANNING

- Discharge/long-range needs, noting who is responsible for each action to be taken.
- Specific referrals made.
- Sources of/maintenance for assistive devices.

SAMPLE NURSING OUTCOMES & INTERVENTIONS CLASSIFICATIONS (NOC/NIC)

NOC—Body Position: Self-Initiated
NIC—Bed Rest Care

impaired physical Mobility

Taxonomy II: Activity/Rest—Class 2 Activity/Exercise (00085)
[Diagnostic Division: Safety]
Submitted 1973; Nursing Diagnosis Extension and Classification (NDEC) Revision 1998

Definition: Limitation in independent, purposeful physical movement of the body or of one or more extremities

---

Information in brackets added by the authors to clarify and enhance the use of nursing diagnoses.

Related Factors

Sedentary lifestyle; activity intolerance; disuse; deconditioning; decreased endurance; limited cardiovascular endurance

Decreased muscle strength/control/mass; joint stiffness; contractures; loss of integrity of bone structures

Pain/discomfort

Neuromuscular/musculoskeletal impairment

Sensoriperceptual/cognitive impairment; developmental delay

Depressive mood state; anxiety

Malnutrition; altered cellular metabolism; body mass index above 75th age-appropriate percentile

Deficient knowledge regarding value of physical activity; cultural beliefs regarding age-appropriate activity; lack of environmental supports (e.g., physical or social)

Prescribed movement restrictions; medications

Reluctance to initiate movement

Defining Characteristics

SUBJECTIVE

[Report of pain/discomfort on movement; unwillingness to move]

OBJECTIVE

Limited range of motion; limited ability to perform gross/fine motor skills; difficulty turning

Slowed movement; uncoordinated/jerky movements; movement-induced tremor; decreased [slower] reaction time

Postural instability; gait changes

Engages in substitutions for movement (e.g., increased attention to other's activity, controlling behavior, focus on pre-illness disability/activity)

Suggested Functional Level Classification:

0—Completely independent
1—Requires use of equipment or device
2—Requires help from another person for assistance, supervision, or teaching
3—Requires help from another person and equipment device
4—Dependent, does not participate in activity

Information in brackets added by the authors to clarify and enhance the use of nursing diagnoses.

   Cultural   Collaborative 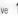 Community/Home Care

Desired Outcomes/Evaluation Criteria—Client Will:

- Verbalize understanding of situation and individual treatment regimen and safety measures.
- Demonstrate techniques/behaviors that enable resumption of activities.
- Participate in ADLs and desired activities.
- Maintain position of function and skin integrity as evidenced by absence of contractures, footdrop, decubitus, and so forth.
- Maintain or increase strength and function of affected and/or compensatory body part.

Actions/Interventions

NURSING PRIORITY NO. **1.** To identify causative/contributing factors:

- Determine diagnosis that contributes to immobility (e.g., MS, arthritis, Parkinson's, hemiplegia/paraplegia, depression).
- Note situations such as surgery, fractures, amputation, tubings (chest, catheter, etc.) **that may restrict movement.**
- Assess degree of pain, listening to client's description.
- Ascertain client's perception of activity/exercise needs.
 • Note decreased motor agility/essential tremor related to age.
- Determine degree of perceptual/cognitive impairment and ability to follow directions.
- Assess nutritional status and client's report of energy level.

NURSING PRIORITY NO. **2.** To assess functional ability:

- Determine degree of immobility in relation to previously suggested scale.
- Observe movement when client is unaware of observation **to note any incongruencies with reports of abilities.**
- Note emotional/behavioral responses to problems of immobility. **Feelings of frustration/powerlessness may impede attainment of goals.**
- Determine presence of complications related to immobility (e.g., pneumonia, elimination problems, contractures, decubitus, anxiety). (Refer to ND risk for Disuse Syndrome.)

NURSING PRIORITY NO. **3.** To promote optimal level of function and prevent complications:

- Assist/have client reposition self on a regular schedule as dictated by individual situation (including frequent shifting of weight when client is wheelchair-bound).

Information in brackets added by the authors to clarify and enhance the use of nursing diagnoses.

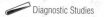 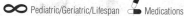

🏠 • Instruct in use of side rails, overhead trapeze, roller pads **for position changes/transfers.**

🏠 • Support affected body parts/joints using pillows/rolls, foot supports/shoes, air mattress, water bed, and so forth **to maintain position of function and reduce risk of pressure ulcers.**

⚙ • Assist with treatment of underlying condition causing pain and/or dysfunction.

💊 • Administer medications prior to activity as needed for pain relief **to permit maximal effort/involvement in activity.**

🏠 • Provide regular skin care to include pressure area management.

• Schedule activities with adequate rest periods during the day **to reduce fatigue.**

🏠 • Encourage participation in self-care, occupational/diversional/recreational activities. **Enhances self-concept and sense of independence.**

🏠 • Provide client with ample time to perform mobility-related tasks.

🏠 • Identify energy-conserving techniques for ADLs. **Limits fatigue, maximizing participation.**

🏠 • Discuss discrepancies in movement when client aware/unaware of observation and methods for dealing with identified problems.

🏠 • Provide for safety measures as indicated by individual situation, including environmental management/fall prevention.

⚙ • Consult with physical/occupational therapist, as indicated, **to develop individual exercise/mobility program and identify appropriate mobility devices.**

🏠 • Encourage adequate intake of fluids/nutritious foods. **Promotes well-being and maximizes energy production.**

NURSING PRIORITY NO. 4. To promote wellness (Teaching/Discharge Considerations):

🏠 • Encourage client's/SO's involvement in decision making as much as possible. **Enhances commitment to plan, optimizing outcomes.**

🏠 • Review safety measures as individually indicated (e.g., use of heating pads, locking wheelchair before transfers, removal or securing of scatter/area rugs).

🏠 • Involve client and SO(s) in care, assisting them to learn ways of managing problems of immobility.

🏠 • Demonstrate use of standing aids and mobility devices (e.g., walkers, strollers, scooters, braces, prosthetics, etc.), and have client/care provider demonstrate knowledge about/safe use of device. Identify appropriate resources for obtaining and

---

Information in brackets added by the authors to clarify and enhance the use of nursing diagnoses.

🌐 Cultural ⚙ Collaborative 🏠 Community/Home Care

maintaining appliances/equipment. **Promotes independence and enhances safety.**

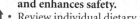 • Review individual dietary needs. Identify appropriate vitamin/herbal supplements.

Documentation Focus

ASSESSMENT/REASSESSMENT

• Individual findings, including level of function/ability to participate in specific/desired activities.

PLANNING

• Plan of care and who is involved in the planning.
• Teaching plan.

IMPLEMENTATION/EVALUATION

• Responses to interventions/teaching and actions performed.
• Attainment/progress toward desired outcome(s).
• Modifications to plan of care.

DISCHARGE PLANNING

• Discharge/long-range needs, noting who is responsible for each action to be taken.
• Specific referrals made.
• Sources of/maintenance for assistive devices.

SAMPLE NURSING OUTCOMES & INTERVENTIONS CLASSIFICATIONS (NOC/NIC)

NOC—Mobility Level
NIC—Exercise Therapy: [specify]

impaired wheelchair Mobility

Taxonomy II: Activity/Rest—Class 2 Activity/Exercise (00089)
[Diagnostic Division: Safety]
Submitted 1998; Revised 2006

Definition: Limitation of independent operation of wheelchair within environment

Related Factors

Neuromuscular/musculoskeletal impairments (e.g., contractures)

Information in brackets added by the authors to clarify and enhance the use of nursing diagnoses.

 Diagnostic Studies   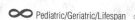 Pediatric/Geriatric/Lifespan   Medications   **461**

Insufficient muscle strength; limited endurance; deconditioning; obesity

Impaired vision

Pain

Depressed mood; cognitive impairment

Deficient knowledge

Environmental constraints (e.g., stairs, inclines, uneven surfaces, unsafe obstacles, distances, lack of assistive devices or persons, wheelchair type)

Defining Characteristics

Impaired ability to operate manual/power wheelchair on even/uneven surface, an incline/decline, curbs

> NOTE: Specify level of independence using a standardized functional scale. [Refer to ND impaired physical Mobility]

Desired Outcomes/Evaluation Criteria—Client Will:

• Move safely within environment, maximizing independence.
• Identify and use resources appropriately.

Caregiver Will:

• Provide safe mobility within environment and community.

Actions/Interventions

NURSING PRIORITY NO. 1. To identify causative/contributing factors:

• Determine diagnosis that contributes to immobility (e.g., ALS, SCI, spastic cerebral palsy, brain injury) and client's functional level/individual abilities.
• Identify factors in environments frequented by the client that contribute to inaccessibility (e.g., uneven floors/surfaces, lack of ramps, steep incline/decline, narrow doorways/spaces).
• Ascertain access to and appropriateness of public and/or private transportation.

NURSING PRIORITY NO. 2. To promote optimal level of function and prevent complications:

 • Determine that client's underlying cognitive, emotional, and physical impairment(s) (e.g., brain injury, pain, depression,

---

Information in brackets added by the authors to clarify and enhance the use of nursing diagnoses.

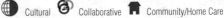 Cultural Collaborative Community/Home Care

vision deficits) are treated/being managed **to maximize desire/motivation to participate in wheelchair activities.**

 • Ascertain that wheelchair provides the base mobility to maximize function.

 • Provide for/instruct client in safety while in a wheelchair (e.g., adaptive cushions, supports for all body parts, repositioning and transfer assistive devices, and height adjustment).

 • Note evenness of surfaces client would need to negotiate and refer to appropriate sources for modifications. Clear pathways of obstructions.

 • Recommend/arrange for modifications to home/work or school/recreational settings frequented by client **to provide safe and suitable environment.**

 • Determine need for and capabilities of assistive persons. Provide training and support as indicated.

 • Monitor client's use of joystick, sip and puff, sensitive mechanical switches, etc., **to provide necessary equipment if condition/capabilities change.**

 • Monitor client for adverse effects of immobility (e.g., contractures, muscle atrophy, DVT, pressure ulcers). (Refer to NDs Disuse Syndrome; risk for Peripheral Vascular Dysfunction, for additional interventions.)

NURSING PRIORITY NO. 3. To promote wellness (Teaching/Discharge Considerations):

 • Identify/refer to medical equipment suppliers **to customize client's wheelchair for size, proper seating angle, positioning aids, incline/decline stability, accessories (e.g., side guards, head rests, heel loops, brake extensions, tool packs) and electronics suited to client's ability (e.g., sip and puff, head movement, sensitive switches).**

 • Encourage client's/SO's involvement in decision making as much as possible. **Enhances commitment to plan, optimizing outcomes.**

 • Involve client/SO(s) in care, assisting them in managing immobility problems. **Promotes independence.**

 • Demonstrate/provide information regarding individually appropriate safety measures.

 • Refer to support groups relative to specific medical condition/disability; independence/political action groups. **Provides role modeling, assistance with problem solving/social change.**

 • Identify community resources **to provide ongoing support.**

Information in brackets added by the authors to clarify and enhance the use of nursing diagnoses.

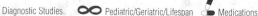

impaired wheelchair MOBILITY

Documentation Focus

ASSESSMENT/REASSESSMENT

- Individual findings, including level of function/ability to participate in specific/desired activities.
- Type of wheelchair/equipment needs.

PLANNING

- Plan of care and who is involved in the planning.
- Teaching plan.

IMPLEMENTATION/EVALUATION

- Responses to interventions/teaching and actions performed.

DISCHARGE PLANNING

- Discharge/long-range needs, noting who is responsible for each action to be taken.
- Specific referrals made.
- Sources of/maintenance for assistive devices.

SAMPLE NURSING OUTCOMES & INTERVENTIONS CLASSIFICATIONS (NOC/NIC)

NOC—Ambulation: Wheelchair
NIC—Positioning: Wheelchair

Nausea

Taxonomy II: Comfort—Class 1 Physical Comfort (00134)
[Diagnostic Division: Food/Fluid]
Submitted 1998; Revised 2002

Definition: A subjective unpleasant, wavelike sensation in the back of the throat, epigastrium, or abdomen that may lead to the urge or need to vomit

Related Factors

TREATMENT

Gastric irritation [e.g., alcohol, blood]
Gastric distention
Pharmaceuticals [e.g., analgesics—aspirin/nonsteroidal anti-inflammatory drugs/opioids, anesthesia, antiviral for HIV, steroids, antibiotics, chemotherapeutic agents]
[Radiation therapy/exposure]

Information in brackets added by the authors to clarify and enhance the use of nursing diagnoses.

 Cultural   Collaborative   Community/Home Care

BIOPHYSICAL

Biochemical disorders (e.g., uremia, diabetic ketoacidosis, pregnancy)

Localized tumors (e.g., acoustic neuroma, primary or secondary brain tumors, bone metastases at base of skull); intra-abdominal tumors

Toxins (e.g., tumor-produced peptides, abdominal metabolites due to cancer)

Esophageal/pancreatic disease; liver/splenetic capsule stretch

Gastric distention [e.g., delayed gastric emptying, pyloric intestinal obstruction, external compression of the stomach, other organ enlargement that slows stomach functioning (squashed stomach syndrome)]

Gastric irritation [e.g., pharyngeal and/or peritoneal inflammation]

Motion sickness; Meniere's disease; labyrinthitis

Increased intracranial pressure; meningitis

SITUATIONAL

Noxious odors/taste; unpleasant visual stimulation

Pain

Psychological factors; anxiety; fear

Defining Characteristics

SUBJECTIVE

Report of nausea ["sick to my stomach"]

OBJECTIVE

Aversion toward food

Increased salivation; sour taste in mouth

Increased swallowing; gagging sensation

Desired Outcomes/Evaluation Criteria—Client Will:

- Be free of nausea.
- Manage chronic nausea, as evidenced by acceptable level of dietary intake.
- Maintain/regain weight as appropriate.

Actions/Interventions

NURSING PRIORITY NO. 1. To determine causative/contributing factors:

Information in brackets added by the authors to clarify and enhance the use of nursing diagnoses.

 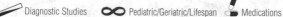

NAUSEA

- Assess for presence of conditions of the GI tract (e.g., peptic ulcer disease, cholecystitis, gastritis, ingestion of "problem" foods). **Dietary changes may be sufficient to decrease frequency of nausea.**
- Note systemic conditions that may result in nausea (e.g., pregnancy, cancer treatment, myocardial infarction [MI], hepatitis, systemic infections, drug toxicity, presence of neurogenic causes [stimulation of the vestibular system], CNS trauma/tumor). **Helps to determine appropriate interventions/need for treatment of underlying condition.**
- Identify situations that client perceives as anxiety-inducing, threatening, or distasteful (e.g., "this is nauseating"). **May be able to limit/control exposure to situations or take medication prophylactically.**
- Note psychological factors, including those that are culturally determined (e.g., eating certain foods considered repulsive in one's own culture).
- Determine if nausea is potentially self-limiting and/or mild (e.g., first trimester of pregnancy, 24-hour GI viral infection) or is severe and prolonged (e.g., cancer treatment, hyperemesis gravidarum). **Indicates degree of effect on fluid/electrolyte balance and nutritional status.**
- Check vital signs, especially for children and older clients, and note signs of dehydration. **Nausea may occur in the presence of postural hypotension/fluid volume deficit.**

NURSING PRIORITY NO. 2. To promote comfort and enhance intake:

- Administer/monitor response to medications used to treat underlying cause of nausea (e.g., vestibular, bowel obstruction, dysmotility of upper gut, infection/inflammation, toxins). **Note: Older individuals are more prone to side effects of antiemitic and anti-anxiety/anti-psychotic medications (e.g., excessive sedation, extrapyramidal movements) and there is increased risk of aspiration in the sedated client.**
- Select route of medication administration best suited to client's needs (i.e., oral, sublingual, injectable, rectal, transdermal).
- Review pain control regimen. **Converting to long-acting opioids or combination drugs may decrease stimulation of the chemotactic trigger zone (CTZ), reducing the occurrence of narcotic-related nausea.**
- Have client try dry foods such as toast, crackers, dry cereal before arising when nausea occurs in the morning, or throughout the day, as appropriate.

Information in brackets added by the authors to clarify and enhance the use of nursing diagnoses.

 Cultural Collaborative Community/Home Care

- Encourage client to begin with ice chips or sips/small amounts of fluids—4 to 8 ounces for adult; 1ounce or less for child.
- Advise client to drink liquids 30 minutes before or after meals, instead of with meals.
- Provide diet and snacks of preferred/bland foods when available (including bland/caffeine-free non-diet carbonated beverages, clear soup broth, non-acidic fruit juice, gelatin, sherbet/ices, skinless cooked chicken) **to reduce gastric acidity and improve nutrient intake.** Avoid milk/dairy products, overly sweet or fried and fatty foods, gas-forming vegetables (e.g., broccoli, cauliflower, cucumbers) **that may increase nausea/be more difficult to digest.**
- Encourage client to eat small meals spaced throughout the day instead of large meals **so stomach does not feel excessively full.**
- Instruct client to eat slowly, chewing food well **to enhance digestion.**
- Recommend client remain seated after meal, or with head well-elevated above feet if in bed.
- Provide clean, peaceful environment and fresh air with fan/open window. Avoid offending odors, such as cooking smells, smoke, perfumes, mechanical emissions when possible, **as they may stimulate or worsen nausea.**
- Provide frequent oral care (especially after vomiting) **to cleanse mouth and minimize "bad tastes."**
- Encourage deep, slow breathing **to promote relaxation and refocus attention away from nausea.**
- Use distraction with music, chatting with family/friends, watching TV **to limit dwelling on unpleasant sensation.**
- Administer antiemetic on regular schedule before/during and after administration of antineoplastic agents **to prevent/control side effects of medication.**
- Time chemotherapy doses **for least interference with food intake.**
- Investigate use of accupressure point therapy (e.g., elastic band worn around wrist with small, hard bump that presses against accupressure point). **Some individuals with chronic nausea/history of motion sickness report this to be helpful and without sedative effect of medication.**

NURSING PRIORITY NO. 3. To promote wellness (Teaching/Discharge Considerations):

- Review individual factors/triggers causing nausea and ways to avoid problem. **Provides necessary information for client to**

Information in brackets added by the authors to clarify and enhance the use of nursing diagnoses.

manage own care. **Some individuals develop anticipatory nausea (a conditioned reflex) that recurs each time he or she encounters the situation that triggers the reflex.**

- Instruct in proper use, side effects, and adverse reactions of antiemetic medications. **Enhances client safety and effective management of condition.**

- Discuss appropriate use of OTC medications/herbal products (e.g., Dramamine, antacids, antiflatulents, ginger), or the use of THC (Marinol).

- Encourage use of nonpharmacologic interventions. **Activites such as self-hypnosis, progressive muscle relaxation, biofeedback, guided imagery, and systemic desensitization promote relaxation, refocus client's attention, increase sense of control, and decrease feelings of helplessness.**

- Advise client to prepare and freeze meals in advance, have someone else cook, or use microwave or oven instead of stove-top cooking **for days when nausea is severe or cooking is impossible.**

- Suggest wearing loose-fitting clothing.

- Recommend recording weight weekly, if appropriate, **to help monitor fluid/nutritional status.**

- Discuss potential complications and possible need for medical follow-up or alternative therapies. **Timely recognition and intervention may limit severity of complications (e.g., dehydration).**

- Review signs of dehydration and stress importance of replacing fluids and/or electrolytes (with products such as Gatorade for adults or Pedialyte for children). **Increases likelihood of preventing potentially serious complications.**

- Identify signs (e.g., emesis appears bloody, black, or like coffee grounds; feeling faint) requiring immediate notification of healthcare provider.

Documentation Focus

ASSESSMENT/REASSESSMENT

- Individual findings, including individual factors causing nausea.
- Baseline/periodic weight, vital signs.
- Specific client preferences for nutritional intake.
- Response to medication.

PLANNING

- Plan of care and who is involved in planning.
- Teaching plan.

Information in brackets added by the authors to clarify and enhance the use of nursing diagnoses.

 Cultural Collaborative 🏠 Community/Home Care

IMPLEMENTATION/EVALUATION

- Response to interventions/teaching and actions performed.
- Attainment/progress toward desired outcome(s).
- Modifications to plan of care.

DISCHARGE PLANNING

- Individual long-term needs, noting who is responsible for actions to be taken.
- Specific referrals made.

SAMPLE NURSING OUTCOMES & INTERVENTIONS CLASSIFICATIONS (NOC/NIC)

NOC—Symptom Severity
NIC—Nausea Management

unilateral Neglect

Taxonomy II: Perception/Cognition—Class 1 Attention (00123)
[Diagnostic Division: Neurosensory]
Submitted 1986; Revised 2006

Definition: Impairment in sensory and motor response, mental representation, and spatial attention to body and the corresponding environment characterized by inattention to one side and overattention to the opposite side. Left side neglect is more severe and persistent than right side neglect.

Related Factors

Brain injury from: cerebrovascular problems; neurological illness; trauma; tumor
Left hemiplegia from CVA of the right hemisphere
Hemianopsia

Defining Characteristics

SUBJECTIVE

[Reports feeling that part does not belong to own self]

OBJECTIVE

Marked deviation of the eyes/head/trunk (as if drawn magnetically) to the non-neglected side to stimuli and activities on that side

---

Information in brackets added by the authors to clarify and enhance the use of nursing diagnoses.

 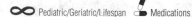

Failure to move eyes/head/limbs/trunk in the neglected hemisphere despite being aware of a stimulus in that space; failure to notice people approaching from the neglected side

Displacement of sounds to the non-neglected side

Appears unaware of positioning of neglected limb

Lack of safety precautions with regard to the neglected side

Failure to: eat food from portion of the plate on the neglected side; dress/groom neglected side

Difficulty remembering details of internally represented familiar scenes that are on the neglected side

Use of only vertical half of page when writing; failure to cancel lines on the half of the page on the neglected side; substitution of letters to form alternative words that are similar to the original in length when reading

Distortion/omission of drawing on the half of the page on the neglected side

Perseveration of visual motor tasks on non-neglected side

Transfer of pain sensation to the non-neglected side

Desired Outcomes/Evaluation Criteria—Client/Caregiver Will:

• Acknowledge presence of sensory-perceptual impairment.
• Identify adaptive/protective measures for individual situation.
• Demonstrate behaviors, lifestyle changes necessary to promote physical safety.

Client Will:

• Verbalize positive realistic perception of self incorporating the current dysfunction.
• Perform self-care within level of ability.

Actions/Interventions

NURSING PRIORITY NO. 1. To assess the extent of altered perception and the related degree of disability:

• Identify underlying reason for alterations in sensory/motor/behavioral perceptions as noted in Related Factors.
• Ascertain client/SO's perception of problem/changes, noting differences in perceptions.
• Measure visual acuity and field of vision.
• Assess sensory awareness (e.g., response to stimulus of hot/cold, dull/sharp); note problems with awareness of motion and proprioception.
• Observe client's behavior (as noted in Defining Characteristics) **to determine the extent of impairment.**

Information in brackets added by the authors to clarify and enhance the use of nursing diagnoses.

 Cultural Collaborative Community/Home Care

- Assess ability to distinguish between right and left.
- Note physical signs of neglect (e.g., disregard for position of affected limb(s), skin irritation/injury).
- Explore and encourage verbalization of feelings **to identify meaning of loss/dysfunction/change to the client and impact it may have on assuming ADLs.**
- Review results of testing performed to determine cause and/or type of neglect syndrome (e.g., sensory, motor, representational, personal, spatial, behavioral inattention). **Aids in distinguishing neglect from visual field cuts, impaired attention, and planning or visuospatial abilities.**

NURSING PRIORITY NO. 2. To promote optimal comfort and safety for the client in the environment:
- Collaborate in treatment strategies focused on training of attention to the neglected hemispace:
  Approach client from the unaffected side during acute phase. Explain to client that one side is being neglected; repeat, as needed.
  Remove excess stimuli from the environment when working with the client **to reduce distractions.**
  Encourage client to turn head and eyes in full rotation and "scan" the environment **to compensate for visual field loss.**
  Position bedside table and objects (such as call bell/telephone, tissues) within functional field of vision.
  Position furniture and equipment so travel path is not obstructed. Keep doors wide open or completely closed.
  Remove articles in the environment that may create a safety hazard (e.g., footstool, throw rug).
  Orient to environment as often as needed and ensure adequate lighting in the environment **to improve client's interpretation of environmental stimuli.**
  Monitor affected body part(s) for positioning/anatomic alignment, pressure points/skin irritation/injury, and dependent edema. **Increased risk of injury/ulcer formation necessitates close observation and timely intervention.**
  Describe where affected areas of body are when moving the client.
  Protect affected body part(s) from pressure/injury/burns, and help client learn to assume this responsibility.
  Assist with ADLs, maximizing self-care potential. Help client to bathe, apply lotion, and so forth to affected side.
  Refer to ND disturbed Sensory Perception for additional interventions, as needed.

Information in brackets added by the authors to clarify and enhance the use of nursing diagnoses.

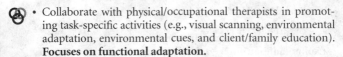

- Collaborate with physical/occupational therapists in promoting task-specific activities (e.g., visual scanning, environmental adaptation, environmental cues, and client/family education). **Focuses on functional adaptation.**

NURSING PRIORITY NO. 3. To promote wellness (Teaching/Discharge Considerations):

- Encourage client to look at and handle affected side **to stimulate awareness.**
- Bring the affected limb across the midline **for client to visualize during care.**
- Provide tactile stimuli to the affected side by touching/manipulating, stroking, and communicating about the affected side by itself rather than stimulating both sides simultaneously.
- Provide objects of various weight, texture, and size for client to handle **to provide tactile stimulation**.
- Assist client to position the affected extremity carefully and teach to routinely visualize placement of the extremity. Remind with visual cues. If client completely ignores one side of the body, use positioning **to improve perception (e.g., position client facing/looking at the affected side).**
- Encourage client to accept affected limb/side as part of self even when it no longer feels like it belongs.
- Use a mirror to help client adjust position **by visualizing both sides of the body.**
- Use descriptive terms to identify body parts rather than "left" and "right;" for example, "Lift this leg" (point to leg) or "Lift your affected leg."
- Encourage client/SO/family members to discuss situation and impact on life/future.
- Acknowledge and accept feelings of despondency, grief, and anger. **When feelings are openly expressed, client can deal with them and move forward.** (Refer to ND Grieving, as appropriate.)
- Reinforce to client the reality of the dysfunction and need to compensate.
- Avoid participating in the client's use of denial.
- Encourage family members and SO(s) to treat client normally and not as an invalid, including client in family activities.
- Place nonessential items (e.g., TV, pictures, hairbrush) on affected side during postacute phase once client begins to cross midline **to encourage continuation of behavior.**
- Refer to/encourage client to use rehabilitative services **to enhance independence in functioning.**
- Identify additional community resources to meet individual needs (e.g., Meals on Wheels, home-care services) **to**

Information in brackets added by the authors to clarify and enhance the use of nursing diagnoses.

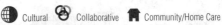 Cultural   Collaborative   Community/Home Care

maximize independence, allow client to return to community setting.

 • Provide informational material/websites **to reinforce teaching and promote self-paced learning.**

Documentation Focus

ASSESSMENT/REASSESSMENT

• Individual findings, including extent of altered perception, degree of disability, effect on independence/participation in ADLs.
• Results of testing.

PLANNING

• Plan of care and who is involved in the planning.
• Teaching plan.

IMPLEMENTATION/EVALUATION

• Responses to intervention/teaching and actions performed.
• Attainment/progress toward desired outcome(s).
• Modifications to plan of care.

DISCHARGE PLANNING

• Long-term needs and who is responsible for actions to be taken.
• Available resources, specific referrals made.

SAMPLE NURSING OUTCOMES & INTERVENTIONS CLASSIFICATIONS (NOC/NIC)

NOC—Self-Care: Activities of Daily Living (ADL)
NIC—Unilateral Neglect Management

Noncompliance
[ineffective Adherence] [Specify]

Taxonomy II: Life Principles—Class 3 Value/Belief/Action Congruence (00079)
[Diagnostic Division: Teaching/Learning]
Submitted 1973; Revised 1996, 1998

Definition: Behavior of person and/or caregiver that fails to coincide with a health-promoting or therapeutic plan agreed on by the person (and/or family and/or community) and healthcare professional. In the presence of an agreed-on health-promoting or therapeutic plan, person's or caregiver's behavior is fully or partially nonadherent and may lead to clinically ineffective or partially ineffective outcomes

---

Information in brackets added by the authors to clarify and enhance the use of nursing diagnoses.

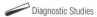 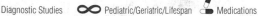

NOTE: When the plan of care is reviewed with client/SO, use of the term *noncompliance* may create a negative response and sense of conflict between healthcare providers and client. Labeling the client noncompliant may also lead to problems with third-party reimbursement. Where possible, use of the ND ineffective Therapeutic Regimen Management is recommended.

Related Factors

HEALTHCARE PLAN

Duration
Cost; financial flexibility of plan; intensity; complexity

INDIVIDUAL

Personal/developmental abilities; knowledge/skill relevant to the regimen behavior; motivational forces
Individual's value system; health beliefs; cultural influences; spiritual values
[Altered thought processes, such as depression, paranoia]
[Difficulty changing behavior, as in addictions]
[Denial; issues of secondary gain]

HEALTH SYSTEM

Individual health coverage
Credibility of provider; client-provider relationships; provider continuity/regular follow-up; provider reimbursement; communication/teaching skills of the provider
Access/convenience of care; satisfaction with care

NETWORK

Involvement of members in health plan; social value regarding plan
Perceived beliefs of significant others

Defining Characteristics

OBJECTIVE

Behavior indicative of failure to adhere
Objective tests (e.g., physiological measures, detection of physiological markers)
Failure to progress
Evidence of development of complications/exacerbation of symptoms
Failure to keep appointments

Information in brackets added by the authors to clarify and enhance the use of nursing diagnoses.

  Cultural Collaborative Community/Home Care

Desired Outcomes/Evaluation Criteria—Client Will:

- Verbalize accurate knowledge of condition and understanding of treatment regimen.
- Make choices at level of readiness based on accurate information.
- Verbalize commitment to mutually agreed upon goals and treatment plan.
- Access resources appropriately.
- Demonstrate progress toward desired outcomes/goals.

Actions/Interventions

NURSING PRIORITY NO. 1. To determine reason for alteration/disregard of therapeutic regimen/instructions:

- Determine client's/SO's perception/understanding of the situation (illness/treatment).
- Listen to/active-listen client's complaints, comments. **Helps to identify client's thinking about the treatment regimen (e.g., may be concerned about side effects of medications or success of procedures/transplantation).**
- Note language spoken, read, and understood.
- Be aware of developmental level as well as chronological age of client.
- Assess level of anxiety, locus of control, sense of powerlessness, and so forth.
- Determine who (e.g., client, SO, other) manages the medication regimen and whether individual knows what the medications are and why they are prescribed.
- Ascertain how client remembers to take medications and how many doses have been missed in the last 72 hours, last week, last two weeks, and last month.
- Identify factors that interfere with taking medications or lead to lack of adherence (e.g., depression, active alcohol/other drug use, low literacy, lack of support, lack of belief in treatment efficacy). **Forgetfulness is the most common reason given for not complying with the treatment plan.**
- Note length of illness. **Individuals tend to become passive and dependent in long-term, debilitating illnesses.**
- Clarify value system: cultural/religious values, health/illness beliefs of the client/SO(s).
- Determine social characteristics, demographic and educational factors, as well as personality of the client.
- Verify psychological meaning of the behavior (e.g., may be denial). Note issues of secondary gain—**family dynamics,**

Information in brackets added by the authors to clarify and enhance the use of nursing diagnoses.

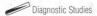 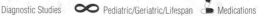

school/workplace issues, involvement in legal system may unconsciously affect client's decision making.

- Assess availability/use of support systems and resources.
- Be aware of nurses'/healthcare providers' attitudes and behaviors toward the client. (Do they have an investment in the client's compliance/recovery? What is the behavior of the client and nurse when client is labeled "noncompliant"?) **Some care providers may be enabling client, whereas others' judgmental attitudes may impede treatment progress.**

NURSING PRIORITY NO. 2. To assist client/SO(s) to develop strategies for dealing effectively with the situation:

- Develop therapeutic nurse-client relationship. **Promotes trust, provides atmosphere in which client/SO(s) can freely express views/concerns. Adherence assessment is most successful when conducted in a positive, nonjudgmental atmosphere.**
- Explore client involvement in or lack of mutual goal setting. **Client will be more likely to follow-through on goals he or she participated in developing.**
- Review treatment strategies. Identify which interventions in the plan of care are most important in meeting therapeutic goals and which are least amenable to compliance. **Sets priorities and encourages problem solving areas of conflict.**
- Contract with the client for participation in care. **Enhances commitment to follow-through.**
- Encourage client to maintain self-care, providing for assistance when necessary. Accept client's evaluation of own strengths/limitations while working with client to improve abilities.
- Provide for continuity of care in and out of the hospital/care setting, including long-range plans. **Supports trust, facilitates progress toward goals.**
- Provide information and help client to know where and how to find it on own. **Promotes independence and encourages informed decision making.**
- Give information in manageable amounts, using verbal, written, and audiovisual modes at level of client's ability. **Using client's style of learning facilitates learning, enabling client to understand diagnosis and treatment regimen.**
- Have client paraphrase instructions/information heard. **Helps validate client's understanding and reveals misconceptions.**
- Accept the client's choice/point of view, even if it appears to be self-destructive. Avoid confrontation regarding beliefs **to maintain open communication.**

Information in brackets added by the authors to clarify and enhance the use of nursing diagnoses.

 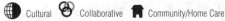 Cultural   Collaborative   Community/Home Care

- Establish graduated goals or modified regimen, as necessary (e.g., client with COPD who smokes a pack of cigarettes a day may be willing to reduce that amount). **May improve quality of life, encouraging progression to more advanced goals.**

NURSING PRIORITY NO. 3. To promote wellness (Teaching/Discharge Considerations):

- Stress importance of the client's knowledge and understanding of the need for treatment/medication, as well as consequences of actions/choices.
- Develop a system for self-monitoring **to provide a sense of control and enable client to follow own progress and assist with making choices.**
- Suggest using a medication reminder system. **These have been shown to improve client adherence by a significant percentage.**
- Provide support systems **to reinforce negotiated behaviors.** Encourage client to continue positive behaviors, especially if client is beginning to see benefit.
- Refer to counseling/therapy and/or other appropriate resources.
- Refer to NDs ineffective Coping; compromised family Coping; deficient Knowledge, (specify); Anxiety; ineffective Therapeutic Regimen Management.

Documentation Focus

ASSESSMENT/REASSESSMENT

- Individual findings/deviation from prescribed treatment plan and client's reasons in own words.
- Consequences of actions to date.

PLANNING

- Plan of care and who is involved in planning.
- Teaching plan.

IMPLEMENTATION/EVALUATION

- Response to interventions/teaching and actions performed.
- Attainment/progress toward desired outcome(s).
- Modifications to plan of care.

DISCHARGE PLANNING

- Long-term needs and who is responsible for actions to be taken.
- Specific referrals made.

Information in brackets added by the authors to clarify and enhance the use of nursing diagnoses.

 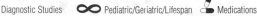

SAMPLE NURSING OUTCOMES & INTERVENTIONS CLASSIFICATIONS (NOC/NIC)

NOC—Compliance Behavior
NIC—Mutual Goal Setting

imbalanced Nutrition: less than body requirements

Taxonomy II: Nutrition—Class 1 Ingestion (00002)
[Diagnostic Division: Food/Fluid]
Submitted 1975; Revised 2000

Definition: Intake of nutrients insufficient to meet metabolic needs

Related Factors

Inability to ingest/digest food; inability to absorb nutrients
Biological/psychological/economic factors
[Increased metabolic demands, e.g., burns]
[Lack of information, misinformation, misconceptions]

Defining Characteristics

SUBJECTIVE

Reported food intake less than RDA (recommended daily allowances); lack of food
Lack of interest in food; aversion to eating; reported altered taste sensation; perceived inability to digest food
Satiety immediately after ingesting food
Abdominal pain/cramping
Lack of information, misinformation, misconceptions [Note: The authors view these as related factors rather than defining characteristics.]

OBJECTIVE

Body weight 20% or more under ideal [for height and frame]; [decreased subcutaneous fat/muscle mass]
Loss of weight with adequate food intake
Hyperactive bowel sounds; diarrhea; steatorrhea
Weakness of muscles required for swallowing or mastication; poor muscle tone
Sore buccal cavity; pale mucous membranes; capillary fragility
Excessive loss of hair [or increased growth of hair on body (lanugo)]; [cessation of menses]

Information in brackets added by the authors to clarify and enhance the use of nursing diagnoses.

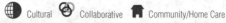 Cultural Collaborative Community/Home Care

[Abnormal laboratory studies (e.g., decreased albumin, total proteins; iron deficiency; electrolyte imbalances)]

Desired Outcomes/Evaluation Criteria—Client Will:

- Demonstrate progressive weight gain toward goal.
- Display normalization of laboratory values and be free of signs of malnutrition as reflected in Defining Characteristics.
- Verbalize understanding of causative factors when known and necessary interventions.
- Demonstrate behaviors, lifestyle changes to regain and/or maintain appropriate weight.

Actions/Interventions

NURSING PRIORITY NO. 1. To assess causative/contributing factors:

- Identify client at risk for malnutrition (e.g., institutionalized elderly; client with chronic illness; child or adult living in poverty/low income area; client with jaw/facial injuries; intestinal surgery/post malabsorptive/restrictive surgical interventions for weight loss; hypermetabolic states [e.g., burns, hyperthroidism]; malabsorption syndromes/lactose intolerance; cystic fibrosis; pancreatic disease; prolonged time of restricted intake; prior nutritional deficiencies).
- Determine client's ability to chew, swallow, and taste food. Evaluate teeth and gums for poor oral health, and note denture fit, as indicated. **All factors that can affect ingestion and/or digestion of nutrients.**
- Ascertain understanding of individual nutritional needs **to determine informational needs of client/SO.**
- Note availability/use of financial resources and support systems. Determine ability to acquire and store various types of food.
- Discuss eating habits, including food preferences, intolerances/aversions **to appeal to client's likes/dislikes.**
- Assess drug interactions, disease effects, allergies, use of laxatives, diuretics **that may be affecting appetite, food intake, or absorption.**
- Evaluate impact of cultural, ethnic, or religious desires/influences **that may affect food choices.**
- Determine psychological factors/perform psychological assessment, as indicated, **to assess body image and congruency with reality.**
- Note occurrence of amenorrhea, tooth decay, swollen salivary glands, and report of constant sore throat, **suggesting bulimia/affecting ability to eat.**

Information in brackets added by the authors to clarify and enhance the use of nursing diagnoses.

 Diagnostic Studies   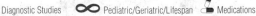 Pediatric/Geriatric/Lifespan   Medications   **479**

imbalanced NUTRITION: less than body requirements

- Review usual activities/exercise program noting repetitive activities (e.g., constant pacing)/inappropriate exercise (e.g., prolonged jogging). **May reveal obsessive nature of weight-control measures.**

NURSING PRIORITY NO. 2. To evaluate degree of deficit:

- Assess weight; measure/calculate body fat and muscle mass via triceps skin fold and midarm muscle circumference or other anthropometric measurements **to establish baseline parameters.**
- Observe for absence of subcutaneous fat/muscle wasting, loss of hair, fissuring of nails, delayed healing, gum bleeding, swollen abdomen, etc., **that indicate protein-energy malnutrition.**
- Auscultate bowel sounds. Note characteristics of stool (color, amount, frequency, etc.).
- Assist in nutritional assessment, using screening tools (e.g., Mini Nutritional Assessment [MNA]/similar tool).
- Review indicated laboratory data (e.g., serum albumin/prealbumin, transferrin, amino acid profile, iron, BUN, nitrogen balance studies, glucose, liver function, electrolytes, total lymphocyte count, indirect calorimetry).
- Assist with diagnostic procedures (e.g., Schilling's test, D-xylose test, 72-hour stool fat, GI series).

NURSING PRIORITY NO. 3. To establish a nutritional plan that meets individual needs:

- Note age, body build, strength, activity/rest level, etc. **Helps determine nutritional needs.**
- Evaluate total daily food intake. Obtain diary of calorie intake, patterns and times of eating, **to reveal possible cause of malnutrition/changes that could be made in client's intake.**
- Calculate basal energy expenditure (BEE) using Harris-Benedict (or similar) formula and estimate energy and protein requirements.
- Assist in treating/managing underlying causative factors (e.g., cancer, malabsorption syndrome, impaired cognition, depression, medications that decrease appetite, fad diets, anorexia).
- Consult dietitian/nutritional team, as indicated, **to implement interdisciplinary team management.**
- Provide diet modifications, as indicated. For example:
  Refer to nutritional resources to determine suitable ways to optimize client's intake of protein, carbohydrates, fats, calories within eating style/needs
  Several small meals and snacks daily
  Mechanical soft or blenderized tube feedings

Information in brackets added by the authors to clarify and enhance the use of nursing diagnoses.

     Cultural   Collaborative   Community/Home Care

    Appetite stimulants (e.g., wine), if indicated

    High-calorie, nutrient-rich dietary supplements, such as meal replacement shake

    Formula tube feedings; parenteral nutrition infusion

 • Administer pharmaceutical agents, as indicated:

    Digestive drugs/enzymes

    Vitamin/mineral (iron) supplements, including chewable multivitamin

    Medications (e.g., antacids, anticholinergics, antiemetics, antidiarrheals)

• Determine whether client prefers/tolerates more calories in a particular meal.

• Use flavoring agents (e.g., lemon and herbs) if salt is restricted **to enhance food satisfaction and stimulate appetite.**

• Encourage use of sugar/honey in beverages if carbohydrates are tolerated well.

• Encourage client to choose foods/have family member bring foods that seem appealing **to stimulate appetite.**

• Avoid foods that cause intolerances/increase gastric motility (e.g., foods that are gas-forming, hot/cold, or spicy; caffeinated beverages; milk products; and so forth), according to individual needs.

• Limit fiber/bulk, if indicated, **because it may lead to early satiety.**

• Promote pleasant, relaxing environment, including socialization when possible **to enhance intake.**

• Prevent/minimize unpleasant odors/sights. **May have a negative effect on appetite/eating.**

• Assist with/provide oral care before and after meals and at bedtime.

• Encourage use of lozenges and so forth **to stimulate salivation when dryness is a factor.**

• Promote adequate/timely fluid intake. Limit fluids 1 hour prior to meal **to reduce possibility of early satiety.**

• Weigh regularly/graph results **to monitor effectiveness of efforts.**

• Develop individual strategies when problem is mechanical (e.g., wired jaws or paralysis following stroke). Consult occupational therapist **to identify appropriate assistive devices,** or speech therapist **to enhance swallowing ability.** (Refer to ND impaired Swallowing.)

• Refer to structured (behavioral) program of nutrition therapy (e.g., documented time/length of eating period, blenderized food/tube feeding, administered parenteral nutritional

---

Information in brackets added by the authors to clarify and enhance the use of nursing diagnoses.

 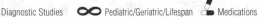

therapy, etc.) per protocol, **particularly when problem is anorexia nervosa or bulimia.**

- Recommend/support hospitalization **for controlled environment in severe malnutrition/life-threatening situations.**
- Refer to social services/other community resources **for possible assistance with client's limitations in buying/preparing foods.**

NURSING PRIORITY NO. 4. To promote wellness (Teaching/Discharge Considerations):

- Emphasize importance of well-balanced, nutritious intake. Provide information regarding individual nutritional needs and ways to meet these needs within financial constraints.
- Develop behavior modification program with client involvement appropriate to specific needs.
- Provide positive regard, love, and acknowledgment of "voice within" guiding client with eating disorder.
- Develop consistent, realistic weight goal with client.
- Weigh at regular intervals and document results **to monitor effectiveness of dietary plan.**
- Consult with dietitian/nutritional support team, as necessary, **for long-term needs.**
- Develop regular exercise/stress reduction program.
- Review drug regimen, side effects, and potential interactions with other medications/over-the-counter drugs.
- Review medical regimen and provide information/assistance, as necessary.
- Assist client to identify/access resources, such as way to obtain nutrient-dense low budget foods, food stamps, Meals on Wheels, community food banks, and/or other appropriate assistance programs.
- Refer for dental hygiene/professional care, counseling/psychiatric care, family therapy, as indicated.
- Provide/reinforce client teaching regarding preoperative and postoperative dietary needs when surgery is planned.
- Assist client/SO(s) to learn how to blenderize food and/or perform tube feeding.
- Refer to home health resources **for initiation/supervision of home nutrition therapy when used.**

Documentation Focus

ASSESSMENT/REASSESSMENT

- Baseline and subsequent assessment findings to include signs/symptoms as noted in Defining Characteristics and laboratory diagnostic findings.

Information in brackets added by the authors to clarify and enhance the use of nursing diagnoses.

 Cultural Collaborative Community/Home Care

- Caloric intake.
- Individual cultural/religious restrictions, personal preferences.
- Availability/use of resources.
- Personal understanding/perception of problem.

PLANNING

- Plan of care and who is involved in planning.
- Teaching plan.

IMPLEMENTATION/EVALUATION

- Client's responses to interventions/teaching and actions performed.
- Results of periodic weigh-in.
- Attainment/progress toward desired outcome(s).
- Modifications to plan of care.

DISCHARGE PLANNING

- Long-term needs/who is responsible for actions to be taken.
- Specific referrals made.

SAMPLE NURSING OUTCOMES & INTERVENTIONS CLASSIFICATIONS (NOC/NIC)

NOC—Nutritional Status
NIC—Nutrition Management

imbalanced Nutrition: more than body requirements

Taxonomy II: Nutrition—Class 1 Ingestion (00001)
[Diagnostic Division: Food/Fluid]
Submitted 1975; Revised 2000

Definition: Intake of nutrients that exceeds metabolic needs

Related Factors

Excessive intake in relationship to metabolic need

Defining Characteristics

SUBJECTIVE

Dysfunctional eating patterns (e.g., pairing food with other activities)

Information in brackets added by the authors to clarify and enhance the use of nursing diagnoses.

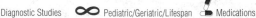
 Diagnostic Studies   ∞ Pediatric/Geriatric/Lifespan   Medications   **483**

Eating in response to external cues (e.g., time of day, social situation)

Concentrating food intake at end of day

Eating in response to internal cues other than hunger (e.g., anxiety)

Sedentary activity level

OBJECTIVE

Weight 20% over ideal for height and frame [obese]

Triceps skin fold >25 mm in women, >15 mm in men

[Percentage of body fat greater than 22% for trim women and 15% for trim men]

Desired Outcomes/Evaluation Criteria—Client Will:

- Verbalize a realistic self-concept/body image (congruent mental and physical picture of self).
- Demonstrate acceptance of self as is rather than an idealized image.
- Demonstrate appropriate changes in lifestyle and behaviors, including eating patterns, food quantity/quality, and exercise program.
- Attain desirable body weight with optimal maintenance of health.

Actions/Interventions

NURSING PRIORITY NO. 1. To identify causative/contributing factors:

- **Assess risk/presence of conditions associated with obesity** (e.g., familial pattern of obesity; slow metabolism/hypothyroidism; type 2 diabetes; high blood pressure; high cholesterol; or history of stroke, heart attack, gallstones, gout/arthritis, sleep apnea) to ascertain treatments/interventions that may be needed in addition to weight management.
- Review daily activity and exercise program. **Sedentary lifestyle is frequently associated with obesity and is a primary focus for modification.**
- Ascertain how client perceives food and the act of eating.
- Review diary of foods/fluids ingested; times and patterns of eating; activities/place; whether alone or with other(s); and feelings before, during, and after eating.
- Calculate total calorie intake.
- Ascertain previous dieting history.

Information in brackets added by the authors to clarify and enhance the use of nursing diagnoses.

 Cultural Collaborative 🏠 Community/Home Care

- Discuss client's view of self, including what being heavy does for the client. **Familial traits/cultural beliefs or life goals may place high importance on food and intake as well as large body size (e.g., Samoan, wrestler/football lineman).**
- Note negative/positive monologues (self-talk) of the individual.
- Obtain comparative body drawing by having client draw self on wall with chalk, then standing against it and having actual body outline drawn. **Determines whether client's view of self-body image is congruent with reality.**
- Ascertain occurrence of negative feedback from SO(s). **May reveal control issues, impact motivation for change.**
- Review results of body fat measurement (e.g., skin calipers, bioelectric impedance analysis [BIA], dual-energy x-ray absorptonmetry [DEXA] scanning, dydrostatic weighing, etc.) **to determine presence/severity of obesity.**

NURSING PRIORITY NO. 2. To establish weight reduction program:

- Discuss client's motivation for weight loss (e.g., for own satisfaction/self-esteem, or to gain approval from another person). **Helps client determine realistic motivating factors for individual situation (e.g., acceptance of self "as is," improvement of health status).**
- Obtain commitment/contract for weight loss.
- Record height, weight, body build, gender, and age. **Provides comparative baseline and helps determine nutritional needs.**
- Calculate calorie requirements based on physical factors and activity level.
- Provide information regarding specific nutritional needs. **Obese individual may be deficient in needed nutrients.**
- Set realistic goals for weekly weight loss.
- Discuss eating behaviors (e.g., eating over sink, "nibbling," kinds of activities associated with eating) and identify necessary modifications.
- Encourage client to start with small changes (e.g., adding one more vegetable/day, introducing healthier versions of favorite foods, learning to read/understand nutrition labels) **to slowly change eating habits.**
- Develop carbohydrate/fat portion control and appetite-reduction plan **to support continuation of behavioral changes.**
- Stress need for adequate fluid intake and taking fluids between meals rather than with meals **to meet fluid requirements and reduce possibility of early satiety resulting in feelings of hunger.**

Information in brackets added by the authors to clarify and enhance the use of nursing diagnoses.

imbalanced NUTRITION: more than body requirements *(left margin, vertical)*

 • Discuss smart snacks (e.g., low-fat yogurt with fruit, nuts, apple slices with peanut butter, low-fat string cheese, etc.) **to assist client in finding healthy options.**

 • Collaborate with physician/dietitian/nutrition team **in creating/evaluating effective nutritional program.**

 • Encourage involvement in planned exercise program of client's choice and within physical abilities.

• Monitor individual drug regimen (e.g., appetite suppressants, hormone therapy, vitamin/mineral supplements).

• Provide positive reinforcement/encouragement for efforts as well as actual weight loss. **Enhances commitment to program.**

 • Refer to bariatric specialist for additional interventions (e.g., extremely low-calorie diet, surgical weight loss procedures).

NURSING PRIORITY NO. 3. To promote wellness (Teaching/Discharge Considerations):

 • Discuss reality of obesity and health consequences as well as myths client/SO(s) may have about weight and weight loss.

 • Assist client to choose nutritious foods that reflect personal likes, meet individual needs, and are within financial budget.

• Encourage parent to model good nutritional choices (e.g., offer vegetables, fruits, and low-fat foods at daily meals and snacks) **to assist child in adopting healthy eating habits.**

 • Identify ways to manage stress/tension during meals. **Promotes relaxation to permit focus on act of eating and awareness of satiety.**

 • Review and discuss strategies to deal appropriately with stressful events/feelings **instead of overeating.**

 • Encourage variety and moderation in dietary plan **to decrease boredom.**

 • Advise client to plan for special occasions (birthday/holidays) by reducing intake before event and/or eating "smart" **to redistribute/reduce calories and allow for participation in food events.**

 • Discuss importance of an occasional treat by planning for inclusion in diet **to avoid feelings of deprivation arising from self-denial.**

 • Recommend client weigh only once per week, same time/clothes, and graph on chart. Measure/monitor body fat when possible (**more accurate measure**).

 • Discuss normalcy of ups and downs of weight loss: plateauing, set point (at which weight is not being lost), hormonal influences, and so forth. **Prevents discouragement when progress stalls.**

Information in brackets added by the authors to clarify and enhance the use of nursing diagnoses.

 Cultural Collaborative Community/Home Care

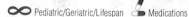 • Encourage buying personal items/clothing as a reward for weight loss or other accomplishments. Suggest disposing of "fat clothes" **to encourage positive attitude of permanent change and remove "safety valve" of having wardrobe available "just in case" weight is regained.**

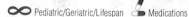 • Involve SO(s) in treatment plan as much as possible **to provide ongoing support and increase likelihood of success.**

• Refer to community support groups/psychotherapy, as indicated.

• Provide contact number for dietitian, bibliography/Internet sites for resources **to address ongoing nutrition concerns/dietary needs.**

• Refer to NDs disturbed Body Image; ineffective Coping.

Documentation Focus

ASSESSMENT/REASSESSMENT

• Individual findings, including current weight, dietary pattern; perceptions of self, food, and eating; motivation for loss, support/feedback from SO(s).
• Results of laboratory/diagnostic testing.
• Results of weekly weigh-in.

PLANNING

• Plan of care/interventions and who is involved in planning.
• Teaching plan.

IMPLEMENTATION/EVALUATION

• Responses to interventions, weekly weight, and actions performed.
• Attainment/progress toward desired outcome(s).
• Modifications to plan of care.

DISCHARGE PLANNING

• Long-term needs and who is responsible for actions to be taken.
• Specific referrals made.

SAMPLE NURSING OUTCOMES & INTERVENTIONS CLASSIFICATIONS (NOC/NIC)

NOC—Weight Control
NIC—Weight Reduction Assistance

Information in brackets added by the authors to clarify and enhance the use of nursing diagnoses.

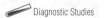 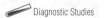

imbalanced Nutrition: risk for more than body requirements

Taxonomy II: Nutrition—Class 1 Ingestion (00003)
[Diagnostic Division: Food/Fluid]
Submitted 1980; Revised 2000

Definition: At risk for an intake of nutrients that exceeds metabolic needs

Risk Factors

Dysfunctional eating patterns; pairing food with other activities; eating in response to external cues other than hunger (e.g., time of day, social situation)/internal cues other than hunger (e.g., anxiety); concentrating food intake at end of day

Parental obesity

Rapid transition across growth percentiles in children; reported use of solid food as major food source before 5 months of age

Higher baseline weight at beginning of each pregnancy

Observed use of food as reward/comfort measure

[Frequent/repeated dieting]

[Alteration in usual activity patterns; sedentary lifestyle]

[Alteration in usual coping patterns; socially/culturally isolated; lacking other outlets]

[Majority of foods consumed are concentrated, high-calorie/fat sources]

[Significant/sudden decline in financial resources, lower socioeconomic status]

> NOTE: A risk diagnosis is not evidenced by signs and symptoms, as the problem has not occurred; and nursing interventions are directed at prevention.

Desired Outcomes/Evaluation Criteria—Client Will:

- Verbalize understanding of body and energy needs.
- Identify lifestyle/cultural factors that predispose to obesity.
- Demonstrate behaviors, lifestyle changes to reduce risk factors.
- Acknowledge responsibility for own actions and need to "act, not react" to stressful situations.
- Maintain weight at a satisfactory level for height, body build, age, and gender.

Information in brackets added by the authors to clarify and enhance the use of nursing diagnoses.

  Cultural Collaborative 🏠 Community/Home Care

Actions/Interventions

NURSING PRIORITY NO. 1. To assess potential factors for undesired weight gain:

• Note presence of factors as listed in Risk Factors. **A high correlation exists between obesity in parents and children. When one parent is obese, 40% of the children may be overweight; when both are obese, the proportion may be as high as 80%.**

• Determine age and activity level/exercise patterns.

• Calculate growth percentiles in infants/children.

• Review laboratory data **for indicators of endocrine/metabolic disorders.**

• Identify cultural factors/lifestyle that may predispose to weight gain. **Socioeconomic group, familial eating patterns, amount of money available for purchasing food, proximity of grocery store, and available storage space for food are all factors that may impact food choices and intake.**

• Assess eating patterns in relation to risk factors. Note patterns of hunger and satiety. **Patterns differ in those who are predisposed to weight gain. Skipping meals decreases the metabolic rate.**

• Determine weight change patterns, history of dieting/kinds of diets used. Determine whether yo-yo dieting or bulimia is a factor.

• Identify personality characteristics that may indicate potential for obesity (e.g., rigid thinking patterns, external locus of control, negative body image/self-concept, negative monologues [self-talk], dissatisfaction with life).

• Determine psychological significance of food to the client.

• Listen to concerns and assess motivation to prevent weight gain.

NURSING PRIORITY NO. 2. To assist client to develop preventive program to avoid weight gain:

• Provide information on balancing calorie intake and energy expenditure.

• Help client develop new eating patterns/habits (e.g., eating slowly, eating only when hungry, controlling portion size, stopping when full, not skipping meals).

• Discuss importance/help client develop a program of exercise and relaxation techniques. **Encourages client to incorporate plan into lifestyle.**

• Assist client to develop strategies for reducing stressful thinking/actions. **Promotes relaxation, reduces likelihood of stress/comfort eating.**

Information in brackets added by the authors to clarify and enhance the use of nursing diagnoses.

 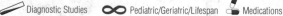

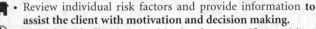

NURSING PRIORITY NO. 3. To promote wellness (Teaching/Discharge Considerations):

 • Review individual risk factors and provide information **to assist the client with motivation and decision making.**

• Consult with dietitian/nutritionist about specific nutrition/dietary issues.

• Provide information to new mothers about nutrition for developing babies.

 • Encourage client to make a decision to lead an active life and control food habits.

 • Assist client in learning to be in touch with own body and to identify feelings that may provoke "comfort eating," such as anger, anxiety, boredom, sadness.

 • Develop a system for self-monitoring **to provide a sense of control and enable the client to follow own progress and assist with making choices.**

• Refer to support groups and appropriate community resources for education/behavior modification, as indicated.

Documentation Focus

ASSESSMENT/REASSESSMENT

• Findings related to individual situation, risk factors, current caloric intake/dietary pattern, activity level.
• Baseline height/weight, growth percentile.
• Results of laboratory tests.
• Motivation to reduce risks/prevent weight problems.

PLANNING

• Plan of care and who is involved in the planning.
• Teaching plan.

IMPLEMENTATION/EVALUATION

• Response to interventions/teaching and actions performed.
• Attainment/progress toward desired outcome(s).
• Modifications to plan of care.

DISCHARGE PLANNING

• Long-range needs, noting who is responsible for actions to be taken.
• Specific referrals made.

Information in brackets added by the authors to clarify and enhance the use of nursing diagnoses.

 Cultural  Collaborative Community/Home Care

SAMPLE NURSING OUTCOMES & INTERVENTIONS CLASSIFICATIONS (NOC/NIC)

NOC—Weight Control
NIC—Weight Management

readiness for enhanced Nutrition

Taxonomy II: Health Awareness—Class 2 Health
  Management (00163)
[Diagnostic Division: Food/Fluid]
Submitted 2002

Definition: A pattern of nutrient intake that is sufficient
for meeting metabolic needs and can be strengthened

Related Factors

To be developed

Defining Characteristics

SUBJECTIVE

Expresses knowledge of healthy food and fluid choices/willingness
  to enhance nutrition
Eats regularly
Attitude toward eating/drinking is congruent with health goals

OBJECTIVE

Consumes adequate food/fluid
Follows an appropriate standard for intake (e.g., the food pyramid
  or American Diabetic Association Guidelines)
Safe preparation/storage for food/fluids

Desired Outcomes/Evaluation
Criteria—Client Will:

• Demonstrate behaviors to attain/maintain appropriate weight.
• Be free of signs of malnutrition.
• Be able to safely prepare and store foods.

Actions/Interventions

NURSING PRIORITY NO. 1. To determine current nutritional status
and eating patterns:
• Review client's knowledge of current nutritional needs and
  ways client is meeting these needs. **Provides baseline for further teaching and interventions.**

Information in brackets added by the authors to clarify and enhance
the use of nursing diagnoses.

 Diagnostic Studies 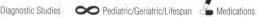 ∞ Pediatric/Geriatric/Lifespan Medications **491**

- Assess eating patterns and food/fluid choices in relation to any health-risk factors and health goals. **Helps to identify specific strengths and weaknesses that can be addressed.**
- Verify that age-related and developmental needs are met. **These factors are constantly present throughout the lifespan, although differing for each age group. For example, older adults need same nutrients as younger adults, but in smaller amounts, and with attention to certain components, such as calcium, fiber, vitamins, protein, and water. Infants/children require small meals and constant attention to needed nutrients for proper growth/development while dealing with child's food preferences and eating habits.**

- Evaluate influence of cultural/religious factors **to determine what client considers to be normal dietary practices, as well as to identify food preferences/restrictions, and eating patterns that can be strengthened and/or altered, if indicated.**
- Assess how client perceives food, food preparation, and the act of eating **to determine client's feeling and emotions regarding food and self-image.**
- Ascertain occurrence of/potential for negative feedback from SO(s). **May reveal control issues that could impact client's commitment to change.**
- Determine patterns of hunger and satiety. **Helps identify strengths and weaknesses in eating patterns and potential for change (e.g., person predisposed to weight gain may need a different time for a big meal than evening, or need to learn what foods reinforce feelings of satisfaction).**
- Assess client's ability to safely store and prepare foods **to determine if health information or resources might be needed.**

NURSING PRIORITY NO. 2. To assist client/SO(s) to develop plan to meet individual needs:

- Determine motivation/expectation for change.
- Assist in obtaining/review results of individual testing (e.g., weight/height, body fat percent, lipids, glucose, complete blood count, total protein, etc.) **to determine that client is healthy and/or identify dietary changes that may be helpful in attaining health goals.**

- Encourage client's beneficial eating patterns/habits (e.g., controlling portion size, eating regular meals, reducing high-fat or fast-food intake, following specific dietary program, drinking water and healthy beverages). **Positive feedback promotes continuation of healthy lifestyle habits and new behaviors.**

Information in brackets added by the authors to clarify and enhance the use of nursing diagnoses.

  Cultural Collaborative 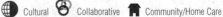 Community/Home Care

- Discuss use of non-food rewards.
- Provide instruction/reinforce information regarding special needs. **Enhances decision-making process and promotes responsibility for meeting own needs.**
- Encourage reading of food labels and instruct in meaning of labeling, as indicated, **to assist client/SO(s) in making healthful choices.**
- Review safe preparation and storage of food **to avoid food-borne illnesses.**
- Consult with/refer to dietitian/physician, as indicated. **Client/SO(s) may benefit from advice regarding specific nutrition/dietary issues or may require regular follow-up to determine that needs are being met when following a medically prescribed program.**
- Develop a system for self-monitoring **to provide a sense of control and enable the client to follow own progress, and assist in making choices.**

NURSING PRIORITY NO. 3. To promote optimum wellness:

- Review individual risk factors and provide additional information/response to concerns. **Assists the client with motivation and decision making.**
- Provide bibliotherapy and help client/SO(s) identify and evaluate resources they can access on their own. **When referencing the Internet or nontraditional/unproven resources, the individual must exercise some restraint and determine the reliability of the source/information before acting on it.**
- Encourage variety and moderation in dietary plan **to decrease boredom and encourage client in efforts to make healthy choices about eating and food.**
- Discuss use of nutritional supplements, OTC/herbal products. **Confusion may exist regarding the need for/use of these products in a balanced dietary regimen.**
- Assist client to identify/access community resources when indicated. **May benefit from assistance such as food stamps, WIC, budget counseling, Meals on Wheels, community food banks, and/or other assistance programs.**

Documentation Focus

ASSESSMENT/REASSESSMENT

- Assessment findings, including client perception of needs and desire/expectations for improvement.
- Individual cultural/religious restrictions, personal preferences.
- Availability/use of resources.

Information in brackets added by the authors to clarify and enhance the use of nursing diagnoses.

 Diagnostic Studies   ∞ Pediatric/Geriatric/Lifespan   Medications

PLANNING

- Individual goals for enhancement.
- Plan for growth and who is involved in planning.

IMPLEMENTATION/EVALUATION

- Response to activities/learning and actions performed.
- Attainment/progress toward desired outcome(s).
- Modifications to plan.

DISCHARGE PLANNING

- Long-range needs/expectations and plan of action.
- Available resources and specific referrals made.

SAMPLE NURSING OUTCOMES & INTERVENTIONS CLASSIFICATIONS (NOC/NIC)

NOC—Health Promoting Behavior
NIC—Nutrition Management

---

impaired Oral Mucous Membrane

Taxonomy II: Safety/Protection—Class 2 Physical Injury (00045)
[Diagnostic Division: Food/Fluid]
Submitted 1982; Nursing Diagnosis Extension and Classification (NDEC) Revision 1998

Definition: Disruption of the lips and/or soft tissue of the oral cavity

---

Related Factors

Dehydration; NPO for more than 24 hours; malnutrition
Decreased salivation; medication side effects; diminished hormone levels (women); mouth breathing
Deficient knowledge of appropriate oral hygiene
Ineffective oral hygiene; barriers to oral self-care/professional care
Mechanical factors (e.g., ill-fitting dentures; braces; tubes [endotracheal/nasogastric], surgery in oral cavity); loss of supportive structures; trauma; cleft lip/palate
Chemical irritants (e.g., alcohol, tobacco, acidic foods, regular use of inhalers or other noxious agents)
Chemotherapy; immunosuppression; immuncompromised; decreased platelets; infection; radiation therapy
Stress; depression

Information in brackets added by the authors to clarify and enhance the use of nursing diagnoses.

 Cultural 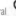 Collaborative 🏠 Community/Home Care

Defining Characteristics

SUBJECTIVE

Xerostomia [dry mouth]

Oral pain/discomfort

Reports bad taste in mouth; diminished taste; difficulty eating/swallowing

OBJECTIVE

Coated tongue; smooth atrophic tongue; geographic tongue

Gingival/mucosal pallor

Stomatitis; hyperemia; gingival hyperplasia; macroplasia; vesicles; nodules; papules

White patches/plaques; spongy patches; white curd-like exudate

Oral lesions/ulcers; fissures; bleeding; cheilitis; desquamation; mucosal denudation

Purulent drainage/exudates; presence of pathogens; enlarged tonsils

Edema

Halitosis; [carious teeth]

Gingival recession, pocketing deeper than 4 mm

Red or bluish masses (e.g., hemangiomas)

Difficult speech

Desired Outcomes/Evaluation Criteria—Client Will:

- Verbalize understanding of causative factors.
- Identify specific interventions to promote healthy oral mucosa.
- Demonstrate techniques to restore/maintain integrity of oral mucosa.
- Report/demonstrate a decrease in symptoms as noted in Defining Characteristics.

Actions/Interventions

NURSING PRIORITY NO. 1. To identify causative/contributing factors affecting oral health:

- Note presence of illness/disease/trauma (e.g., gingivitis/periodontal disease; presence of oral ulcerations; bacterial/viral/fungal oral infections; facial fractures; cancer or cancer therapies; generalized debilitating conditions) **that affect health of oral tissues.**
- Determine nutrition/fluid intake and reported changes (e.g., avoiding eating, change in taste, chews painstakingly, swallows numerous times for even small bites, unexplained weight loss) **that can indicate problems with oral mucosa.**

Information in brackets added by the authors to clarify and enhance the use of nursing diagnoses.

 Diagnostic Studies   ∞ Pediatric/Geriatric/Lifespan   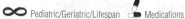 Medications   **495**

impaired ORAL MUCOUS MEMBRANE

- Note use of tobacco (including smokeless) and alcohol **which may predispose mucosa to infection, cell damage, and cancer**.
- Assess for dry mouth, thick or absent saliva, and abnormal tongue surfaces.
- Observe for chipped or sharp-edged teeth. Note fit of dentures or other prosthetic devices when used.
- Assess medication use and possibility of side effects **affecting health or integrity of oral mucous membranes**.
- Determine allergies to food/drugs, other substances.
- Evaluate client's ability to provide self-care and availability of necessary equipment/assistance. **Client's age, as well as current health status, affects ability to provide self-care.**
- Review oral hygiene practices: frequency and type (brush/floss/Water Pik); professional dental care.

NURSING PRIORITY NO. 2. To correct identified/developing problems:

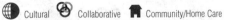 • Routinely inspect oral cavity and throat for inflammation, sores, lesions, and/or bleeding. Determine if client is experiencing pain or painful swallowing.

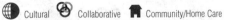 • Encourage adequate fluids **to prevent dry mouth and dehydration.**

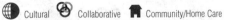 • Encourage use of tart, sour, and citrus foods and drinks; chewing gum; or hard candy **to stimulate saliva.**

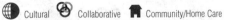 • Lubricate lips and provide commercially prepared oral lubricant solution.

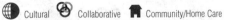 • Provide for increased humidity, if indicated, by vaporizer or room humidifier if client is mouth-breather.

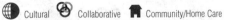 • Provide dietary modifications (e.g., food of comfortable texture, temperature, density) **to reduce discomfort/improve intake,** and adequate nutrients and vitamins **to promote healing**.

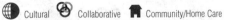 • Avoid irritating foods/fluids, temperature extremes. Provide soft or pureed diet as required.

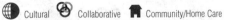 • Use lemon/glycerin swabs with caution; **may be irritating if mucosa is injured.**

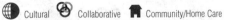 • Assist with/provide oral care, as indicated:

  Offer/provide tap water or saline rinses, diluted alcohol-free mouthwashes.

  Provide gentle gum massage and tongue brushing with soft toothbrush or sponge/cotton-tip applicators (**limits mucosal/gum irritation**).

  Assist with/encourage brushing and flossing **when client is unable to do self-care.**

  Review safe use of electric or battery-powered mouth care devices (e.g., toothbrush, plaque remover, etc.), as indicated.

Information in brackets added by the authors to clarify and enhance the use of nursing diagnoses.

   Cultural   Collaborative   Community/Home Care

Assist with/provide denture care when indicated (e.g., remove and clean after meals and at bedtime).

🏠 • Provide anesthetic lozenges or analgesics such as Stanford solution, viscous lidocaine (Xylocaine), sulfacrate slurry, as indicated, **to provide protection/reduce oral discomfort/pain.**

💊 • Administer antibiotics, as ordered, **when infection is present.**

• Reposition ET tubes and airway adjuncts routinely, carefully padding/protecting teeth/prosthetics **to minimize pressure on tissues.**

🏠 • Emphasize avoiding alcohol, smoking/chewing tobacco if periodontal disease present, or if client has xerostomia/other oral discomforts, **which may further irritate/damage mucosa.**

🔗 • Refer for evaluation of dentures/other prosthetics, structural defects **when impairments are affecting oral health.**

NURSING PRIORITY NO. 3. To promote wellness (Teaching/Discharge Considerations):

🏠 • Review current oral hygiene patterns and provide information about oral health as required/desired **to correct deficiencies/encourage proper care.**

∞ • Instruct parents in oral hygiene techniques and proper dental care for infants/children (e.g., safe use of pacifier, brushing of teeth and gums, avoidance of sweet drinks and candy, recognition and treatment of thrush). **Encourages early initiation of good oral health practices and timely intervention for treatable problems.**

🏠 • Discuss special mouth care required during and after illness/trauma, or following surgical repair (e.g., cleft lip/palate) **to facilitate healing.**

🏠 • Identify need for/demonstrate use of special "appliances" **to perform own oral care.**

🏠 • Listen to concerns about appearance and provide accurate information about possible treatments/outcomes. Discuss effect of condition on self-esteem/body image, noting withdrawal from usual social activities/relationships, and/or expressions of powerlessness.

💊 • Review information regarding drug regimen, use of local anesthetics.

🏠 • Promote general health/mental health habits. (**Altered immune response can affect the oral mucosa.**)

🏠 • Provide nutritional information **to correct deficiencies, reduce irritation/gum disease, prevent dental caries.**

∞ • Stress importance of limiting nighttime regimen of bottle of milk for infant in bed. Suggest pacifier or use of water during night **to prevent bottle syndrome with decaying of teeth.**

Information in brackets added by the authors to clarify and enhance the use of nursing diagnoses.

impaired ORAL MUCOUS MEMBRANE

- Recommend regular dental checkups/professional care.
- Identify community resources (e.g., low-cost dental clinics, smoking cessation resources, cancer information services/support group, Meals on Wheels, food stamps, home care aide).

Documentation Focus

ASSESSMENT/REASSESSMENT

- Condition of oral mucous membranes, routine oral care habits and interferences.
- Availability of oral care equipment/products.
- Knowledge of proper oral hygiene/care.
- Availability/use of resources.

PLANNING

- Plan of care and who is involved in planning.
- Teaching plan.

IMPLEMENTATION/EVALUATION

- Responses to interventions/teaching and actions performed.
- Attainment/progress toward desired outcome(s).
- Modifications to plan of care.

DISCHARGE PLANNING

- Long-term needs and who is responsible for actions to be taken.
- Specific referrals made, resources for special appliances.

SAMPLE NURSING OUTCOMES & INTERVENTIONS CLASSIFICATIONS (NOC/NIC)

NOC—Oral Health
NIC—Oral Health Restoration

acute Pain

Taxonomy II: Comfort—Class 1 Physical Comfort (00132)
[Diagnostic Division: Pain/Comfort]
Submitted 1996

Definition: Unpleasant sensory and emotional experience arising from actual or potential tissue damage or described in terms of such damage (International Association for the Study of Pain); sudden or slow onset of any intensity from mild to severe with an anticipated or predictable end and a duration of less than 6 months

Information in brackets added by the authors to clarify and enhance the use of nursing diagnoses.

 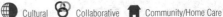

Related Factors

Injuring agents (biological, chemical, physical, psychological)

Defining Characteristics

SUBJECTIVE

Verbal report of pain; coded report [may be less from clients younger than age 40, men, and some cultural groups]

Changes in appetite

OBJECTIVE

Observed evidence of pain

Guarding behavior; protective gestures; positioning to avoid pain

Facial mask; sleep disturbance (eyes lack luster, beaten look, fixed or scattered movement, grimace)

Expressive behavior (e.g., restlessness, moaning, crying, vigilance, irritability, sighing)

Distraction behavior (e.g., pacing, seeking out other people and/or activities, repetitive activities)

Change in muscle tone (may span from listless [flaccid] to rigid)

Diaphoresis; change in blood pressure/heart rate/respiratory rate; pupillary dilation

Self-focusing; narrowed focus (altered time perception, impaired thought process, reduced interaction with people and environment)

Desired Outcomes/Evaluation Criteria—Client Will:

- Report pain is relieved/controlled.
- Follow prescribed pharmacological regimen.
- Verbalize nonpharmacologic methods that provide relief.
- Demonstrate use of relaxation skills and diversional activities, as indicated, for individual situation.

Actions/Interventions

NURSING PRIORITY NO. 1. To assess etiology/precipitating contributory factors:

- Note client's age/developmental level and current condition (e.g., infant/child, critically ill, ventilated/sedated, or cognitively impaired client) affecting ability to report pain parameters.
- Determine/document presence of possible pathophysiological/psychological causes of pain (e.g., inflammation; tissue

Information in brackets added by the authors to clarify and enhance the use of nursing diagnoses.

trauma/fractures; surgery; infections; heart attack/angina; abdominal conditions [e.g., appendicitis, cholecystitis]; burns; grief; fear/anxiety; depression; and personality disorders).

- Note location of surgical procedures, **as this can influence the amount of postoperative pain experienced; for example, vertical/diagonal incisions are more painful than transverse or S-shaped. Presence of known/unknown complication(s) may make the pain more severe than anticipated.**

- Assess for referred pain, as appropriate, **to help determine possibility of underlying condition or organ dysfunction requiring treatment.**

- Note client's attitude toward pain and use of pain medications, including any history of substance abuse.

- Note client's locus of control (internal/external). **Individuals with external locus of control may take little or no responsibility for pain management.**

- Assist in thorough evaluation, including neurological and psychological factors (pain inventory, psychological interview), as appropriate, when pain persists.

NURSING PRIORITY NO. 2. To evaluate client's response to pain:

- Obtain client's assessment of pain to include location, characteristics, onset/duration, frequency, quality, intensity, and precipitating/aggravating factors. Reassess each time pain occurs/is reported. Note and investigate changes from previous reports **to rule out worsening of underlying condition/development of complications.**

- Use pain rating scale appropriate for age/cognition (e.g., 0 to 10 scale; facial expression scale [pediatric, nonverbal]; pain assessment scale for dementing elderly [PADE]; behavioral pain scale [BPS]).

- Accept client's description of pain. Acknowledge the pain experience and convey acceptance of client's response to pain. **Pain is a subjective experience and cannot be felt by others.**

- Observe nonverbal cues/pain behaviors (e.g., how client walks, holds body, sits; facial expression; cool fingertips/toes, which can mean constricted blood vessels) and other objective Defining Characteristics, as noted, especially in persons who cannot communicate verbally. **Observations may/may not be congruent with verbal reports or may be only indicator present when client is unable to verbalize.**

- Ask others who know client well (e.g., spouse, parent) to identify behaviors that may indicate pain **when client is unable to verbalize.**

Information in brackets added by the authors to clarify and enhance the use of nursing diagnoses.

 Cultural Collaborative 🏠 Community/Home Care

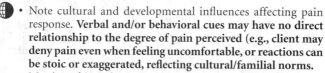
- Note cultural and developmental influences affecting pain response. **Verbal and/or behavioral cues may have no direct relationship to the degree of pain perceived (e.g., client may deny pain even when feeling uncomfortable, or reactions can be stoic or exaggerated, reflecting cultural/familial norms.**
- Monitor skin color/temperature and vital signs (e.g., heart rate, blood pressure, respirations), **which are usually altered in acute pain.**
- Ascertain client's knowledge of and expectations about pain management.
- Review client's previous experiences with pain and methods found either helpful or unhelpful for pain control in the past.

NURSING PRIORITY NO. 3. To assist client to explore methods for alleviation/control of pain:

- Determine client's acceptable level of pain/pain control goals. **Varies with individual and situation.**
- **Determine factors in client's lifestyle (e.g., alcohol/other drug use/abuse)** that can affect responses to analgesics and/or choice of interventions for pain management.
- Note when pain occurs (e.g., only with ambulation, every evening) **to medicate prophylactically, as appropriate.**
- Collaborate in treatment of underlying condition/disease processes causing pain and proactive management of pain (e.g., epidural analgesia, nerve blockade for postoperative pain).
- Provide comfort measures (e.g., touch, repositioning, use of heat/cold packs, nurse's presence), quiet environment, and calm activities **to promote nonpharmacological pain management.**
- Instruct in/encourage use of relaxation techniques, such as focused breathing, imaging, CDs/tapes (e.g., "white" noise, music, instructional) **to distract attention and reduce tension.**
- Encourage diversional activities (e.g., TV/radio, socialization with others).
- Review procedures/expectations and tell client when treatment may cause pain **to reduce concern of the unknown and associated muscle tension.**
- Encourage verbalization of feelings about the pain.
- Use puppets to demonstrate procedure for child **to enhance understanding and reduce level of anxiety/fear.**
- Suggest parent be present during procedures **to comfort child.**
- Identify ways of avoiding/minimizing pain (e.g., splinting incision during cough; using firm mattress/proper supporting shoes for low back pain; good body mechanics).

Information in brackets added by the authors to clarify and enhance the use of nursing diagnoses.

- Work with client to prevent pain. Use flow sheet to document pain, therapeutic interventions, response, and length of time before pain recurs. Instruct client to report pain as soon as it begins **as timely intervention is more likely to be successful in alleviating pain.**
- Administer analgesics, as indicated, to maximum dosage, as needed, **to maintain "acceptable" level of pain. Notify physician if regimen is inadequate to meet pain control goal.**
- Demonstrate/monitor use of self-administration/patient-controlled analgesia (PCA) for management of severe, persistent pain.
- Evaluate/document client's response to analgesia, and assist in transitioning/altering drug regimen, based on individual needs. **Increasing/decreasing dosage, stepped program (switching from injection to oral route, increased time span as pain lessens) helps in self-management of pain.**
- Instruct client in use of transcutaneous electrical stimulation (TENS) unit, when ordered.

NURSING PRIORITY NO. 4. To promote wellness (Teaching/Discharge Considerations):

- Encourage adequate rest periods **to prevent fatigue.**
- Review ways to lessen pain, including techniques such as Therapeutic Touch (TT), biofeedback, self-hypnosis, and relaxation skills.
- Discuss impact of pain on lifestyle/independence and ways to maximize level of functioning.
- Provide for individualized physical therapy/exercise program that can be continued by the client after discharge. **Promotes active, not passive, role and enhances sense of control.**
- Discuss with SO(s) ways in which they can assist client and reduce precipitating factors that may cause or increase pain (e.g., participating in household tasks following abdominal surgery).
- Identify specific signs/symptoms and changes in pain characteristics requiring medical follow-up.

Documentation Focus

ASSESSMENT/REASSESSMENT

- Individual assessment findings, including client's description of response to pain, specifics of pain inventory, expectations of pain management, and acceptable level of pain.
- Prior medication use; substance abuse.

Information in brackets added by the authors to clarify and enhance the use of nursing diagnoses.

 Cultural Collaborative Community/Home Care

PLANNING

- Plan of care and who is involved in planning.
- Teaching plan.

IMPLEMENTATION/EVALUATION

- Response to interventions/teaching and actions performed.
- Attainment/progress toward desired outcome(s).
- Modifications to plan of care.

DISCHARGE PLANNING

- Long-term needs, noting who is responsible for actions to be taken.
- Specific referrals made.

SAMPLE NURSING OUTCOMES & INTERVENTIONS CLASSIFICATIONS (NOC/NIC)

NOC—Pain Level
NIC—Pain Management

chronic Pain

Taxonomy II: Comfort—Class 1 Physical Comfort (00133) [Diagnostic Division: Pain/Discomfort] Submitted 1986; Revised 1996

Definition: Unpleasant sensory and emotional experience arising from actual or potential tissue damage or described in terms of such damage (International Association for the Study of Pain); sudden or slow onset of any intensity from mild to severe, constant or recurring without an anticipated or predictable end and a duration of greater than 6 months

[Pain is a signal that something is wrong. Chronic pain can be recurrent and periodically disabling (e.g., migraine headaches) or may be unremitting. While chronic pain syndrome includes various learned behaviors, psychological factors become the primary contribution to impairment. It is a complex entity, combining **elements from other NDs,** such as Powerlessness; deficient Diversional Activity; interrupted Family Processes; Self-Care Deficit; and risk for Disuse Syndrome.]

Related Factors

Chronic physical/psychosocial disability

Information in brackets added by the authors to clarify and enhance the use of nursing diagnoses.

 Diagnostic Studies 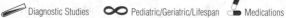 Pediatric/Geriatric/Lifespan Medications **503**

chronic PAIN

Defining Characteristics

SUBJECTIVE

Verbal report of pain; coded report
Fear of reinjury
Altered ability to continue previous activities
Changes in sleep patterns; fatigue; anorexia
[Preoccupation with pain]
[Desperately seeks alternative solutions/therapies for relief/
control of pain]

OBJECTIVE

Observed protective/guarding behavior; irritability; restlessness
Facial mask; self-focusing
Reduced interaction with people; depression
Atrophy of involved muscle group
Sympathetic mediated responses (e.g., temperature, cold, changes
of body position, hypersensitivity)

Desired Outcomes/Evaluation
Criteria—Client Will:

• Verbalize and demonstrate (nonverbal cues) relief and/or
control of pain/discomfort.
• Verbalize recognition of interpersonal/family dynamics and
reactions that affect the pain problem.
• Demonstrate/initiate behavioral modifications of lifestyle and
appropriate use of therapeutic interventions.

Family/SO(s) Will:

• Cooperate in pain management program. (Refer to ND readiness for enhanced family Coping.)

Actions/Interventions

NURSING PRIORITY NO. 1. To assess etiology/precipitating factors:

• Assess for conditions associated with long-term pain (e.g., low
back pain, arthritis, fibromyalgia, neuropathies, multiple/slow
healing traumatic musculoskeletal injuries, amputation
[phantom limb pain], etc.) **to identify client with potential
for pain lasting beyond normal healing period.**

• Assist in thorough diagnosis, including neurological, psychological evaluation (Minnesota Multiphasic Personality Inventory—
MMPI, pain inventory, psychological interview).

Information in brackets added by the authors to clarify and enhance
the use of nursing diagnoses.

 Cultural Collaborative Community/Home Care

- Evaluate emotional/physical components of individual situation. Note codependent components, enabling behaviors of caregivers/family members **that support continuation of the status quo.**
- Determine cultural factors for the individual situation (e.g., how expression of pain is accepted—moaning aloud or enduring in stoic silence; magnification of symptoms to convince others of reality of pain).
- Note gender and age of client. **Current literature suggests there may be differences between women and men as to how they perceive and/or respond to pain. Sensitivity to pain is likely to decline as one gets older.**
- Discuss use of nicotine, sugar, caffeine, white flour, as appropriate (**some holistic practitioners believe these items need to be eliminated from the client's diet**).
- Evaluate current and past analgesic/opioid drug use (including alcohol).
- Determine issues of secondary gain for the client/SO(s) (e.g., financial/insurance, marital/family concern, work issues). **May interfere with progress in pain management/resolution of situation.**
- Make home visit when possible, observing such factors as safety equipment, adequate room, colors, plants, family interactions. Note impact of home environment on the client.

NURSING PRIORITY NO. 2. To determine client response to chronic pain situation:

- Acknowledge and assess pain matter-of-factly, avoiding undue expressions of concern while conveying compassionate regard for client's feelings and situation of living with pain and coping with an often ill-defined disability.
- Evaluate pain behaviors. **May be exaggerated because client's perception of pain is not believed or because client believes caregivers are discounting reports of pain.**
- Determine individual client threshold for pain (physical examination, pain profile, and the like).
- Ascertain duration of pain problem, who has been consulted, and what drugs and therapies (including alternative/complementary) have been used.
- Note lifestyle effects of pain (e.g., decreased activity/deconditioning, severe fatigue, weight loss or gain, sleep difficulties, depression).
- Assess degree of personal maladjustment of the client, such as isolationism, anger, irritability, loss of work time/job.
- Note availability/use of personal and community resources.

Information in brackets added by the authors to clarify and enhance the use of nursing diagnoses.

NURSING PRIORITY NO. 3. To assist client to deal with pain:

* Review client pain management goals/expectations versus reality. **Pain may not be completely resolved, but may be significantly lessened to "acceptable level" or managed to the degree that client can participate in desired/needed life activities.**

* Apply pain management interventions, as appropriate (e.g., extended-relief oral pain medications and patches, nerve blocking injection, implanted pump, electrical stimulation/TENS unit) **to medically intervene, as indicated, in all aspects of long-term pain.**

* Encourage use of nonpharmacological methods of pain control (e.g., heat/cold applications, splinting or exercises, hydrotherapy, deep breathing, meditation, visualization/guided imagery, Therapeutic Touch [TT], posture correction and muscle strengthening exercises, progressive muscle relaxation, biofeedback, massage).

* Assist client to learn breathing techniques (e.g., diaphragmatic breathing) **to assist in muscle and generalized relaxation.**

* Discuss the physiological dynamics of tension/anxiety and how this affects pain.

* Include client and SO(s) in establishing pattern of discussing pain for specified length of time **to limit focusing on pain.**

* Encourage client to use positive affirmations: "I am healing." "I am relaxed." "I love this life." Have client be aware of internal-external dialogue. Say "cancel" when negative thoughts develop.

* Use tranquilizers, opioids, and analgesics sparingly. **These drugs are physically and psychologically addicting and promote sleep disturbances—especially interfering with deep REM (rapid eye movement) sleep. Client may need to be detoxified if many medications are currently used. Note: Antidepressants have an added benefit with analgesic effects because perception of pain decreases as depression is lessened.**

* Encourage right-brain stimulation with activities such as love, laughter, and music **to release endorphins, enhancing sense of well-being.**

* Suggest use of subliminal tapes **to bypass logical part of the brain by saying: "I am becoming a more relaxed person." "It is all right for me to relax."**

* Assist family in developing a program of coping strategies (e.g., staying active even when modified activities are required, living a healthy lifestyle, implementing positive reinforcement

---

Information in brackets added by the authors to clarify and enhance the use of nursing diagnoses.

for all persons, encouraging client to use own control, and diminishing attention given to pain behavior).

- Be alert to changes in pain. **May indicate a new physical problem.**

NURSING PRIORITY NO. 4. To promote wellness (Teaching/Discharge Considerations):

- Provide anticipatory guidance to client with condition in which pain is common and educate about when, where, and how to seek intervention/treatments.
- Assist client and SO(s) to learn how to heal by developing sense of internal control, by being responsible for own treatment, and by obtaining the information and tools to accomplish this.
- Discuss potential for developmental delays in child with chronic pain. Identify current level of function and review appropriate expectations for individual child.
- Review safe use of medications, management of minor side effects, and adverse effects requiring medical intervention.
- Assist client to learn to change pain behavior to wellness behavior: "Act as if you are well."
- Encourage and assist family member/SO(s) to learn massage techniques.
- Recommend that client and SO(s) take time for themselves. **Provides opportunity to re-energize and refocus on tasks at hand.**
- Identify and discuss potential hazards of unproved and/or nonmedical therapies/remedies.
- Identify community support groups/resources to meet individual needs (e.g., yard care, home maintenance, alternative transportation). **Proper use of resources may reduce negative pattern of "overdoing" heavy activities, then spending several days in bed recuperating.**
- Refer for individual/family counseling and/or marital therapy, parent effectiveness classes, etc., as needed. **Presence of chronic pain affects all relationships/family dynamics.**
- Refer to NDs ineffective Coping; compromised family Coping.

Documentation Focus

ASSESSMENT/REASSESSMENT

- Individual findings, including duration of problem/specific contributing factors, previously/currently used interventions.
- Perception of pain, effects on lifestyle, and expectations of therapeutic regimen.
- Family's/SO's response to client, and support for change.

Information in brackets added by the authors to clarify and enhance the use of nursing diagnoses.

PLANNING

- Plan of care and who is involved in planning.
- Teaching plan.

IMPLEMENTATION/EVALUATION

- Responses to interventions/teaching and actions performed.
- Attainment/progress toward desired outcome(s).
- Modifications to plan of care.

DISCHARGE PLANNING

- Long-term needs and who is responsible for actions to be taken.
- Specific referrals made.

SAMPLE NURSING OUTCOMES & INTERVENTIONS CLASSIFICATIONS (NOC/NIC)

NOC—Pain Control
NIC—Pain Management

impaired Parenting

Taxonomy II: Role Relationships—Class 1 Caregiving
   Roles (00056)
[Diagnostic Division: Social Interaction]
Submitted 1998; Nursing Diagnosis Extension and
   Classification (NDEC) Revision 1998

Definition: Inability of the primary caretaker to create,
maintain, or regain an environment that promotes the
optimum growth and development of the child

[NOTE: It is important to reaffirm that adjustment to parenting in
general is a normal maturational process that elicits nursing behaviors to prevent potential problems and to promote health.]

Related Factors

INFANT OR CHILD

Premature birth; multiple births; not desired gender
Illness; separation from parent
Difficult temperament; temperamental conflicts with parental
   expectations
Handicapping condition; developmental delay; altered percep-
   tual abilities; attention-deficit hyperactivity disorder

Information in brackets added by the authors to clarify and enhance
the use of nursing diagnoses.

KNOWLEDGE

Deficient knowledge about child/development health maintenance, parenting skills; inability to respond to infant cues

Unrealistic expectations [for self, infant, partner]

Lack of education; limited cognitive functioning; lack of cognitive readiness for parenthood

Poor communication skills

Preference for physical punishment

PHYSIOLOGICAL

Physical illness

PSYCHOLOGICAL

Young parental age

Lack of prenatal care; difficult birthing process; high number of/closely spaced pregnancies

Sleep disruption/deprivation; depression

History of mental illness/substance abuse

Disability

SOCIAL

Presence of stress (e.g., financial, legal, recent crisis, cultural move [from another country/cultural group within same country]); job problems; unemployment; financial difficulties; relocations; poor home environment

Situational/chronic low self-esteem

Lack of family cohesiveness; marital conflict; change in family unit; inadequate childcare arrangements

Role strain; single parent; father/mother of child not involved

Lack of/poor parental role model; lack of valuing of parenthood; inability to put child's needs before own

Unplanned/unwanted pregnancy

Low socioeconomic class; poverty; lack of resources; lack of transportation

Poor problem-solving skills; maladaptive coping strategies

Lack of social support networks; social isolation

History of being abusive/being abused; legal difficulties

Defining Characteristics

SUBJECTIVE

Parental

Statements of inability to meet child's needs; verbalization of inability to control child

---

Information in brackets added by the authors to clarify and enhance the use of nursing diagnoses.

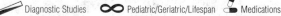

Negative statements about child
Verbalization of frustration/role inadequacy

OBJECTIVE

Infant or Child
Frequent accidents/illness; failure to thrive
Poor academic performance/cognitive development
Poor social competence; behavioral disorders
Incidence of trauma (e.g., physical and psychological)/abuse
Lack of attachment/separation anxiety; runaway

Parental
Maternal-child interaction deficit; poor parent-child interaction; little cuddling; inadequate attachment
Inadequate child health maintenance; unsafe home environment; inappropriate childcare arrangements; inappropriate stimulation (e.g., visual, tactile, auditory)
Inappropriate caretaking skills; inconsistent care/behavior management
Inflexibility in meeting needs of child
Frequently punitive; rejection of/hostility to child; child abuse/neglect; abandonment

Desired Outcomes/Evaluation Criteria—Parents Will:

• Verbalize realistic information and expectations of parenting role.
• Verbalize acceptance of the individual situation.
• Participate in appropriate classes, e.g., parenting class.
• Identify own strengths, individual needs, and methods/resources to meet them.
• Demonstrate appropriate attachment/parenting behaviors.

Actions/Interventions

NURSING PRIORITY NO. 1. To assess causative/contributing factors:

 • Note family constellation; for example, two-parent, single, extended family, or child living with other relative, such as grandparent.
• Determine developmental stage of the family (e.g., new child, adolescent, child leaving/returning home).
• Assess family relationships between individual members and with others.
• Assess parenting skill level, taking into account the individual's intellectual, emotional, and physical strengths and weaknesses.

Information in brackets added by the authors to clarify and enhance the use of nursing diagnoses.

 Cultural Collaborative Community/Home Care

Parents with significant impairments may need more education/support.

- Observe attachment behaviors between parental figure and child. Determine cultural significance of behaviors. (Refer to ND risk for impaired parent/infant/child Attachment.)

- Note presence of factors in the child (e.g., birth defects, hyperactivity) **that may affect attachment and caretaking needs.**

- Identify physical challenges/limitations of the parents (e.g., visual/hearing impairment, quadriplegia, severe depression). **May affect ability to care for child and suggests individual needs for assistance/support.**

- Determine presence/effectiveness of support systems, role models, extended family, and community resources available to the parent(s).

- Note absence from home setting/lack of child supervision by parent (e.g., working long hours/out of town, multiple responsibilities, such as working and attending educational classes).

NURSING PRIORITY NO. 2. To foster development of parenting skills:

- Create an environment in which relationships can be developed and needs of each individual met. **Learning is more effective when individuals feel safe.**

- Make time for listening to concerns of the parent(s).

- Emphasize positive aspects of the situation, maintaining a hopeful attitude toward the parent's capabilities and potential for improving the situation.

- Note staff attitudes toward parent/child and specific problem/disability; for example, needs of disabled parent(s) to be seen as an individual and evaluated apart from a stereotype. **Negative attitudes are detrimental to promoting positive outcomes.**

- Encourage expression of feelings, such as helplessness, anger, frustration. Set limits on unacceptable behaviors. **Individuals who lose control develop feelings of low self-esteem.**

- Acknowledge difficulty of situation and normalcy of feelings. **Enhances feelings of acceptance.**

- Recognize stages of grieving process when the child is disabled or other than anticipated (e.g., girl instead of boy, misshapen head/prominent birthmark). Allow time for parents to express feelings and deal with the "loss."

- Encourage attendance at skill classes (e.g., parent effectiveness). **Assists in improving parenting skills by developing communication and problem-solving techniques.**

Information in brackets added by the authors to clarify and enhance the use of nursing diagnoses.

• Emphasize parenting functions rather than mothering/fathering skills. **By virtue of gender, each person brings something to the parenting role; however, nurturing tasks can be done by both parents.**

NURSING PRIORITY NO. 3. To promote wellness (Teaching/Discharge Considerations):

• Involve all available members of the family in learning.

• Provide information appropriate to the situation, including time management, limit setting, and stress-reduction techniques. **Facilitates satisfactory implementation of plan/new behaviors.**

• Discuss parental beliefs about child-rearing, punishment and rewards, teaching. **Identifying these beliefs allows opportunity to provide new information regarding not using spanking and/or yelling and what actions can be substituted for more effective parenting.**

• Develop support systems appropriate to the situation (e.g., extended family, friends, social worker, home-care services).

• Assist parent to plan time and conserve energy in positive ways. **Enables individual to cope more effectively with difficulties as they arise.**

• Encourage parents to identify positive outlets for meeting their own needs (e.g., going out for dinner, making time for their own interests and each other/dating). **Promotes general well-being, helps parents to be more effective and reduces burnout.**

• Refer to appropriate support/therapy groups, as indicated.

• Identify community resources (e.g., childcare services, respite house) **to assist with individual needs, provide respite and support.**

• Report and take necessary actions, as legally/professionally indicated, if child's safety is a concern. **Family may believe corporal punishment is the best way to have children behave.**

• Refer to NDs ineffective Coping; compromised family Coping; risk for Violence [specify]; Self-Esteem [specify]; and interrupted Family Processes.

Documentation Focus

ASSESSMENT/REASSESSMENT

• Individual findings, including parenting skill level, deviations from normal parenting expectations, family makeup, and developmental stages.

• Availability/use of support systems and community resources.

Information in brackets added by the authors to clarify and enhance the use of nursing diagnoses.

  Cultural Collaborative Community/Home Care

PLANNING

- Plan of care and who is involved in planning.
- Teaching plan.

IMPLEMENTATION/EVALUATION

- Parent(s')/child's responses to interventions/teaching and actions performed.
- Attainment/progress toward desired outcome(s).
- Modification to plan of care.

DISCHARGE PLANNING

- Long-range needs and who is responsible for actions to be taken.
- Specific referrals made.

SAMPLE NURSING OUTCOMES & INTERVENTIONS CLASSIFICATIONS (NOC/NIC)

NOC—Role Performance
NIC—Parenting Promotion

readiness for enhanced Parenting

Taxonomy II: Role Relationships—Class 1 Caregiving Roles (00164)
[Diagnostic Divisions: Social Interaction]
Submitted 2002

Definition: A pattern of providing an environment for children or other dependent person(s) that is sufficient to nurture growth and development and can be strengthened

Related Factors

To be developed

Defining Characteristics

SUBJECTIVE

Expresses willingness to enhance parenting
Children or other dependent person(s) express(es) satisfaction with home environment

OBJECTIVE

Emotional support of children [/dependent person(s)]; evidence of attachment

---

Information in brackets added by the authors to clarify and enhance the use of nursing diagnoses.

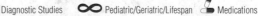

Needs of children [/dependent person(s)] are met (e.g., physical and emotional)

Exhibits realistic expectations of children [/dependent person(s)]

Desired Outcomes/Evaluation Criteria—Parents Will:

- Verbalize realistic information and expectations of parenting role.
- Identify own strengths, individual needs, and methods/resources to meet them.
- Participate in activities to enhance parenting skills.
- Demonstrate improved parenting behaviors.

Actions/Interventions

NURSING PRIORITY NO. 1. To determine need/motivation for improvement:

- Ascertain motivation/expectation for change.
- Note family constellation: for example, two-parent; single parent; extended family; child living with other relative, such as grandparent; or relationship of dependent person. **Understanding makeup of the family provides information about needs to assist them in improving their family connections.**
- Determine developmental stage of the family (e.g., new child, adolescent, child leaving/returning home, retirement). **These maturational crises bring changes in the family, which can provide opportunity for enhancing parenting skills and improving family interactions.**
- Assess family relationships and identify needs of individual members, noting any special concerns that exist, such as birth defects, illness, hyperactivity. **The family is a system and when members make decisions to improve parenting skills, the changes affect all parts of the system. Identifying needs, special situations, and relationships can help to develop plan to bring about effective change.**
- Assess parenting skill level, taking into account the individual's intellectual, emotional, and physical strengths and weaknesses. **Identifies areas of need for education, skill training, and information on which to base plan for enhancing parenting skills.**
- Observe attachment behaviors between parent(s) and child(ren), recognizing cultural background which may influence expected behaviors. **Behaviors such as eye-to-eye contact, use of en-face position, talking to infant in high-pitched**

Information in brackets added by the authors to clarify and enhance the use of nursing diagnoses.

  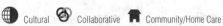 Cultural   Collaborative   Community/Home Care

voice, are indicative of attachment behaviors in American culture, but may not be appropriate in another culture. Failure to bond is thought to affect subsequent parent-child interactions.

- Determine presence/effectiveness of support systems, role models, extended family, and community resources available to the parent(s). **Parents desiring to enhance abilities and improve family life can benefit by role models that help them develop their own style of parenting.**
- Note cultural/religious influences on parenting, expectations of self/child, sense of success or failure. **Expectations may vary with different cultures (e.g., Arab-Americans hold children to be sacred, but child-rearing is based on negative rather than positive reinforcements, and parents are more strict with girls than boys). These beliefs may interfere with desire to improve parenting skills when there is conflict between the two.**

NURSING PRIORITY NO. 2. To foster improvement of parenting skills:

- Create an environment in which relationships can be strengthened. **A safe environment in which individuals can freely express their thoughts and feelings optimizes learning and positive interactions among family members, thus enhancing relationships.**
- Make time for listening to concerns of the parent(s). **Promotes sense of importance and of being heard and identifies accurate information regarding needs of the family for enhancing relationships.**
- Encourage expression of feelings, such as frustration/anger, while setting limits on unacceptable behaviors. **Identification of feelings promotes understanding of self and enhances connections with others in the family. Unacceptable behaviors result in diminished self-esteem and can lead to problems in the family relationships.**
- Emphasize parenting functions rather than mothering/fathering skills. **By virtue of gender, each person brings something to the parenting role; however, nurturing tasks can be done by both parents, enhancing family relationships.**
- Encourage attendance at skill classes, such as Parent/Family Effectiveness Training. **Assists in developing communication skills of active-listening, I-messages, and problem-solving techniques to improve family relationships and promote a win-win environment.**

Information in brackets added by the authors to clarify and enhance the use of nursing diagnoses.

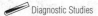 Diagnostic Studies ∞ Pediatric/Geriatric/Lifespan Medications **515**

NURSING PRIORITY NO. 3. To promote optimal wellness:

• Involve all members of the family in learning. **The family system benefits from all members participating in learning new skills to enhance family relationships.**

• Encourage parents to identify positive outlets for meeting their own needs. **Activities, such as going out for dinner/dating, making time for their own interests and each other, promote general well-being and can enhance family relationships and improve family functioning.**

• Provide information, as indicated, including time management, stress-reduction techniques. **Learning about positive parenting skills, understanding growth and developmental expectations, and discovering ways to reduce stress and anxiety promote the individual's ability to deal with problems that may arise in the course of family relationships.**

• Discuss current "family rules," identifying areas of needed change. **Rules may be imposed by adults, rather than through a democratic process involving all family members, leading to conflict and angry confrontations. Setting positive family rules with all family members participating can promote an effective, functional family.**

• Discuss need for long-term planning and ways in which family can maintain desired positive relationships. **Each stage of life brings its own challenges and understanding and preparing for each stage enables family members to move through them in positive ways, promoting family unity and resolving inevitable conflicts with win-win solutions.**

Documentation Focus

ASSESSMENT/REASSESSMENT

• Individual findings, including parenting skill level, parenting expectations, family makeup, and developmental stages.
• Availability/use of support systems and community resources.
• Motivation and expectations for change.

PLANNING

• Plan for enhancement, who is involved in planning.

IMPLEMENTATION/EVALUATION

• Family members' responses to interventions/teaching and actions performed.
• Attainment/progress toward desired outcome(s).
• Modifications to plan.

Information in brackets added by the authors to clarify and enhance the use of nursing diagnoses.

   Cultural   Collaborative   Community/Home Care

DISCHARGE PLANNING

- Long-range needs and who is responsible for actions to be taken.
- Modification to plan.

SAMPLE NURSING OUTCOMES & INTERVENTIONS CLASSIFICATIONS (NOC/NIC)

NOC—Parenting
NIC—Parenting Education: Childbearing Family

risk for impaired Parenting

Taxonomy II: Role Relationships—Class 1 Caregiving Roles (00057)
[Diagnostic Division: Social Interaction]
Submitted 1978; Nursing Diagnosis Extension and Classification (NDEC) Revision 1998

Definition: Rick for inability of the primary caretaker to create, maintain, or regain an environment that promotes the optimum growth and development of the child

[NOTE: It is important to reaffirm that adjustment to parenting in general is a normal maturational process that elicits nursing behaviors to prevent potential problems and to promote health.]

Risk Factors

INFANT OR CHILD

Altered perceptual abilities; attention deficit hyperactivity disorder
Difficult temperament; temperament conflicts with parental expectation
Premature birth; mulitple births; not gender desired
Handicapping condition; developmental delay
Illness; prolonged separation from parent

KNOWLEDGE

Unrealistic expectations of child; deficient knowledge about child development/health maintenance, parenting skills
Low educational level or attainment; lack of cognitive readiness for parenthood; low cognitive functioning

---

Information in brackets added by the authors to clarify and enhance the use of nursing diagnoses.

 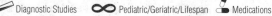

Poor communication skills
Inability to respond to infant cues
Preference for physical punishment

PHYSIOLOGICAL

Physical illness

PSYCHOLOGICAL

Young parental age
Closely spaced pregnancies; high number of pregnancies; difficult birthing process
Sleep disruption/deprivation
Depression; history of mental illness/substance abuse
Disability

SOCIAL

Stress; job problems; unemployment; financial difficulties; poor home environment; relocation
Situational/chronic low self-esteem
Lack of family cohesiveness; marital conflict; change in family unit; inadequate childcare arrangements
Role strain; single parent; father/mother of child not involved; parent-child separation
Poor/lack of parental role model; lack of valuing of parenthood
Unplanned/unwanted pregnancy; late/lack of prenatal care
Low socioeconomic class; poverty; lack of resources/access to resources; lack of transportation
Poor problem-solving skills; maladaptive coping strategies
Lack of social support network; social isolation
History of being abused/being abusive; legal difficulties

> NOTE: A risk diagnosis is not evidenced by signs and symptoms, as the problem has not occurred and nursing interventions are directed at prevention.

Desired Outcomes/Evaluation Criteria—Parents Will:

- Verbalize awareness of individual risk factors.
- Identify own strengths, individual needs, and methods/resources to meet them.
- Demonstrate behavior/lifestyle changes to reduce potential for development of problem or reduce/eliminate effects of risk factors.

Information in brackets added by the authors to clarify and enhance the use of nursing diagnoses.

  Cultural Collaborative 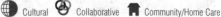 Community/Home Care

- Participate in activities, classes to promote growth.
- Refer to NDs impaired Parenting; risk for impaired parent/infant/child Attachment for interventions and documentation focus.

SAMPLE NURSING OUTCOMES & INTERVENTIONS CLASSIFICATIONS (NOC/NIC)

NOC—Parenting
NIC—Parenting Promotion

risk for Peripheral Neurovascular Dysfunction

Taxonomy II: Safety/Protection—Class 2 Physical Injury (00086)
[Diagnostic Division: Neurosensory]
Submitted 1992

Definition: At risk for disruption in circulation, sensation, or motion of an extremity

Risk Factors

Fractures; trauma; vascular obstruction
Mechanical compression (e.g., tourniquet, cane, cast, brace, dressing, restraint)
Orthopedic surgery; immobilization
Burns

> NOTE: A risk diagnosis is not evidenced by signs and symptoms, as the problem has not occurred and nursing interventions are directed at prevention.

Desired Outcomes/Evaluation Criteria—Client Will:

- Maintain function as evidenced by sensation/movement within normal range for the individual.
- Identify individual risk factors.
- Demonstrate/participate in behaviors and activities to prevent complications.
- Relate signs/symptoms that require medical reevaluation.

Information in brackets added by the authors to clarify and enhance the use of nursing diagnoses.

 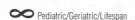

Actions/Interventions

NURSING PRIORITY NO. 1. To determine significance/degree of potential for compromise:

- Assess for individual risk factors: 1) trauma to extremity(ies) that cause internal tissue damage (e.g., high-velocity and penetrating trauma); fractures (especially long-bone fractures) with hemorrhage; or external pressures from burn eschar; 2) immobility (e.g., long-term bedrest, tight dressings, splints or casting); 3) presence of conditions affecting peripheral circulation, such as atherosclerosis, Raynaud's disease, or diabetes; and 4) smoking, obesity, and sedentary lifestyle **that potentiate risk of circulation insufficiency and occulusion.**
- Assess presence, location, and degree of swelling/edema formation. Measure affected extremity and compare with unaffected extremity.
- Monitor for tissue bleeding and spread of hematoma formation **that can compress blood vessels and raise compartment pressures.**
- Note position/location of casts, braces, traction apparatus **to ascertain potential for pressure on tissues**.
- Review recent/current drug regimen, noting use of anticoagulants and vasoactive agents.

NURSING PRIORITY NO. 2. To prevent deterioration/maximize circulation of affected limb(s):

- Perform neurovascular assessment in person immobilized for any reason (e.g., surgery, diabetic neuropathy, fractures) or individuals with suspected neruovascular problems. **Provides baseline for future comparisons.**
- Evaluate for differences between affected extremity and unaffected extremity, noting pain, pulses, pallor, parasthesia, paralysis, changes in motor/sensory function.
- Ask client to localize pain/discomfort and to report numbness and tingling or presence of pain with exercise or rest (atherosclerotic changes). (Refer to ND ineffective peripheral Tissue Perfusion, as appropriate.)
- Monitor presence/quality of peripheral pulse distal to injury or impairment via palpation/Doppler. **Occasionally a pulse may be palpated even though circulation is blocked by a soft clot through which pulsations may be felt; or perfusion through larger arteries may continue after increased compartment pressure has collapsed the arteriole/venule circulation in the muscle.**

Information in brackets added by the authors to clarify and enhance the use of nursing diagnoses.

 Cultural Collaborative Community/Home Care

- Assess capillary return, skin color, and warmth in the limb(s) at risk and compare with unaffected extremities. **Peripheral pulses, capillary refill, skin color, and sensation may be normal initially even in the presence of compartmental syndrome, because superficial circulation is usually not compromised.**
- Test sensation of peroneal nerve by pinch/pinprick in the dorsal web between first and second toe, and assess ability to dorsiflex toes if indicated (e.g., presence of leg fracture).
- Minimize edema formation/elevated tissue pressure:
  Remove jewelry from affected limb.
  Limit/avoid use of restraints. Pad limb and evaluate status frequently, if restraints are required.
  Observe position/location of supporting ring of splints/sling. Readjust, as indicated.
  Maintain elevation of injured extremity(ies), unless contraindicated by confirmed presence of compartment syndrome. **In presence of increased compartment pressure, elevation of extremity actually impedes arterial flow, decreasing perfusion.**
  Apply ice bags around injury/fracture site, as indicated, for initial 24 to 48 hours.
- Maximize circulation:
  Use techniques, such as repositioning/padding, **to relieve pressure.**
  Encourage client to routinely exercise digits/joints distal to injury. Encourage ambulation as soon as possible.
  Apply antiembolic hose/sequential pressure device, as indicated.
  Administer IV fluids, blood products, as needed, **to maintain circulating volume/tissue perfusion.**
  Administer anticoagulants, as indicated, **to prevent deep vein thrombosis (DVT)/treat thrombotic vascular obstructions.**
  Split/bivalve cast, reposition traction/restraints, as appropriate, **to release pressure.**
  Prepare for surgical intervention (e.g., fibulectomy/fasciotomy), as indicated, **to relieve pressure/restore circulation.**
- Monitor for development of complications:
  Inspect tissues around cast edges for rough places, pressure points. Investigate reports of "burning sensation" under cast.
  Evaluate for tenderness, swelling, pain on dorsiflexion of foot (positive Homans' sign).

Information in brackets added by the authors to clarify and enhance the use of nursing diagnoses.

Monitor Hb/Hct, coagulation studies (e.g., prothrombin time).

Investigate sudden signs of limb ischemia (e.g., decreased skin temperature, pallor, increased pain), reports of pain that are extreme for type of injury, increased pain on passive movement of extremity, development of paresthesia, muscle tension/tenderness with erythema, change in pulse quality distal to injury. Place limb in neutral position, avoiding elevation. Report symptoms to physician at once **to provide for timely intervention/limit severity of problem.**

Assist with measurements of/monitor intracompartmental pressures, as indicated. **Provides for early intervention/ evaluates effectiveness of therapy.**

NURSING PRIORITY NO. **3.** To promote wellness (Teaching/ Discharge Considerations):

- Review proper body alignment, elevation of limbs, as appropriate.
- Keep linens off affected extremity with bed cradle/cut-out box, as indicated.
- Discuss necessity of avoiding constrictive clothing, sharp angulation of legs/crossing legs.
- Demonstrate proper application of antiembolic hose.
- Review safe use of heat/cold therapy, as indicated.
- Instruct client/SO(s) to check shoes/socks for proper fit and/or wrinkles.
- Demonstrate/recommend continuation of exercises **to maintain function and circulation of limbs.**

Documentation Focus

ASSESSMENT/REASSESSMENT

- Specific risk factors, nature of injury to limb.
- Assessment findings, including comparison of affected/ unaffected limb, characteristics of pain in involved area.

PLANNING

- Plan of care and who is involved in the planning.
- Teaching plan.

IMPLEMENTATION/EVALUATION

- Response to interventions/teaching and actions performed.
- Attainment/progress toward desired outcome(s).
- Modification of plan of care.

Information in brackets added by the authors to clarify and enhance the use of nursing diagnoses.

 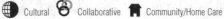 Cultural Collaborative Community/Home Care

- Long-term needs/referrals and who is responsible for actions to be taken.
- Specific referrals made.

SAMPLE NURSING OUTCOMES & INTERVENTIONS CLASSIFICATIONS (NOC/NIC)

NOC—Tissue Perfusion: Peripheral
NIC—Peripheral Sensation Management

risk for Poisoning

Taxonomy II: Safety/Protection—Class 4 Environmental Hazards (00037)
[Diagnostic Division: Safety]
Submitted 1980; Revised 2006

Definition: Accentuated risk of accidental exposure to, or ingestion of, drugs or dangerous products in doses sufficient to cause poisoning [or the adverse effects of prescribed medication/drug use]

Risk Factors

INTERNAL

Reduced vision
Lack of safety/drug education
Lack of proper precaution; [unsafe habits, disregard for safety measures, lack of supervision]
Verbalization that occupational setting is without adequate safeguards
Cognitive/emotional difficulties
[Age (e.g., young child, elderly person)]
[Chronic disease state, disability]
[Cultural or religious beliefs/practices]

EXTERNAL

Large supplies of drugs in house
Medicines stored in unlocked cabinets accessible to children/confused individuals
Availability of illicit drugs potentially contaminated by poisonous additives
Dangerous products placed within reach of children/confused individuals

---

Information in brackets added by the authors to clarify and enhance the use of nursing diagnoses.

[Therapeutic margin of safety of specific drugs (e.g., therapeutic versus toxic level, half-life, method of uptake and degradation in body, adequacy of organ function)]

[Use of multiple herbal supplements or megadosing]

> NOTE: A risk diagnosis is not evidenced by signs and symptoms, as the problem has not occurred and nursing interventions are directed at prevention.

Desired Outcomes/Evaluation Criteria—Client Will:

- Verbalize understanding of dangers of poisoning.
- Identify hazards that could lead to accidental poisoning.
- Correct external hazards as identified.
- Demonstrate necessary actions/lifestyle changes to promote safe environment.
- Refer to NDs Contamination; risk for Contamination for additional interventions related to poisoning associated with environmental contaminants.

Actions/Interventions

NURSING PRIORITY NO. 1. To assess causative/contributing factors:

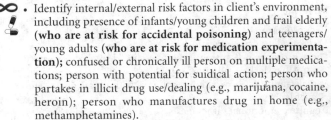

- Identify internal/external risk factors in client's environment, including presence of infants/young children and frail elderly **(who are at risk for accidental poisoning)** and teenagers/young adults **(who are at risk for medication experimentation);** confused or chronically ill person on multiple medications; person with potential for suicidal action; person who partakes in illicit drug use/dealing (e.g., marijuana, cocaine, heroin); person who manufactures drug in home (e.g., methamphetamines).

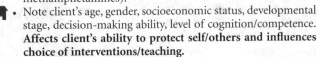

- Note client's age, gender, socioeconomic status, developmental stage, decision-making ability, level of cognition/competence. **Affects client's ability to protect self/others and influences choice of interventions/teaching.**
- Assess mood, coping abilities, personality styles (e.g., temperament, impulsive behavior, level of self-esteem) **that may result in carelessness/increased risk-taking without consideration of consequences.**
- Assess client's knowledge of safe use of drugs/herbal supplements, safety hazards in the environment, and ability to respond to potential threat.

Information in brackets added by the authors to clarify and enhance the use of nursing diagnoses.

 Cultural Collaborative Community/Home Care

- Review results of laboratory tests/toxicology screening, as indicated.

NURSING PRIORITY NO. 2. To assist in correcting factors that can lead to accidental poisoning:

- Discuss medication safety with client/SO(s) to:
  Prevent accidental ingestion:
  Stress importance of supervising infant/child, frail elderly, or individuals with cognitive limitations.
  Keep medicines and vitamins out of sight/reach of children or cognitively impaired persons.
  Use child-resistant/tamper-resistant caps and lock medication cabinets.
  Recap medication containers immediately after obtaining current dosage.
  Code medicines for the visually impaired.
  Administer children's medications as drugs, not candy.
- Prevent duplication/possible overdose:
  Keep updated list of all medications (prescription, OTC, herbals, supplements) and review with healthcare providers when medications are changed, new ones added, or new healthcare providers are consulted.
  Keep prescription medication in original bottle with label. Do not mix with other medication/place in unmarked containers.
  Have responsible SO(s)/home health nurse supervise medication regimen/prepare medications for the cognitively or visually impaired, or obtain prefilled medication box from pharmacy.
  Take prescription medications, as prescribed on label.
  Do not adjust medication dosage.
  Retain and read safety information that accompanies prescriptions about expected effects, minor side effects, reportable/adverse affects that require medical intervention, and how to manage forgotten dose.
- Prevent taking medications that interact with one another or OTC/herbals/other supplements in an undesired or dangerous manner:
  Keep list of/reveal medication allergies, including type of reaction to healthcare providers/pharmacist.
  Wear medical alert bracelet/necklace, as appropriate.
  Do not take outdated/expired medications. Do not save partial prescriptions to use another time.
  Encourage discarding outdated/unused drug safely (disposing in hazardous waste collection areas, not down drain/toilet).

Information in brackets added by the authors to clarify and enhance the use of nursing diagnoses.

 Diagnostic Studies ∞ Pediatric/Geriatric/Lifespan ⚕ Medications

Do not take medications prescribed for another person.

Coordinate care when multiple healthcare providers are involved to limit number of prescriptions/dosage levels.

NURSING PRIORITY NO. 3. To promote wellness (Teaching/Discharge Considerations):

- Review drug side effects/potential interactions with client/SO(s). Discuss use of OTC drugs/herbal supplements and possibilities of misuse, drug interactions, and overdosing as with vitamin megadosing, and so forth.

- Obtain lab tests (e.g., prothrombin time/INR for Coumadin; drug levels for dilantin, digoxin) at regular intervals **to ascertain that circulating blood levels are within therapeutic range.**

- Review periodic lab tests performed to monitor for adverse drug effect (e.g., liver function tests when lipid-lowering agents [statins] are prescribed, or renal/thyroid function and serum glucose levels for antimanics [lithium]).

- Discuss vitamins (especially those containing iron) that can be poisonous to children if taken in large doses.

- Review common analgesic safety (e.g., acetaminophen is an ingredient in many OTC medications and unintentional overdose can occur).

- Ask healthcare provider/pharmacist about any considered medications if pregnant, nursing, or planning to become pregnant **as some drugs are dangerous to fetus or nursing infant.**

- Provide list of emergency numbers (i.e., local/national poison control numbers, physician's office) to be placed by telephone **for use if poisoning occurs.**

- Encourage parent to place safety stickers on drugs/chemicals **to warn children of harmful contents.**

- Discuss use of ipecac syrup in home. **The use of ipecac is controversial as it may delay appropriate medical treatment (e.g., reduce the effectiveness of activated charcoal/oral antidotes) or be used inappropriately with adverse effects. Therefore, use in the home without direct advice from poison control professionals is not recommended.**

- Refer substance abuser to detoxification programs, inpatient/outpatient rehabilitation, counseling, support groups, and psychotherapy.

- Encourage emergency measures, awareness, and education (e.g., CPR/first aid class, community safety programs, ways to access emergency medical personnel).

- Institute community programs to assist individuals **to identify and correct risk factors in own environment.**

Information in brackets added by the authors to clarify and enhance the use of nursing diagnoses.

  Cultural Collaborative Community/Home Care

Documentation Focus

ASSESSMENT/REASSESSMENT

- Identified risk factors noting internal/external concerns.

PLANNING

- Plan of care and who is involved in the planning.
- Teaching plan.

IMPLEMENTATION/EVALUATION

- Response to interventions/teaching and actions performed.
- Attainment/progress toward desired outcome(s).
- Modification to plan of care.

DISCHARGE PLANNING

- Long-term needs and who is responsible for actions to be taken.
- Specific referrals made.

SAMPLE NURSING OUTCOMES & INTERVENTIONS CLASSIFICATIONS (NOC/NIC)

NOC—Risk Control: Drug Use
NIC—Medication Management

Post-Trauma Syndrome
[Specify Stage]

Taxonomy II: Coping/Stress Tolerance—Class 1 Post-Trauma Responses (00141)
[Diagnostic Division: Ego Integrity]
Submitted 1986; Nursing Diagnosis Extension and Classification (NDEC) Revision 1998

Definition: Sustained maladaptive response to a traumatic, overwhelming event

Related Factors

Events outside the range of usual human experience
Serious threat to self/loved ones
Serious injury to self/loved ones; serious accidents (e.g., industrial, motor-vehicle)
Abuse (physical and psychosocial); criminal victimization; rape
Witnessing mutilation/violent death; tragic occurrence involving multiple deaths

---

Information in brackets added by the authors to clarify and enhance the use of nursing diagnoses.

 Diagnostic Studies 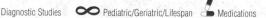 Pediatric/Geriatric/Lifespan Medications

Disasters; sudden destruction of one's home/community; epidemics

Wars; being held prisoner of war; torture

Defining Characteristics

SUBJECTIVE

Intrusive thoughts/dreams; nightmares; flashbacks; [excessive verbalization of the traumatic event]

Palpitations; headaches; [loss of interest in usual activities, loss of feeling of intimacy/sexuality]

Hopelessness; shame; guilt; [verbalization of survival guilt or guilt about behavior required for survival]

Anxiety; fear; grieving; depression

Reports feeling numb

Gastric irritability; [change in appetite; sleep disturbance/insomnia; chronic fatigue/easy fatigability]

Difficulty in concentrating

OBJECTIVE

Hypervigilance; exaggerated startle response; irritability; neurosensory irritability

Anger; rage; aggression

Avoidance; repression; alienation; denial; detachment; psychogenic amnesia

Altered mood states; [poor impulse control/explosiveness]; panic attacks; horror

Substance abuse; compulsive behavior

Enuresis (in children)

[Difficulty with interpersonal relationships; dependence on others; work/school failure]

[Stages:

ACUTE: Begins within 6 months and does not last longer than 6 months.

CHRONIC: Lasts more than 6 months.

DELAYED ONSET: Period of latency of 6 months or more before onset of symptoms.]

Desired Outcomes/Evaluation
Criteria—Client Will:

- Express own feelings/reactions, avoiding projection.
- Verbalize a positive self-image.
- Report reduced anxiety/fear when memories occur.

Information in brackets added by the authors to clarify and enhance the use of nursing diagnoses.

 Cultural Collaborative Community/Home Care

- Demonstrate ability to deal with emotional reactions in an individually appropriate manner.
- Demonstrate appropriate changes in behavior/lifestyle (e.g., share experiences with others, seek/get support from SO[s] as needed, change in job/residence).
- Report absence of physical manifestations (such as pain, chronic fatigue).
- Refer to ND Rape-Trauma Syndrome for additional outcomes when trauma is the result of rape.

Actions/Interventions

NURSING PRIORITY NO. 1. To assess causative factor(s) and individual reaction:

ACUTE

- Observe for and elicit information about physical or psychological injury and note associated stress-related symptoms (e.g., "numbness," headache, tightness in chest, nausea, pounding heart).
- Identify psychological responses: anger, shock, acute anxiety, confusion, denial. Note laughter, crying, calm or agitated/excited (hysterical) behavior, expressions of disbelief, guilt/self-blame, labile emotions.
- Assess client's knowledge of and anxiety related to the situation. Note ongoing threat to self (e.g., contact with perpetrator and/or associates).
- Identify social aspects of trauma/incident (e.g., disfigurement, chronic conditions/permanent disabilities, loss of home or community).
- Ascertain ethnic background/cultural and religious perceptions and beliefs about the occurrence (e.g., retribution from God).
- Determine degree of disorganization (e.g., task-oriented activity is not goal directed, organized, or effective; individual is overwhelmed by emotion most of the time).
- Identify whether incident has reactivated preexisting or coexisting situations (physical/psychological). **Affects how the client views the trauma.**
- Determine disruptions in relationships (e.g., family, friends, coworkers, SOs). **Support persons may not know how to deal with client/situation (e.g., may be oversolicitous or withdraw).**
- Note withdrawn behavior, use of denial, and use of chemical substances or impulsive behaviors (e.g., chain-smoking, overeating).

Information in brackets added by the authors to clarify and enhance the use of nursing diagnoses.

• Be aware of signs of increasing anxiety (e.g., silence, stuttering, inability to sit still). **Increasing anxiety may indicate risk for violence.**

 • Note verbal/nonverbal expressions of guilt or self-blame when client has survived trauma in which others died. Validate congruency of observations with verbalizations.

 • Assess signs/stage of grieving for self and others.

 • Identify development of phobic reactions to ordinary articles (e.g., knives); situations (e.g., walking in groups of people, strangers ringing doorbell).

CHRONIC (IN ADDITION TO ABOVE)

 • Evaluate continued somatic complaints (e.g., gastric irritation, anorexia, insomnia, muscle tension, headache). Investigate reports of new/changes in symptoms.

 • Note manifestations of chronic pain or pain symptoms in excess of degree of physical injury.

 • Be aware of signs of severe/prolonged depression. Note presence of flashbacks, intrusive memories, nightmares; panic attacks; poor impulse control; problems with memory/concentration, thoughts/perceptions; and conflict/aggression/rage.

 • Assess degree of dysfunctional coping (e.g., use of alcohol/other drugs/substance abuse; suicidal/homicidal ideation) and consequences.

NURSING PRIORITY NO. 2. To assist client to deal with situation that exists:

ACUTE

• Provide a calm, safe environment. **Promotes sense of trust and safety.**

• Assist with documentation for police report, as indicated, and stay with the client.

• Listen to/investigate physical complaints. **Emotional reactions may limit client's ability to recognize physical injury.**

 • Identify supportive persons for the individual (e.g., loved ones, counselor, spiritual advisor/pastor).

• Remain with client, listen as client recounts incident/concerns—possibly repeatedly. (If client does not want to talk, accept silence.) **Provides psychological support.**

• Provide environment in which client can talk freely about feelings, fear (including concerns about relationship with/response of SO), and experiences/sensations (e.g., loss of control, "near-death experience").

Information in brackets added by the authors to clarify and enhance the use of nursing diagnoses.

  Cultural 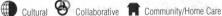 Collaborative Community/Home Care

- Help child to express feelings about event using techniques appropriate to developmental level (e.g., play for young child, stories/puppets for preschooler, peer group for adolescent). **Children are more likely to express in play what they may not be able to verbalize directly.**
- Assist with practical realities (e.g., temporary housing, money, notifications of family members, or other needs).
- Be aware of and assist client to use ego strengths in a positive way by acknowledging ability to handle what is happening. **Enhances self-concept, supports self-esteem, and reduces sense of helplessness.**
- Allow the client to work through own kind of adjustment. If the client is withdrawn or unwilling to talk, do not force the issue.
- Listen for expressions of fear of crowds and/or people.
- Administer anti-anxiety or sedative/hypnotic medications with caution.

CHRONIC

- Continue listening to expressions of concern. May need to continue to talk about the incident.
- Permit free expression of feelings (may continue from the crisis phase). Avoid rushing client through expressions of feelings too quickly and refrain from providing reassurance inappropriately. **Client may believe pain and/or anguish is misunderstood and may be depressed. Statements such as "You don't understand" or "You weren't there" are a defense, a way of pushing others away.**
- Encourage client to talk out experience when ready, expressing feelings of fear, anger, loss/grief. (Refer to ND complicated Grieving.)
- Ascertain/monitor sleep pattern of children as well as adults. **Sleep disturbances/nightmares may develop, delaying resolution, impairing coping abilities.**
- Encourage client to become aware of and accept own feelings and reactions as being normal reactions in an abnormal situation.
- Acknowledge reality of loss of self that existed before the incident. Help client to move toward a state of acceptance as to the potential for growth that still exists within client.
- Continue to allow client to progress at own pace.
- Give "permission" to express/deal with anger at the assailant/situation in acceptable ways.
- Avoid prompting discussion of issues that cannot be resolved. Keep discussion on practical and emotional level rather than

---

Information in brackets added by the authors to clarify and enhance the use of nursing diagnoses.

intellectualizing the experience, **which allows client to deal with reality while taking time to work out feelings.**

* Assist in dealing with practical concerns and effects of the incident, such as court appearances, altered relationships with SO(s), employment problems.
* Provide for sensitive, trained counselors/therapists and engage in therapies, such as psychotherapy, Implosive Therapy (flooding), hypnosis, relaxation, rolfing, memory work, cognitive restructuring, Eye Movement Desensitization and Reprocessing (EMDR), physical and occupational therapies.
* Administer psychotropic medications, as indicated.

NURSING PRIORITY NO. 3. To promote wellness (Teaching/Discharge Considerations):

* Assist client to identify and monitor feelings while therapy is occurring.
* Provide information about what reactions client may expect during each phase. **Helps reduce fear of the unknown.** Let client know these are common reactions. Be sure to phrase in neutral terms of "You may or you may not..."
* Assist client to identify factors that may have created a vulnerable situation and that he or she may have power to change **to protect self in the future.**
* Avoid making value judgments.
* Discuss lifestyle changes client is contemplating and how they may contribute to recovery. **Helps client evaluate appropriateness of plans and identify shortcomings (e.g., moving away from effective support group).**
* Assist client to learn stress-management techniques.
* Discuss drug regimen, potential side effects of prescribed medications, and necessity of prompt reporting of untoward effects.
* Discuss recognition of, and ways to manage, "anniversary reactions," reinforcing normalcy of recurrence of thoughts and feelings at this time.
* Suggest support group for SO(s) **to assist with understanding and ways to deal with client.**
* Encourage psychiatric consultation, especially if client is unable to maintain control, is violent, is inconsolable, or does not seem to be making an adjustment.
* Refer for long-term individual/family/marital counseling, if indicated.
* Refer to NDs Powerlessness; ineffective Coping; Grieving; complicated Grieving.

Information in brackets added by the authors to clarify and enhance the use of nursing diagnoses.

  Cultural 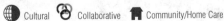 Collaborative 🏠 Community/Home Care

Documentation Focus

ASSESSMENT/REASSESSMENT

- Individual findings, noting current dysfunction and behavioral/emotional responses to the incident.
- Specifics of traumatic event.
- Reactions of family/SO(s).
- Availability/use of resources.

PLANNING

- Plan of care and who is involved in the planning.
- Teaching plan.

IMPLEMENTATION/EVALUATION

- Responses to interventions/teaching and actions performed.
- Emotional changes.
- Attainment/progress toward desired outcome(s).
- Modifications to plan of care.

DISCHARGE PLANNING

- Long-term needs and who is responsible for actions to be taken.
- Specific referrals mades.

SAMPLE NURSING OUTCOMES & INTERVENTIONS CLASSIFICATIONS (NOC/NIC)

NOC—Fear Control
NIC—Support System Enhancement

risk for Post-Trauma Syndrome

Taxonomy II: Coping/Stress Tolerance—Class 1 Post-Trauma Responses (00145)
[Diagnostic Division: Ego Integrity]
Submitted 1998; Nursing Diagnosis Extension and Classification (NDEC) Submission 1998

Definition: At risk for sustained maladaptive response to a traumatic, overwhelming event

Risk Factors

Occupation (e.g., police, fire, rescue, corrections, emergency room staff, mental health worker, [and their family members])

Information in brackets added by the authors to clarify and enhance the use of nursing diagnoses.

 Diagnostic Studies   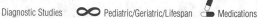 Pediatric/Geriatric/Lifespan   Medications

Perception of event; exaggerated sense of responsibility; diminished ego strength

Survivor's role in the event

Inadequate social support; nonsupportive environment; displacement from home

Duration of the event

> NOTE: A risk diagnosis is not evidenced by signs and symptoms, as the problem has not occurred and nursing interventions are directed at prevention.

Desired Outcomes/Evaluation Criteria—Client Will:

- Verbalize absence of severe anxiety.
- Demonstrate ability to deal with emotional reactions in an individually appropriate manner.
- Report relief/absence of physical manifestations (pain, nightmares/flashbacks, fatigue) associated with event.

Actions/Interventions

NURSING PRIORITY NO. 1. To assess contributing factors and individual reaction:

- Identify client who survived or witnessed traumatic event (e.g, airplane/motor vehicle crash, mass shooting, fire destroying home and lands, robbery at gunpoint/other violent act) **to recognize individual at high-risk for post-trauma syndrome**.
- Note occupation (e.g., police, fire, emergency services personnel/rescue workers, soldiers and support personnel in combat areas, etc.), as listed in Risk Factors. **Studies reveal a moderate to high percentage of post-traumatic stress disorders develop in these populations when they have been exposed to one or more traumatic incidents.**
- Assess client's knowledge of and anxiety related to potential for work-related trauma (e.g., shooting in line of duty, or viewing body of murdered child); and number, duration, and intensity of recurring situations (e.g., EMT exposed to numerous on-the-job traumatic incidents; rescuers searching for victims of natural or man-made disasters).
- Identify how client's past experiences may affect current situation.
- Listen for comments of guilt, humiliation, shame, or taking on responsibility (e.g., "I should have been more careful/gone

---

Information in brackets added by the authors to clarify and enhance the use of nursing diagnoses.

 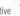

back to get her"; "Don't call me a hero, I couldn't save my partner"; "My kids are the same age as the ones that died").

🏠 • Evaluate for life factors/stressors currently or recently occurring, such as displacement from home due to catastrophic event (e.g., fire/flood/violent storm) happening to individual whose child is dying with cancer, or who suffered abuse as a child. **This individual is at greater risk for developing traumatic symptoms (acute added to delayed onset reactions).**

🏠 • Identify client's general health and coping mechanisms.

🏠 • Determine availability/usefulness of client's support systems, family, social, community, etc. (Note: Family members can also be at risk.)

NURSING PRIORITY NO. 2. To assist client to deal with situation that exists:

🏠 • Educate high-risk persons/families about signs/symptoms of post-trauma response, especially if it is likely to occur in their occupation/life.

🏠 • Identify and discuss client's strengths (e.g., very supportive family, usually copes well with stress, etc.) as well as vulnerabilities (e.g., client tends toward alcohol/other drugs for coping, client has witnessed a murder).

🏠 • Discuss how individual coping mechanisms have worked in past traumatic events. **Client/SO(s) may be able to employ previously successful strategies to deal with current incident.**

🏠 • Evaluate client's perceptions of events and personal significance (e.g., policeman/parent investigating death of a child).

🏠 • Provide emotional and physical presence **to strengthen client's coping abilities.**

🏠 • Encourage expression of feelings and reinforce that feelings/reactions to trauma are common, and not indicators of weakness or failure. Note whether feelings expressed appear congruent with events the client experienced. **Incongruency may indicate deeper conflict and can impede resolution.**

🏠 • Observe for signs and symptoms of stress responses, such as nightmares, reliving an incident, poor appetite, irritability, numbness and crying, family/relationship disruption. **These responses are normal in the early post-incident time frame. If prolonged and persistent, the client may be experiencing post-traumatic stress disorder.**

Information in brackets added by the authors to clarify and enhance the use of nursing diagnoses.

NURSING PRIORITY NO. 3. To promote wellness (Teaching/Discharge Considerations):

• Provide a calm, safe environment **in which client can deal with disruption of life.**

• Encourage client to identify and monitor feelings on an ongoing basis. **Promotes awareness of changes in ability to deal with stressors.**

• Encourage learning stress-management techniques **to help with resolution of situation.**

• Recommend participation in debriefing sessions that may be provided following major events. **Dealing with the stressor promptly may facilitate recovery from event/prevent exacerbation, although issues about best timing of debriefing continue to be debated.**

• Explain that post-traumatic symptoms can emerge months or sometimes years after a traumatic expeirence and that help/support can be obtained when needed/desired if client begins to experience intrusive memories/other symptoms.

• Identify employment, community resource groups (e.g., Assistance Support and Self Help in Surviving Trauma [ASSIST], employee peer assistance programs; Red Cross/other victim support services, Compasionate Friends). **Provides opportunity for ongoing support to deal with recurrent stressors.**

• Refer for individual/family counseling, as indicated.

Documentation Focus

ASSESSMENT/REASSESSMENT

• Identified risk factors noting internal/external concerns.
• Client's perception of event and personal significance.

PLANNING

• Plan of care and who is involved in the planning.
• Teaching plan.

IMPLEMENTATION/EVALUATION

• Response to interventions/teaching and actions performed.
• Attainment/progress toward desired outcome(s).

DISCHARGE PLANNING

• Long-term needs and who is responsible for actions to be taken.
• Specific referrals made.

Information in brackets added by the authors to clarify and enhance the use of nursing diagnoses.

 Cultural Collaborative Community/Home Care

SAMPLE NURSING OUTCOMES & INTERVENTIONS CLASSIFICATIONS (NOC/NIC)

NOC—Grief Resolution
NIC—Crisis Intervention

readiness for enhanced Power

Taxonomy II: Self-Perception—Class 1 Self-Concept (00187)
[Diagnostic Divisions: Ego Integrity]
Submitted 2006

Definition: A pattern of participating knowingly in change that is sufficient for well-being and can be strengthened

Related Factors

To be developed

Defining Characteristics

SUBJECTIVE

Expresses readiness to enhance power; knowledge for participation in change; awareness of possible changes to be made; identification of choices that can be made for change

Expresses readiness to enhance freedom; need to perform actions for change; involvement in creating change; participation in choices for daily living and health

---

NOTE: Even though power (a response) and empowerment (an intervention approach) are different concepts, the literature related to both concepts supports the defining characteristics of this diagnosis.

Desired Outcomes/Evaluation Criteria—Client Will:

- Verbalize knowledge of what changes he or she wants to make.
- Express awareness of own ability to be in charge of changes to be made.
- Participate in classes/group activities to learn new skills.
- State readiness to take power over own life.

Information in brackets added by the authors to clarify and enhance the use of nursing diagnoses.

 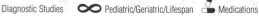

Actions/Interventions

NURSING PRIORITY NO. 1. To determine need/motivation for improvement:

- Determine current situation and circumstances that client is experiencing leading to desire to improve life.
- Ascertain motivation and expectations for change.
- Identify emotional climate in which client and relationships live and work. **The emotional climate has a great impact between people. When a power differential exists in relationships, the atmosphere is largely determined by the person or people who have the power.**
- Identify client locus of control: internal (expressions of responsibility for self and ability to control outcomes) or external (expressions of lack of control over self and environment). **Understanding locus of control can help client work toward positive, internal control as he or she develops ability to freely choose own actions.**
- 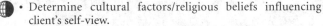 Determine cultural factors/religious beliefs influencing client's self-view.
- Assess degree of mastery client has exhibited in his or her life. **Helps client to understand how he or she has functioned in the past and what is needed to improve.**
- Note presence of family/SO(s) that can, or do, act as support systems for client.
- Determine whether client knows and/or uses assertiveness skills.

NURSING PRIORITY NO. 2. To assist client to clarify needs relative to ability to improve feelings of power:

- Discuss needs and how client is meeting them at this time.
- Listen/active-listen to client's perceptions and beliefs about how power can be gained in his or her life.
- Identify strengths/assets and past coping strategies that were successful and can be built on **to enhance feelings of control.**
- Discuss the importance of assuming personal responsibility for life and relationships. This requires one to be open to new ideas and experiences and different values and beliefs and to be inquisitive.
- Identify things client can and/or cannot control. **Avoids wasting time on things that are not in the control of the client.**
- Treat expressed desires and decisions with respect. Avoid critical parenting expressions.

NURSING PRIORITY NO. 3. To promote optimum wellness, enhancing power (Teaching/Discharge Considerations):

Information in brackets added by the authors to clarify and enhance the use of nursing diagnoses.

- Assist client to set realistic goals for the future.
- Provide accurate verbal and written information about what is happening and discuss with client. **Reinforces learning and promotes self-paced review.**
- Assist client to learn/use assertive communication skills. **These techniques require practice, but as the client becomes more proficient they will help client to develop more effective relationships.**
- Use "I-messages" instead of "You-messages." **"I-messages" acknowledge ownership of what is said, while "You-messages" suggest the other person is wrong or bad, fostering resentment and resistance instead of understanding and cooperation.**
- Discuss importance of client paying attention to nonverbal communication. **Messages are often confusing/misinterpreted when verbal and nonverbal communications are not congruent.**
- Help client learn to problem solve differences. **Promotes win-win solutions.**
- Instruct and encourage use of stress-reduction techniques.
- Refer to support groups/classes, as indicated (assertiveness training, effectiveness for women, "Be your Best")

Documentation Focus

ASSESSMENT/REASSESSMENT

- Individual findings, noting determination to improve sense of power, locus of control.
- Motivation and expectations for change.

PLANNING

- Plan of care/interventions and who is involved in planning.
- Teaching plan.

IMPLEMENTATION/EVALUATION

- Client's responses to interventions/teaching and actions performed.
- Attainment/progress toward desired outcome(s).
- Modifications to plan of care.

DISCHARGE PLANNING

- Long-term needs and who is responsible for actions to be taken.
- Specific referrals made.

Information in brackets added by the authors to clarify and enhance the use of nursing diagnoses.

 Diagnostic Studies   ∞ Pediatric/Geriatric/Lifespan   Medications   **539**

SAMPLE NURSING OUTCOMES & INTERVENTIONS CLASSIFICATIONS (NOC/NIC)

NOC—Health Beliefs: Perceived Control
NIC—Self-Responsibility Facilitation

Powerlessness
[Specify Level]

Taxonomy II: Self-Perception—Class 1 Self-Concept (00125)
[Diagnostic Division: Ego Integrity]
Submitted 1982

Definition: Perception that one's own action will not significantly affect an outcome; a perceived lack of control over a current situation or immediate happening

Related Factors

Healthcare environment [e.g., loss of privacy, personal possessions, control over therapies]
Interpersonal interaction [e.g., misuse of power, force; abusive relationships]
Illness-related regimen [e.g., chronic/debilitating conditions]
Lifestyle of helplessness [e.g., repeated failures, dependency]

Defining Characteristics

SUBJECTIVE

Low
Expressions of uncertainty about fluctuating energy levels

Moderate
Expressions of dissatisfaction/frustration over inability to perform previous tasks/activities
Expressions of doubt regarding role performance
Fear of alienation from caregivers
Reluctance to express true feelings; resentment; anger; guilt

Severe
Verbal expressions of having no control (e.g., over self-care, situation, outcome)
Depression over physical deterioration

OBJECTIVE

Low
Passivity

Information in brackets added by the authors to clarify and enhance the use of nursing diagnoses.

   Cultural   Collaborative   Community/Home Care

Moderate

Dependence on others that may result in irritability

Inability to seek information regarding care

Passivity

Nonparticipation in care/decision making when opportunities are provided; does not monitor progress

Does not defend self-care practices when challenged

Severe

Apathy [withdrawal, resignation, crying]

Desired Outcomes/Evaluation Criteria—Client Will:

- Express sense of control over the present situation and future outcome.
- Make choices related to and be involved in care.
- Identify areas over which individual has control.
- Acknowledge reality that some areas are beyond individual's control.

Actions/Interventions

NURSING PRIORITY NO. 1. To assess causative/contributing factors:

- Identify situational circumstances (e.g., strange environment, immobility, diagnosis of terminal/chronic illness, lack of support system, lack of knowledge about situation).
- Determine client's perception/knowledge of condition and treatment plan.
- Ascertain client response to treatment regimen. Does client see reason(s) and understand it is in the client's best interest or is client compliant and helpless?
- Identify client locus of control: internal (expressions of responsibility for self and ability to control outcomes—"I didn't quit smoking") or external (expressions of lack of control over self and environment—"Nothing ever works out"; "What bad luck to get lung cancer").
- Note cultural factors/religious beliefs that may contribute to how client is handling the situation.
- Assess degree of mastery client has exhibited in life. **Passive individual may have more difficulty being assertive and standing up for rights.**
- Determine if there has been a change in relationships with SO(s). **Conflict in the family, loss of a family member, or divorce can contribute to feelings of powerlessness and lack of ability to manage situation.**

Information in brackets added by the authors to clarify and enhance the use of nursing diagnoses.

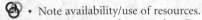

- Note availability/use of resources.
- Investigate caregiver practices. Do they support client control/responsibility?

NURSING PRIORITY NO. 2. To assess degree of powerlessness experienced by client:

- Listen to statements client makes: "They don't care"; "It won't make any difference"; "Are you kidding?"
- Note expressions that indicate "giving up," such as "It won't do any good."
- Note behavioral responses (verbal and nonverbal) including expressions of fear, interest or apathy, agitation, withdrawal.
- Note lack of communication, flat affect, and lack of eye contact.
- Identify the use of manipulative behavior and reactions of client and caregivers. **Manipulation is used for management of powerlessness because of distrust of others, fear of intimacy, search for approval, and validation of sexuality.**

NURSING PRIORITY NO. 3. To assist client to clarify needs relative to ability to meet them:

- Show concern for client as a person.
- Make time to listen to client's perceptions and concerns and encourage questions.
- Accept expressions of feelings, including anger and hopelessness.
- Avoid arguing or using logic with hopeless client. **Client will not believe it can make a difference.**
- Deal with manipulative behavior by being straightforward and honest with your communication and letting client know that this is a better way to get needs met.
- Express hope for the client. (**There is always hope of something.**)
- Identify strengths/assets and past coping strategies that were successful. **Helps client to recognize own ability to deal with difficult situation.**
- Assist client to identify what he or she can do for self. Identify things the client can/cannot control.
- Encourage client to maintain a sense of perspective about the situation.

NURSING PRIORITY NO. 4. To promote independence:

- Use client's locus of control to develop individual plan of care (e.g., for client with internal control, encourage client to take control of own care and for those with external control, begin with small tasks and add, as tolerated).

Information in brackets added by the authors to clarify and enhance the use of nursing diagnoses.

  Cultural Collaborative Community/Home Care

- Develop contract with client specifying goals agreed on. **Enhances commitment to plan, optimizing outcomes.**
- Treat expressed decisions and desires with respect. Avoid critical parenting behaviors and communications.
- Provide client opportunities to control as many events as energy and restrictions of care permit.
- Discuss needs openly with client and set up agreed-on routines for meeting identified needs. **Minimizes use of manipulation.**
- Minimize rules and limit continuous observation to the degree that safety permits **to provide sense of control for the client.**
- Support client efforts to develop realistic steps to put plan into action, reach goals, and maintain expectations.
- Provide positive reinforcement for desired behaviors.
- Direct client's thoughts beyond present state to future when appropriate.
- Schedule frequent brief visits to check on client, deal with client needs, and let client know someone is available.
- Involve SO(s) in client care as appropriate.

NURSING PRIORITY NO. 5. To promote wellness (Teaching/Discharge Considerations):

- Instruct in/encourage use of anxiety and stress-reduction techniques.
- Provide accurate verbal and written information about what is happening and discuss with client/SO(s). Repeat as often as necessary.
- Assist client to set realistic goals for the future.
- Assist client to learn/use assertive communication skills. **Use of I-messages, active-listening, and problem solving encourages client to be more in control of own life.**
- Refer to occupational therapist/vocational counselor, as indicated. **Facilitates return to a productive role in whatever capacity possible for the individual.**
- Encourage client to think productively and positively and take responsibility for choosing own thoughts.
- Problem solve with client/SO(s). **Outcome is more likely to be accepted when arrived at by all parties involved.**
- Suggest periodic review of own needs/goals.
- Refer to support groups, counseling/therapy, and so forth, as indicated.

Documentation Focus

ASSESSMENT/REASSESSMENT

- Individual findings, noting degree of powerlessness, locus of control, individual's perception of the situation.

Information in brackets added by the authors to clarify and enhance the use of nursing diagnoses.

- Specific culteral/religious factors.
- Availability/use of support system and resources.

PLANNING

- Plan of care and who is involved in the planning.
- Teaching plan.

IMPLEMENTATION/EVALUATION

- Responses to interventions/teaching and actions performed.
- Specific goals/expectations.
- Attainment/progress toward desired outcome(s).
- Modifications to plan of care.

DISCHARGE PLANNING

- Long-term needs and who is responsible for actions to be taken.
- Specific referrals made.

SAMPLE NURSING OUTCOMES & INTERVENTIONS CLASSIFICATIONS (NOC/NIC)

NOC—Health Beliefs: Perceived Control
NIC—Self-Responsibility Facilitation

risk for Powerlessness

Taxonomy II: Self-Perception—Class 1 Self-Concept (00125)
[Diagnostic Division: Ego Integrity]
Submitted 2000

Definition: At risk for perceived lack of control over a situation and/or one's ability to significantly affect an outcome

Risk Factors

PHYSIOLOGICAL

Illness [hospitalization, intubation, ventilator, suctioning]; dying
Acute injury; progressive debilitating disease process (e.g., spinal cord injury, multiple sclerosis)
Aging [e.g., decreased physical strength, decreased mobility]

PSYCHOSOCIAL

Deficient knowledge (e.g., of illness or healthcare system)
Lifestyle of dependency

Information in brackets added by the authors to clarify and enhance the use of nursing diagnoses.

Inadequate coping patterns
Absence of integrality (e.g., essence of power)
Situational/chronic low self-esteem; disturbed body image

> NOTE: A risk diagnosis is not evidenced by signs and symptoms, as the problem has not occurred and nursing interventions are directed at prevention.

Desired Outcomes/Evaluation Criteria—Client Will:

- Express sense of control over the present situation and hopefulness about future outcomes.
- Verbalize positive self-appraisal in current situation.
- Make choices related to and be involved in care.
- Identify areas over which individual has control.
- Acknowledge reality that some areas are beyond individual's control.

Actions/Interventions

NURSING PRIORITY NO. 1. To assess causative/contributing factors:

- Identify situational circumstances (e.g., acute illness, sudden hospitalization, diagnosis of terminal or debilitating/chronic illness, very young or aging with decreased physical strength and mobility, lack of knowledge about illness/healthcare system).
- Determine client's perception/knowledge of condition and proposed treatment plan.
- Identify client's locus of control: internal (expressions of responsibility for self and environment) or external (expressions of lack of control over self and environment). **May affect willingness to accept responsibility to manage situation.**
- Assess client's self-esteem and degree of mastery client has exhibited in life situations. **Passive individual may have more difficulty being assertive and standing up for rights.**
- Determine associated cultural values/religious beliefs impacting self-view.
- Note availability and use of resources.
- Listen to statements client makes (e.g., "They can't really help"; "It probably won't make a difference"). **Suggests concerns regarding own power/ability to control situation.**
- Determine congruency of responses (verbal and nonverbal) and note expressions of fear, disinterest or apathy, or withdrawal.

Information in brackets added by the authors to clarify and enhance the use of nursing diagnoses.

- Be alert for signs of manipulative behavior and note reactions of client and caregivers. **Manipulation may be used for management of powerlessness because of fear and distrust.**

NURSING PRIORITY NO. 2. To assist client to clarify needs and ability to meet them:

- Make time to listen to client's perceptions of the situation. **Shows concern for client as a person.**
- Encourage questions.
- Accept expressions of feelings, including anger and reluctance, to try to work things out. **Being able to express feelings freely enables client to sort out what is happening and come to a positive conclusion.**
- Express hope for client and encourage review of past experiences with successful strategies.
- Assist client to identify what he or she can do to help self and what situations can/cannot be controlled.

NURSING PRIORITY NO. 3. To promote wellness (Teaching/ Discharge Considerations):

- Encourage client to think productively and positively and take responsibility for choosing own thoughts and reactions. **Can enhance feelings of power and sense of positive self-esteem.**
- Provide accurate verbal and written instructions about what is happening and what realistically might happen. **Reinforces learning and promotes self-paced review.**
- Involve client/SO(s) in planning process and problem solve using client's locus of control (e.g., for client with internal control, encourage client to take control of own care and for those with external control, begin with small tasks and add, as tolerated).
- Support client efforts to develop realistic steps to put plan into action, reach goals, and maintain expectations.
- Identify resource books/classes for assertiveness training and stress-reduction, as appropriate.
- Encourage client to be active in long-term healthcare management and engage in periodic review of own needs/goals.
- Refer to support groups for chronic conditions/disability (e.g., MS Society, Easter Seals, Alzheimer's, Al-Anon) or counseling/therapy, as appropriate.

Documentation Focus

ASSESSMENT/REASSESSMENT

- Individual findings, noting potential for powerlessness, locus of control, individual's perception of the situation.

Information in brackets added by the authors to clarify and enhance the use of nursing diagnoses.

  Cultural Collaborative ⌂ Community/Home Care

- Cultural values/religious beliefs.
- Availability/use of resources.

PLANNING

- Plan of care and who is involved in the planning.
- Teaching plan.

IMPLEMENTATION/EVALUATION

- Responses to interventions/teaching and actions performed.
- Specific goals/expectations.
- Modifications to plan of care.

DISCHARGE PLANNING

- Long-term needs and who is responsible for actions to be taken.
- Specific referrals made.

SAMPLE NURSING OUTCOMES & INTERVENTIONS CLASSIFICATIONS (NOC/NIC)

NOC—Health Beliefs: Perceived Control
NIC—Self-Responsibility Facilitation

ineffective Protection

Taxonomy II: Safety/Protection—Class 2 Physical Injury (00043)
[Diagnostic Division: Safety]
Submitted 1990

Definition: Decrease in the ability to guard self from internal or external threats such as illness or injury

Related Factors

Extremes of age
Inadequate nutrition
Alcohol abuse
Abnormal blood profiles (e.g., leukopenia, thrombocytopenia, anemia, coagulation)
Drug therapies (e.g., antineoplastic, corticosteroid, immune, anticoagulant, thrombolytic)
Treatments (e.g., surgery, radiation)
Cancer; immune disorders

Information in brackets added by the authors to clarify and enhance the use of nursing diagnoses.

 Diagnostic Studies 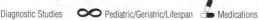 Pediatric/Geriatric/Lifespan   Medications

Defining Characteristics

SUBJECTIVE

Neurosensory alterations
Chilling
Itching
Insomnia; fatigue; weakness
Anorexia

OBJECTIVE

Deficient immunity
Impaired healing; altered clotting
Maladaptive stress response
Perspiring [inappropriately]
Dyspnea; cough
Restlessness; immobility
Disorientation
Pressure sores

NOTE: The purpose of this diagnosis seems to combine multiple NDs under a single heading for ease of planning care when a number of variables may be present. Outcomes/evaluation criteria and interventions are specifically tied to individual related factors that are present, such as:

EXTREMES OF AGE: Concerns may include body temperature/thermoregulation; memory or thought process/sensory-perceptual alterations, as well as impaired mobility, risk for falls, sedentary lifestyle, self-care deficits; risk for trauma, suffocation, or poisoning; risk for skin/tissue integrity; and fluid volume imbalances.

INADEQUATE NUTRITION: Brings up issues of nutrition (less or more than body requirements), risk for unstable blood glucose; risk for infection, delayed surgical recovery; impaired swallowing; disturbed thought processes, impaired skin/tissue integrity; trauma, ineffective coping, and interrupted family processes.

ALCOHOL [OTHER DRUG] ABUSE: May be situational or chronic with problems ranging from ineffective breathing patterns, decreased cardiac output, impaired liver function and fluid volume deficit, to nutritional problems, infection, trauma, disturbed thought processes, and coping/family process difficulties.

ABNORMAL BLOOD PROFILE: Suggests possibility of fluid volume deficit, decreased tissue perfusion, impaired gas exchange, activity intolerance, or risk for infection or injury.

Information in brackets added by the authors to clarify and enhance the use of nursing diagnoses.

 Cultural Collaborative 🏠 Community/Home Care

DRUG THERAPIES, TREATMENTS, AND DISEASE CONCERNS: Would include ineffective tissue perfusion, activity intolerance; cardiovascular, respiratory, and elimination concerns; risk for infection, fluid volume imbalances, impaired skin/tissue integrity, impaired liver function; pain, nutritional problems, fatigue/sleep deprivation, ineffective therapeutic regimen management; and emotional responses (e.g., anxiety, sorrow/grief, coping, etc.). It is suggested that the user refer to specific NDs based on identified related factors and individual concerns for this client to find appropriate outcomes and interventions, and Documentation Focus.

SAMPLE NURSING OUTCOMES & INTERVENTIONS CLASSIFICATIONS (NOC/NIC)

NOC/NICs also depend on the specifics of the client's situation such as:

NOC—Blood Coagulation; Immune Status; Neurological Status: Consciousness

NIC—Bleeding Precautions; Infection Protection; Postanesthesia Care

Rape-Trauma Syndrome
[Specify]

Taxonomy II: Coping/Stress Tolerance—Class 1 Post-Trauma Responses (see A, B, C, following)
[Diagnostic Division: Ego Integrity]
Submitted 1980; Nursing Diagnosis Extension and Classification (NDEC) Revision 1998

Definition: Sustained maladaptive response to a forced, violent sexual penetration against the victim's will and consent. [Rape is not a sexual crime, but a crime of violence and identified as sexual assault. Although attacks are most often directed toward women, men also may be victims.]

NOTE: This syndrome includes the following three subcomponents: [A] Rape-Trauma; [B] Compound Reaction; and [C] Silent Reaction

[A] RAPE-TRAUMA—(00142)

Related Factors

Rape [actual/attempted forced sexual penetration]

Information in brackets added by the authors to clarify and enhance the use of nursing diagnoses.

 Diagnostic Studies   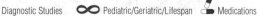 Pediatric/Geriatric/Lifespan   Medications   **549**

Defining Characteristics

SUBJECTIVE

Embarrassment; humiliation; shame; guilt; self-blame
Loss of self-esteem; helplessness; powerlessness
Shock; fear; anxiety; anger; revenge
Nightmares; sleep disturbances
Change in relationships; sexual dysfunction

OBJECTIVE

Physical trauma [e.g., bruising, tissue irritation]; muscle tension/
    spasms
Confusion; disorganization; impaired decision making
Agitation; hyperalertness; aggression
Mood swings; vulnerability; dependence; depression
Substance abuse; suicide attempts
Denial; phobias; paranoia; dissociative disorders

[B] COMPOUND REACTION—(00143)

Definition: Forced violent sexual penetration against the victim's will and consent. The trauma syndrome that develops from this attack or attempted attack includes an acute phase of disorganization of the victim's lifestyle and a long-term process of reorganization of lifestyle.

Related Factors

To be developed

Defining Characteristics

SUBJECTIVE

Acute Phase
Emotional reactions (e.g., anger, embarrassment, fear of physi-
    cal violence and death, humiliation, self-blame, revenge)
Multiple physical symptoms (e.g., gastrointestinal irritability,
    genitourinary discomfort, muscle tension, sleep pattern dis-
    turbance)
Reactivated symptoms of previous conditions (e.g., physical/
    psychiatric illness); substance abuse

Long-Term Phase
Changes in lifestyle (e.g., changes in residence, dealing with
    repetitive nightmares and phobias, seeking family/social net-
    work support)

Information in brackets added by the authors to clarify and enhance the use of nursing diagnoses.

  Cultural Collaborative Community/Home Care

[c] SILENT REACTION—(00141)

Definition: Forced violent sexual penetration against the victim's will and consent. The trauma syndrome that develops from this attack or attempted attack includes an acute phase of disorganization of the victim's lifestyle and a long-term process of reorganization of lifestyle.

Related Factors

To be developed

Defining Characteristics

SUBJECTIVE

Increase in nightmares
Abrupt changes in relationships with men
Pronounced changes in sexual behavior

OBJECTIVE

Increasing anxiety during interview (e.g., blocking of associations, long periods of Silence, minor stuttering, physical distress)
No verbalization of the occurrence of rape
Sudden onset of phobic reactions

Desired Outcomes/Evaluation Criteria—Client Will:

- Deal appropriately with emotional reactions as evidenced by behavior and expression of feelings.
- Report absence of physical complications, pain, and discomfort.
- Verbalize a positive self-image.
- Verbalize recognition that incident was not of own doing.
- Identify behaviors/situations within own control that may reduce risk of recurrence.
- Deal with practical aspects (e.g., court appearances).
- Demonstrate appropriate changes in lifestyle (e.g., change in job/residence) as necessary and seek/obtain support from SO(s) as needed.
- Interact with individuals/groups in desired and acceptable manner.

Actions/Interventions

NURSING PRIORITY NO. 1. To assess trauma and individual reaction, noting length of time since occurrence of event:

Information in brackets added by the authors to clarify and enhance the use of nursing diagnoses.

- Observe for and elicit information about physical injury and assess stress-related symptoms, such as numbness, headache, tightness in chest, nausea, pounding heart, and so forth.
- Identify psychological responses: anger, shock, acute anxiety, confusion, denial. Note laughter, crying, calm or agitated state, excited (hysterical) behavior, expressions of disbelief, and/or self-blame.
- Note signs of increasing anxiety (e.g., silence, stuttering, inability to sit still). **Indicates need for immediate interventions to prevent panic reaction.**
- Determine degree of disorganization. **May need help to manage ADLs and other aspects of life.**
- Identify whether incident has reactivated preexisting or coexisting situations (physical/psychological). **Can affect how the client views the trauma.**
- Ascertain cultural values/religious beliefs that may affect how client views incident, self, and expectations of SO/family reaction.
- Determine disruptions in relationships with men and with others (e.g., family, friends, coworkers, SO[s])
- Identify development of phobic reactions to ordinary articles (e.g., knives) and situations (e.g., walking in groups of people, strangers ringing doorbell).
- Note degree of intrusive repetitive thoughts, sleep disturbances.
- Assess degree of dysfunctional coping (e.g., use of alcohol, other drugs, suicidal/homicidal ideation, marked change in sexual behavior).

NURSING PRIORITY NO. 2. To assist client to deal with situation that exists:

- Explore own feelings (nurse/caregiver) regarding rape/incest issue prior to interacting with the client. **Need to recognize own biases to prevent imposing them on the client.**

ACUTE PHASE

- Stay with the client/do not leave child unattended. Provides reassurance/sense of safety.
- Involve rape response team where available. Provide same-sex examiner when appropriate.
- Evaluate infant/child/adolescent as dictated by age, sex, and developmental level.
- Assist with documentation of incident for police/child-protective services reports, maintain sequencing and collection of evidence (chain of evidence), label each specimen, and store/package properly. **Protecting the evidence is important to the judicial process when offender goes to trial.**

Information in brackets added by the authors to clarify and enhance the use of nursing diagnoses.

  Cultural Collaborative 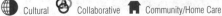 Community/Home Care

- Provide environment in which client can talk freely about feelings and fears, including concerns about relationship with/response of SO(s), pregnancy, sexually transmitted diseases.
- Provide psychological support by listening and remaining with client. If client does not want to talk, accept silence. **May indicate Silent Reaction.**
- Listen to/investigate physical complaints. Assist with medical treatments, as indicated. **Emotional reactions may limit client's ability to recognize physical injury.**
- Assist with practical realities (e.g., safe temporary housing, money, or other needs).
- Determine client's ego strengths and assist client to use them in a positive way by acknowledging client's ability to handle what is happening.
- Identify support persons for this individual. **The client's partner can be important to her or his recovery by being patient and comforting. When partners talk through the incident, the relationship can be strengthened.**

POST-ACUTE PHASE

- Allow the client to work through own kind of adjustment. May be withdrawn or unwilling to talk; do not force the issue, but be available, if needed .
- Listen for expressions of fear of crowds, men, and so forth. **May reveal developing phobias.**
- Discuss specific concerns/fears. Identify appropriate actions (e.g., diagnostic testing for pregnancy, sexually transmitted diseases) and provide information, as indicated.
- Include written instructions that are concise and clear regarding medical treatments, crisis support services, and so forth. **Reinforces teaching, provides opportunity to deal with information at own pace.**

LONG-TERM PHASE

- Continue listening to expressions of concern. May need to continue to talk about the assault. Note persistence of somatic complaints (e.g., nausea, anorexia, insomnia, muscle tension, headache).
- Permit free expression of feelings (may continue from the crisis phase). Refrain from rushing client through expressions of feelings and avoid reassuring inappropriately. **Client may believe pain and/or anguish is misunderstood and depression may limit responses.**

Information in brackets added by the authors to clarify and enhance the use of nursing diagnoses.

• Acknowledge reality of loss of self that existed before the incident. Assist client to move toward an acceptance of the potential for growth that exists within individual.

 • Continue to allow client to progress at own pace.

 • Give "permission" to express/deal with anger at the perpetrator/situation in acceptable ways. Set limits on destructive behaviors. **Facilitates resolution of feelings without diminishing self-concept.**

 • Keep discussion on practical and emotional level rather than intellectualizing the experience, **which allows client to avoid dealing with feelings.**

 • Assist in dealing with ongoing concerns about and effects of the incident, such as court appearance, pregnancy, sexually transmitted disease, relationship with SO(s), and so forth.

 • Provide for sensitive, trained counselors, considering individual needs. (**Male/female counselors may be best determined on an individual basis as counselor's gender may be an issue for some clients, affecting ability to disclose.**)

NURSING PRIORITY NO. 3. To promote wellness (Teaching/Discharge Considerations):

 • Provide information about what reactions client may expect during each phase. Let client know these are common reactions and phrase in neutral terms of "You may or may not..." (Be aware that, although male rape perpetrators are usually heterosexual, the male victim may be concerned about his own sexuality and may exhibit a homophobic response.)

 • Assist client to identify factors that may have created a vulnerable situation and that she or he may have power to change **to protect self in the future.**

 • Avoid making value judgments.

 • Discuss lifestyle changes client is contemplating and how they will contribute to recovery. **Helps client evaluate appropriateness of plans and make decisions that will be helpful to eventual recovery.**

 • Encourage psychiatric consultation if client is violent, inconsolable, or does not seem to be making an adjustment. **Participation in a group may be helpful.**

 • Refer to family/marital counseling, as indicated.

• Refer to NDs Powerlessness; ineffective Coping; Grieving; complicated Grieving; Anxiety; Fear.

Information in brackets added by the authors to clarify and enhance the use of nursing diagnoses.

   Cultural   Collaborative   Community/Home Care

Documentation Focus

ASSESSMENT/REASSESSMENT

- Individual findings, including nature of incident, individual reactions/fears, degree of trauma (physical/emotional), effects on lifestyle.
- Cultural/religious factors.
- Reactions of family/SO(s).
- Samples gathered for evidence and disposition/storage (chain of evidence).

PLANNING

- Plan of action and who is involved in planning.
- Teaching plan.

IMPLEMENTATION/EVALUATION

- Responses to interventions/teaching and actions performed.
- Attainment/progress toward desired outcome(s).
- Modifications to plan of care.

DISCHARGE PLANNING

- Long-term needs and who is responsible for actions to be taken.
- Specific referrals made.

SAMPLE NURSING OUTCOMES & INTERVENTIONS CLASSIFICATIONS (NOC/NIC)—RAPE-TRAUMA SYNDROME

NOC—Abuse Recovery: Emotional
NIC—Rape Trauma Treatment

COMPOUND REACTION

NOC—Coping
NIC—Crises Intervention

SILENT REACTION

NOC—Abuse Recovery: Sexual
NIC—Counseling

Information in brackets added by the authors to clarify and enhance the use of nursing diagnoses.

 Diagnostic Studies 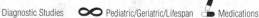 Pediatric/Geriatric/Lifespan   Medications

impaired Religiosity

Taxonomy II: Life Principles—Class 3 Value/Belief/Action
   Conguence (00169)
[Diagnostic Division: Ego Integrity]
Submitted 2004

Definition: Impaired ability to exercise reliance on
beliefs and/or participate in rituals of a particular
faith tradition

NOTE: NANDA recognizes that the term "religiosity" may be culture specific; however, the term is useful in the United States and is
well-supported in the U.S. literature.

Related Factors

DEVELOPMENTAL AND SITUATIONAL

Life transitons; aging; end-stage life crises

PHYSICAL

[Sickness/]illness; pain

PSYCHOLOGICAL FACTORS

Ineffective support/coping
Anxiety; fear of death
Personal crisis [/disaster], lack of security
Use of religion to manipulate

SOCIOCULTURAL

Cultural/environmental barriers to practicing religion
Lack of social integration; lack of sociocultural interaction

SPIRITUAL

Spiritual crises; suffering

Defining Characteristics

SUBJECTIVE

Expresses emotional distress because of separation from faith
   community
Expresses a need to reconnect with previous belief patterns/
   customs
Questions religious belief patterns/customs

Information in brackets added by the authors to clarify and enhance
the use of nursing diagnoses.

 Cultural   Collaborative   Community/Home Care

Difficulty adhering to prescribed religious beliefs and rituals (e.g., religious ceremonies, dietary regulations, clothing, prayer, worship/religious services, private religious behaviors/reading religious materials/media, holiday observances, meetings with religious leaders)

Desired Outcomes/Evaluation Criteria—Client Will:

• Express ability to once again participate in beliefs and rituals of desired religion.
• Discuss beliefs/values about spiritual/religious issues.
• Attend religious/worship services of choice as desired.
• Verbalize concerns about end-of-life issues and fear of death.

Actions/Interventions

NURSING PRIORITY NO. 1. To assess causative/contributing factors:

• Determine client's usual religious/spiritual beliefs, values, past spiritual commitment. **Provides a baseline for understanding current problem.**
• Note client's/SO's reports and expressions of anger/concern, alienation from God, sense of guilt or retribution. **Perception of guilt may cause spiritual crisis/suffering resulting in rejection of religious symbols.**
• Determine sense of futility, feelings of hopelessness, lack of motivation to help self. **Indicators that client may see no, or only limited, options/alternatives or personal choices.**
• Assess extent of depression client may be experiencing. **Some studies suggest that a focus on religion may protect against depression.**
• Note recent changes in behavior (e.g., withdrawal from others/religious activities, dependence on alcohol or medications). **Lack of connectedness with self/others impairs ability to trust others or feel worthy of trust from others/God.**

NURSING PRIORITY NO. 2. To assist client/SO(s) to deal with feelings/situation:

• Use therapeutic communication skills of reflection and active-listening. **Communicates acceptance and enables client to find own solutions to concerns.**
• Encourage expression of feelings about illness/condition, death.
• Suggest use of journaling/reminiscence. **Promotes life review and can assist in clarifying values/ideas, recognizing and resolving feelings/situation.**

Information in brackets added by the authors to clarify and enhance the use of nursing diagnoses.

Diagnostic Studies   Pediatric/Geriatric/Lifespan   Medications   **557**

- Discuss differences between grief and guilt and help client to identify and deal with each. Point out consequences of actions based on guilt.
- Encourage client to identify individuals (e.g., spiritual advisor, parish nurse) who can provide needed support.
- Review client's religious affiliation, associated rituals, and beliefs. **Helps client examine what has been important in the past.**
- Provide opportunity for nonjudgmental discussion of philosophical issues related to religious belief patterns and customs. **Open communication can assist client to check reality of perceptions and identify personal options and willingness to resume desired activities.**
- Discuss desire to continue/reconnect with previous belief patterns and customs and current barriers.
- Involve client in refining heathcare goals and therapeutic regimen, as appropriate. **Identifies role illness is playing in current concerns about ability to participate/appropriateness of participating in desired religious activities.**

NURSING PRIORITY NO. 3. To promote wellness (Teaching/Discharge Considerations):

- Assist client to identify spiritual resources that could be helpful (e.g., contacting spiritual advisor who has qualifications/experience in dealing with specific problems individual is concerned about). **Provides answers to spiritual questions, assists in the journey of self-discovery, and can help client learn to accept/forgive self.**
- Provide privacy for meditation/prayer, performance of rituals, as appropriate.
- Explore alternatives/modifications of ritual based on setting and individual needs/limitations.

Documentation Focus

ASSESSMENT/REASSESSMENT

- Individual findings, including nature of spiritual conflict, effects of participation in treatment regimen.
- Physical/emotional responses to conflict.

PLANNING

- Plan of care and who is involved in planning.
- Teaching plan.

IMPLEMENTATION/EVALUATION

- Responses to interventions/teaching and actions performed.

Information in brackets added by the authors to clarify and enhance the use of nursing diagnoses.

 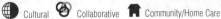

- Attainment/progress toward desired outcome(s).
- Modifications to plan of care.

DISCHARGE PLANNING

- Long-term needs and who is responsible for actions to be taken.
- Available resources, specific referrals made.

SAMPLE NURSING OUTCOMES & INTERVENTIONS CLASSIFICATIONS (NOC/NIC)

NOC—Spiritual Health
NIC—Religious Ritual Enhancement

readiness for enhanced Religiosity

Taxonomy II: Life Principles— Class 3 Value/Belief/Action Conguence (00171)
[Diagnostic Division: Ego Integrity]
Submitted 2004

Definition: Ability to increase reliance on religious beliefs and/or participate in rituals of a particular faith tradition

NOTE: NANDA recognizes that the term "religiosity" may be culture specific; however, the term is useful in the United States and is well-supported in the U.S. literature.

Related Factors

To be developed

Defining Characteristics

SUBJECTIVE

Expresses desire to strengthen religious belief patterns/customs that had provided comfort/religion in the past
Request for assistance to increase participation in prescribed religious beliefs (e.g., religious ceremonies, dietary regulations/rituals, clothing, prayer, worship/religious services, private religious behaviors, reading religious materials/media, holiday observances)
Requests assistance expanding religious options/religious materials/experiences

---

Information in brackets added by the authors to clarify and enhance the use of nursing diagnoses.

 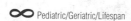

Requests meeting with religious leaders/facilitators
Requests forgiveness/reconciliation
Questions/rejects belief patterns/customs that are harmful

Desired Outcomes/Evaluation Criteria—Client Will:

• Acknowledge need to strengthen religious affiliations and continue/resume previously comforting rituals.
• Verbalize willingness to seek help to enhance desired religious beliefs.
• Become involved in spiritually based programs of own choice.
• Recognize the difference between belief patterns and customs that are helpful and those that may be harmful.

Actions/Interventions

NURSING PRIORITY NO. 1. To determine spiritual state/motivation for growth:

 • Determine client's current thinking about desire to learn more about religious beliefs and actions.
 • Ascertain religious beliefs of family of origin and climate in which client grew up. **Early religious training deeply affects children and is carried on into adulthood. Conflict between family's beliefs and client's current learning may need to be addressed.**
 • Discuss client's spiritual commitment, beliefs, and values. **Enables examination of these issues and helps client learn more about self and what he or she desires/believes.**
 • Explore how spirituality/religious practices have affected client's life.
 • Ascertain motivation and expectations for change.

NURSING PRIORITY NO. 2. To assist client to integrate values and beliefs to strengthen sense of wholeness and achieve optimum balance in daily living:

 • Establish nurse/client relationship in which dialogue can occur. **Client can feel safe to say anything and know it will be accepted.**
 • Identify barriers and beliefs that might hinder growth and/or self-discovery. **Previous practices and beliefs may need to be considered and accepted or discarded in new search for religious beliefs.**
 • Discuss cultural beliefs of family of origin and how they have influenced client's religious practices. **As client expands options for learning new/other religious beliefs**

Information in brackets added by the authors to clarify and enhance the use of nursing diagnoses.

and practices, these influences will provide information for comparing/contrasting new information.

- Explore connection of desire to strengthen belief patterns and customs to daily life. **Becoming aware of how these issues affect the individual's daily life can enhance ability to incorporate them into everything he or she does.**
- Identify ways in which individual can develop a sense of harmony with self and others.

NURSING PRIORITY NO. 3. To enhance optimum wellness:

- Encourage client to seek out and experience different religious beliefs, services, and ceremonies. **Trying out different religions will give client more information to contrast and compare what will fit his or her belief system.**
- Provide bibliotherapy/reading materials pertaining to spiritual issues client is interested in learning about.
- Help client learn about stress-reducing activities, e.g., meditation, relaxation exercises, mindfulness. **Promotes general well-being and sense of control over self and ability to choose religious activities desired. Mindfulness is a method of being in the moment.**
- Encourage participation in religious activities, worship/religious services, reading religious materials/media, study groups, volunteering in church choir, or other needed duties.
- Refer to community resources, e.g., parish nurse, religion classes, other support groups.

Documentation Focus

ASSESSMENT/REASSESSMENT

- Assessment findings, including client perception of needs and desire/expectations for growth/enhancement.
- Motivation/expectations for change.

PLANNING

- Plan for growth and who is involved in planning.

IMPLEMENTATION/EVALUATION

- Response to activities/learning and actions performed.
- Attainment/progress toward desired outcome(s).
- Modifications to plan.

DISCHARGE PLANNING

- Long-range needs/expectations and plan of action.
- Specific referrals made.

Information in brackets added by the authors to clarify and enhance the use of nursing diagnoses.

readiness for enhanced RELIGIOSITY

SAMPLE NURSING OUTCOMES & INTERVENTIONS CLASSIFICATIONS (NOC/NIC)

NOC—Spiritual Well-Being
NIC—Spiritual Growth Facilitation

risk for impaired Religiosity

Taxonomy II: Life Principles—Class 3 Value/Belief/
    Action Conguence (00170)
[Diagnostic Division: Ego Integrity]
Submitted 2004

Definition: At risk for an impaired ability to exercise reliance on religious beliefs and/or participate in rituals of a particular faith tradition

NOTE: NANDA recognizes that the term "religiosity" may be culture specific; however, the term is useful in the United States and is well-supported in the U.S. literature.

Risk Factors

DEVELOPMENTAL

Life transitions

ENVIRONMENTAL

Lack of transportation
Barriers to practicing religion

PHYSICAL

Illness; hospitalization; pain

PSYCHOLOGICAL

Ineffective support/coping/caregiving
Depression
Lack of security

SOCIOCULTURAL

Lack of social interaction; social isolation
Cultural barrier to practicing religion

SPIRITUAL

Suffering

Information in brackets added by the authors to clarify and enhance the use of nursing diagnoses.

 Cultural Collaborative Community/Home Care

NOTE: A risk diagnosis is not evidenced by signs and symptoms, as the problem has not occurred and nursing interventions are directed at prevention.

Desired Outcomes/Evaluation Criteria—Client Will:

- Express understanding of relation of situation/health status to thoughts and feelings of concern about ability to participate in desired religious activities.
- Seek solutions to individual factors that may interfere with reliance on religious beliefs/participation in religious rituals.
- Identify and use resources appropriately.

Actions/Interventions

NURSING PRIORITY NO. 1. To assess causative/contributing factors:

- Ascertain current situation, e.g., illness, hospitalization, prognosis of death, depression, lack of support systems, financial concerns. **Identifies problems client is dealing with in the moment that may be affecting desire to be involved with religious activities.**
- Note client's concerns/expressions of anger, belief that illness/condition is result of lack of faith. **Individual may blame himself or herself for what has happened and could reject religious beliefs and/or God.**
- Determine client's usual religious/spiritual beliefs, past or current involvement in specific church activities.
- Identify cultural values/expectations regarding religious beliefs and/or practices.
- Note quality of relationships with significant others and friends. **Individual may withdraw from others in relation to the stress of illness, pain, and suffering. Others may be encouraging client to rely on religious beliefs at a time when individual is questioning own beliefs in the current situation.**
- Assess lack of transportation/environmental barriers to participation in desired religious activities.
- Ascertain substance use/abuse. **Individuals often turn to use of various substances in distress, and this can affect the ability to deal with problems in a positive manner.**

NURSING PRIORITY NO. 2. To assist client to deal with feelings/situation:

- Develop nurse/client relationship. **Individual can express feelings and concerns freely when he or she feels safe to do so.**

Information in brackets added by the authors to clarify and enhance the use of nursing diagnoses.

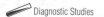

- Use therapeutic communications skills of active-listening, reflection, and I-messages. **Helps client to find own solutions to problems and concerns and promotes sense of control.**
- Have client identify and prioritize current/immediate needs. **Dealing with current needs is easier than trying to predict the future.**
- Provide time for nonjudgmental discussion of individual's spiritual beliefs and fears about impact of current illness and/or treatment regimen. **Helps to clarify thoughts and promote ability to deal with stresses of what is happening.**
- Review with client past difficulties in life and coping skills that were used at that time.
- Encourage client to discuss feelings about death and end-of-life issues when illness/prognosis is grave.

NURSING PRIORITY NO. 3. To promote wellness (Teaching/Discharge Considerations):

- Have client identify support systems available.
- Help client learn relaxation techniques, meditation, guided imagery, and mindfulness/living in the moment and enjoying it.
- Take the lead from the client in initiating participation in religious activities, prayer, other activities. **Client may be vulnerable in current situation and must be allowed to decide own participation in these actions.**
- Refer to appropriate resources (e.g., crisis counselor, governmental agencies, spiritual advisor) who has qualifications/experience dealing with specific problems, such as death/dying, relationship problems, substance abuse, suicide, hospice, psychotherapy, Alcoholics/Narcotics Anonymous.

Documentation Focus

ASSESSMENT/REASSESSMENT

- Individual findings, including risk factors, nature of current distress.
- Physical/emotional response to distress.
- Access to/use of resources.

PLANNING

- Plan of care and who is involved in planning.
- Teaching plan.

IMPLEMENTATION/EVALUATION

- Responses to interventions/teaching and actions performed.
- Attainment/progress toward desired outcome(s).

Information in brackets added by the authors to clarify and enhance the use of nursing diagnoses.

    Cultural   Collaborative   🏠 Community/Home Care

- Modifications to plan of care.

DISCHARGE PLANNING

- Long-term needs and who is responsible for actions to be taken.
- Available resources, specific referrals made.

SAMPLE NURSING OUTCOMES & INTERVENTIONS CLASSIFICATIONS (NOC/NIC)

NOC Spiritual Well-Being
NIC—Spiritual Support

Relocation Stress Syndrome

Taxonomy II: Coping/Stress Tolerance—Class 1 Post-
  Trauma Responses (00114)
[Diagnostic Division: Ego Integrity]
Submitted 1992; Revised 2000

Definition: Physiological and/or psychosocial disturbance following transfer from one environment to
another

Related Factors

Losses; feeling of powerlessness
Lack of adequate support system; lack of predeparture counsel-
  ing; unpredictability of experience
Isolation; language barrier
Impaired psychosocial health; passive coping
Decreased health status

Defining Characteristics

SUBJECTIVE

Anxiety (e.g., separation); anger
Insecurity; worry; fear
Loneliness; depression
Unwillingness to move; concern over relocation
Sleep disturbance

OBJECTIVE

Move from one environment to another
Increased [frequency of] verbalization of needs

Information in brackets added by the authors to clarify and enhance
the use of nursing diagnoses.

Pessimism; frustration
Increased physical symptoms/illness
Withdrawal; aloneness; alienation; [hostile behavior/outbursts]
Loss of identity/self-worth/self-esteem; dependency
[Increased confusion/cognitive impairment]

Desired Outcomes/Evaluation Criteria—Client Will:

- Verbalize understanding of reason(s) for change.
- Demonstrate appropriate range of feelings and lessened fear.
- Participate in routine and special/social events as able.
- Verbalize acceptance of situation.
- Experience no catastrophic event.

Actions/Interventions

NURSING PRIORITY NO. 1. To assess degree of stress as perceived/experienced by client and determine issues of safety:

- **Determine situation/cause for relocation** (e.g., planned move for new job, loss of home/community due to natural or man-made disaster such as fire, earthquake, flood, war/act of terror; older adult unable to care for self/caregiver burnout; change in marital or health status). **Influences needs/choice of plans/interventions.**
- Ascertain if client participated in the decision to relocate and perceptions about change(s) and expectations for the future. **Decision may have been made with/without client's input or understanding of event or consequences, which can impact adjustment.**
- ∞ Note client's age, developmental level, role in family. **Child can be traumatized by transfer to new school/loss of peers; elderly persons may be affected by loss of long-term home/neighborhood setting and support persons.**
- Determine presence of cultural and/or religious concerns/conflicts.
- Monitor behavior, noting presence of anxiety, suspiciousness/paranoia, irritability, defensiveness. Compare with SO's/staff's description of customary responses. **May temporarily exacerbate mental deterioration (cognitive inaccessibility) and impair communication (social inaccessibility).**
- Note signs of increased stress (e.g., irritability, withdrawal, crying, moodiness, problems sleeping, increased use of alcohol/other drugs), reports of "new" physical discomfort/pain

---

Information in brackets added by the authors to clarify and enhance the use of nursing diagnoses.

(e.g., stomach aches, headaches, back pain); change in appetite; greater susceptiblilty to colds, fatigue.
- Determine involvement of family/SO(s). Note availability/use of support systems and resources.
- Identify issues of safety that may be involved.

NURSING PRIORITY NO. 2. To assist client to deal with situation/changes:

- Encourage visit to new community/surroundings/school prior to transfer when possible. **Provides opportunity to "get acquainted" with new situation, reducing fear of unknown.**
- Encourage free expression of feelings about reason for relocation, including venting of anger, grief, loss of personal space/belongings/friends, financial strains, powerlessness, etc. Acknowledge reality of situation and maintain hopeful attitude regarding move/change. Refer to NDs relating to client's particular situation (e.g., Grieving; ineffective Coping) for additional interventions.
- Identify strengths/successful coping behaviors the individual has used previously. **Incorporating these into problem solving builds on past successes.**
- Orient to surroundings/schedules. Introduce to neighbors, staff members, roommate/residents. Provide clear, honest information about actions/events.
- Encourage individual/family to personalize area with pictures, own belongings, and the like as possible/appropriate. **Enhances sense of belonging/personal space.**
- Determine client's usual schedule of activities and incorporate into routine as possible. **Reinforces sense of importance of individual.**
- Introduce planned diversional activities, such as movies, meals with new acquantances, art therapy, music, religious activities, etc. **Involvement increases opportunity to interact with others, decreasing isolation.**
- Place in private facility room, if appropriate, and include SO(s)/family into care activities, meal time, etc.
- Encourage hugging and use of touch unless client is paranoid or agitated at the moment. **Human connection reaffirms acceptance of individual.**
- Deal with aggressive behavior by imposing calm, firm limits. Control environment and protect others from client's disruptive behavior. **Promotes safety for client/others.**
- Remain calm, place in a quiet environment, providing time-out, **to prevent escalation into panic state and violent behavior.**

Information in brackets added by the authors to clarify and enhance the use of nursing diagnoses.

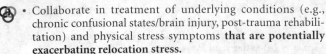

- Collaborate in treatment of underlying conditions (e.g., chronic confusional states/brain injury, post-trauma rehabilitation) and physical stress symptoms **that are potentially exacerbating relocation stress.**
- Refer to social worker, financial resources, mental healthcare provider, minister/spiritual advisor for additional assessment/interventions, as indicated. **May be useful/needed if client has special needs and/or persistent problems with adaptation.**

NURSING PRIORITY NO. 3. To promote wellness (Teaching/Discharge Considerations):

- Involve client in formulating goals and plan of care when possible. **Supports independence and commitment to achieving outcomes.**
- Discuss benefits of adequate nutrition, rest, and exercise **to maintain physical well-being.**
- Involve in anxiety- and stress-reduction activities (e.g., meditation, progressive muscle relaxation, group socialization), as able, to enhance psychological well-being.
- Encourage participation in activities/hobbies/personal interactions as appropriate. **Promotes creative endeavors, stimulating the mind.**
- Identify community supports/cultural or ethnic groups client can access.
- Support self-responsibility and coping strategies. Foster sense of control and self-worth.

Documentation Focus

ASSESSMENT/REASSESSMENT

- Assessment findings, individual's perception of the situation/changes, specific behaviors.
- Cultural/religious concerns.
- Safety issues.

PLANNING

- Note plan of care, who is involved in planning, and who is responsible for proposed actions.
- Teaching plan.

IMPLEMENTATION/EVALUATION

- Response to interventions (especially time-out/seclusion)/teaching and actions performed.
- Sentinel events.

Information in brackets added by the authors to clarify and enhance the use of nursing diagnoses.

    Cultural   Collaborative   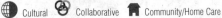 Community/Home Care

- Attainment/progress toward desired outcome(s).
- Modifications to plan of care.

DISCHARGE PLANNING

- Long-term needs and who is responsible for actions to be taken.
- Specific referrals made.

SAMPLE NURSING OUTCOMES & INTERVENTIONS CLASSIFICATIONS (NOC/NIC)

NOC—Psychosocial Adjustment: Life Change
NIC—Coping Enhancement

risk for Relocation Stress Syndrome

Taxonomy II: Coping/Stress Tolerance—Class 1 Post-Trauma Responses (00149)
[Diagnostic Division: Ego Integrity]
Submitted 2000

Definition: At risk for physiological and/or psychosocial disturbance following transfer from one environment to another

Risk Factors

Move from one environment to another
Moderate to high degree of environmental change [e.g., physical, ethnic, cultural]
Lack of adequate support system/group; lack of predeparture counseling
Passive coping; feelings of powerlessness; losses
Moderate mental competence
Unpredictability of experiences
Decreased health status

NOTE: A risk diagnosis is not evidenced by signs and symptoms, as the problem has not occurred and nursing interventions are directed at prevention.

Desired Outcomes/Evaluation Criteria—Client Will:

- Verbalize understanding of reason(s) for change.

Information in brackets added by the authors to clarify and enhance the use of nursing diagnoses.

 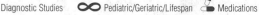

- Express feelings and concerns openly and appropriately.
- Experience no catastrophic event.

Actions/Interventions

NURSING PRIORITY NO. 1. To assess causative/contributing factors:

- Determine situation/cause for relocation (e.g., planned move for new job, loss of home/community due to natural or man-made disaster such as fire, earthquake, war; older adult unable to care for self/caregiver burnout; change in marital or health status). **Influences needs/choice of plans/interventions.**
- Determine presence of cultural and/or religious concerns/conflicts.
- Ascertain if client participated in the decision to relocate and perceptions about change(s) and expectations for the future. **Decision can be made with/without client's input or understanding of event or consequences, which can impact adjustment/sense of control over life.**
- Note client's age, developmental level, role in family. **Child can be traumatized by transfer to new school/loss of peers; elderly persons may be affected by loss of long-term home/neighborhood setting and support persons.**
- Determine physical/emotional health status. **Stress associated with move, even if desired, can exacerbate health problems.**
- Note whether relocation will be temporary (e.g., extended care for rehabilitation therapies, moving in with family while house is being repaired after fire, etc.) or long-term/permanent (e.g., move from home of many years, placement in nursing home).
- Evaluate client/caregiver's resources and coping abilities. Determine family's/SO's degree of involvement and willingness to be involved.
- Identify issues of safety that may be involved.

NURSING PRIORITY NO. 2. To prevent/minimize adverse response to change:

- Involve client in formulating goals and plan of care when possible. **Supports independence and commitment to achieving outcomes.**
- Encourage client/SO(s) to accept that relocation is an adjustment and that it takes time to adapt to new circumstances/environment.
- Allow as much time as possible for move preparation and provide information and support in planning.

Information in brackets added by the authors to clarify and enhance the use of nursing diagnoses.

  Cultural 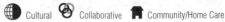 Collaborative ⌂ Community/Home Care

- Support self-responsibility and coping strategies **to foster sense of control and self-worth.**
- Encourage visit to new community/surroundings prior to transfer when possible. **Provides opportunity to "get acquainted" with new situation, thus reducing fear of unknown.**
- Refer to ND Relocation Stress Syndrome for additional Action/Interventions and Documentation Focus.

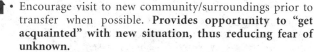

ineffective Role Performance

Taxonomy II: Role Relationships—Class 3 Role Performance (00055)
[Diagnostic Division: Social Interaction]
Submitted 1978; Revised 1996, 1998

Definition: Patterns of behavior and self-expression that do not match the environmental context, norms, and expectations

[NOTE: There is a typology of roles: sociopersonal (friendship, family, marital, parenting, community), home management, intimacy (sexuality, relationship building), leisure/exercise/recreation, self-management, socialization (developmental transitions), community contributor, and religious]

Related Factors

KNOWLEDGE

Inadequate/lack of role model
Inadequate role preparation (e.g., role transition, skill rehearsal, validation)
Lack of education
[Developmental transitions]
Unrealistic role expectations

PHYSIOLOGICAL

Body image alteration; cognitive deficits; neurological deficits; physical illness; mental illness; depression; low self-esteem
Fatigue; pain; substance abuse

SOCIAL

Inadequate role socialization [e.g., role model, expectations, responsibilities]

Information in brackets added by the authors to clarify and enhance the use of nursing diagnoses.

Young age, developmental level
Lack of resources; low socioeconomic status
Stress; conflict; job schedule demands
[Family conflict]; domestic violence
Inadequate support system; lack of rewards
Inappropriate linkage with the healthcare system

Defining Characteristics

SUBJECTIVE

Altered role perceptions; change in self-/other's perception of role

Change in usual patterns of responsibility/capacity to resume role

Inadequate opportunities for role enactment

Role dissatisfaction/overload/denial

Discrimination [by others]; powerlessness

OBJECTIVE

Deficient knowledge; inadequate role competency/skills

Inadequate adaptation to change; inappropriate developmental expectations

Inadequate confidence/motivation/self-management/coping

Inadequate external support for role enactment

Role strain/conflict/confusion/ambivalence; [failure to assume role]

Uncertainty; anxiety; depression; pessimism

Domestic violence; harassment; system conflict

Desired Outcomes/Evaluation Criteria—Client Will:

• Verbalize understanding of role expectations/obligations.
• Verbalize realistic perception and acceptance of self in changed role.
• Talk with family/SO(s) about situation and changes that have occurred and limitations imposed.
• Develop realistic plans for adapting to new role/role changes.

Actions/Interventions

NURSING PRIORITY NO. 1. To assess causative/contributing factors:

 • Identify type of role dysfunction; for example, developmental (adolescent to adult); situational (husband to father, gender identity); health–illness transitions.

Information in brackets added by the authors to clarify and enhance the use of nursing diagnoses.

 Cultural Collaborative Community/Home Care

🏠 • Determine client role in family constellation.

🏠 • Identify how client sees self as a man/woman in usual lifestyle/role functioning.

🏠 • Ascertain client's view of sexual functioning (e.g., loss of childbearing ability following hysterectomy).

🌐 • Identify cultural factors relating to individual's sexual roles. **Different cultures define male/female roles strictly (e.g., Muslim culture demands that the woman adopts a subservient role, whereas the man is seen as the powerful one in the relationship.)**

🏠 • Determine client's perceptions/concerns about current situation. **May believe current role is more appropriate for the opposite sex (e.g., passive role of the patient may be somewhat less threatening for women).**

🏠 • Interview SO(s) regarding their perceptions and expectations. **May influence client's view of self.**

NURSING PRIORITY NO. 2. To assist client to deal with existing situation:

🏠 • Discuss perceptions and significance of the situation as seen by client.

🏠 • Maintain positive attitude toward the client.

🏠 • Provide opportunities for client to exercise control over as many decisions as possible. **Enhances self-concept and promotes commitment to goals.**

🏠 • Offer realistic assessment of situation while communicating sense of hope.

🌐 • Discuss and assist the client/SO(s) to develop strategies for dealing with changes in role related to past transitions, cultural expectations, and value/belief challenges. **Helps those involved deal with differences between individuals (e.g., adolescent task of separation in which parents clash with child's choices; individual's decision to change religious affiliation).**

🏠 • Acknowledge reality of situation related to role change and help client to express feelings of anger, sadness, and grief. Encourage celebration of positive aspects of change and expressions of feelings.

🏠 • Provide open environment for client to discuss concerns about sexuality. **Embarrassment can block discussion of sensitive subject.** (Refer to NDs Sexual Dysfunction; ineffective Sexuality Pattern.)

🏠 • Identify role model for the client. Educate about role expectations using written and audiovisual materials.

Information in brackets added by the authors to clarify and enhance the use of nursing diagnoses.

ineffective ROLE PERFORMANCE

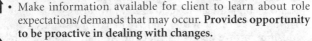

ineffective ROLE PERFORMANCE

 • Use the techniques of role rehearsal to help the client develop new skills **to cope with changes.**

NURSING PRIORITY NO. **3.** To promote wellness (Teaching/Discharge Considerations):

 • Make information available for client to learn about role expectations/demands that may occur. **Provides opportunity to be proactive in dealing with changes.**

 • Accept client in changed role. Encourage and give positive feedback for changes and goals achieved. **Provides reinforcement and facilitates continuation of efforts.**

 • Refer to support groups, employment counselors, parent effectiveness classes, counseling/psychotherapy, as indicated by individual need(s). **Provides ongoing support to sustain progress.**

• Refer to NDs Self-Esteem [specify] and the Parenting diagnoses.

Documentation Focus

ASSESSMENT/REASSESSMENT

• Individual findings, including specifics of predisposing crises/situation, perception of role change.
• Expectations of SO(s).

PLANNING

• Plan of care and who is involved in planning.
• Teaching plan.

IMPLEMENTATION/EVAULATION

• Responses to interventions/teaching and actions performed.
• Attainment/progress toward desired outcome(s).
• Modifications plan of care.

DISCHARGE PLANNING

• Long-term needs and who is responsible for actions to be taken.
• Specific referrals made.

SAMPLE NURSING OUTCOMES & INTERVENTIONS CLASSIFICATIONS (NOC/NIC)

NOC—Role Performance
NIC—Role Enhancement

Information in brackets added by the authors to clarify and enhance the use of nursing diagnoses.

   Cultural   Collaborative   Community/Home Care

Self-Care Deficit: bathing/hygiene, dressing/grooming, feeding, toileting

Taxonomy II: Activity/Rest—Class 5 Self-Care
(Bathing/Hygiene 00108, Dressing/Grooming 00109,
Feeding 00102, Toileting 00110)
[Diagnostic Division: Hygiene]
Submitted 1980; Nursing Diagnosis Extension and
Classification (NDEC) Revision 1998

Definition: Impaired ability to perform or complete
feeding, bathing/hygiene, dressing and grooming, or
toileting activities for oneself

[NOTE: Self-care also may be expanded to include the practices
used by the client to promote health, the individual responsibility
for self, a way of thinking. Refer to NDs impaired Home Maintenance; ineffective Health Maintenance.]

Related Factors

Weakness; fatigue; decreased motivation
Neuromuscular/musculoskeletal impairment
Environmental barriers
Severe anxiety
Pain, discomfort
Perceptual/cognitive impairment
Inability to perceive body part/spatial relationship [bathing/
hygiene]
Impaired transfer ability [self-toileting]
Impaired mobility status [self-toileting]
[Mechanical restrictions such as cast, splint, traction, ventilator]

Defining Characteristics

SELF-FEEDING DEFICIT

Inability to:
Prepare food for ingestion; open containers
Handle utensils; get food onto utensil; bring food from a recep-
tacle to the mouth
Ingest food safely; manipulate food in mouth; chew/swallow
food
Pick up cup or glass
Use assistive device

Information in brackets added by the authors to clarify and enhance
the use of nursing diagnoses.

 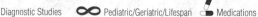

Ingest sufficient food; complete a meal
Ingest food in a socially acceptable manner

SELF-BATHING/HYGIENE DEFICIT

Inability to:
Get bath supplies
Wash body
Obtain water source; regulate bath water
Access bathroom [tub]
Dry body

SELF-DRESSING/GROOMING DEFICIT

Inability to:
Choose clothing; pick up clothing
Put clothing on upper/lower body; put on socks/shoes; remove
   clothing
Use zippers/assistive devices
Maintain appearance at a satisfactory level
Impaired ability to obtain clothing; put on/take off necessary
   items of clothing; fasten clothing

SELF-TOILETING DEFICIT

Inability to:
Get to toilet or commode
Manipulate clothing for toileting
Sit on/rise from toilet or commode
Carry out proper toilet hygiene
Flush toilet or [empty] commode

Desired Outcomes/Evaluation Criteria—Client Will:

- Identify individual areas of weakness/needs.
- Verbalize knowledge of healthcare practices.
- Demonstrate techniques/lifestyle changes to meet self-care
  needs.
- Perform self-care activities within level of own ability.
- Identify personal/community resources that can provide
  assistance.

Actions/Interventions

NURSING PRIORITY NO. 1. To identify causative/contributing factors:

 • Determine age/developmental issues **affecting ability of individual to participate in own care.**

Information in brackets added by the authors to clarify and enhance
the use of nursing diagnoses.

 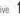

- Note concomitant medical problems/existing conditions that may be factors for care (e.g., high BP, heart disease, renal failure, spinal cord injury, CVA, MS, malnutrition, pain, Alzheimer's disease).
- Review medication regimen for possible effects on alertness/mentation, energy level, balance, perception.
- Note other etiological factors present, including language barriers, speech impairment, visual acuity/hearing problem, emotional stability/ability. (Refer to NDs impaired verbal Communication; impaired Environmental Interpretation; risk for unilateral Neglect; disturbed Sensory Percption (specify) for related interventions.)
- Assess barriers to participation in regimen (e.g., lack of information, insufficient time for discussion; psychological and/or intimate family problems that may be difficult to share; fear of appearing stupid or ignorant; social/economic, work/home environment problems).

NURSING PRIORITY NO. 2. To assess degree of disability:

- Identify degree of individual impairment/functional level according to scale (as listed in ND impaired physical Mobility).
- Assess memory/intellectual functioning. Note developmental level to which client has regressed/progressed.
- Determine individual strengths and skills of the client.
- Note whether deficit is temporary or permanent, should decrease or increase with time.

NURSING PRIORITY NO. 3. To assist in correcting/dealing with situation:

- Perform/assist with meeting client's needs when he or she is unable to meet own needs (e.g., personal care assistance is part of nursing care and should not be neglected while promoting and integrating self-care independence).
- Promote client's/SO's participation in problem identification and desired goals and decision making. **Enhances commitment to plan, optimizing outcomes, and supporting recovery and/or health promotion.**
- Develop plan of care appropriate to individual situation, scheduling activities to conform to client's usual/desired schedule.
- Plan time for listening to the client's/SO's feelings/concerns **to discover barriers to participation in regimen and to work on problem solutions.**
- Practice and promote short-term goal setting and achievement **to recognize that today's success is as important as any**

Information in brackets added by the authors to clarify and enhance the use of nursing diagnoses.

SELF-CARE DEFICIT: bathing/hygiene, dressing/grooming, feeding, toileting

long-term goal, accepting ability to do one thing at a time, and conceputalization of self-care in a broader sence.

 • Provide for communication among those who are involved in caring for/assisting the client. **Enhances coordination and continuity of care.**

 • Establish remotivation/resocialization programs when indicated.

 • Establish "contractual" partnership with client/SO(s) **if appropriate/indicated for motivation/behavioral modification**.

• Assist with rehabilitation program **to enhance capabilities/ promote independence.**

 • Provide privacy and equipment within easy reach during personal care activities.

 • Allow sufficient time for client to accomplish tasks to fullest extent of ability. Avoid unnecessary conversation/interruptions.

 • Assist with necessary adaptations to accomplish ADLs. Begin with familiar, easily accomplished tasks **to encourage client and build on successes.**

• Collaborate with rehabilitation professionals to identify/ obtain assistive devices, mobility aids, and home modification as necessary (e.g., adequate lighting/visual aids; bedside commonde; raised toilet seat/grab bars for bathroom; modified clothing; modified eating utensils).

 • Identify energy-saving behaviors (e.g., sitting instead of standing when possible). (Refer to NDs Activity Intolerance; Fatigue for additional interventions.)

 • Implement bowel or bladder training/retraining program, as indicated. (Refer to Constipation; Bowel Incontinence; impaired Urinary Elimination for appropriate interventions.)

 • Encourage food and fluid choices reflecting individual likes and abilities that meet nutritional needs. Provide assistive devices/alternate feeding methods, as appropriate. (Refer to ND impaired Swallowing for related interventions.)

• Assist with medication regimen as necessary, encouraging timely use of medications (e.g., taking diuretics in morning when client is more awake/able to manage toileting, use of pain relievers prior to activity to facilitate movement, postponing intake of medications that cause sedation until self-care activites completed).

 • Make home visit **to assess environmental/discharge needs.**

NURSING PRIORITY NO. 4. To promote wellness (Teaching/ Discharge Considerations):

 • Assist the client to become aware of rights and responsibilities in health/healthcare and to assess own health strengths— physical, emotional, and intellectual.

Information in brackets added by the authors to clarify and enhance the use of nursing diagnoses.

 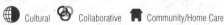 Cultural Collaborative Community/Home Care

- Support client in making health-related decisions and assist in developing self-care practices and goals that promote health.
- Provide for ongoing evaluation of self-care program, identifying progress and needed changes.
- Review/modify program periodically to accommodate changes in client's abilities. **Assists client to adhere to plan of care to fullest extent.**
- Encourage keeping a journal of progress and practicing of independent living skills **to foster self-care and self-determination**.
- Review safety concerns. Modify activities/environment **to reduce risk of injury and promote successful community functioning.**
- Refer to home care provider, social services, physical/occupational therapy, rehabilitation, and counseling resources, as indicated.
- Identify additional community resources (e.g., senior services, Meals on Wheels).
- Review instructions from other members of the healthcare team and provide written copy. **Provides clarification, reinforcement, and periodic review by client/caregivers.**
- Give family information about respite/other care options. **Allows them free time away from the care situation to renew themselves.** (Refer to ND Caregiver Role Strain for additional interventions.)
- Assist/support family with alternative placements as necessary. **Enhances likelihood of finding individually appropriate situation to meet client's needs.**
- Be available for discussion of feelings about situation (e.g., grieving, anger).
- Refer to NDs risk for Falls; Injury/Trauma; ineffective Coping; compromised family Coping; risk for Disuse Syndrome; situational low Self-Esteem; impaired physical Mobility; Powerlessness, as appropriate.

Documentation Focus

ASSESSMENT/REASSESSMENT

- Individual findings, functional level, and specifics of limitation(s).
- Needed resources/adaptive devices.
- Availability/use of community resources.
- Who is involved in care/provides assistance.

PLANNING

- Plan of care and who is involved in planning.
- Teaching plan.

Information in brackets added by the authors to clarify and enhance the use of nursing diagnoses.

IMPLEMENTATION/EVALUATION

- Response to interventions/teaching and actions performed.
- Attainment/progress toward desired outcome(s).
- Modifications of plan of care.

DISCHARGE PLANNING

- Long-term needs and who is responsible for actions to be taken.
- Type of and source for assistive devices.
- Specific referrals made.

SAMPLE NURSING OUTCOMES & INTERVENTIONS CLASSIFICATIONS (NOC/NIC)

BATHING/HYGIENE DEFICIT

NOC—Self-Care Bathing
NIC—Self-Care Assistance: Bathing/Hygiene

DRESSING/GROOMING DEFICIT

NOC—Self-Care Dressing
NIC—Self-Care Assistance: Dressing/Grooming

FEEDING DEFICIT

NOC—Self-Care Eating
NIC—Self-Care Assistance: Feeding

TOILETING DEFICIT

NOC—Self-Care Toileting
NIC—Self-Care Assistance: Toileting

---

readiness for enhanced Self-Care

Taxonomy II: Activity/Rest—Class 5 Self-Care (00182)
[Diagnostic Divisions: Teaching/Learning]
Submitted 2006

Definition: A pattern of performing activities for oneself that helps to meet health-related goals and can be strengthened

Related Factors

To be developed

Information in brackets added by the authors to clarify and enhance the use of nursing diagnoses.

 Cultural Collaborative Community/Home Care

Defining Characteristics

SUBJECTIVE

Expresses desire to enhance independence in maintaining: life/health/personal development/well-being

Expresses desire to enhance self-care/knowledge for strategies for self-care/responsibility for self-care

> [NOTE: Based on the definition and defining characteristics of this ND, the focus appears to be broader than simply meeting routine basic ADLs and addresses independence in maintaining overall health, personal development, and general well-being.]

Desired Outcomes/Evaluation Criteria—Client Will:

- Maintain responsibility for planning and achieving self-care goals/general well-being.
- Demonstrate proactive management of chronic conditions/ potential complications or changes in capabilities.
- Identify/use resources appropriately.
- Remain free of preventable complications.

Actions/Interventions

NURSING PRIORITY NO. 1. To determine current self-care status and motivation for growth:

- Determine individual strengths and skills of the client.
- Ascertain motivation and expectations for change.
- Note availability/use of resources, supportive person(s), assistive devices.
- Determine age/developmental issues, presence of medical conditions **that could impact potential for growth/interrupt client's ability to meet own needs.**
- Assess for potential barriers to enhanced participation in self-care (e.g., lack of information, insufficient time for discussion, sudden/progressive change in health status, catastrophic events).

NURSING PRIORITY NO. 2. To assist client's/SO's plan to meet individual needs:

- Discuss client's understanding of situation.
- Provide accurate/relevant information regarding current/ future needs **so that client can incorporate into self-care plans while minimizing problems associated with change.**

Information in brackets added by the authors to clarify and enhance the use of nursing diagnoses.

 Diagnostic Studies 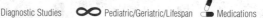 Pediatric/Geriatric/Lifespan Medications

readiness for enhanced SELF-CARE

readiness for enhanced SELF-CARE

 • Promote client's/SO's participation in problem identification and decision making. **Optimizes outcomes and supports health promotion.**

 • Active-listen client's/SO's concerns **to exhibit regard for client's values and beliefs, to support positive responses, and to address questions/concerns.**

 • Encourage communication among those who are involved in the client's health promotion. **Periodic review allows for clarification of issues, reinforcement of successful interventions, and possibility for early intervention (where needed) to manage chronic conditions.**

NURSING PRIORITY NO. 3. To promote optimum wellness (Teaching/Discharge Considerations):

 • Assist client to set realistic goals for the future.

 • Support client in making health-related decisions and pursuit of self-care practices that promote health **to foster self-esteem and support positive self-concept.**

 • Identify reliable reference sources regarding individual needs/strategies for self-care. **Reinforces learning and promotes self-paced review.**

 • Provide for ongoing evaluation of self-care program **to identify progress and needed changes for continuation of health, adaptation in management of limiting conditions.**

 • Review safety concerns and modification of medical therapies or activities/environment, as needed, **to prevent injury and enhance successful functioning.**

 • Refer to home care provider, social services, physical/occupational therapy, rehabilitation, and counseling resources, as indicated/requested, **for education, assistance, adaptive devices, and modifications that may be desired.**

 • Identify additional community resources (e.g., senior services, handicap transportation van for appointments, accessible/safe locations for social/sports activities, Meals on Wheels, etc.).

Documentation Focus

ASSESSMENT/REASSESSMENT

• Individual findings including strengths, health status, and any limitation(s).
• Availability/use of community resources, support person(s), assistive devices.
• Motivation and expectations for change.

Information in brackets added by the authors to clarify and enhance the use of nursing diagnoses.

Cultural Collaborative Community/Home Care

PLANNING

- Plan of care/interventions and who is involved in planning.
- Teaching plan.

IMPLEMENTATION/EVALUATION

- Client's responses to interventions/teaching and actions performed.
- Attainment/progress toward desired outcome(s).
- Modifications to plan.

DISCHARGE PLANNING

- Long-term needs and who is responsible for actions to be taken.
- Type of and source for assistive devices.
- Specific referrals made.

SAMPLE NURSING OUTCOMES & INTERVENTIONS CLASSIFICATIONS (NOC/NIC)

NOC—Self-Care Status
NIC—Self-Modification Assistance

readiness for enhanced Self-Concept

Taxonomy II: Self-Perception—Class 1 Self-Concept
(00167)
[Diagnostic Divisions: Ego Integrity]
Submitted 2002

Definition: A pattern of perceptions or ideas about the self that is sufficient for well-being and can be strengthened

Related Factors

To be developed

Defining Characteristics

SUBJECTIVE

Expresses willingness to enhance self-concept
Accepts strengths/limitations
Expresses confidence in abilities
Expresses satisfaction with thoughts about self/sense of worthiness

---

Information in brackets added by the authors to clarify and enhance the use of nursing diagnoses.

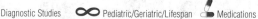

Expresses satisfaction with body image/personal identity/role performance

OBJECTIVE

Actions are congruent with expressed feelings and thoughts

Desired Outcomes/Evaluation Criteria—Client Will:

- Verbalize understanding of own sense of self-concept.
- Participate in programs and activities to enhance self-esteem.
- Demonstrate behaviors/lifestyle changes to promote positive self-esteem.
- Participate in family/group/community activities to enhance self-concept.

Actions/Interventions

NURSING PRIORITY NO. 1. To assess current situation and desire for improvement:

 • Determine current status of individual's belief about self. **Self-concept consists of the physical self (body image) and the personal self (identity) and self-esteem. Information about client's current thinking about self provides a beginning for making changes to improve self.**

 • Determine availability/quality of family/SO(s) support. **Presence of supportive people who reflect positive attitudes regarding the individual promotes a positive sense of self.**

 • Identify family dynamics—present and past. **Self-esteem begins in early childhood and is influenced by the perceptions of how the individual is viewed by significant others. Provides information about family functioning that will help to develop plan of care for enhancing client's self-concept.**

 • Note willingness to seek assistance/motivation for change. **Individuals who have a sense of their own self-image and are willing to look at themselves realistically will be able to progress in the desire to improve.**

 • Determine client's concept of self in relation to cultural/religious ideals/beliefs. **Cultural characteristics are learned in the family of origin and shape how the individual views self.**

 • Observe nonverbal behaviors and note congruence with verbal expressions. Discuss cultural meanings of nonverbal communication. **Incongruencies between verbal and nonverbal communication require clarification. Interpretation of**

Information in brackets added by the authors to clarify and enhance the use of nursing diagnoses.

 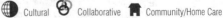

nonverbal expressions is culturally determined and needs to be clarified to avoid misinterpretation.

NURSING PRIORITY NO. 2. To facilitate personal growth:

- Develop therapeutic relationship. Be attentive, maintain open communication, use skills of active-listening and I-messages. **Promotes trusting situation in which client is free to be open and honest with self and others.**

- Validate client's communication, provide encouragement for efforts.

- Accept client's perceptions/view of current status. **Avoids threatening existing self-esteem and provides opportunity for client to develop realistic plan for improving self-concept.**

- Be aware that people are not programmed to be rational. **Individuals must seek information—choosing to learn; to think rather than merely accepting/reacting in order to have respect for self, facts, honesty, and to develop positive self-esteem.**

- Discuss client perception of self, confronting misconceptions and identifying negative self-talk. Address distortions in thinking, such as self-referencing (beliefs that others are focusing on individual's weaknesses/limitations); filtering (focusing on negative and ignoring positive); catastrophizing (expecting the worst outcomes). **Addressing these issues openly allows client to identify things that may negatively affect self-esteem and provides opportunity for change.**

- Have client list current/past successes and strengths. **Emphasizes fact that client is and has been successful in many actions taken.**

- Use positive I-messages rather than praise. **Praise is a form of external control, coming from outside sources, whereas I-messages allow the client to develop internal sense of self-esteem.**

- Discuss what behavior does for client (positive intention). Ask what options are available to the client/SO(s). **Encourages thinking about what inner motivations are and what actions can be taken to enhance self-esteem.**

- Give reinforcement for progress noted. **Positive words of encouragement support development of effective coping behaviors.**

- Encourage client to progress at own rate. **Adaptation to a change in self-concept depends on its significance to the individual and disruption to lifestyle.**

Information in brackets added by the authors to clarify and enhance the use of nursing diagnoses.

Diagnostic Studies   ∞ Pediatric/Geriatric/Lifespan   Medications   **585**

• Involve in activities/exercise program of choice, promote socialization. **Enhances sense of well-being/can help to energize client.**

NURSING PRIORITY NO. 3. To promote optimum sense of self-worth and happiness:

 • Assist client to identify goals that are personally achievable. Provide positive feedback for verbal and behavioral indications of improved self-view. **Increases likelihood of success and commitment to change.**

 • Refer to vocational/employment counselor, educational resources, as appropriate. **Assists with improving development of social/vocational skills.**

 • Encourage participation in classes/activities/hobbies that client enjoys or would like to experience. **Provides opportunity for learning new information/skills that can enhance feelings of success, improving self-esteem.**

 • Reinforce that current decision to improve self-concept is ongoing. **Continued work and support are necessary to sustain behavior changes/personal growth.**

 • Discuss ways to develop optimism. **Optimism is a key ingredient in happiness and can be learned.**

 • Suggest assertiveness training classes. **Enhances ability to interact with others and develop more effective relationships, enhancing one's self-concept.**

 • Emphasize importance of grooming and personal hygiene and assist in developing skills to improve appearance and dress for success as needed. **Looking one's best improves sense of self-esteem and presenting a positive appearance enhances how others see you.**

Documentation Focus

ASSESSMENT/REASSESSMENT

• Individual findings, including evaluations of self and others, current and past successes.
• Interactions with others/lifestyle.
• Motivation for/willingness to change.

PLANNING

• Plan of care and who is involved in planning.
• Educational plan.

IMPLEMENTATION/EVALUATION

• Responses to interventions/teaching and actions performed.

Information in brackets added by the authors to clarify and enhance the use of nursing diagnoses.

 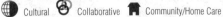 Cultural Collaborative Community/Home Care

- Attainment/progress toward desired outcome(s).
- Modifications to plan of care.

DISCHARGE PLANNING

- Long-term needs and who is responsible for actions to be taken.
- Specific referrals made.

SAMPLE NURSING OUTCOMES & INTERVENTIONS CLASSIFICATIONS (NOC/NIC)

NOC—Self-Esteem
NIC—Self-Modification Assistance

chronic low Self-Esteem

Taxonomy II: Self-Perception—Class 2 Self-Esteem
 (00119)
[Diagnostic Division: Ego Integrity]
Submitted 1988; Revised 1996

Definition: Long-standing negative self-evaluation/
feelings about self or self-capabilities

Related Factors

To be developed
[Fixation in earlier level of development]
[Personal vulnerability]
[Life choices perpetuating failure; ineffective social/occupational
 functioning]
[Feelings of abandonment by SO; willingness to tolerate possibly
 life-threatening domestic violence]
[Chronic physical/psychiatric conditions; antisocial behaviors]

Defining Characteristics

SUBJECTIVE

Self-negating verbalization
Expressions of shame/guilt
Evaluates self as unable to deal with events
Rejects positive/exaggerates negative feedback about self

OBJECTIVE

Hesitant to try new things/situations
Frequent lack of success in work/in life events

Information in brackets added by the authors to clarify and enhance
the use of nursing diagnoses.

 Diagnostic Studies   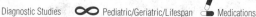 ∞ Pediatric/Geriatric/Lifespan   Medications   **587**

Overly conforming; dependent on others' opinions
Lack of eye contact
Nonassertive; passive; indecisive
Excessively seeks reassurance

Desired Outcomes/Evaluation Criteria—Client Will:

- Verbalize understanding of negative evaluation of self and reasons for this problem.
- Participate in treatment program to promote change in self-evaluation.
- Demonstrate behaviors/lifestyle changes to promote positive self-image.
- Verbalize increased sense of self-worth in relation to current situation.
- Participate in family/group/community activities to enhance change.

Actions/Interventions

NURSING PRIORITY NO. 1. To assess causative/contributing factors:

- Determine factors of low self-esteem related to current situation (e.g., family crises, physical disfigurement, social isolation), noting age and developmental level of individual. **Current crises may exacerbate long-standing feelings and self-evaluation as not being worthwhile.**
- Assess content of negative self-talk. Note client's perceptions of how others view him or her.
- Determine availability/quality of family/SO(s) support.
- Identify family dynamics—present and past—and cultural influences. **Family may engage in "put-downs" or "teasing" in ways that give client the message that he or she is worthless.**
- Be alert to client's concept of self in relation to cultural/religious ideal(s).
- Note nonverbal behavior (e.g., nervous movements, lack of eye contact). **Incongruencies between verbal/nonverbal communication require clarification.**
- Determine degree of participation and cooperation with therapeutic regimen (e.g., maintaining scheduled medications such as antidepressants/antipsychotics).
- Note willingness to seek assistance, motivation for change.

NURSING PRIORITY NO. 2. To promote client sense of self-esteem in dealing with current situation:

Information in brackets added by the authors to clarify and enhance the use of nursing diagnoses.

 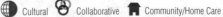 Cultural Collaborative Community/Home Care

- Develop therapeutic relationship. Be attentive, validate client's communication, provide encouragement for efforts, maintain open communication, use skills of active-listening and I-messages. **Promotes trusting situation in which client is free to be open and honest with self and therapist.**
- Address presenting medical/safety issues.
- Accept client's perceptions/view of situation. Avoid threatening existing self-esteem.
- Be aware that people are not programmed to be rational. **They must seek information—choosing to learn; to think rather than merely accepting/reacting—in order to have respect for self, facts, honesty, and to develop positive self-esteem.**
- Discuss client perceptions of self related to what is happening; confront misconceptions and negative self-talk. Address distortions in thinking, such as self-referencing (belief that others are focusing on individual's weaknesses/limitations), filtering (focusing on negative and ignoring positive), catastrophizing (expecting the worst outcomes). **Addressing these issues openly provides opportunity for change.**
- Emphasize need to avoid comparing self with others. Encourage client to focus on aspects of self that can be valued.
- Have client list current/past successes and strengths. **May help client see that he or she can develop an internal locus of control (a belief that one's successes and failures is the result of one's efforts) by recognizing these aspects of themselves.**
- Use positive I-messages rather than praise. **Assists client to develop internal sense of self-esteem.**
- Discuss what behavior does for client (positive intention). What options are available to the client/SO(s)?
- Assist client to deal with sense of powerlessness. (Refer to ND Powerlessness.)
- Set limits on aggressive or problem behaviors such as acting out, suicide preoccupation, or rumination. Put self in client's place (empathy not sympathy). **These negative behaviors diminish sense of self-concept.**
- Give reinforcement for progress noted. **Positive words of encouragement promote continuation of efforts, supporting development of coping behaviors.**
- Encourage client to progress at own rate. **Adaptation to a change in self-concept depends on its significance to individual, disruption to lifestyle, and length of illness/debilitation.**
- Assist client to recognize and cope with events, alterations, and sense of loss of control by incorporating changes accurately into self-concept.

Information in brackets added by the authors to clarify and enhance the use of nursing diagnoses.

Diagnostic Studies   ∞ Pediatric/Geriatric/Lifespan   Medications   **589**

• Involve in activities/exercise program, promote socialization. **Enhances sense of well-being/can help energize client.**

NURSING PRIORITY NO. 3. To promote wellness (Teaching/Discharge Considerations):

 • Discuss inaccuracies in self-perception with client/SO(s).

 • Model behaviors being taught, involving client in goal setting and decision making. **Facilitates client's developing trust in own unique strengths.**

 • Prepare client for events/changes that are expected, when possible.

 • Provide structure in daily routine/care activities.

 • Emphasize importance of grooming and personal hygiene. Assist in developing skills as indicated (e.g., makeup classes, dressing for success). **People feel better about themselves when they present a positive outer appearance.**

 • Assist client to identify goals that are personally achievable. Provide positive feedback for verbal and behavioral indications of improved self-view. **Increases likelihood of success and commitment to change.**

 • Refer to vocational/employment counselor, educational resources, as appropriate. **Assists with development of social/vocational skills, enhancing sense of self-concept and inner locus of control.**

 • Encourage participation in classes/activities/hobbies that client enjoys or would like to experience.

 • Reinforce that this therapy is a brief encounter in overall life of the client/SO(s), with continued work and ongoing support being necessary **to sustain behavior changes/personal growth.**

 • Refer to classes (e.g., assertiveness training, positive self-image, communication skills) **to assist with learning new skills to promote self-esteem.**

 • Refer to counseling/therapy, mental health, and special needs support groups, as indicated.

Documentation Focus

ASSESSMENT/REASSESSMENT

• Individual findings, including early memories of negative evaluations (self and others), subsequent/precipitating failure events.
• Effects on interactions with others/lifestyle.
• Specific medical/safety issues.
• Motivation for/willingness to change.

Information in brackets added by the authors to clarify and enhance the use of nursing diagnoses.

⊕ Cultural   Collaborative   Community/Home Care

PLANNING

• Plan of care and who is involved in planning.
• Teaching plan.

IMPLEMENTATION/EVALUATION

• Responses to interventions/teaching and actions performed.
• Attainment/progress toward desired outcome(s).
• Modifications to plan of care.

DISCHARGE PLANNING

• Long-term needs and who is responsible for actions to be taken.
• Specific referrals made.

SAMPLE NURSING OUTCOMES & INTERVENTIONS CLASSIFICATIONS (NOC/NIC)

NOC—Self-Esteem
NIC—Self-Esteem Enhancement

situational low Self-Esteem

Taxonomy II: Self-Perception—Class 2 Self-Esteem
   (00120)
[Diagnostic Division: Ego Integrity]
Submitted 1988; Revised 1996, 2000

Definition: Development of a negative perception of self-worth in response to a current situation (specify)

Related Factors

Developmental changes [e.g., maturational transitions, adolescence, aging]
Functional impairment; disturbed body image
Loss [e.g., loss of health status, body part, independent functioning; memory deficit/cognitive impairment]
Social role changes
Failures/rejections; lack of recognition[/rewards; feelings of abandonment by SO]
Behavior inconsistent with values

Defining Characteristics

SUBJECTIVE

Verbally reports current situational challenge to self-worth

Information in brackets added by the authors to clarify and enhance the use of nursing diagnoses.

 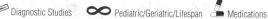

Expressions of helplessness/uselessness
Evaluation of self as unable to deal with situations or events

OBJECTIVE

Self-negating verbalizations
Indecisive/nonassertive behavior

Desired Outcomes/Evaluation Criteria—Client Will:

- Verbalize understanding of individual factors that precipitated current situation.
- Identify feelings and underlying dynamics for negative perception of self.
- Express positive self-appraisal.
- Demonstrate behaviors to restore positive self-esteem.
- Participate in treatment regimen/activities to correct factors that precipitated crisis.

Actions/Interventions

NURSING PRIORITY NO. 1. To assess causative/contributing factors:

- Determine individual situation (e.g., family crisis, termination of a relationship, loss of employment, physical disfigurement) related to low self-esteem in the present circumstances.
- Identify client's basic sense of self-esteem and image client has of self: existential, physical, psychological.
- Assess degree of threat/perception of client in regard to crisis. **Some people view a major situation as manageable, while another person may be overly concerned about a minor problem.**
- Ascertain sense of control client has (or perceives to have) over self and situation. Note client's locus of control (internal/external). **Locus of control is important in determining whether the client believes he or she has control over the situation, or whether one is at the mercy of fate or luck.**
- Determine client's awareness of own responsibility for dealing with situation, personal growth, and so forth. **When client is aware of and accepts own responsibility, may indicate internal locus of control.**
- Verify client's concept of self in relation to cultural/religious ideals. **May provide client with support or reinforce negative self-evaluation.**
- Review past coping skills in relation to current episode.
- Assess negative attitudes and/or self-talk.

Information in brackets added by the authors to clarify and enhance the use of nursing diagnoses.

 Cultural Collaborative 🏠 Community/Home Care

- Note nonverbal body language. **Incongruencies between verbal/nonverbal communication requires clarification.**
- Assess for self-destructive/suicidal behavior. (Refer to ND risk for Suicide, as appropriate.)
- Identify previous adaptations to illness/disruptive events in life. **May be predictive of current outcome.**
- Assess family/SO(s) dynamics and support of client.
- Note availability/use of resources.

NURSING PRIORITY NO. 2. To assist client to deal with loss/change and recapture sense of positive self-esteem:

- Assist with treatment of underlying condition when possible. **For example, cognitive restructuring and improved concentration in mild brain injury often result in restoration of positive self-esteem.**
- Encourage expression of feelings, anxieties. **Facilitates grieving the loss.**
- Active-listen client's concerns/negative verbalizations without comment or judgment.
- Identify individual strengths/assets and aspects of self that remain intact, can be valued. Reinforce positive traits, abilities, self-view.
- Help client identify own responsibility and control or lack of control in situation. **When able to acknowledge what is out of his or her control, client can focus attention on area of own responsibility.**
- Assist client to problem solve situation, developing plan of action and setting goals to achieve desired outcome. **Enhances commitment to plan, optimizing outcomes.**
- Convey confidence in client's ability to cope with current situation.
- Mobilize support systems.
- Provide opportunity for client to practice alternative coping strategies, including progressive socialization opportunities.
- Encourage use of visualization, guided imagery, and relaxation **to promote positive sense of self.**
- Provide feedback of client's self-negating remarks/behavior, using I-messages, **to allow the client to experience a different view.**
- Encourage involvement in decisions about care when possible.

NURSING PRIORITY NO. 3. To promote wellness (Teaching/Discharge Considerations):

- Encourage client to set long-range goals for achieving necessary lifestyle changes. **Supports view that this is an ongoing process.**

Information in brackets added by the authors to clarify and enhance the use of nursing diagnoses.

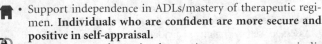

- Support independence in ADLs/mastery of therapeutic regimen. **Individuals who are confident are more secure and positive in self-appraisal.**
- Promote attendance in therapy/support group, as indicated.
- Involve extended family/SO(s) in treatment plan. **Increases likelihood they will provide appropriate support to client.**
- Provide information to assist client in making desired changes. **Appropriate books, DVDs, or other resources allow client to learn at own pace.**
- Suggest participation in group/community activities (e.g., assertiveness classes, volunteer work, support groups).

Documentation Focus

ASSESSMENT/REASSESSMENT

- Individual findings, noting precipitating crisis, client's perceptions, effects on desired lifestyle/interaction with others.
- Cultural values/religious beliefs, locus of control.
- Family support, availability/use of resources.

PLANNING

- Plan of care and who is involved in planning.
- Teaching plan.

IMPLEMENTATION/EVALUATION

- Responses to interventions/teaching, actions performed, and changes that may be indicated.
- Attainment/progress toward desired outcome(s).
- Modifications to plan of care.

DISCHARGE PLANNING

- Long-term needs/goals and who is responsible for actions to be taken.
- Specific referrals made.

SAMPLE NURSING OUTCOMES & INTERVENTIONS CLASSIFICATIONS (NOC/NIC)

NOC—Self-Esteem
NIC—Self-Esteem Enhancement

Information in brackets added by the authors to clarify and enhance the use of nursing diagnoses.

 Cultural Collaborative Community/Home Care

risk for situational low Self-Esteem

Taxonomy II: Self-Perception—Class 2 Self-Esteem
(00153)
[Diagnostic Division: Ego Integrity]
Submitted 2000

Definition: At risk for developing negative perception of
self-worth in response to a current situation (specify)

Risk Factors

Developmental changes
Disturbed body image; functional impairment
Loss [e.g., loss of health status, body part, independent func-
tioning; memory deficit/cognitive impairment]
Social role changes
Unrealistic self-expectations; history of learned helplessness
History of neglect/abuse/abandonment
Behavior inconsistent with values
Lack of recognition; failures; rejections
Decreased control over environment
Physical illness

> NOTE: A risk diagnosis is not evidenced by signs and symptoms, as
> the problem has not occurred and nursing interventions are
> directed at prevention.

Desired Outcomes/Evaluation Criteria—Client Will:

- Acknowledge factors that lead to possibility of feelings of low
  self-esteem.
- Verbalize view of self as a worthwhile, important person who
  functions well both interpersonally and occupationally.
- Demonstrate self-confidence by setting realistic goals and
  actively participating in life situation.

Actions/Interventions

NURSING PRIORITY NO. 1. To assess causative/contributing factors:

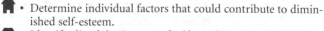
- Determine individual factors that could contribute to dimin-
  ished self-esteem.
- Identify client's basic sense of self-worth and image client has
  of self: existential, physical, psychological.

Information in brackets added by the authors to clarify and enhance
the use of nursing diagnoses.

 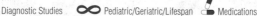

• Note client's perception of threat to self in current situation.

 • Ascertain sense of control client has (or perceives to have) over self and situation.

 • Determine client awareness of own responsibility for dealing with situation, personal growth, and so forth.

 • Verify client's concept of self in relation to cultural/religious ideals. **Conflict between current situation and these ideals may contribute to risk of low self-esteem.**

 • Assess negative attitudes and/or self-talk. **Contributes to view of situation as hopeless, difficult.**

 • Note nonverbal body language. **Incongruencies between verbal/nonverbal communication require clarification.**

 • Listen for self-destructive/suicidal verbalizations, noting behaviors that indicate these thoughts. **Necessitates intervention to prevent client following through on thoughts.**

 • Identify previous adaptations to illness/disruptive events in life. **May be predictive of current outcome.**

 • Assess family/SO(s) dynamics and support of client.

 • Note availability/use of resources.

• Refer to NDs situational low Self-Esteem; chronic low Self-Esteem, as appropriate, for additional nursing priorities/interventions.

Documentation Focus

ASSESSMENT/REASSESSMENT

• Individual findings, including individual expressions of lack of self-esteem, effects on interactions with others/lifestyle.
• Underlying dynamics and duration (situational or situational exacerbating chronic).
• Cultural values/religious beliefs, locus of control.
• Family support, availability/use of resources.

PLANNING

• Plan of care and who is involved in planning.
• Teaching plan.

IMPLEMENTATION/EVALUATION

• Responses to interventions/teaching, actions performed, and changes that may be indicated.
• Attainment/progress toward desired outcome(s).
• Modifications to plan of care.

Information in brackets added by the authors to clarify and enhance the use of nursing diagnoses.

Cultural   Collaborative   Community/Home Care

DISCHARGE PLANNING

- Long-term needs/goals and who is responsible for actions to be taken.
- Specific referrals made.

SAMPLE NURSING OUTCOMES & INTERVENTIONS CLASSIFICATIONS (NOC/NIC)

NOC—Self-Esteem
NIC—Self-Esteem Enhancement

Self-Mutilation

Taxonomy II: Safety/Protection—Class 3 Violence (00151)
[Diagnostic Division: Safety]
Submitted 2000

Definition: Deliberate self-injurious behavior causing tissue damage with the intent of causing nonfatal injury to attain relief of tension

Related Factors

Adolescence; peers who self-mutilate; isolation from peers

Dissociation; depersonalization; psychotic state (e.g., command hallucinations); character disorder; borderline personality disorders; emotionally disturbed; developmentally delayed/autistic individual

History of: self-injurious behavior, inability to plan solutions, inability to see long-term consequences

Childhood illness/surgery/sexual abuse; battered child

Disturbed body image; eating disorders

Ineffective coping; perfectionism

Negative feelings (e.g., depression, rejection, self-hatred, separation anxiety, guilt, depersonalization); low self-esteem; unstable self-esteem/body image

Poor communication between parent and adolescent; lack of family confidant

Feels threated with loss of significant relationship [loss of parent/parental relationship]

Disturbed interpersonal relationships; use of manipulation to obtain nurturing relationship with others

Family alcoholism/divorce; violence between parental figures; family history of self-destructive behaviors

---

Information in brackets added by the authors to clarify and enhance the use of nursing diagnoses.

 Diagnostic Studies 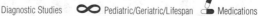 Pediatric/Geriatric/Lifespan Medications **597**

Living in nontraditional settings (e.g., foster, group, or institutional care); incarceration

Inability to express tension verbally; mounting tension that is intolerable; needs quick reduction of stress

Irresistable urge to cut/damage self; impulsivity; labile behavior

Sexual identity crisis

Substance abuse

Defining Characteristics

SUBJECTIVE

Self-inflicted burns [e.g., eraser, cigarette]

Ingestion/inhalation of harmful substances

OBJECTIVE

Cuts/scratches on body

Picking at wounds

Biting; abrading; severing

Insertion of object into body orifice

Hitting

Constricting a body part

Desired Outcomes/Evaluation Criteria—Client Will:

- Verbalize understanding of reasons for occurrence of behavior.
- Identify precipitating factors/awareness of arousal state that occurs prior to incident.
- Express increased self-concept/self-esteem.
- Seek help when feeling anxious and having thoughts of harming self.

Actions/Interventions

NURSING PRIORITY NO. 1. To assess causative/contributing factors:

 • Determine underlying dynamics of individual situation as listed in Related Factors. Note presence of inflexible, maladaptive personality traits that reflect personality/character disorder (e.g., impulsive, unpredictable, inappropriate behaviors, intense anger, or lack of control of anger).

• Evaluate history of mental illness (e.g., borderline personality, identity disorder, bipolar disorder).

• Identify previous episodes of self-mutilation behavior. **Note: Although some body piercing (e.g., ears) is generally accepted as decorative, and while piercing of multiple sites**

Information in brackets added by the authors to clarify and enhance the use of nursing diagnoses.

 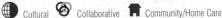

often is an attempt to establish individuality, addressing issues of separation and belonging, it is not considered as self-injury behavior.

🏠 • Determine relationship of previous self-mutilative behavior to stressful events. **Self-injury is considered to be an attempt to alter a mood state.**

💊 • Note use/abuse of addicting substances.

🧪 • Review laboratory findings (e.g., blood alcohol, polydrug screen, glucose, and electrolyte levels). **Drug use may affect self-injury behavior.**

NURSING PRIORITY NO. 2. To structure environment to maintain client safety:

🏠 • Assist client to identify feelings leading up to desire for self-mutilation. **Early recognition of recurring feelings provides opportunity to seek and learn other ways of coping.**

🏠 • Provide external controls/limit setting. **May decrease the opportunity to self-mutilate.**

🏠 • Include client in development of plan of care. **Commitment to plan increases likelihood of adherence.**

🏠 • Encourage appropriate expression of feelings. **Identifies feelings and promotes understanding of what leads to development of tension.**

🏠 • Note feelings of healthcare providers/family, such as frustration, anger, defensiveness, need to rescue. **Client may be manipulative, evoking defensiveness and conflict. These feelings need to be identified, recognized, and dealt with openly with staff/family and client.**

🔗 • Provide care for client's wounds, when self-mutilation occurs, in a matter-of-fact manner **that conveys empathy/concern.** Refrain from offering sympathy or additional attention **that could provide reinforcement for maladaptive behavior and may encourage its repetition.**

NURSING PRIORITY NO. 3. To promote movement toward positive changes:

🏠 • Involve client in developing goals for stopping behavior. **Enhances commitment, optimizing outcomes.**

🏠 • Develop a contract between client and counselor **to enable the client to stay physically safe, such as "I will not cut or harm myself for the next 24 hours."** Renew contract on a regular basis and have both parties sign and date each contract.

🏠 • Provide avenues of communication **for times when client needs to talk to avoid cutting or damaging self.**

Information in brackets added by the authors to clarify and enhance the use of nursing diagnoses.

• Assist client to learn assertive behavior. Include the use of effective communication skills, focusing on developing self-esteem by replacing negative self-talk with positive comments.

• Use interventions that help the client to reclaim power in own life (e.g., experiential and cognitive).

NURSING PRIORITY NO. 4. To promote wellness (Teaching/Discharge Considerations):

• Discuss commitment to safety and ways in which client will deal with precursors to undesired behavior. **Provides opportunity for client to assume responsibility for self.**

• Promote the use of healthy behaviors, identifying the consequences and outcomes of current actions.

• Identify support systems.

• Discuss living arrangements when client is discharged/relocated. **May need assistance with transition to changes required to avoid recurrence of self-mutilating behaviors.**

• Involve family/SO(s) in planning for discharge and in group therapies, as appropriate. **Promotes coordination and continuation of plan, commitment to goals.**

• Discuss information about the role neurotransmitters play in predisposing an individual to beginning this behavior. **It is believed that problems in the serotonin system may make the person more aggressive and impulsive, combined with a home where he or she learned that feelings are bad or wrong, leading to turning aggression on self.**

• Provide information and discuss the use of medication, as appropriate. **Antidepressant medications may be useful, but they need to be weighed against the potential for overdosing.**

• Refer to NDs Anxiety; impaired Social Interaction; Self-Esteem (specify).

Documentation Focus

ASSESSMENT/REASSESSMENT

• Individual findings, including risk factors present, underlying dynamics, prior episodes.
• Cultural/religious practices.
• Laboratory test results.
• Substance use/abuse.

PLANNING

• Plan of care and who is involved in planning.
• Teaching plan.

Information in brackets added by the authors to clarify and enhance the use of nursing diagnoses.

 Cultural Collaborative Community/Home Care

IMPLEMENTATION/EVALUATION

- Response to interventions/teaching and actions performed.
- Attainment/progress toward desired outcome(s).
- Modifications to plan of care.

DISCHARGE PLANNING

- Long-range needs and who is responsible for actions to be taken.
- Community resources, referrals made.

SAMPLE NURSING OUTCOMES & INTERVENTIONS CLASSIFICATIONS (NOC/NIC)

NOC—Self-Mutilation Restraint
NIC—Behavior Management: Self-Harm

risk for Self-Mutilation

Taxonomy II: Safety/Protection—Class 3 Violence (00139)
[Diagnostic Division: Safety]
Submitted 1992; Revised 2000

Definition: At risk for deliberate self-injurious behavior causing tissue damage with the intent of causing nonfatal injury to attain relief of tension

Risk Factors

Adolescence; peers who self-mutilate; isolation from peers

Dissociation; depersonalization; psychotic state (e.g., command hallucinations); character disorders; borderline personality disorders; emotionally disturbed child; developmentally delayed/autistic individuals

History of: self-injurious behavior, inability to plan solutions, inability to see long-term consequences

Childhood illness/surgery/sexual abuse; battered child

Disturbed body image; eating disorders

Ineffective coping; loss of control over problem-solving situations; perfectionism

Negative feelings (e.g., depression, rejection, self-hatred, separation anxiety, guilt); low/unstable self-esteem

Feels threatened with loss of significant relationship; loss of significant relationship; lack of family confidant

Disturbed interpersonal relationships; use of manipulation to obtain nurturing relationship with others

---

Information in brackets added by the authors to clarify and enhance the use of nursing diagnoses.

 Diagnostic Studies 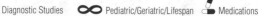 Pediatric/Geriatric/Lifespan   Medications **601**

Family alcoholism/divorce; violence between parental figures; family history of self-destructive behaviors

Living in nontraditional settings (e.g., foster, group, or institutional care); incarceration

Inability to express tension verbally; mounting tension that is intolerable; needs quick reduction of stress; irresistable urge to damage self; impulsivity

Sexual identity crisis

Substance abuse

> NOTE: A risk diagnosis is not evidenced by signs and symptoms, as the problem has not occurred and nursing interventions are directed at prevention.

Desired Outcomes/Evaluation Criteria—Client Will:

- Verbalize understanding of reasons for wanting to cut self.
- Identify precipitating factors/awareness of arousal state that occurs prior to incident.
- Express increased self-concept/self-esteem.
- Demonstrate self-control as evidenced by lessened (or absence of) episodes of self-injury.
- Engage in use of alternative methods for managing feelings/individuality.

Actions/Interventions

NURSING PRIORITY NO. 1. To assess causative/contributing factors:

 • Determine underlying dynamics of individual situation as listed in Risk Factors. Note presence of inflexible, maladaptive personality traits (e.g., impulsive, unpredictable, inappropriate behaviors; intense anger or lack of control of anger) **reflecting personality/character disorder or mental illness (e.g., bipolar disorder)** or conditions that may interfere with ability to control own behavior (e.g., psychotic state, mental retardation, autism).

 • Identify previous episodes of self-mutilating behavior (e.g., cutting, scratching, bruising). **Note: Although some body piercing (e.g., ears) is generally accepted as decorative, and while piercing of multiple sites often is an attempt to establish individuality, addressing issues of separation and belonging, it is not considered as self-injury behavior.**

 • Note beliefs, cultural/religious practices that may be involved in choice of behavior. **Growing up in a family that did not**

Information in brackets added by the authors to clarify and enhance the use of nursing diagnoses.

    Cultural   Collaborative   Community/Home Care

allow feelings to be expressed, individuals learn that feelings are bad or wrong. Family dynamics may come out of religious or cultural expectations that believe in strict punishment for transgressions.

- Determine use/abuse of addictive substances. **May be trying to resist impulse to self-injure by turning to drugs.**
- Review laboratory findings (e.g., blood alcohol, polydrug screen, glucose, electrolyte levels).
- Note degree of impairment in social and occupational functioning. **May dictate treatment setting (e.g., specific outpatient program, short-stay inpatient).**

NURSING PRIORITY NO. 2. To structure environment to maintain client safety:

- Assist client to identify feelings and behaviors that precede desire for mutilation. **Early recognition of recurring feelings provides client opportunity to seek other ways of coping.**
- Provide external controls/limit setting **to decrease the need to mutilate self.**
- Include client in development of plan of care. **Being involved in own decisions can help to reestablish ego boundaries and strengthen commitment to goals and participation in therapy.**
- Encourage client to recognize and appropriately express feelings verbally.
- Keep client in continuous staff view and provide special observation checks during inpatient therapy **to promote safety.**
- Structure inpatient milieu to maintain positive, clear, open communication among staff and clients, with an understanding that "secrets are not tolerated" and will be confronted.
- Develop schedule of alternative, healthy, success-oriented activities, including involvement in such groups as Overeaters Anonymous (OA) or similar 12-step program based on individual needs; self-esteem activities include positive affirmations, visiting with friends, and exercise.
- Note feelings of healthcare providers/family, such as frustration, anger, defensiveness, distraction, despair and powerlessness, and need to rescue. **Client may be manipulative, evoking defensiveness and conflict. These feelings need to be identified, recognized, and dealt with openly with staff/family and client.**

NURSING PRIORITY NO. 3. To promote movement toward positive actions:

- Involve client in developing goals for preventing undesired behavior. **Enhances commitment, optimizing outcomes.**

Information in brackets added by the authors to clarify and enhance the use of nursing diagnoses.

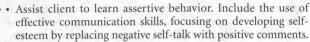

risk for SELF-MUTILATION

- Assist client to learn assertive behavior. Include the use of effective communication skills, focusing on developing self-esteem by replacing negative self-talk with positive comments.

- Develop a contract between client and counselor **to enable the client to stay physically safe, such as "I will not cut or harm myself for the next 24 hours."** Renew contract on a regular basis and have both parties sign and date each contract. Make contingency arrangements **so client can talk to counselor, as needed.**

- Discuss with client/family normalcy of adolescent task of separation and ways of achieving.

- Promote the use of healthy behaviors, identifying the consequences and outcomes of current actions: "Does this get you what you want?" "How does this behavior help you achieve your goals?" **Dialectical Behavior Therapy is an effective therapy in reducing self-injurious behavior along with appropriate medication.**

- Provide reinforcement for use of assertive behavior rather than nonassertive/aggressive behavior.

- Use interventions that help the client to reclaim power in own life (e.g., experiential and cognitive).

- Involve client/family in group therapies as appropriate.

NURSING PRIORITY NO. 4. To promote wellness (Teaching/Discharge Considerations):

- Discuss commitment to safety and ways in which client will deal with precursors to undesired behavior.

- Mobilize support systems.

- Involve family/SO(s) in planning for discharge, as appropriate. **Promotes coordination and continuation of plan, commitment to goals.**

- Identify living circumstances client will be going to once discharged/relocated. **May need assistance with transition to changes required to reduce risk/avoid recurrence of self-mutilating behaviors.**

- Arrange for continued involvement in group therapy(ies).

- Discuss and provide information about the use of medication, as appropriate. **Antidepressant medications may be useful, but use needs to be weighed against potential for overdosing/adverse side effects (e.g., the antidepressant Effexor can cause hostility, suicidal ideas, and self-harm). Medications that stabilize moods, ease depression, and calm anxiety may be tried to reduce the urge to self-harm.**

- Refer to NDs Anxiety; impaired Social Interaction; Self-Esteem (specify).

Information in brackets added by the authors to clarify and enhance the use of nursing diagnoses.

 Cultural Collaborative 🏠 Community/Home Care

Documentation Focus

ASSESSMENT/REASSESSMENT

- Individual findings, including risk factors present, underlying dynamics, prior episodes.
- Cultural/religious practices.
- Laboratory test results.
- Substance use/abuse.

PLANNING

- Plan of care and who is involved in planning.
- Teaching plan.

IMPLEMENTATION/EVALUATION

- Response to interventions/teaching and actions performed.
- Attainment/progress toward desired outcome(s).
- Modifications to plan of care.

DISCHARGE PLANNING

- Long-range needs and who is responsible for actions to be taken.
- Community resources, referrals made.

SAMPLE NURSING OUTCOMES & INTERVENTIONS CLASSIFICATIONS (NOC/NIC)

NOC—Self-Mutilation Restraint
NIC—Behavior Management: Self-Harm

disturbed Sensory Perception
(Specify: Visual, Auditory, Kinesthetic, Gustatory, Tactile, Olfactory)

Taxonomy II: Perception/Cognition—Class 3
  Sensation/Perception (00122)
[Diagnostic Division: Neurosensory]
Submitted 1978; Revised 1980, 1998 (by small group work 1996)

Definition: Change in the amount or patterning of incoming stimuli accompanied by a diminished, exaggerated, distorted, or impaired response to such stimuli

Related Factors

Insufficient environmental stimuli: [therapeutically restricted environments (e.g., isolation, intensive care, bedrest, traction,

---

Information in brackets added by the authors to clarify and enhance the use of nursing diagnoses.

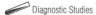 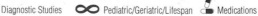

confining illnesses, incubator); socially restricted environment (e.g., institutionalization, homebound, aging, chronic/terminal illness, infant deprivation); stigmatized (e.g., mentally ill/developmentally delayed/handicapped)]

Excessive environmental stimuli: [excessive noise level, such as work environment, client's immediate environment (ICU with support machinery and the like)]

Altered sensory reception/transmission/integration: [neurological disease, trauma, or deficit; altered status of sense organs]

Biochemical imbalances [e.g., elevated BUN, elevated ammonia, hypoxia]; electrolyte imbalance; [drugs, e.g., stimulants or depressants, mind-altering drugs]

Psychological stress; [sleep deprivation]

Defining Characteristics

SUBJECTIVE

[Reported] change in sensory acuity [e.g., photosensitivity, hypoesthesias/hyperesthesias, diminished/altered sense of taste, inability to tell position of body parts (proprioception)]
Sensory distortions

OBJECTIVE

[Measured] change in sensory acuity
Change in usual response to stimuli [e.g., rapid mood swings, exaggerated emotional responses, anxiety/panic state]
Change in behavior pattern; restlessness; irritability
Change in problem-solving abilities; poor concentration
Disorientation; hallucinations; [illusions]; [bizarre thinking]
Impaired communication
[Motor incoordination, altered sense of balance/falls (e.g., Ménière's syndrome)]

Desired Outcomes/Evaluation Criteria—Client Will:

• Regain/maintain usual level of cognition.
• Recognize and correct/compensate for sensory impairments.
• Verbalize awareness of sensory needs and presence of overload and/or deprivation.
• Identify/modify external factors that contribute to alterations in sensory/perceptual abilities.
• Use resources effectively and appropriately.
• Be free of injury.

Information in brackets added by the authors to clarify and enhance the use of nursing diagnoses.

 Cultural Collaborative   Community/Home Care

Actions/Interventions

NURSING PRIORITY NO. 1. To assess causative/contributing factors and degree of impairment:

- Identify client with condition that can affect sensing, interpreting, and communicating stimuli (e.g., stroke, brain injury, cognitive impairment/dementia; pain, surgery, or trauma involving sensory organs; central nervous system disorders [e.g., spinal cord injury, cerebral palsy, Parkinson's disease, etc.]; peripheral neuropathies).
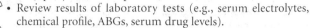
- Review results of laboratory tests (e.g., serum electrolytes, chemical profile, ABGs, serum drug levels).
- Assist with/review diagnostic studies and sensory/motor neurological testing.
- Monitor drug regimen **to identify medications with effects or drug interactions that may cause/exacerbate sensory/ perceptual problems.**
- Assess ability to speak, hear, interpret and respond to simple commands **to obtain an overview of client's mental/cognitive status and ability to interpret stimuli**.
- Evaluate sensory awareness: Stimulus of hot/cold, dull/sharp, smell, taste, visual acuity and hearing; gait/mobility, and location/function of body parts.
- Determine response to painful stimuli **to note whether response is appropriate to stimulus, immediate, or delayed.**
- Observe for behavioral responses (e.g., illusions/hallucinations, delusions, withdrawal, hostility, crying, inappropriate affect, confusion/disorientation).
- Ascertain client's/SO's perception of problem/changes in activities of daily living. Listen to and respect client's expressions of deprivation and take these into consideration in planning care.

NURSING PRIORITY NO. 2. To promote normalization of response to stimuli:

- Provide means of communication, as indicated.
- Encourage use of listening devices (e.g., hearing aid, audiovisual amplifier, closed-caption TV, signing interpreter) **to assist in managing auditory impairment.**
- Avoid isolation of client, physically or emotionally, **to prevent sensory deprivation/limit confusion.**
- Promote a stable environment with continuity of care by same personnel as much as possible.
- Interpret stimuli/offer feedback **to assist client to separate reality from fantasy/altered perception.**
- Reorient to person, place, time, and events, as necessary.

Information in brackets added by the authors to clarify and enhance the use of nursing diagnoses.

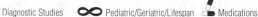

- Explain procedures/activities, expected sensations, and outcomes.
- Limit/carefully monitor use of sedation, especially in older population.
- Minimize discussion of negatives (e.g., client and personnel problems) within client's hearing. **Client may misinterpret and believe references are to himself or herself.**
- Eliminate extraneous noise/stimuli, including nonessential equipment, alarms/audible monitor signals when possible.
- Provide undisturbed rest/sleep periods.
- Speak to visually impaired or unresponsive client during care **to provide auditory stimulation and prevent startle reflex.**
- Provide tactile stimulation as care is given. **Touching is an important part of caring and a deep psychological need communicating presence/connection with another human being.**
- Encourage SO(s) to bring in familiar objects, talk to, and touch the client frequently.
- Provide sensory stimulation, including familiar smells/ sounds, tactile stimulation with a variety of objects, changing of light intensity and other cues (e.g., clocks, calendars).
- Provide diversional activities, as able (e.g., TV/radio, conversation, large-print or talking books). (Refer to ND deficient Diversional Activity.)
- Promote meaningful socialization. (Refer to ND Social Isolation.)
- Collaborate with/involve other health-team members in providing rehabilitative therapies and stimulating modalities (e.g., music therapy, sensory training, remotivation therapy) **to achieve maximal gains in function and psychosocial well-being.**
- Identify and encourage use of resources/prosthetic devices (e.g., hearing aids, computerized visual aid/glasses with a level plumbline for balance). **Useful for augmenting senses.**

NURSING PRIORITY NO. 3. To prevent injury/complications:

- Record perceptual deficit on chart **so that caregivers are aware.**
- Place call bell/other communication device within reach and be sure client knows where it is/how to use it.
- Provide safety measures, as needed (e.g., side rails, bed in low position, adequate lighting; assistance with walking; use of vision/hearing devices).
- Review basic and specific safety information (e.g., "I am on your right side"; "This water is hot"; "Swallow now"; "Stand up"; "You cannot drive").
- Position doors and furniture so they are out of travel path for client with impaired vision, or strategically place items/grab bars **to aid in maintaining balance.**

Information in brackets added by the authors to clarify and enhance the use of nursing diagnoses.

  Cultural Collaborative Community/Home Care

- Ambulate with assistance/devices **to enhance balance.**
- Describe where affected areas of body are when moving client.
- Monitor use of heating pads/ice packs; use thermometer to measure temperature of bath water **to protect from thermal injury**.
- Refer to NDs risk for Injury; risk for Trauma; risk for Falls.

NURSING PRIORITY NO. 4. To promote wellness (Teaching/Discharge Considerations):

- Assist client/SO(s) to learn effective ways of coping with and managing sensory disturbances, anticipating safety needs according to client's sensory deficits and developmental level.
- Identify alternative ways of dealing with perceptual deficits (e.g., vision and hearing aids; augmentative communication devices; computer technologies; specific deficit-compensation techniques).
- Provide explanations of and plan care with client, involving SO(s) as much as possible. **Enhances commitment to and continuation of plan, optimizing outcomes.**
- Review home safety measures pertinent to deficits.
- Discuss drug regimen, noting possible toxic side effects of both prescription and OTC drugs. **Prompt recognition of side effects allows for timely intervention/change in drug regimen.**
- Demonstrate use/care of sensory prosthetic devices (e.g., assistive vision or listening devices, etc.).
- Identify resources/community programs for acquiring and maintaining assistive devices.
- Discuss with client/SO ways to prevent/limit exposure to conditions affecting sensory functions (e.g., how exposure to loud noise and toxic side effects of some drugs can impair hearing; early childhood screening for speech and language disorders; vaccines to prevent measles, mumps, meningitis [**once known to be major causes of hearing loss**]).
- Refer to appropriate helping resources, such as Society for the Blind, Self-Help for the Hard of Hearing (SHHH), or local support groups, screening programs, etc.

Documentation Focus

ASSESSMENT/REASSESSMENT

- Individual findings, noting specific deficit/associated symptoms, perceptions of client/SO(s).
- Assistive device needs.

PLANNING

- Plan of care, including who is involved in planning.
- Teaching plan.

Information in brackets added by the authors to clarify and enhance the use of nursing diagnoses.

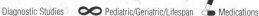

IMPLEMENTATION/EVALUATION

- Responses to interventions/teaching and actions performed.
- Attainment/progress toward desired outcome(s).
- Modifications to plan of care.

DISCHARGE PLANNING

- Long-term needs and who is responsible for actions to be taken.
- Available resources; specific referrals made.

SAMPLE NURSING OUTCOMES & INTERVENTIONS CLASSIFICATIONS (NOC/NIC)

AUDITORY

NOC—Hearing Compensation Behavior
NIC—Communication Enhancement: Hearing Deficit

VISUAL

NOC—Vision Compensation Behavior
NIC—Communication Enhancement: Visual Deficit

GUSTATORY/OLFACTORY

NOC—Distorted Thought Control
NIC—Nutrition Management

KINESTHETIC

NOC—Balance
NIC—Body Mechanics Promotion

TACTILE

NOC—Sensory Function: Cutaneous
NIC—Peripheral Sensation Management

Sexual Dysfunction

Taxonomy II: Sexuality—Class 2 Sexual Function (00059)
[Diagnostic Division: Sexuality]
Submitted 1980; Revised 2006

Definition: The state in which an individual experiences a change in sexual function during the sexual response phases of desire, excitation, and/or orgasm, which is viewed as unsatisfying, unrewarding, or inadequate

---

Information in brackets added by the authors to clarify and enhance the use of nursing diagnoses.

 Cultural   Collaborative   Community/Home Care

Related Factors

Ineffectual/absent role models; lack of SO
Lack of privacy
Misinformation or lack of knowledge
Vulnerability
Physical abuse; psychosocial abuse (e.g., harmful relationships)
Altered body function/structure (e.g., pregnancy, recent child-birth, drugs, surgery, anomalies, disease process, trauma, radiation, [effects of aging])
Biopsychosocial alteration of sexuality
Values conflict

Defining Characteristics

SUBJECTIVE

Verbalization of problem [e.g., loss of sexual desire, disruption of sexual response patterns such as premature ejaculation, dyspareunia, vaginismus], alterations in achieving percieved sex role
Actual/perceived limitation imposed by disease/therapy
Alterations in achieving sexual satisfaction; inability to achieve desired satisfaction
Perceived deficiency of sexual desire/alteration in sexual excitation
Seeking confirmation of desirability [concern about body image]
Change of interest in self/others; [alteration in relationship with SO]

Desired Outcomes/Evaluation
Criteria—Client Will:

- Verbalize understanding of sexual anatomy/function and alterations that may affect function.
- Verbalize understanding of individual reasons for sexual problems.
- Identify stressors in lifestyle that may contribute to the dysfunction.
- Identify satisfying/acceptable sexual practices and alternative ways of dealing with sexual expression.
- Discuss concerns about body image, sex role, desirability as a sexual partner with partner/SO.

Actions/Interventions

NURSING PRIORITY NO. 1. To assess causative/contributing factors:

- Do a complete history and physical, including a sexual history, which would include usual pattern of functioning and

---

Information in brackets added by the authors to clarify and enhance the use of nursing diagnoses.

 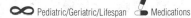

level of desire. Note vocabulary used by the individual to maximize communication/understanding.

🏠 • Have client describe problem in own words.

🏠 • Determine importance of sex to individual/partner and client's motivation for change. **Interpersonal problems (marital and relationship), lack of trust and open communication between partners can contribute to client's concern.**

🏠 • Be alert to comments of client **as sexual concerns are often disguised as humor, sarcasm, and/or offhand remarks.**

🏠 • Assess knowledge of client/SO regarding sexual anatomy/function and effects of current situation/condition. **Individuals are often ignorant of anatomy of sexual system and how it works, impacting client's understanding of situation and expectations.**

🏠 • Determine preexisting problems that may be factors in current situation (e.g., marital/job stress, role conflicts).

🏠 • Identify current stress factors in individual situation. **These factors may be producing enough anxiety to cause depression or other psychological reaction(s) leading to physiological symptoms.**

🌐 • Discuss cultural values/religious beliefs or conflicts present. **Client may have anxiety and guilt as a result of family beliefs about sex and genital area of the body because of how sexuality was communicated to the client as he or she was growing up.**

🏠 • Determine pathophysiology, illness/surgery/trauma involved, and impact on (perception of) individual/SO. **The client may be more concerned about these issues when the sexual parts of the body are involved (e.g., mastectomy, hysterectomy, prostatectomy).**

💊 • Review medication regimen/drug use (prescriptions, OTC, illegal, alcohol) and cigarette use. **Antihypertensives may cause erectile dysfunction; MAO inhibitors and tricyclics can cause erection/ejaculation problems and anorgasmia in women; narcotics/alcohol produce impotence and inhibit orgasm; smoking creates vasoconstriction and may be a factor in erectile dysfunction.**

🏠 • Observe behavior/stage of grieving when related to body changes or loss of a body part (e.g., pregnancy, obesity, amputation, mastectomy).

• Discuss client's view of body, concern about penis size, failure with performance.

🧪 • Assist with diagnostic studies to determine cause of erectile dysfunction. **More than half of the cases have a physical**

Information in brackets added by the authors to clarify and enhance the use of nursing diagnoses.

cause such as diabetes, vascular problems. Monitor penile tumescence during REM sleep **to assist in determining physical ability.**

🏠 • Explore with client the meaning of client's behavior. **Masturbation, for instance, may have many meanings/purposes, such as for relief of anxiety, sexual deprivation, pleasure, a nonverbal expression of need to talk, way of alienating.** (Note: Nurse needs to be aware of and be in control of own feelings and response to client expressions/self-revelation.)

🏠 • Avoid making value judgments **as they do not help the client to cope with the situation.**

NURSING PRIORITY NO. 2. To assist client/SO to deal with individual situation:

🏠 • Establish therapeutic nurse-client relationship **to promote treatment and facilitate sharing of sensitive information/ feelings.**

☯ • Assist with treatment of underlying medical conditions, including changes in medication regimen, weight management, cessation of smoking, and so forth.

🏠 • Provide factual information about individual condition involved. **Promotes informed decision making.**

🏠 • Determine what client wants to know **to tailor information to client needs.** Note: Information affecting client safety/consequences of actions may need to be reviewed/reinforced.

🏠 • Encourage and accept expressions of concern, anger, grief, fear. **Client needs to talk about these feelings to begin resolution.**

🏠 • Assist client to be aware/deal with stages of grieving for loss/ change.

🏠 • Encourage client to share thoughts/concerns with partner and to clarify values/impact of condition on relationship.

🏠 • Provide for/identify ways to obtain privacy **to allow for sexual expression for individual and/or between partners without embarrassment and/or objections of others.**

🏠 • Assist client/SO to problem solve alternative ways of sexual expression. **When client is unable to perform in usual manner, there are many ways the couple can learn to satisfy sexual needs.**

💊 • Provide information about availability of corrective measures such as medication (e.g., papaverine or sildenafil—Viagra— for erectile dysfunction) or reconstructive surgery (e.g., penile/breast implants) when indicated.

☯ • Refer to appropriate resources as need indicates (e.g., health-care coworker with greater comfort level and/or knowledgeable

---

Information in brackets added by the authors to clarify and enhance the use of nursing diagnoses.

clinical nurse specialist or professional sex therapist, family counseling).

NURSING PRIORITY NO. 3. To promote wellness (Teaching/Discharge Considerations):

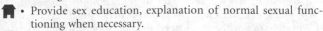

• Provide sex education, explanation of normal sexual functioning when necessary.

• Provide written material appropriate to individual needs (include list of books related to client's concerns) **for reinforcement at client's leisure/readiness to deal with sensitive materials.**

• Encourage ongoing dialogue and take advantage of teachable moments that occur. **Nurse needs to become comfortable with talking about sexual issue so he or she can recognize these moments and be willing to discuss the client's concerns.**

• Demonstrate and assist client to learn relaxation and/or visualization techniques.

• Encourage client to engage in regular self-examination, as indicated (e.g., breast/testicular examinations).

• Identify community resources for further assistance (e.g., Reach for Recovery, CanSurmount, Ostomy Association, family/sex therapist).

• Refer for further professional assistance concerning relationship difficulties, low sexual desire/other sexual concerns (such as premature ejaculation, vaginismus, painful intercourse).

• Identify resources for assistive devices/sexual "aids."

Documentation Focus

ASSESSMENT/REASSESSMENT

• Individual findings including nature of dysfunction, predisposing factors, perceived effect on sexuality/relationships.
• Cultural/religious factors, conflicts.
• Response of SO.
• Motivation for change.

PLANNING

• Plan of care and who is involved in planning.
• Teaching plan.

IMPLEMENTATION/EVALUATION

• Response to interventions/teaching and actions performed.
• Attainment/progress toward desired outcome(s).
• Modifications to plan of care.

Information in brackets added by the authors to clarify and enhance the use of nursing diagnoses.

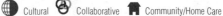 Cultural Collaborative Community/Home Care

DISCHARGE PLANNING

• Long-term needs/referrals and who is responsible for actions to be taken.
• Community resources, specific referrals made.

SAMPLE NURSING OUTCOMES & INTERVENTIONS CLASSIFICATIONS (NOC/NIC)

NOC—Sexual Functioning
NIC—Sexual Counseling

ineffective Sexuality Pattern

Taxonomy II: Sexuality—Class 2 Sexual Function (00065)
[Diagnostic Division: Sexuality]
Submitted 1986; Revised 2006

Definition: Expressions of concern regarding own sexuality

Related Factors

Knowledge/skill deficit about alternative responses to health-related transitions, altered body function or structure, illness, or medical treatment
Lack of privacy
Impaired relationship with a SO; lack of SO
Ineffective/absent role models
Conflicts with sexual orientation or variant preferences
Fear of pregnancy/acquiring a sexually transmitted disease

Defining Characteristics

SUBJECTIVE

Reported difficulties/limitations/changes in sexual behaviors/ activities
Alteration in relationship with SO
Alterations in achieving perceived sex role
Conflicts involving values
[Expressions of feeling alienated, lonely, loss, powerless, angry]

Desired Outcomes/Evaluation Criteria—Client Will:

• Verbalize understanding of sexual anatomy and function.

Information in brackets added by the authors to clarify and enhance the use of nursing diagnoses.

 Diagnostic Studies 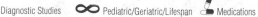 Pediatric/Geriatric/Lifespan Medications **615**

- Verbalize knowledge and understanding of sexual limitations, difficulties, or changes that have occurred.
- Verbalize acceptance of self in current (altered) condition.
- Demonstrate improved communication and relationship skills.
- Identify individually appropriate method of contraception.

Actions/Interventions

NURSING PRIORITY NO. 1. To assess causative/contributing factors:

- Obtain complete physical, and sexual history, as indicated, including perception of normal function. **Sexuality is multifaceted beginning with one's body, biological sex, and gender (biological, social, and legal status as girls/boys, women/men).**
- Note use of vocabulary (assessing basic knowledge) and comments/concerns about sexual identity. **Components of sexual identity include one's gender identity (how one feels about his or her gender) as well as one's sexual orientation (straight, lesbian, gay, bisexual, transgendered).**
- Determine importance of sex and a description of the problem in the client's own words. Be alert to comments of client/SO (e.g., discount of overt or covert sexual expressions such as "He's just a dirty old man"). **Sexual concerns are often disguised as sarcasm, humor, or in offhand remarks.**
- Elicit impact of perceived problem on SO/family. **One's values about life, love, and the people in one's life are also components of one's sexuality.**
- Note cultural values/religious beliefs and conflicts that may exist. **Individuals are enculturated as they grow up and, depending on particular family views and taboos, may harbor feelings of shame and guilt about their sexual feelings.**
- Assess stress factors in client's environment that might cause anxiety or psychological reactions (e.g., power issues involving SO, adult children, aging, employment, loss of prowess).
- Explore knowledge of effects of altered body function/limitations precipitated by illness (e.g., MS, arthritis, mutilating cancer surgery) or medical treatment of alternative sexual responses and expressions (e.g., undescended testicle in young male, gender change/reassignment procedure).
- Review history of substance use (prescription medications, OTC drugs, alcohol, and illicit drugs). **May be used by client to treat underlying feelings/anxiety.**
- Explore issues and fears associated with sex (pregnancy, sexually transmitted diseases, trust/control issues, inflexible beliefs, preference confusion, altered performance).

Information in brackets added by the authors to clarify and enhance the use of nursing diagnoses.

    Cultural   Collaborative   Community/Home Care

- Determine client's interpretation of the altered sexual activity or behavior (e.g., a way of controlling, relief of anxiety, pleasure, lack of partner). **These behaviors (when related to body changes, including pregnancy or weight loss/gain, or loss of body part) may reflect a stage of grieving.**
- Assess lifecycle issues, such as adolescence, young adulthood, menopause, aging. **All people are sexual beings from birth to death. Each transition has its own concerns and needs specific education to help the client deal with it in a healthy manner.**

NURSING PRIORITY NO. 2. To assist client/SO to deal with individual situation:

- Provide atmosphere in which discussion of sexual problems is encouraged/permitted. **Sense of trust/comfort enhances ability to discuss sensitive matters.**
- Avoid value judgments—**they do not help the client to cope with the situation.**
- Provide information about individual situation, determining client needs and desires.
- Encourage discussion of individual situation with opportunity for expression of feelings without judgment. **Sexuality also includes feelings, attitudes, relationships, self-image, ideals, and behaviors, and influences how one experiences the world.** (Note: Nurse needs to be aware of and in control of own feelings and responses to the client's expressions and/or concerns.)
- Provide specific information and suggestions about interventions directed toward the identified problems.
- Identify alternative forms of sexual expression that might be acceptable to both partners. **When illness or trauma (rheumatoid arthritis, paraplegia) interferes with usual sexual pattern, there are many different methods that can be used to obtain sexual satisfaction.**
- Discuss ways to manage individual devices/appliances (e.g., ostomy bag, breast prostheses, urinary collection device) **when change in body image/medical condition is involved.**
- Provide anticipatory guidance about losses that are to be expected (e.g., loss of known self when transsexual surgery is planned).
- Introduce client to individuals who have successfully managed a similar problem. **Provides positive role model/support for problem solving.**

Information in brackets added by the authors to clarify and enhance the use of nursing diagnoses.

NURSING PRIORITY NO. 3. To promote wellness (Teaching/Discharge Considerations):

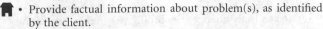

* Provide factual information about problem(s), as identified by the client.
* Engage in ongoing dialogue with the client and SO(s), as situation permits.
* Discuss methods/effectiveness/side effects of contraceptives, if indicated. **Assists individual/couple to make an informed decision on a method which meets own values/religious beliefs.**
* Refer to community resources (e.g., Planned Parenthood; gender-identity clinic; social services; Parents, Families and Friends of Lesbians and Gays [PFLAG]), as indicated.
* Refer for intensive individual/group psychotherapy, which may be combined with couple/family and/or sex therapy, as appropriate.
* Refer to NDs Sexual Dysfunction; disturbed Body Image; Self-Esteem [specify].

Documentation Focus

ASSESSMENT/REASSESSMENT

* Individual findings, including nature of concern, perceived difficulties/limitations or changes, specific needs/desires.
* Cultural/religious beliefs, conflicts.
* Response of SO(s).

PLANNING

* Plan of care and who is involved in the planning.
* Teaching plan.

IMPLEMENTATION/EVALUATION

* Response to interventions/teaching and actions performed.
* Attainment/progress toward desired outcome(s).
* Modifications to plan of care.

DISCHARGE PLANNING

* Long-term needs/teaching and referrals and who is responsible for actions to be taken.
* Community resources, specific referrals made.

SAMPLE NURSING OUTCOMES & INTERVENTIONS CLASSIFICATIONS (NOC/NIC)

NOC—Sexual Identity: Acceptance
NIC—Teaching: Sexuality

Information in brackets added by the authors to clarify and enhance the use of nursing diagnoses.

 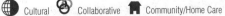 Cultural Collaborative Community/Home Care

impaired Skin Integrity

Taxonomy II: Safety/Protection—Class 2 Physical Injury (00046)
[Diagnostic Division: Safety]
Submitted 1975; Revised 1998 (by small group work 1996)

Definition: Altered epidermis and/or dermis

Related Factors

EXTERNAL

Hyperthermia; hypothermia
Chemical substance; radiation; medications
Physical immobilization
Humidity; moisture; [excretions/secretions]
Mechanical factors (e.g., shearing forces, pressure, restraint); [trauma: injury/surgery]
Extremes in age

INTERNAL

Imbalanced nutritional state (e.g., obesity, emaciation); impaired metabolic state; changes in fluid status
Skeletal prominence; changes in turgor; [presence of edema]
Impaired circulation/sensation; changes in pigmentation
Developmental factors
Immunological deficit
[Psychogenetic factors]

Defining Characteristics

SUBJECTIVE

[Reports of itching, pain, numbness of affected/surrounding area]

OBJECTIVE

Disruption of skin surface [epidermis]
Destruction of skin layers [dermis]
Invasion of body structures

Desired Outcomes/Evaluation Criteria—Client Will:

• Display timely healing of skin lesions/wounds/pressure sores without complication.
• Maintain optimal nutrition/physical well-being.

Information in brackets added by the authors to clarify and enhance the use of nursing diagnoses.

 Diagnostic Studies   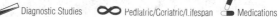 Pediatric/Geriatric/Lifespan   Medications   **619**

- Participate in prevention measures and treatment program.
- Verbalize feelings of increased self-esteem and ability to manage situation.

Actions/Interventions

NURSING PRIORITY NO. 1. To assess causative/contributing factors:

- Identify underlying condition/pathology involved (e.g., skin and other cancers, burns, scleroderma, lupus, psoriasis, acne, allergic reaction, diabetes, occupational hazards, familial history, trauma, surgical incision/amputation, communicable diseases).
- Note general debilitation, reduced mobility, changes in skin/muscle mass associated with aging/chronic disease, presence of incontinence/problems with self-care.
- Assess blood supply and sensation (nerve damage) of affected area. Calculate ankle-brachial index **to evaluate actual/potential for impairment of circulation to lower extremities. Result less than 0.9 indicates need for close monitoring/ more aggressive intervention (e.g., tighter blood glucose and weight control in diabetic client).**
- Determine nutritional status and potential for delayed healing or tissue injury exacerbated by malnutrition (e.g., pressure points on emaciated and/or elderly client).
- Review medication/therapy regimen (e.g., steroid use, chemotherapy, radiation).
- Evaluate client with impaired cognition, developmental delay, need for/use of restraints, long-term immobility **to identify risk for injury/safety requirements**.
- Review laboratory results pertinent to causative factors (e.g., studies such as Hb/Hct, blood glucose, infectious agents [viral/bacterial/fungal], albumin/protein). **Albumin less than 3.5 correlates to decreased wound healing/increased pressure ulcers.**
- Obtain specimen from draining wounds when appropriate for culture/sensitivities/Gram's stain **to determine appropriate therapy**.

NURSING PRIORITY NO. 2. To assess extent of involvement/injury:

- Obtain a history of condition, including age at onset, date of first episode, original site/characteristics of lesions, duration of problem, and changes that have occurred over time.
- Note skin color, texture, and turgor. Assess areas of least pigmentation for color changes (e.g., sclera, conjunctiva, nailbeds, buccal mucosa, tongue, palms, and soles of feet).

Information in brackets added by the authors to clarify and enhance the use of nursing diagnoses.

- Palpate skin lesions for size, shape, consistency, texture, temperature, and hydration.
- Determine degree/depth of injury/damage to integumentary system (i.e., involves epidermis, dermis, and/or underlying tissues).
- Measure length, width, depth of ulcers/wounds. Note extent of tunneling/undermining, if present.
- Inspect surrounding skin for erythema, induration, maceration.
- Photograph lesion(s)/burns, as appropriate, **to document status/provide visual baseline for future comparisons.**
- Note odors emitted from the skin/lesion/wound.
- Classify ulcer using tool such as Wagner Ulcer Classification System. **Provides consistent terminology for documentation.**

NURSING PRIORITY NO. 3. To determine impact of condition:

- Ascertain attitudes of individual/SO(s) about condition (e.g., cultural values, stigma). Note misconceptions. **Identifies areas to be addressed in teaching plan and potential referral needs.**
- Determine impact on life (e.g., work, leisure, increased caregiver requirements).
- Obtain psychological assessment of client's emotional status, as indicated, noting potential for sexual problems arising from presence of condition.
- Note presence of compromised vision, hearing, or speech. **Skin is a particularly important avenue of communication for this population and, when compromised, may affect responses.**

NURSING PRIORITY NO. 4. To assist client with correcting/minimizing condition and promote optimal healing:

- Inspect skin on a daily basis, describing wound/lesion characteristics and changes observed.
- Periodically remeasure/photograph wound and observe for complications (e.g., infection, dehiscence) **to monitor progress of wound healing.**
- Keep the area clean/dry, carefully dress wounds, support incision (e.g., use of Steri-Strips, splinting when coughing), prevent infection, manage incontinence, and stimulate circulation to surrounding areas **to assist body's natural process of repair.**
- Assist with débridement/enzymatic therapy, as indicated (e.g., burns, severe pressure sores), **to remove nonviable, contaminated, or infected tissue**.
- Use appropriate barrier dressings, wound coverings, drainage appliances, wound vac, and skin-protective agents for

---

Information in brackets added by the authors to clarify and enhance the use of nursing diagnoses.

open/draining wounds and stomas **to protect the wound and/or surrounding tissues.**

- Apply appropriate dressing (e.g., adhesive/nonadhesive film, hydrofiber or gel, acrylics, hydropolymers) **for wound healing and to best meet needs of client and caregiver/care setting.**

- Maintain appropriate moisture environment for particular wound (e.g., expose lesions/ulcer to air and light if excess moisture is impeding healing, or use occlusive dressings to maintain a moist environment for autolytic debridement of wound), as indicated.

- Limit/avoid use of plastic material (e.g., plastic-backed linen savers). Remove wet/wrinkled linens promptly. **Moisture potentiates skin breakdown.**

- Use paper tape or nonadherent dressing on frail skin and remove gently. Use stockinette, gauze wrap, or any other similar type of wrap instead of tape to secure dressings and drains.

- Reposition client on regular schedule, involving client in reasons for and decisions about times and positions **to enhance understanding and cooperation.**

- Use appropriate padding devices (e.g., air/water mattress, gel pad, waffle boots), when indicated, **to reduce pressure on/enhance circulation to compromised tissues.** Avoid use of sheepskin **that may retain heat/moisture.**

- Encourage early ambulation/mobilization. **Promotes circulation and reduces risks associated with immobility.**

- Provide optimum nutrition, including vitamins (e.g., A, C, D, E) and increased protein intake, **to provide a positive nitrogen balance to aid in skin/tissue healing and to maintain general good health.**

- Monitor periodic laboratory studies relative to general well-being and status of specific problem.

- Consult with wound/stoma specialist, as indicated, **to assist with developing plan of care for problematic or potentially serious wounds.**

NURSING PRIORITY NO. 5. To promote wellness (Teaching/Discharge Considerations):

- **Review importance of skin and measures to maintain proper skin functioning.** The integumentary system is the largest multifunctional organ of the body.

- Discuss importance of early detection of skin changes and/or complications.

- Assist the client/SO(s) in understanding and following medical regimen and developing program of preventive care and

---

Information in brackets added by the authors to clarify and enhance the use of nursing diagnoses.

  Cultural Collaborative 🏠 Community/Home Care

daily maintenance. **Enhances commitment to plan, optimizing outcomes.**

 • Review measures to avoid spread/reinfection of communicable disease/conditions.

• Emphasize importance of proper fit of clothing/shoes, use of specially lined shock-absorbing socks or pressure-reducing insoles for shoes **in presence of reduced sensation/circulation.**

• Identify safety factors for use of equipment/appliances (e.g., heating pad, ostomy appliances, padding straps of braces).

• Encourage client to verbalize feelings and discuss how/if condition affects self-concept/self-esteem. (Refer to NDs disturbed Body Image; situational low Self-Esteem.)

• Assist client to work through stages of grief and feelings associated with individual condition.

• Lend psychological support and acceptance of client, using touch, facial expressions, and tone of voice.

• Assist client to learn stress reduction and alternate therapy techniques **to control feelings of helplessness and deal with situation.**

• Refer to dietitian or certified diabetes educator, as appropriate, **to enhance healing, reduce risk of recurrence of diabetic ulcers.**

Documentation Focus

ASSESSMENT/REASSESSMENT

• Characteristics of lesion(s)/condition, ulcer classification.
• Causative/contributing factors.
• Impact of condition.

PLANNING

• Plan of care and who is involved in planning.
• Teaching plan.

IMPLEMENTATION/EVALUATION

• Responses to interventions/teaching and actions performed.
• Attainment/progress toward desired outcome(s).
• Modifications to plan of care.

DISCHARGE PLANNING

• Long-term needs/referrals and who is responsible for actions to be taken.
• Specific referrals made.

Information in brackets added by the authors to clarify and enhance the use of nursing diagnoses.

SAMPLE NURSING OUTCOMES & INTERVENTIONS CLASSIFICATIONS (NOC/NIC)

NOC—Tissue Integrity: Skin & Mucous Membranes
NIC—Wound/Pressure Ulcer Care

risk for impaired Skin Integrity

Taxonomy II: Safety/Protection—Class 2 Physical Injury (00047)
[Diagnostic Division: Safety]
Submitted 1975; Revised 1998 (by small group work 1996)

Definition: At risk for skin being adversely altered

NOTE: Risk should be determined by use of a standardized risk assessment tool [e.g., Braden Scale]

Risk Factors

EXTERNAL

Chemical substance; radiation
Hypothermia; hyperthermia
Physical immobilization
Excretions; secretions; humidity; moisture
Mechanical factors (e.g., shearing forces, pressure, restraint)
Extremes of age

INTERNAL

Medications
Imbalanced nutritional state (e.g., obesity, emaciation); impaired metabolic state; [fluid status]
Skeletal prominence; changes in skin turgor; [presence of edema]
Impaired circulation/sensation; changes in pigmentation
Developmental factors
Psychogenetic factors
Immunologic factors

NOTE: A risk diagnosis is not evidenced by signs and symptoms as the problem has not occurred; rather, nursing interventions are directed at prevention.

Information in brackets added by the authors to clarify and enhance the use of nursing diagnoses.

 Cultural Collaborative Community/Home Care

Desired Outcomes/Evaluation Criteria—Client Will:

- Identify individual risk factors.
- Verbalize understanding of treatment/therapy regimen.
- Demonstrate behaviors/techniques to prevent skin breakdown.

Actions/Interventions

NURSING PRIORITY NO. 1. To assess causative/contributing factors:

- Assess skin routinely, noting moisture, color, and elasticity. Review with client/SO history of past skin problems (e.g., allergic reactions, rashes, easy bruising/skin tears) **that may indicate particular vulnerability.**
- Note presence of conditions/situations **that may impair skin integrity** (e.g., age-related changes in skin and muscle mass, general debilitation, impaired mobility, poor nutritional status, presence of chronic conditions/immunosuppression, incontinence, problems of self-care, side/adverse effects of medication or therapy).
- Assess for diminished circulation in lower extremities. Calculate ankle-brachial index (ABI), as appropriate (diabetic clients or others with impaired circulation to lower extremities). **Result less than 0.9 indicates need for more aggressive preventive interventions (e.g., stricter blood glucose and weight control).**
- Review pertinent laboratory results (e.g., studies such as Hb/Hct, blood glucose, infectious agents [viral/bacterial/fungal], albumin/protein). **Note: Albumin less than 3.5 correlates to decreased wound healing/increased pressure ulcers.**

NURSING PRIORITY NO. 2. To maintain skin integrity at optimal level:

- Handle client gently (particularly infant, young child, elderly). **Epidermis of infants and very young children is thin and lacks subcutaneous depth that will develop with age. Skin of the older client is also thin, less elastic, and prone to injury, such as bruising and skin tears.**
- Inspect skin surfaces/pressure points routinely, especially in mobility-impaired client.
- Observe for reddened/blanched areas or skin rashes, and institute treatment immediately. **Reduces likelihood of progression to skin breakdown.**
- Maintain meticulous skin hygiene, using mild nondetergent soap, drying gently and thoroughly, and lubricating with lotion or emollient, as indicated.

Information in brackets added by the authors to clarify and enhance the use of nursing diagnoses.

 Diagnostic Studies 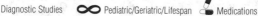 Pediatric/Geriatric/Lifespan   Medications **625**

- Massage bony prominences and use proper positioning, turning, lifting, and transferring techniques when moving client **to prevent friction or shear injury.**
- Change position in bed/chair on a regular schedule. Encourage client participation in early ambulation, active and assistive range-of-motion exercises.
- Provide adequate clothing/covers; protect from drafts **to prevent vasoconstriction.**
- Keep bedclothes dry and wrinkle-free, use nonirritating linens.
- Provide protection by use of pads, pillows, foam mattress, water bed, etc., **to increase circulation and limit/eliminate excessive tissue pressure.**
- Use paper tape or a nonadherent dressing on frail skin and remove it gently. Or use stockinette, gauze wrap, or any other similar type of wrap instead of tape to secure dressings and drains.
- Provide for safety measures during ambulation and other therapies that might cause dermal injury (e.g., use of properly fitting hose/footwear, safe use of heating pads/lamps, restraints).
- Provide preventative skin care to incontinent client: Change continence pads/diapers frequently; cleanse perineal skin daily and after each incontinence episode apply skin protectant ointment **to minimize contact with irritants (urine, stool, excessive moisture)**

NURSING PRIORITY NO. 3. To promote wellness (Teaching/Discharge Considerations):

- Provide information to client/SO(s) about the importance of regular observation and effective skin care in preventing problems.
- Emphasize importance of adequate nutritional/fluid intake **to maintain general good health and skin turgor.**
- Encourage continuation of regular exercise program (active/assistive) **to enhance circulation.**
- Recommend elevation of lower extremities when sitting **to enhance venous return and reduce edema formation.**
- Encourage restriction/abstinence from tobacco, **which can cause vasoconstriction.**
- Suggest use of ice, colloidal bath, lotions **to decrease irritable itching.**
- Recommend keeping nails short or wearing gloves **to reduce risk of dermal injury when severe itching is present.**
- Discuss importance of avoiding exposure to sunlight in specific conditions (e.g., systemic lupus, tetracycline/psychotropic drug use, radiation therapy) as well as potential for development of skin cancer.

Information in brackets added by the authors to clarify and enhance the use of nursing diagnoses.

  Cultural Collaborative Community/Home Care

- Advise regular use of sunscreen, particularly on young child, client with fair skin (prone to burn), or client using multiple medications, etc., **to limit skin damage (immediate and over time) associated with sun exposure**.
- Counsel diabetic and neurologically impaired client about importance of skin care, especially of lower extremities.
- Perform periodic assessment using a tool such as the Braden Scale **to determine changes in risk status and need for alterations in the plan of care.**
- Refer to dietitian or certified diabetes educator, as appropriate, **to identify nutritional needs/maintain proper diabetic control.**

Documentation Focus

ASSESSMENT/REASSESSMENT

- Individual findings, including individual risk factors.

PLANNING

- Plan of care and who is involved in planning.
- Teaching plan.

IMPLEMENTATION/EVALUATION

- Responses to interventions/teaching and actions performed.
- Attainment/progress toward desired outcome(s).
- Modifications to plan of care.

DISCHARGE PLANNING

- Long-term needs and who is responsible for actions to be taken.

SAMPLE NURSING OUTCOMES & INTERVENTIONS CLASSIFICATIONS (NOC/NIC)

NOC—Risk Control
NIC—Pressure Management

readiness for enhanced Sleep

Taxonomy II: Activity/Rest—Class 1 Sleep/Rest (00165)
[Diagnostic Division: Activity/Rest]
Submitted 2002

Definition: A pattern of natural, periodic suspension of consciousness that provides adequate rest, sustains a desired lifestyle, and can be strengthened

---

Information in brackets added by the authors to clarify and enhance the use of nursing diagnoses.

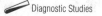 Diagnostic Studies 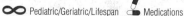 Pediatric/Geriatric/Lifespan Medications **627**

Related Factors

To be developed

Defining Characteristics

SUBJECTIVE

Expresses willingness to enhance sleep
Expresses a feeling of being rested after sleep
Follows sleep routines that promote sleep habits

OBJECTIVE

Amount of sleep and REM sleep is congruent with developmental needs
Occasional use of medications to induce sleep

Desired Outcomes/Evaluation Criteria—Client Will:

- Identify individually appropriate interventions to promote sleep.
- Verbalize feeling rested after sleep.
- Adjust lifestyle to accommodate routines that promote sleep.

Actions/Interventions

NURSING PRIORITY NO. 1. To determine motivation for continued growth:

- Listen to client's reports of sleep quantity and quality. Determine client's/SO's perception of adequate sleep. **Reveals client's experience and expectations. Provides opportunity to address misconceptions/unrealistic expectations and plan for interventions.**
- Observe and/or obtain feedback from client/SO(s) regarding usual bedtime, desired rituals and routines, number of hours of sleep, time of arising, and environmental needs **to determine usual sleep pattern and provide comparative baseline for improvements.**
- Ascertain motivation and expectation for change.
- Note client report of potential for alteration of habitual sleep time (e.g., change of work pattern/rotating shifts) or change in normal bedtime (e.g., hospitalization). **Helps identify circumstances that are known to interrupt sleep patterns and that could disrupt the person's biological rhythms.**

Information in brackets added by the authors to clarify and enhance the use of nursing diagnoses.

🌐 Cultural 🅐 Collaborative 🏠 Community/Home Care

NURSING PRIORITY NO. 2. To assist client to enhance sleep/rest:

🏠 • Recommend limiting intake of chocolate and caffeine/alcoholic beverages (especially prior to bedtime), **which are substances known to impair falling or staying asleep. Use of alcohol at bedtime may help individual initially fall asleep, but ensuing sleep is then fragmented.**

🏠 • Limit fluid intake in evening if nocturia or bedwetting is a problem **to reduce need for nighttime elimination.**

• Recommend appropriate changes to usual bedtime rituals:
Provide quiet environment and comfort measures (e.g., back rub, washing hands/face, cleaning and straightening sheets). **Promotes relaxation and readiness for sleep.**

🏠 Explore/implement use of warm bath, comfortable room temperature, use of soothing music, favorite calming TV show. **Nonpharmaceutical aids may enhance falling asleep.**

∞ Discuss/implement effective age-appropriate bedtime rituals for infant/child (e.g., soothing bath, rocking, story reading, cuddling, favorite blanket/toy). **Rituals can enhance ability to fall asleep, reinforce that bed is a place to sleep, and promote sense of security for child.**

🏠 • Assist client in use of necessary equipment, instructing as necessary. **Client may use oxygen or CPAP system to improve sleep/rest if hypoxia or sleep apnea diagnosed.**

🏠 • Investigate use of sleep mask, darkening shades/curtains, earplugs, low-level background (white) noise. **Aids in blocking out light and disturbing noise.**

• Arrange care **to provide for uninterrupted periods for rest.** Explain necessity of disturbances for monitoring vital signs and/or other care when client is hospitalized. Do as much care as possible without waking client during night. **Allows for longer periods of uninterrupted sleep, especially during night.**

NURSING PRIORITY NO. 3. To promote optimum wellness:

🏠 • Assure client that occasional sleeplessness should not threaten health. **Knowledge that occasional insomnia is universal and usually not harmful may promote relaxation and relief from worry.**

🏠 • Encourage regular exercise during day **to aid in stress control/release of energy. Note: Exercise at bedtime may stimulate rather than relax client and actually interfere with sleep.**

💊 • Advise using barbiturates and/or other sleeping medications sparingly. **These medications, while useful for promoting sleep in the short-term, can interfere with REM sleep.**

Information in brackets added by the authors to clarify and enhance the use of nursing diagnoses.

readiness for enhanced SLEEP

Documentation Focus

ASSESSMENT/REASSESSMENT

- Assessment findings, including specifics of sleep pattern (current and past) and effects on lifestyle/level of functioning.
- Medications/interventions, previous therapies.

PLANNING

- Plan of care and who is involved in planning.
- Teaching plan.

IMPLEMENTATION/EVALUATION

- Client's response to interventions/teaching and actions performed.
- Attainment/progress toward desired outcome(s).
- Modifications to plan of care.

DISCHARGE PLANNING

- Long-term needs and who is responsible for actions to be taken.
- Specific referrals made.

SAMPLE NURSING OUTCOMES & INTERVENTIONS CLASSIFICATIONS (NOC/NIC)

NOC—Sleep
NIC—Sleep Enhancement

Sleep Deprivation

Taxonomy II: Activity/Rest—Class 1 Sleep/Rest (00096)
[Diagnostic Division: Activity/Rest]
Nursing Diagnosis Extension and Classification (NDEC)
  Submission 1998

Definition: Prolonged periods of time without sleep
(sustained natural, periodic suspension of relative
consciousness)

Related Factors

Sustained environmental stimulation/uncomfortable sleep
  environment
Inadequate daytime activity; sustained circadian asynchrony;
  aging-related sleep stage shifts; non–sleep-inducing parenting practices

---

Information in brackets added by the authors to clarify and enhance
the use of nursing diagnoses.

Sustained inadequate sleep hygiene; prolonged use of pharmacologic or dietary antisoporifics

Prolonged discomfort (e.g., physical, psychological); periodic limb movement (e.g., restless leg syndrome, nocturnal myoclonus); sleep-related enuresis/painful erections

Nightmares; sleepwalking; sleep terror

Sleep apnea

Sundowner's syndrome; dementia

Idiopathic CNS hypersomnolence; narcolepsy; familial sleep paralysis

Defining Characteristics

SUBJECTIVE

Daytime drowsiness; decreased ability to function

Malaise; lethargy; fatigue

Anxiety

Perceptual disorders (e.g., disturbed body sensation, delusions, feeling afloat); heightened sensitivity to pain

OBJECTIVE

Restlessness; irritability

Inability to concentrate; slowed reaction

Listlessness; apathy

Fleeting nystagmus; hand tremors

Acute confusion; transient paranoia; agitation; combativeness; hallucinations

Desired Outcomes/Evaluation Criteria—Client Will:

- Identify individually appropriate interventions to promote sleep.
- Verbalize understanding of sleep disorder.
- Adjust lifestyle to accommodate chronobiological rhythms.
- Report improvement in sleep/rest pattern.

Family Will:

- Deal appropriately with parasomnias.

Actions/Interventions

NURSING PRIORITY NO. 1. To assess causative/contributing factors:

- Determine presence of physical or psychological stressors, including night-shift working hours/rotating shifts, pain, advanced age, current/recent illness, death of a spouse.

Information in brackets added by the authors to clarify and enhance the use of nursing diagnoses.

- Note medical diagnoses that affect sleep (e.g., dementia, encephalitis, brain injury, narcolepsy, depression, asthma, sleep-induced respiratory disorders/obstructive sleep apnea, nocturnal myoclonus [jerking of legs causing repeated awakening]).

- Evaluate for use of medications and/or other drugs affecting sleep (e.g., diet pills, antidepressives, antihypertensives, stimulants, sedatives, diuretics, opioids, alcohol).
- Note environmental factors affecting sleep (e.g., unfamiliar or uncomfortable sleep environment, excessive noise and light, uncomfortable temperature, roommate irritations/actions— e.g., snoring, watching TV late at night).
- Determine presence of parasomnias: nightmares/terrors or somnambulism (e.g., sitting, sleepwalking, or other complex behavior during sleep).
- Note reports of terror, brief periods of paralysis, sense of body being disconnected from the brain. **Occurrence of sleep paralysis, though not widely recognized in the United States, has been well-documented elsewhere and may result in feelings of fear/reluctance to go to sleep.**

NURSING PRIORITY NO. 2. To assess degree of impairment:

- Determine client's usual sleep pattern and expectations. **Provides comparative baseline.**
- Ascertain duration of current problem and effect on life/functional ability.
- Listen to client's/SO's subjective reports of client's sleep quality and family concerns.
- Observe for physical signs of fatigue (e.g., frequent yawning, restlessness, irritability; inability to tolerate stress; disorientation; problems with concentration/memory; behavioral, learning, or social problems).
- Determine interventions client has tried in the past. **Helps identify appropriate options.**
- Distinguish client's beneficial bedtime habits from detrimental ones (e.g., drinking late-evening milk versus drinking late-evening coffee).
- Instruct client and/or bed partner to keep a sleep-wake log **to document symptoms and identify factors that are interfering with sleep.**
- Do a chronological chart **to determine peak performance rhythms.**

NURSING PRIORITY NO. 3. To assist client to establish optimal sleep pattern:

Information in brackets added by the authors to clarify and enhance the use of nursing diagnoses.

  Cultural Collaborative Community/Home Care

- Encourage client to develop plan to restrict caffeine, alcohol, and other stimulating substances from late afternoon/evening intake and avoid eating large evening/late-night meals. **These factors are known to disrupt sleep patterns.**
- Recommend bedtime snack (protein, simple carbohydrate, and low fat) for young children 15 to 30 minutes before retiring. **Sense of fullness and satiety promotes sleep and reduces likelihood of gastric upset.**
- Promote adequate physical exercise activity during day. **Enhances expenditure of energy/release of tension so that client feels ready for sleep/rest.**
- Review medications being taken and their effect on sleep, suggesting modifications in regimen **if medications are found to be interfering.**
- Suggest abstaining from daytime naps **because they impair ability to sleep at night.**
- Investigate anxious feelings **to help determine basis and appropriate anxiety-reduction techniques.**
- Recommend quiet activities, such as reading/listening to soothing music in the evening, **to reduce stimulation so client can relax.**
- Instruct in relaxation techniques, music therapy, meditation, etc., **to decrease tension, prepare for rest/sleep.**
- Limit evening fluid intake if nocturia is present **to reduce need for nighttime elimination.**
- Discuss/implement effective age-appropriate bedtime rituals (e.g., going to bed at same time each night, drinking warm milk, soothing bath, rocking, story reading, cuddling, favorite blanket/toy) **to enhance client's ability to fall asleep, reinforce that bed is a place to sleep, and promote sense of security for child.**
- Provide calm, quiet environment and manage controllable sleep-disrupting factors (e.g., noise, light, room temperature).
- Administer sedatives/other sleep medications, when indicated, noting client's response. Time pain medications for peak effect/duration **to reduce need for redosing during prime sleep hours.**
- Instruct client to get out of bed, leave bedroom, engage in relaxing activities if unable to fall asleep, and not return to bed until feeling sleepy.
- Review with client the physician's recommendations for medications or surgery (alteration of facial structures/tracheotomy) and/or apneic oxygenation therapy—continuous positive airway pressure (CPAP) such as Respironics—

Information in brackets added by the authors to clarify and enhance the use of nursing diagnoses.

when sleep apnea is severe, as documented by sleep disorder studies.

NURSING PRIORITY NO. 4. To promote wellness (Teaching/Discharge Considerations):

 • Review possibility of next-day drowsiness/"rebound" insomnia and temporary memory loss **that may be associated with prescription sleep medications.**
• Discuss use/appropriateness of OTC sleep medications/herbal supplements. Note possible side effects and drug interactions.
 • Refer to support group/counselor **to help deal with psychological stressors (e.g., grief, sorrow).** (Refer to NDs Grieving; chronic Sorrow.)
 • Encourage family counseling **to help deal with concerns arising from parasomnias.**
• Refer to sleep specialist/laboratory **when problem is unresponsive to interventions.**

Documentation Focus

ASSESSMENT/REASSESSMENT

• Assessment findings, including specifics of sleep pattern (current and past) and effects on lifestyle/level of functioning.
• Medications/interventions, previous therapies.
• Family history of similar problem.

PLANNING

• Plan of care and who is involved in planning.
• Teaching plan.

IMPLEMENTATION/EVALUATION

• Client's response to interventions/teaching and actions performed.
• Attainment/progress toward desired outcome(s).
• Modifications to plan of care.

DISCHARGE PLANNING

• Long-term needs and who is responsible for actions to be taken.
• Specific referrals made.

SAMPLE NURSING OUTCOMES & INTERVENTIONS CLASSIFICATIONS (NOC/NIC)

NOC—Sleep
NIC—Sleep Enhancement

Information in brackets added by the authors to clarify and enhance the use of nursing diagnoses.

 Cultural   Collaborative   Community/Home Care

impaired Social Interaction

Taxonomy II: Role Relationship—Class 3 Role
 Performance (00052)
[Diagnostic Division: Social Interaction]
Submitted 1986

Definition: Insufficient or excessive quantity or
ineffective quality of social exchange

Related Factors

Deficit about ways to enhance mutuality (e.g., knowledge, skills)
Communication barriers [including head injury, stroke, other
 neurological conditions affecting ability to communicate]
Self-concept disturbance
Absence of significant others
Limited physical mobility [e.g., neuromuscular disease]
Therapeutic isolation
Sociocultural dissonance
Environmental barriers
Disturbed thought processes

Defining Characteristics

SUBJECTIVE

Discomfort in social situations
Inability to communicate/receive a satisfying sense of social
 engagement (e.g., belonging, caring, interest, or shared history)
Family report of changes in interaction (e.g., style, pattern)

OBJECTIVE

Use of unsuccessful social interaction behaviors
Dysfunctional interaction with others

Desired Outcomes/Evaluation
Criteria—Client Will:

• Verbalize awareness of factors causing or promoting impaired
 social interactions.
• Identify feelings that lead to poor social interactions.
• Express desire/be involved in achieving positive changes in
 social behaviors and interpersonal relationships.
• Give self positive reinforcement for changes that are achieved.
• Develop effective social support system; use available
 resources appropriately.

 Information in brackets added by the authors to clarify and enhance
the use of nursing diagnoses.

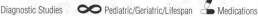

Actions/Interventions

NURSING PRIORITY NO. 1. To assess causative/contributing factors:

- Review social history with client/SO(s) going back far enough in time to note when changes in social behavior or patterns of relating occurred/began, for example, loss or long-term illness of loved one; failed relationships; loss of occupation, financial, or social/political (power) position; change in status in family hierarchy (job loss, aging, illness); poor coping/adjustment to developmental stage of life, as with marriage, birth/adoption of child, or children leaving home.

- Ascertain ethnic/cultural or religious implications for the client **because these impact choice of behaviors/may even script interactions with others.**

- Review medical history noting stressors of physical/long-term illness (e.g., stroke, cancer, MS, head injury, Alzheimer's disease); mental illness (e.g., schizophrenia); medications/drugs, debilitating accidents, learning disabilities (e.g., sensory integration difficulties, Asperger's disorder, autism spectrum disorder); and emotional disabilities.

- Determine family patterns of relating and social behaviors. Explore possible family scripting of behavioral expectations in the children and how the client was affected. **May result in conforming or rebellious behaviors. Parents are important in teaching their children social skills (e.g., sharing, taking turns, and allowing others to talk without interrupting).**

- Observe client while relating to family/SO(s) **to note prevalent interaction patterns.**

- Encourage client to verbalize feeling of discomfort about social situations. Identify causative factors, if any, recurring precipitating patterns, and barriers to using support systems.

NURSING PRIORITY NO. 2. To assess degree of impairment:

- Encourage client to verbalize perceptions of problem and causes. Active-listen noting indications of hopelessness, powerlessness, fear, anxiety, grief, anger, feeling unloved or unlovable, problems with sexual identity, hate (directed or not).

- Observe and describe social/interpersonal behaviors in objective terms, noting speech patterns, body language—in the therapeutic setting and in normal areas of daily functioning (if possible)—such as in family, job, social/entertainment settings. **Helps identify the kinds and extent of problems client is exhibiting.**

- Determine client's use of coping skills and defense mechanisms. **Affects ability to be involved in social situations.**

Information in brackets added by the authors to clarify and enhance the use of nursing diagnoses.

 Cultural Collaborative 🏠 Community/Home Care

- Evaluate possibility of client being the victim of or using destructive behaviors against self or others. (Refer to NDs risk for other-/self-directed Violence.) **Problems with communication lead to frustration and anger, leaving the individual with few coping skills, and may result in destructive behaviors.**
- Interview family, SO(s), friends, spiritual leaders, coworkers, as appropriate, **to obtain observations of client's behavioral changes and effect on others.**
- Note effects of changes on socioeconomic level, ethnic/religious practices.

NURSING PRIORITY NO. 3. To assist client/SO(s) to recognize/make positive changes in impaired social and interpersonal interactions:

- Establish therapeutic relationship using positive regard for the client, active-listening, and providing safe environment for self-disclosure.
- Have client list behaviors that cause discomfort. **Once recognized, client can choose to change as he or she learns to listen and communicate in socially acceptable ways.**
- Have family/SO(s) list client's behaviors that are causing discomfort for them. **Family needs to understand that the client is unable to use social skills that have not been learned.**
- Review/list negative behaviors observed previously by caregivers, coworkers, and so forth.
- Compare lists and validate reality of perceptions. Help client prioritize those behaviors needing change.
- Explore with client and role play means of making agreed upon changes in social interactions/behaviors.
- Role play random social situations in therapeutically controlled environment with "safe" therapy group. Have group note behaviors, both positive and negative, and discuss these and any changes needed.
- Role play changes and discuss impact. Include family/SO(s), as indicated. **Enhances comfort with new behaviors.**
- Provide positive reinforcement for improvement in social behaviors and interactions. **Encourages continuation of desired behaviors/efforts for change.**
- Participate in multidisciplinary client-centered conferences to evaluate progress. Involve everyone associated with client's care, family members, SO(s), and therapy group.
- Work with client to alleviate underlying negative self-concepts **because they often impede positive social interactions. Attempts at trying to connect with another can**

Information in brackets added by the authors to clarify and enhance the use of nursing diagnoses.

become devastating to self-esteem and emotional well-being.

- Involve neurologically impaired client in individual and/or group interactions/special classes, as situation allows.
- Refer for family therapy, as indicated, **because social behaviors and interpersonal relationships involve more than the individual.**

NURSING PRIORITY NO. 4. To promote wellness (Teaching/Discharge Considerations):

- Encourage client to keep a daily journal in which social interactions of each day can be reviewed and the comfort/discomfort experienced noted with possible causes/precipitating factors. **Helps client to identify responsibility for own behavior(s) and learn new skills that can be used to enhance social interactions.**
- Assist the client to develop positive social skills through practice of skills in real social situations accompanied by a support person. Provide positive feedback during interactions with client.
- Seek community programs for client involvement that promote positive behaviors the client is striving to achieve.
- Encourage classes, reading materials, community support groups, and lectures for self-help in alleviating negative self-concepts that lead to impaired social interactions.
- Involve client in a music-based program, if available (e.g., The Listening Program). **There is a direct correlation between the musical portion of the brain and the language area, and the use of these programs may result in better communication skills.**
- Encourage ongoing family or individual therapy as long as it is promoting growth and positive change. (However, be alert to possibility of therapy being used as a crutch.)
- Provide for occasional follow-up **for reinforcement of positive behaviors after professional relationship has ended.**
- Refer to/involve psychiatric clinical nurse specialist for additional assistance when indicated.

Documentation Focus

ASSESSMENT/REASSESSMENT

- Individual findings, including factors affecting interactions, nature of social exchanges, specifics of individual behaviors, type of learning disability present.

Information in brackets added by the authors to clarify and enhance the use of nursing diagnoses.

- Cultural/religious beliefs and expectations.
- Perceptions/response of others.

PLANNING

- Plan of care and who is involved in the planning.
- Teaching plan.

IMPLEMENTATION/EVALUATION

- Responses to interventions/teaching and actions performed.
- Attainment/progress toward desired outcome(s).
- Modifications to plan of care.

DISCHARGE PLANNING

- Long-term needs and who is responsible for actions to be taken.
- Community resources, specific referrals made.

SAMPLE NURSING OUTCOMES & INTERVENTIONS CLASSIFICATIONS (NOC/NIC)

NOC—Social Interaction Skills
NIC—Socialization Enhancement

Social Isolation

Taxonomy II: Comfort—Class 3 Social Comfort (00053)
[Diagnostic Division: Social Interaction]
Submitted 1982

Definition: Aloneness experienced by the individual and perceived as imposed by others and as a negative or threatened state

Related Factors

Factors contributing to the absence of satisfying personal relationships (e.g., delay in accomplishing developmental tasks); immature interests
Alterations in physical appearance/mental status
Altered state of wellness
Unaccepted social behavior/values
Inadequate personal resources
Inability to engage in satisfying personal relationships
[Traumatic incidents or events causing physical and/or emotional pain]

Information in brackets added by the authors to clarify and enhance the use of nursing diagnoses.

 Diagnostic Studies   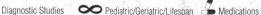 Pediatric/Geriatric/Lifespan   Medications   **639**

SOCIAL ISOLATION

Defining Characteristics

SUBJECTIVE

Expresses feelings of: aloneness imposed by others, differences from others, rejection,
Expresses values unacceptable to the dominant cultural group
Inability to meet expectations of others
Inadequate purpose in life
Developmentally inappropriate interests
Insecurity in public

OBJECTIVE

Absence of supportive significant other(s)—[family, friends, group]
Sad/dull affect
Developmentally inappropriate behaviors
Projects hostility
Evidence of handicap (e.g., physical/mental); illness
Uncommunicative; withdrawn; no eye contact
Preoccupation with own thoughts; repetitive/meaningless actions
Seeks to be alone; exists in a subculture
Shows behavior unaccepted by dominant cultural group

Desired Outcomes/Evaluation Criteria—Client Will:

- Identify causes and actions to correct isolation.
- Verbalize willingness to be involved with others.
- Participate in activities/programs at level of ability/desire.
- Express increased sense of self-worth.

Actions/Interventions

NURSING PRIORITY NO. 1. To assess causative/contributing factors:

- Determine presence of factors as listed in Related Factors and other concerns (e.g., elderly, female, adolescent, ethnic/racial minority, economically/educationally disadvantaged).
- Note onset of physical/mental illness and whether recovery is anticipated or condition is chronic/progressive. **May affect client's desire to isolate self.**
- Do physical exam, paying particular attention to any illnesses that are identified. **Individuals who are isolated appear to be susceptible to health problems, especially coronary heart disease, although little is understood about why this is true.**

Information in brackets added by the authors to clarify and enhance the use of nursing diagnoses.

  Cultural Collaborative Community/Home Care

- Identify blocks to social contacts (e.g., physical immobility, sensory deficits, housebound, incontinence). **Client may be unable to go out, embarrassed to be with others, and reluctant to solve these problems.**
- Ascertain implications of cultural values/religious beliefs for the client **because these impact choice of behaviors and may even script interactions with others.**
- Assess factors in client's life that may contribute to sense of helplessness (e.g., loss of spouse/parent). **Client may withdraw and fail to seek out friends who may have been in his or her life previously.**
- Ascertain client's perception regarding sense of isolation. Differentiate isolation from solitude and loneliness **which may be acceptable or by choice.**
- Assess client's feelings about self, sense of ability to control situation, sense of hope.
- Note use/effectiveness of coping skills.
- Identify support systems available to the client, including presence of/relationship with extended family.
- Determine drug use (legal/illicit). **Possibility of a relationship between unhealthy behaviors and social isolation or the influence others have on the individual.**
- Identify behavior response of isolation (e.g., excessive sleeping/daydreaming, substance use), **which also may potentiate isolation.**
- Review history and elicit information about traumatic events that may have occurred. (Refer to ND Post-Trauma Syndrome.)

NURSING PRIORITY NO. 2. To alleviate conditions contributing to client's sense of isolation:

- Establish therapeutic nurse-client relationship. **Promotes trust, allowing client to feel free to discuss sensitive matters.**
- Spend time visiting with client, and identify other resources available (e.g., volunteer, social worker, chaplain).
- Develop plan of action with client: Look at available resources, support risk-taking behaviors, financial planning, appropriate medical care/self-care, and so forth.
- Introduce client to those with similar/shared interests and other supportive people. **Provides role models, encourages problem solving, and possibly making friends that will relieve client's sense of isolation.**
- Provide positive reinforcement when client makes move(s) toward others. **Encourages continuation of efforts.**
- Provide for placement in sheltered community when necessary.

Information in brackets added by the authors to clarify and enhance the use of nursing diagnoses.

- Assist client to problem solve solutions to short-term/imposed isolation (e.g., communicable disease measures, including compromised host).
- Encourage open visitation when possible and/or telephone contacts **to maintain involvement with others.**
- Provide environmental stimuli (e.g., open curtains, pictures, TV, and radio).
- Promote participation in recreational/special interest activities in setting that client views as safe.
- 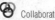 Identify foreign-language resources, such as interpreter, newspaper, radio programming, as appropriate.

NURSING PRIORITY NO. 3. To promote wellness (Teaching/Discharge Considerations):

- Assist client to learn/enhance skills (e.g., problem solving, communication, social skills, self-esteem, ADLs).
- Encourage/assist client to enroll in classes, as desired (e.g., assertiveness, vocational, sex education).
- Involve children and adolescents in programs/activities **to promote socialization skills and peer contact.**
- Help client differentiate between isolation and loneliness/aloneness and about ways to prevent slipping into an undesired state.
- Involve client in programs directed at correction and prevention of identified causes of problem (e.g., senior citizen services, daily telephone contact, house sharing, pets, day-care centers, church resources). **Social isolation seems to be growing and may be related to time stressors, TV/Internet, or fatigue, resulting in individuals finding they don't have a close friend they can share intimate thoughts with.**
- Refer to therapists, as appropriate, **to facilitate grief work, relationship building, and so forth.**

Documentation Focus

ASSESSMENT/REASSESSMENT

- Individual findings, including precipitating factors, effect on lifestyle/relationships, and functioning.
- Client's perception of situation.
- Cultural/religious factors.
- Availability/use of resources and support systems.

PLANNING

- Plan of care and who is involved in planning.
- Teaching plan.

Information in brackets added by the authors to clarify and enhance the use of nursing diagnoses.

 Cultural 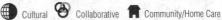 Collaborative Community/Home Care

IMPLEMENTATION/EVALUATION

- Responses to interventions/teaching and actions performed.
- Attainment/progress toward desired outcome(s).
- Modifications to plan of care.

DISCHARGE PLANNING

- Long-term needs/referrals and who is responsible for actions to be taken.
- Available resources, specific referrals made.

SAMPLE NURSING OUTCOMES & INTERVENTIONS CLASSIFICATIONS (NOC/NIC)

NOC—Social Involvement
NIC—Social Enhancement

chronic Sorrow

Taxonomy II: Coping/Stress Tolerance   Class 2 Coping Responses (00137)
[Diagnostic Division: Ego Integrity]
Submitted 1998

Definition: Cyclical, recurring, and potentially progressive pattern of pervasive sadness experienced (by a parent, caregiver, individual with chronic illness or disability) in response to continual loss, throughout the trajectory of an illness or disability

Related Factors

Death of a loved one
Experiences chronic illness/disability (e.g., physical or mental); crises in management of the illness
Crises related to developmental stages; missed opportunities/milestones
Unending caregiving

Defining Characteristics

SUBJECTIVE

Expresses negative feelings (e.g., anger, being misunderstood, confusion, depression, disappointment, emptiness, fear, frustration, guilt, self-blame, helplessness, hopelessness, loneliness, low self-esteem, recurring loss, overwhelmed)

Information in brackets added by the authors to clarify and enhance the use of nursing diagnoses.

 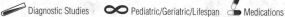

Expresses feelings of sadness (e.g., periodic, recurrent)
Expresses feelings that interfere with ability to reach highest level of personal/social well-being

Desired Outcomes/Evaluation Criteria—Client Will:

- Acknowledge presence/impact of sorrow.
- Demonstrate progress in dealing with grief.
- Participate in work and/or self-care ADLs as able.
- Verbalize a sense of progress toward resolution of sorrow and hope for the future.

Actions/Interventions

NURSING PRIORITY NO. 1. To assess causative/contributing factors:

- Determine current/recent events or conditions contributing to client's state of mind, as listed in Related Factors (e.g., death of loved one, chronic physical or mental illness, disability).
- Look for cues of sadness (e.g., sighing, faraway look, unkempt appearance, inattention to conversation, refusing food, etc.). **Chronic sorrow has a cyclical effect, ranging from times of deepening sorrow to times of feeling somewhat better.**
- Determine level of functioning, ability to care for self.
- Note avoidance behaviors (e.g., anger, withdrawal, denial).
- Identify cultural factors/religious conflicts. **Family may experience conflict between the feelings of sorrow and anger because of change in expectation that has occurred (e.g., newborn with a disability when the expectation was for a perfect child, while religious belief is that all children are gifts from God and that the individual/parent is never "given" more than he or she can handle).**
- Ascertain response of family/SO(s) to client's situation. Assess needs of family/SO. **Family may have difficulty dealing with child/ill person because of their own feelings of sorrow/loss and will do better when their needs are met.**
- Refer to dysfunctional Grieving; Caregiver Role Strain; ineffective Coping, as appropriate.

NURSING PRIORITY NO. 2. To assist client to move through sorrow:

- Encourage verbalization about situation (**helpful in beginning resolution and acceptance**). Active-listen feelings and be available for support/assistance.
- Encourage expression of anger/fear/anxiety. Refer to appropriate NDs.

Information in brackets added by the authors to clarify and enhance the use of nursing diagnoses.

 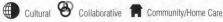

- Acknowledge reality of feelings of guilt/blame, including hostility toward spiritual power. (Refer to ND Spiritual Distress.) **When feelings are validated, client is free to take steps toward acceptance.**
- Provide comfort and availability as well as caring for physical needs.
- Discuss ways individual has dealt with previous losses. Reinforce use of previously effective coping skills.
- Instruct/encourage use of visualization and relaxation skills.
- Discuss use of medication when depression is interfering with ability to manage life. **Client may benefit from the short-term use of an antidepressant medication to help with dealing with situation.**
- Assist SO to cope with client response. **Family/SO may not be dysfunctional but may be intolerant.**
- Include family/SO in setting realistic goals for meeting individual needs.

NURSING PRIORITY NO. 3. To promote wellness (Teaching/Discharge Considerations):

- Discuss healthy ways of dealing with difficult situations.
- Have client identify familial, religious, and cultural factors that have meaning for him or her. **May help bring loss or distressing situation into perspective and facilitate grief/sorrow resolution.**
- Encourage involvement in usual activities, exercise, and socialization within limits of physical and psychological state. **Maintaining usual activities may keep individuals from deepening sorrow/depression.**
- Introduce concept of mindfulness (living in the moment). **Promotes feelings of capability and belief that this moment can be dealt with.**
- Refer to other resources (e.g., pastoral care, counseling, psychotherapy, respite-care providers, support groups). **Provides additional help when needed to resolve situation, continue grief work.**

Documentation Focus

ASSESSMENT/REASSESSMENT

- Physical/emotional response to conflict, expressions of sadness.
- Cultural issues/religious conflicts.
- Reactions of family/SO.

Information in brackets added by the authors to clarify and enhance the use of nursing diagnoses.

 Diagnostic Studies   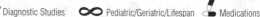 Pediatric/Geriatric/Lifespan   Medications   **645**

PLANNING

- Plan of care and who is involved in planning.
- Teaching plan.

IMPLEMENTATION/EVALUATION

- Response to interventions/teaching and actions performed.
- Attainment/progress toward desired outcome(s).
- Modifications to plan of care.

DISCHARGE PLANNING

- Long-term needs and who is responsible for actions to be taken.
- Available resources, specific referrals made.

SAMPLE NURSING OUTCOMES & INTERVENTIONS CLASSIFICATIONS (NOC/NIC)

NOC—Depression Level
NIC—Hope Instillation

Spiritual Distress

Taxonomy II: Life Principles—Class 3 Value/Belief/Action Congruence (00066)
[Diagnostic Division: Ego Integrity]
Submitted 1978; Revised 2002

Definition: Impaired ability to experience and integrate meaning and purpose in life through connectedness with self, others, art, music, literature, nature, and/or a power greater than oneself

Related Factors

Active dying
Loneliness; social alienation; self-alienation; sociocultural deprivation
Anxiety; pain
Life change
Chronic illness [of self or others]; death
[Challenged belief/value system (e.g., moral/ethical implications of therapy)]

Information in brackets added by the authors to clarify and enhance the use of nursing diagnoses.

  Cultural Collaborative Community/Home Care

Defining Characteristics

SUBJECTIVE

Connections to Self
Expresses lack of: hope, meaning/purpose in life, serenity (e.g., peace), love, acceptance, forgiveness of self, courage
[Expresses] anger; guilt

Connections with Others
Refuses interactions with SO(s)/spiritual leaders
Verbalizes being separated from support system
Expresses alienation

Connections with Art, Music, Literature, Nature
Inability to express previous state of creativity (e.g., singing/ listening to music, writing)
Disinterested in nature/reading spiritual literature

Connections with Power Greater Than Self
Sudden changes in spiritual practices
Inability to pray/participate in religious activities/to experience the transcendent
Expresses hopelessness/suffering/having anger toward God
Expresses being abandoned
Request to see a religious leader

OBJECTIVE

Connections to Self
Poor coping

Connections with Power Greater Than Self
Inability to be introspective

Desired Outcomes/Evaluation Criteria—Client Will:

- Verbalize increased sense of connectedness and hope for future.
- Demonstrate ability to help self/participate in care.
- Participate in activities with others, actively seek relationships.
- Discuss beliefs/values about spiritual issues.
- Verbalize acceptance of self as not deserving illness/situation, "no one is to blame."

Actions/Interventions

NURSING PRIORITY NO. 1. To assess causative/contributing factors:

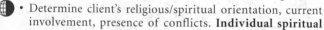 • Determine client's religious/spiritual orientation, current involvement, presence of conflicts. **Individual spiritual**

Information in brackets added by the authors to clarify and enhance the use of nursing diagnoses.

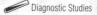 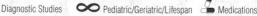

practices/restrictions may affect client care or create conflict between spiritual beliefs and treatment.

- Listen to client's/SO's reports/expressions of concern, anger, alienation from God, belief that illness/situation is a punishment for wrongdoing, and so forth. **Suggests need for spiritual advisor to address client's belief system, if desired.**

- Determine sense of futility, feelings of hopelessness and helplessness, lack of motivation to help self. **Indicators that client may see no, or only limited, options/alternatives or personal choices available and lacks energy to deal with situation.**

- Note expressions of inability to find meaning in life, reason for living. Evaluate suicidal ideation. **Crisis of the spirit/loss of will-to-live places client at increased risk for inattention to personal well-being/harm to self.**

- Note recent changes in behavior (e.g., withdrawal from others/ creative or religious activities, dependence on alcohol/ medications). **Helpful in determining severity/duration of situation and possible need for additional referrals, such as substance withdrawal.**

- Assess sense of self-concept, worth, ability to enter into loving relationships. **Lack of connectedness with self/others impairs client's ability to trust others or feel worthy of trust from others.**

- Observe behavior indicative of poor relationships with others (e.g., manipulative, nontrusting, demanding). **Manipulation is used for management of client's sense of powerlessness because of distrust of others.**

- Determine support systems available to client/SO(s) and how they are used. **Provides insight to client's willingness to pursue outside resources.**

- Be aware of influence of care provider's belief system. **(It is still possible to be helpful to client while remaining neutral/ not espousing own beliefs.)**

NURSING PRIORITY NO. 2. To assist client/SO(s) to deal with feelings/ situation:

- Develop therapeutic nurse–client relationship. Ascertain client's views as to how care provider(s) can be most helpful. Convey acceptance of client's spiritual beliefs/concerns. **Promotes trust and comfort, encouraging client to be open about sensitive matters.**

- Establish environment that promotes free expression of feelings and concerns.

- Suggest use of journaling. **Can assist in clarifying values/ ideas, recognizing and resolving feelings/situation.**

Information in brackets added by the authors to clarify and enhance the use of nursing diagnoses.

• Encourage client/family to ask questions. **Demonstrates support for individual's willingness to learn.**

 • Identify inappropriate coping behaviors currently being used and associated consequences. **Recognizing negative consequences of actions may enhance desire to change.**

 • Ascertain past coping behaviors **to determine approaches used previously that may be more effective in dealing with current situation.**

 • Problem solve solutions/identify areas for compromise **that may be useful in resolving possible conflicts.**

 • Provide calm, peaceful setting when possible. **Promotes relaxation and enhances opportunity for reflection on situation/discussions with others, meditation.**

 • Set limits on acting-out behavior that is inappropriate/destructive. **Promotes safety for client/others and helps prevent loss of self-esteem.**

 • Make time for nonjudgmental discussion of philosophic issues/questions about spiritual impact of illness/situation and/or treatment regimen. **Open communication can assist client in reality checks of perceptions and identifying personal options.**

NURSING PRIORITY NO. 3. To facilitate setting goals and moving forward:

 • Involve client in refining healthcare goals and therapeutic regimen, as appropriate. **Enhances commitment to plan, optimizing outcomes.**

 • Discuss difference between grief and guilt and help client to identify and deal with each. Point out consequences of actions based on guilt. **Aids client in assuming responsibility for own actions and avoiding acting out of false guilt.**

 • Use therapeutic communication skills of reflection and active-listening. **Helps client find own solutions to concerns.**

 • Identify role models (e.g., nurse, individual experiencing similar situation). **Provides opportunities for sharing of experiences/hope and identifying options to deal with situation.**

 • Assist client to learn use of meditation/prayer and forgiveness **to heal past hurts.**

 • Provide information that anger with God is a normal part of the grieving process. **Realizing these feelings are not unusual can reduce sense of guilt, encourage open expression, and facilitate resolution of conflict.**

 • Provide time and privacy to engage in spiritual growth/religious activities (e.g., prayer, meditation, scripture reading, listening to music). **Allows client to focus on self and seek connectedness.**

Information in brackets added by the authors to clarify and enhance the use of nursing diagnoses.

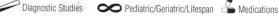 Diagnostic Studies ∞ Pediatric/Geriatric/Lifespan   Medications **649**

- Encourage/facilitate outings to neighborhood park/nature walks, when able. **Sunshine, fresh air, and activity can stimulate release of endorphins, promoting sense of well-being.**
- Provide play therapy for child that encompasses spiritual data. **Interactive pleasurable activity promotes open discussion and enhances retention of information. Also provides opportunity for child to practice what has been learned.**
- Abide by parents' wishes in discussing and implementing child's spiritual support. **Limits confusion for child and prevents conflict of values/beliefs.**
- Refer to appropriate resources (e.g., pastoral/parish nurse or religious counselor, crisis counselor, hospice; psychotherapy; Alcoholics/Narcotics Anonymous). **Useful in dealing with immediate situation and identifying long-term resources for support to help foster sense of connectedness.**
- Refer to NDs ineffective Coping; Powerlessness; Self-Esteem [specify]; Social Isolation; risk for Suicide.

NURSING PRIORITY NO. 4. To promote wellness (Teaching/ Discharge Considerations):

- Assist client to develop goals for dealing with life/illness situation. **Enhances commitment to goal, optimizing outcomes.**
- Encourage life-review by client. Help client find a reason for living. **Promotes sense of hope and willingness to continue efforts to improve situation.**
- Assist in developing coping skills **to deal with stressors of illness/necessary changes in lifestyle.**
- Assist client to identify SO(s) and people who could provide support as needed. **Ongoing support is required to enhance sense of connectedness and continue progress toward goals.**
- Encourage family to provide a quiet, calm atmosphere. Be willing to just "be" there and not have a need to "do" something. **Helps client to think about self in the context of current situation.**
- Assist client to identify spiritual resources that could be helpful (e.g., contact spiritual advisor who has qualifications/experience in dealing with specific problems, such as death/dying, relationship problems, substance abuse, suicide). **Provides answers to spiritual questions, assists in the journey of self-discovery, and can help client learn to accept and forgive self.**

Documentation Focus

ASSESSMENT/REASSESSMENT

- Individual findings, including nature of spiritual conflict, effects of participation in treatment regimen.

Information in brackets added by the authors to clarify and enhance the use of nursing diagnoses.

- Physical/emotional responses to conflict.

PLANNING

- Plan of care and who is involved in planning.
- Teaching plan.

IMPLEMENTATION/EVALUATION

- Responses to interventions/teaching and actions performed.
- Attainment/progress toward desired outcome(s).
- Modifications to plan of care.

DISCHARGE PLANNING

- Long-term needs and who is responsible for actions to be taken.
- Available resources, specific referrals made.

SAMPLE NURSING OUTCOMES & INTERVENTIONS CLASSIFICATIONS (NOC/NIC)

NOC—Spiritual Well-Being
NIC—Spiritual Support

risk for Spiritual Distress

Taxonomy II: Life Principles—Class 3 Value/Belief/Action
  Congruence (00067)
[Diagnostic Division: Ego Integrity]
Nursing Diagnosis Extension and Classification (NDEC)
  Submission 1998; Revised 2004

Definition: At risk for an impaired ability to experience
and integrate meaning and purpose in life through
connectedness with self, others, art, music, literature,
nature, and/or a power greater than oneself

Risk Factors

PHYSICAL

Physical/chronic illness, substance abuse

PSYCHOSOCIAL

Stress; anxiety; depression
Low self-esteem; poor relationships; blocks to experiencing
  love; inability to forgive; loss; separated support systems;
  racial/cultural conflict
Change in religious rituals/spiritual practices

Information in brackets added by the authors to clarify and enhance
the use of nursing diagnoses.

 Diagnostic Studies 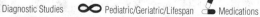 Pediatric/Geriatric/Lifespan   Medications   **651**

DEVELOPMENTAL

Life changes

ENVIRONMENTAL

Environmental changes; natural disasters

> NOTE: A risk diagnosis is not evidenced by signs and symptoms, as the problem has not occurred and nursing interventions are directed at prevention.

Desired Outcomes/Evaluation Criteria—Client Will:

- Identify meaning and purpose in own life that reinforces hope, peace, and contentment.
- Verbalize acceptance of self as being worthy, not deserving of illness/situation, and so forth.
- Identify and use resources appropriately.

Actions/Interventions

NURSING PRIORITY NO. 1. To assess causative/contributing factors:

- Ascertain current situation (e.g., natural disaster, death of a spouse, personal injustice).
- Listen to client's/SO's reports/expressions of anger/concern, belief that illness/situation is a punishment for wrongdoing, and so forth. **May indicate possibility of becoming distressed about spiritual and religious beliefs.**
- Note client's reason for living and whether it is directly related to situation (e.g., home and business washed away in a flood, parent whose only child is terminally ill). **Questioning meaning or purpose of life may indicate inner conflict about previous religious beliefs and rituals.**
- Determine client's religious/spiritual orientation, current involvement, presence of conflicts, especially in current circumstances.
- Assess sense of self-concept, worth, ability to enter into loving relationships. **Feelings of abandonment may accompany sense of "not being good enough" in face of illness, disaster.**
- Observe behavior indicative of poor relationships with others (e.g., manipulative, nontrusting, demanding).
- Determine support systems available to and used by client/SO(s).

Information in brackets added by the authors to clarify and enhance the use of nursing diagnoses.

  Cultural Collaborative Community/Home Care

- Ascertain substance use/abuse. **Affects ability to deal with problems in a positive manner.**

NURSING PRIORITY NO. 2. To assist client/SO(s) to deal with feelings/situation:

- Establish environment that promotes free expression of feelings and concerns. **Listening, and a quiet demeanor can convey acceptance to the client.**

- Have client identify and prioritize current/immediate needs. **Helps client focus on what needs to be done and identify manageable steps to take.**

- Make time for nonjudgmental discussion of philosophical issues/questions about spiritual impact of illness/situation and/or treatment regimen. **Client may believe that illness is the result of being sinful, bad, or that God has abandoned him or her.**

- Discuss difference between grief and guilt and help client to identify and deal with each, assuming responsibility for own actions, expressing awareness of the consequences of acting out of false guilt. **Client needs to decide whether guilt is deserved or not. Cultural and religious beliefs may lead client to feel guilty when in fact nothing has been done to feel guilty about.**

- Use therapeutic communication skills of reflection and active-listening. **Helps client find own solutions to concerns.**

- Review coping skills used and their effectiveness in current situation. **Identifies strengths to incorporate into plan and techniques needing revision.**

- Provide role model (e.g., nurse, individual experiencing similar situation/disease). **Sharing of experiences/hope assists client to deal with reality.**

- Suggest use of journaling. **Can assist in clarifying values/ideas, recognizing and resolving feelings/situation.**

- Discuss client's interest in the arts, music, literature. **Provides insight into meaning of these issues and how they are integrated into the individual's life.**

- Refer to appropriate resources for help (e.g., crisis counselor, governmental agencies; pastoral/parish nurse or spiritual advisor who has qualifications/experience dealing with specific problems [such as death/dying, relationships, substance abuse, suicide]; hospice, psychotherapy, Alcoholics/Narcotics Anonymous).

NURSING PRIORITY NO. 3. To promote wellness (Teaching/Discharge Considerations):

Information in brackets added by the authors to clarify and enhance the use of nursing diagnoses.

Diagnostic Studies   Pediatric/Geriatric/Lifespan   Medications

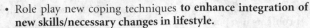

risk for SPIRITUAL DISTRESS

- Role play new coping techniques **to enhance integration of new skills/necessary changes in lifestyle.**
- Encourage individual to become involved in cultural activities of his or her choosing. **Art, music, plays, and other cultural activities provide a means of connecting with self and others.**
- Discuss possibilities of taking classes, being involved in discussion groups, community programs.
- Assist client to identify SO(s) and individuals/support groups that could provide ongoing support **because this is a daily need requiring lifelong commitment.**
- Abide by parents' wishes in discussing and implementing child's spiritual support.
- Discuss benefit of family counseling, as appropriate. **Issues of this nature (e.g., situational losses, natural disasters, difficult relationships) affect family dynamics.**

Documentation Focus

ASSESSMENT/REASSESSMENT

- Individual findings, including risk factors, nature of current distress.
- Physical/emotional responses to distress.
- Access to/use of resources.

PLANNING

- Plan of care and who is involved in planning.
- Teaching plan.

IMPLEMENTATION/EVALUATION

- Responses to interventions/teaching and actions performed.
- Attainment/progress toward desired outcome(s).
- Modifications to plan of care.

DISCHARGE PLANNING

- Long-term needs and who is responsible for actions to be taken.
- Available resources, specific referrals made.

SAMPLE NURSING OUTCOMES & INTERVENTIONS CLASSIFICATIONS (NOC/NIC)

NOC—Spiritual Well-Being
NIC—Spiritual Support

Information in brackets added by the authors to clarify and enhance the use of nursing diagnoses.

  Cultural 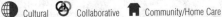 Collaborative   Community/Home Care

readiness for enhanced Spiritual Well-Being

Taxonomy II: Life Principles—Class 2 Beliefs (00068)
[Diagnostic Division: Ego Integrity]
Submitted 1994; Revised 2002

Definition: Ability to experience and integrate meaning and purpose in life through connectedness with self, others, art, music, literature, nature, and/or a power greater than oneself that can be strengthened

Defining Characteristics

SUBJECTIVE

Connections to Self
Expresses desire for enhanced acceptance; coping; courage; forgiveness of self; hope; joy; love; meaning/purpose in life; satisfying philosophy of life; surrender
Expresses lack of serenity (e.g., peace)
Meditation

Connections with Others
Requests interactions with significant others/spiritual leaders
Requests forgiveness of others

Connections with Powers Greater Than Self
Participates in religious activities; prays
Expresses reverence/awe; reports mystical experiences

OBJECTIVE

Connections with Others
Provides service to others

Connections with Art, Music, Literature, Nature
Displays creative energy (e.g., writing poetry, singing); listens to music; reads spiritual literature; spends time outdoors

Desired Outcomes/Evaluation Criteria—Client Will:

- Acknowledge the stabilizing and strengthening forces in own life needed for balance and well-being of the whole person.
- Identify meaning and purpose in own life that reinforces hope, peace, and contentment.
- Verbalize a sense of peace/contentment and comfort of spirit.

Information in brackets added by the authors to clarify and enhance the use of nursing diagnoses.

 Diagnostic Studies 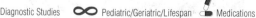 Pediatric/Geriatric/Lifespan Medications

- Demonstrate behavior congruent with verbalizations that lend support and strength for daily living.

Actions/Interventions

NURSING PRIORITY NO. 1. To determine spiritual state/motivation for growth:

- Ascertain client's perception of current state/degree of connectedness and expectations. **Provides insight as to where client is currently and what his or her hopes for the future may be.**
- Identify motivation and expectations for change.
- Review spiritual/religious history, activities/rituals and frequency of participation. **Provides basis to build on for growth/change.**
- Determine relational values of support systems to one's spiritual centeredness. **The client's family of origin may have differing beliefs from those espoused by the individual that may be a source of conflict for the client. Comfort can be gained when family and friends share client's beliefs and support search for spiritual knowledge.**
- Explore meaning/interpretation and relationship of spirituality, life/death, and illness to life's journey. **Identifying the meaning of these issues is helpful for the client to use the information in forming a belief system that will enable him or her to move forward and live life to the fullest.**
- Clarify the meaning of one's spiritual beliefs/religious practice and rituals to daily living. **Discussing these issues allows client to explore spiritual needs and decide what fits own view of the world to enhance life.**
- Explore ways that spirituality/religious practices have affected one's life and given meaning and value to daily living. Note consequences as well as benefits. **Understanding that there is a difference between spirituality and religion and how each can be useful will help client begin to view the information in a new way.**
- Discuss life's/God's plan for the individual, if client desires. **Helpful in determining individual goals/choosing specific options.**

NURSING PRIORITY NO. 2. To assist client to integrate values and beliefs to achieve a sense of wholeness and optimum balance in daily living:

- Explore ways beliefs give meaning and value to daily living. **As client develops understanding of these issues, they will provide support for dealing with current/future concerns.**

Information in brackets added by the authors to clarify and enhance the use of nursing diagnoses.

Cultural   Collaborative   Community/Home Care

- Clarify reality/appropriateness of client's self-perceptions and expectations. **Necessary to provide firm foundation for growth.**
- Determine influence of cultural beliefs/values. **Most individuals are strongly influenced by the spiritual/religious orientation of their family of origin, which can be a very strong determinate for client's choice of activities/receptiveness to various options.**
- Discuss the importance and value of connections to one's daily life. **The contact that one has with others maintains a feeling of belonging and connection and promotes feelings of wholeness and well-being.**
- Identify ways to achieve connectedness or harmony with self, others, nature, higher power (e.g., meditation, prayer, talking/sharing oneself with others; being out in nature/gardening/walking; attending religious activities). **This is a highly individual and personal decision, and no action is too trivial to be considered.**

NURSING PRIORITY NO. 3. To enhance optimum wellness:

- Encourage client to take time to be introspective in the search for peace and harmony. **Finding peace within oneself will carry over to relationships with others and own outlook on life.**
- Discuss use of relaxation/meditative activities (e.g., yoga, tai chi, prayer). **Helpful in promoting general well-being and sense of connectedness with self/nature/spiritual power.**
- Suggest attendance/involvement in dream-sharing group **to develop/enhance learning of the characteristics of spiritual awareness and facilitate the individual's growth.**
- Identify ways for spiritual/religious expression. **There are multiple options for enhancing spirituality through connectedness with self/others (e.g., volunteering time to community projects, mentoring, singing in the choir, painting, or spiritual writings).**
- Encourage participation in desired religious activities, contact with minister/spiritual advisor. **Validating own beliefs in an external way can provide support and strengthen the inner self.**
- Discuss and role play, as necessary, ways to deal with alternative view/conflict that may occur with family/SO(s)/society/cultural group. **Provides opportunity to try out different behaviors in a safe environment and be prepared for potential eventualities.**
- Provide bibliotherapy, list of relevant resources (e.g., study groups, parish nurse, poetry society), and possible websites

---

Information in brackets added by the authors to clarify and enhance the use of nursing diagnoses.

Diagnostic Studies   Pediatric/Geriatric/Lifespan   Medications   **657**

for later reference/self-paced learning and ongoing support.

Documentation Focus

ASSESSMENT/REASSESSMENT

- Assessment findings, including client perception of needs and desire for growth/enhancement.
- Motivation/expectations for change.

PLANNING

- Plan for growth and who is involved in planning.

IMPLEMENTATION/EVALUATION

- Response to activities/learning and actions performed.
- Attainment/progress toward desired outcome(s).
- Modifications to plan.

DISCHARGE PLANNING

- Long-range needs/expectations and plan of action.
- Specific referrals made.

SAMPLE NURSING OUTCOMES & INTERVENTIONS CLASSIFICATIONS (NOC/NIC)

NOC—Spiritual Well-Being
NIC—Spiritual Growth Facilitation

Stress Overload

Taxonomy II: Coping/Stress Tolerance—Class 2 Coping
   Responses (00177)
[Diagnostic Division: Ego Intregrity]
Submitted 2006

Definition: Excessive amounts and types of demands that require action

Related Factors

Inadequate resources (e.g., financial, social, education/knowledge level)

Intense, repeated stressors (e.g., family violence, chronic illness, terminal illness)

Multiple coexisting stressors (e.g., environmental threats/demands; physical threats/demands; social threats/demands)

Information in brackets added by the authors to clarify and enhance the use of nursing diagnoses.

  Cultural Collaborative Community/Home Care

Defining Characteristics

SUBJECTIVE

Expresses difficulty in functioning/problems with decision making

Expresses a feeling of pressure/tension/increased feelings of impatience/anger

Reports negative impact from stress (e.g., physical symptoms, psychological distress, feeling of "being sick" or of "going to get sick")

Reports situational stress as excessive (e.g., rates stress level as a seven or above on a 10-point scale)

OBJECTIVE

Demonstrates increased feelings of impatience/anger

Desired Outcomes/Evaluation Criteria—Client Will:

- Assess current situation accurately.
- Identify ineffective stress-management behaviors and consequences.
- Meet psychological needs as evidenced by appropriate expression of feelings, identification of options and use of resources.
- Verbalize or demonstrate reduced stress reaction.

Actions/Interventions

NURSING PRIORITY NO. 1. To identify causative/precipitating factors and degree of impairment:

- Ascertain what events have occurred (e.g., family violence; death of loved one; chronic/terminal illness; work place stress/loss of job; catastrophic natural or man-made event) over remote and recent past **to assist in determining number, duration, and intensity of events causing perception of overwhelming stress.**
- Determine client's/SO's understanding of events, noting differences in viewpoints.
- Note client's gender, age, and developmental level of functioning. **Women, children, young adults, and divorced and separated persons tend to have higher stress levels. Multiple stressors can weaken the immune system and tax physical and emotional coping mechanisms in persons of any age, but particulary the elderly.**
- Note cultural values/religious beliefs that may affect client's expectation for self in dealing with situation and expectations placed on client by SO(s)/family. **For example, in dealing**

Information in brackets added by the authors to clarify and enhance the use of nursing diagnoses.

 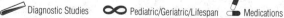

with Navajo parents, it is important to look at how they **define family (can be nuclear, extended, or clan), who are the primary caregivers, and what are their social goals.**

- Identify client locus of control: internal (expressions of responsibility for self and ability to control outcomes "I didn't quit smoking") or external (expressions of lack of control over self and environment "Nothing ever works out"). **Knowing client's locus of control will help in developing a plan of care reflecting client's ability to realistically make changes that will help to manage stress better.**
- Assess emotional responses and coping mechanisms being used.
- Determine stress feelings and self-talk client is engaging in. **Negative self-talk, all or nothing/pessimistic thinking, exaggeration, or unrealistic expectations all contribute to stress overload.**
- Assess degree of mastery client has exhibited in life. **Passive individual may have more difficulty being assertive and standing up for rights.**
- Determine presence/absence/nature of resources (e.g., whether family/SO(s) are supportive, lack of money, problems with relationship/social functioning).
- Note change in relationships with SO(s). **Conflict in the family, loss of a family member, divorce can result in a change in support client is accustomed to and impair ability to manage situation.**
- Evaluate stress level using appropriate tool (e.g., Stress & Depression, Self-Assessment Tool, etc.) to help identify areas of most distress. **While most stress seems to come from disasterous events in individual's life, positive events can also be stressful.**

NURSING PRIORITY NO. 2. To assist client to deal with current situation:

- Active-listen concerns and provide empathetic presence, using talk and silence as needed.
- Provide/encourage restful environment where possible.
- Discuss situation/condition in simple, concise manner. Devote time for listening. **May help client to express emotions, grasp situation, and feel more in control.**
- Deal with the immediate issues first (e.g., treatment of acute physical/psychological illness, meet safety needs, removal from traumatic/violent environment).
- Assist client in determining whether or not he or she can change stressor or response. **May help client to sort out things over which he or she has control, and/or determine responses that can be modified.**

Information in brackets added by the authors to clarify and enhance the use of nursing diagnoses.

  Cultural Collaborative 🏠 Community/Home Care

🏠 • Allow client to react in own way without judgment. **Provide support and diversion, as indicated.**

🏠 • Help client to set limits on acting-out behaviors and learn ways to express emotions in an acceptable manner. **Promotes internal locus of control, enabling client to maintain self-concept and feel more positive about self.**

🔟 • Address use of ineffective/dangerous coping mechanisms (e.g., substance use/abuse, self/other-directed violence) and refer for counseling as indicated.

🔟 • Collaborate in treatment of underlying conditions (e.g., physical injury, depression, anger management).

NURSING PRIORITY NO. 3. To promote wellness (Teaching/Discharge Considerations):

🏠 • Use client's locus of control to develop individual plan of care **(e.g., for client with internal control, encourage client to take control of own care and for those with external control, begin with small tasks and add as tolerated).**

🏠 • Incorporate strengths/assets and past coping strategies that were successful for client. **Reinforces that client is able to deal with difficult situations.**

🏠 • Provide information about stress and exhaustion phase, which occurs when person is experiencing chronic/unresolved stress. **Release of cortisol can contribute to reduction in immune function, resulting in physical illness, mental disability, and life dysfunction.**

🏠 • Review stress management/coping skills that client can use:
  Practice behaviors that may help reduce negative consequences—change thinking by focusing on positives, reframing thoughts, changing lifestyle.
  Take a step back, simplify life; learn to say "no" **to reduce sense of being overwhelmed.**
  Learn to control and redirect anger.
  Develop and practice positive self-esteem skills.
  Rest, sleep, and exercise **to recuperate and rejuvenate self.**
  Participate in self-help actions (e.g., deep breathing, find time to be alone, get involved in recreation or desired activity, plan something fun/develop humor) **to actively relax.**
  Eat right; avoid junk food, excessive caffeine, alcohol, and nicotine **to support general health.**
  Develop spiritual self (e.g., meditate/pray, block negative thoughts, learn to give and take, speak and listen, forgive and move on).
  Interact socially, reach out, nurture self and others **to reduce loneliness/sense of isolation.**

Information in brackets added by the authors to clarify and enhance the use of nursing diagnoses.

🧪 Diagnostic Studies ∞ Pediatric/Geriatric/Lifespan 💊 Medications **661**

- Review proper medication use to manage exacerbating conditions (e.g., depression, mood disorders).
- Identify community resources (e.g., vocational counseling, educational programs, child/elder care, WIC/food stamps, home/respite care) **that can help client manage lifestyle/ environmental stress.**
- Refer for therapy as indicated (e.g., medical treatment, psychological counseling, hypnosis, massage, biofeedback).

Documentation Focus

ASSESSMENT/REASSESSMENT

- Individual findings, noting specific stressors, individual's perception of the situation, locus of control.
- Specific cultural/religious factors.
- Availability/use of support systems and resources.

PLANNING

- Plan of care and who is involved in planning.
- Teaching plan.

IMPLEMENTATION/EVALUATION

- Responses to interventions/teaching and actions performed.
- Attainment/progress toward desired outcome(s).
- Modifications to plan of care.

DISCHARGE PLANNING

- Long-term needs/referrals and who is responsible for actions to be taken.
- Specific referrals made.

SAMPLE NURSING OUTCOMES & INTERVENTIONS CLASSIFICATIONS (NOC/NIC)

NOC—Stress Level
NIC—Coping Enhancement

risk for Suffocation

Taxonomy II: Safety/Protection—Class 2 Physical Injury
    (00036)
[Diagnostic Division: Safety]
Submitted 1980

Definition: Accentuated risk of accidental suffocation
(inadequate air available for inhalation)

Information in brackets added by the authors to clarify and enhance the use of nursing diagnoses.

  Cultural Collaborative Community/Home Care

Risk Factors

INTERNAL

Reduced olfactory sensation
Reduced motor abilities
Lack of safety education/precautions
Cognitive/emotional difficulties [e.g., altered consciousness/ mentation]
Disease/injury process

EXTERNAL

Pillow/propped bottle placed in an infant's crib
Hanging a pacifier around infant's neck
Playing with plastic bags; inserting small objects into airway
Leaving children unattended in water
Discarded refrigerators without removed doors
Vehicle warming in closed garage [/faulty exhaust system]; use of fuel-burning heaters not vented to outside
Household gas leaks; smoking in bed
Low-strung clothesline
Eating large mouthfuls [or pieces] of food

> NOTE: A risk diagnosis is not evidenced by signs and symptoms, as the problem has not occurred and nursing interventions are directed at prevention.

Desired Outcomes/Evaluation Criteria—Client/Caregiver Will:

- Verbalize knowledge of hazards in the environment.
- Identify interventions appropriate to situation.
- Correct hazardous situations to prevent/reduce risk of suffocation.
- Demonstrate CPR skills and how to access emergency assistance.

Actions/Interventions

NURSING PRIORITY NO. 1. To assess causative/contributing factors:

- Note presence of internal/external factors in individual situation (e.g., seizure activity; asthma; frail elderly; impaired cognition/consciousness; risky teen behavior, such as playing suffocation game, sniffing inhalants; hazards in or around home [e.g., abandoned large appliances, swimming pool]; inadequate supervision of infants/small children, etc.).

Information in brackets added by the authors to clarify and enhance the use of nursing diagnoses.

 Diagnostic Studies   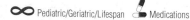 Pediatric/Geriatric/Lifespan   Medications   **663**

- Determine client's/SO's knowledge of safety factors/hazards present in the environment.
- Identify level of concern/awareness and motivation of client/SO(s) to correct safety hazards and improve individual situation.
- Assess neurological status and note factors that have potential to compromise airway or affect ability to swallow (e.g., stroke, cerebral palsy, MS, ALS).
- Determine use of antiepileptics and how well epilepsy is controlled.
- Note reports of sleep disturbance and fatigue; **may be indicative of sleep apnea (airway obstruction).**
- Assess for allergies (e.g., medications, foods, environmental) **to which individual could have severe/anaphylactic reaction resulting in respiratory arrest.**

NURSING PRIORITY NO. 2. To reverse/correct contributing factors:

- Identify/encourage relevant safety measures (e.g., seizure precautions; close supervision of toddler; avoiding smoking in bed, propping baby bottle, or running automobile in closed garage) **to prevent/minimize risk of injury.**
- Recommend storing small toys, coins, cords/drawstrings, and plastic bags out of reach of infants/young children. Avoid use of plastic mattress or crib covers, comforter, or fluffy pillows in cribs **to reduce risk of accidental suffocation.**
- Use proper positioning, suctioning, use of airway adjuncts, as indicated, for comatose individual or client with swallowing impairment or obstructive sleep apnea **to protect/maintain airway.**
- Provide diet modifications as indicated by specific needs (e.g., developmental level, presence/degree of swallowing disability, impaired cognition) **to reduce risk of aspiration.**
- Monitor medication regimen (e.g., anticonvulsants, analgesics, sedatives), noting potential for oversedation.
- Discuss with client/SO(s) identified environmental/work-related safety hazards and problem solve methods for resolution.
- Emphasize importance of periodic evaluation and repair of gas appliances/furnace, automobile exhaust system **to prevent exposure to carbon monoxide.**

NURSING PRIORITY NO. 3. To promote wellness (Teaching/Discharge Considerations):

- Review safety factors identified in individual situation and methods for remediation.

Information in brackets added by the authors to clarify and enhance the use of nursing diagnoses.

  Cultural Collaborative 🏠 Community/Home Care

- Develop plan with client/caregiver for long-range management of situation to avoid injuries. **Enhances commitment to plan, optimizing outcomes.**
- Review importance of chewing carefully, taking small amounts of food, using caution when talking or drinking while eating. Discuss possibility of choking **because of throat muscle relaxation and impaired judgment when drinking alcohol and eating.**
- Emphasize the importance of getting help when beginning to choke; instead of leaving table, remain calm and make gesture across throat, making sure someone recognizes the emergency.
- Promote public education in techniques for clearing blocked airways, backblows, Heimlich maneuver, CPR.
- Collaborate in community public health education regarding hazards for children (e.g., appropriate toy size for young child) discussing dangers of "huffing" [inhalants] and playing choking/hanging games with pre-teens; fire safety drills; bathtub rules; how to spot potential for depression/risk of suidical gestures in adolescent **to reduce potential for accidental/ intentional suffocation.**
- Assist individuals to learn to read package labels and identify safety hazards.
- Promote pool safety, use of approved flotation devices, proper fencing enclosure/alarm system for home pools.
- Discuss safety measures regarding use of heaters, household gas appliances, old/discarded appliances.
- Refer to NDs ineffective Airway Clearance; risk for Aspiration; ineffective Breathing Pattern; impaired Parenting.

Documentation Focus

ASSESSMENT/REASSESSMENT

- Individual risk factors, including individual's cognitive status and level of knowledge.
- Level of concern/motivation for change.
- Equipment/airway adjunct needs.

PLANNING

- Plan of care and who is involved in planning.
- Teaching plan.

IMPLEMENTATION/EVALUATION

- Responses to interventions/teaching and actions performed.
- Attainment/progress toward desired outcome(s).
- Modifications to plan of care.

Information in brackets added by the authors to clarify and enhance the use of nursing diagnoses.

Diagnostic Studies   Pediatric/Geriatric/Lifespan   Medications   **665**

DISCHARGE PLANNING

- Long-term needs/referrals, appropriate preventive measures, and who is responsible for actions to be taken.
- Specific referrals made.

SAMPLE NURSING OUTCOMES & INTERVENTIONS CLASSIFICATIONS (NOC/NIC)

NOC—Risk Control
NIC—Airway Management

risk for Suicide

Taxonomy II: Safety/Protection—Class 3 Violence (00150)
[Diagnostic Division: Safety]
Submitted 2000

Definition: At risk for self-inflicted, life-threatening injury

Risk Factors/[Indicators]

BEHAVIORAL

History of prior suicide attempt
Buying a gun; stockpiling medicines
Making/changing a will; giving away possessions
Sudden euphoric recovery from major depression
Impulsiveness; marked changes in behavior/attitude/school performance

VERBAL

Threats of killing oneself; states desire to die[/end it all]

SITUATIONAL

Living alone; retired; economic instability; relocation; institutionalization
Loss of autonomy/indepednence
Presence of gun in home
Adolescents living in nontraditional settings (e.g., juvenile detention center, prison, half-way house, group home)

PSYCHOLOGICAL

Family history of suicide; childhood abuse
Substance abuse
Psychiatric illness/disorder (e.g., depression, schizophrenia, bipolar disorder)

Information in brackets added by the authors to clarify and enhance the use of nursing diagnoses.

 Cultural Collaborative Community/Home Care

Guilt
Gay or lesbian youth

DEMOGRAPHIC

Age (e.g., elderly, young adult males, adolescents)
Race (e.g., Caucasian, Native American)
Male gender
Divorced; widowed

PHYSICAL

Physical/terminal illness; chronic pain

SOCIAL

Loss of important relationship; disrupted family life; poor support systems; social isolation
Grief; loneliness
Hopelessness; helplessness
Legal/disciplinary problem
Cluster suicides

NOTE: A risk diagnosis is not evidenced by signs and symptoms, as the problem has not occurred and nursing interventions are directed at prevention.

Desired Outcomes/Evaluation Criteria—Client Will:

- Acknowledge difficulties perceived in current situation.
- Identify current factors that can be dealt with.
- Be involved in planning course of action to correct existing problems.
- Make decision that suicide is not the answer to the perceived problems.

Actions/Interventions

NURSING PRIORITY NO. 1. To assess causative/contributing factors:

- Identify degree of risk/potential for suicide and seriousness of threat. Use a scale of 1 to 10 and prioritize according to severity of threat, availability of means.
- Note behaviors indicative of intent (e.g., gestures; presence of means, such as guns; threats; giving away possessions; previous attempts; and presence of hallucinations or delusions). **Many people signal their intent, particularly to healthcare providers.**

Information in brackets added by the authors to clarify and enhance the use of nursing diagnoses.

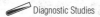 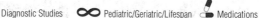

- Ask directly if person is thinking of acting on thoughts/feelings. **Determines intent. Most people will answer honestly because they actually want help.**
- Note age and gender. **Risk of suicide is greater in males, teens, and the elderly, but there is a rising awareness of risk in early childhood.**
- Review family history for suicidal behavior. **Individual risk is increased, especially when the person who commited suicide was close to the client.**
- Identify conditions, such as acute/chronic brain syndrome, panic state, hormonal imbalance (e.g., PMS, postpartum psychosis, drug-induced) **that may interfere with ability to control own behavior and will require specific interventions to promote safety.**
- Review laboratory findings (e.g., blood alcohol, blood glucose, ABGs, electrolytes, renal function tests), **to identify factors that may affect reasoning ability.**
- Note withdrawal from usual activities, lack of social interactions.
- Assess physical complaints (e.g., sleeping difficulties, lack of appetite).
- Determine drug use/"self" medication.
- Note history of disciplinary problems/involvement with judicial system.
- Assess coping behaviors presently used. Note: Client may believe there is no alternative except suicide.
- Determine presence of SO(s)/friends who are available for support.

NURSING PRIORITY NO. 2. To assist clients to accept responsibility for own behavior and prevent suicide:

- Develop therapeutic nurse–client relationship, providing consistent caregiver. **Promotes sense of trust, allowing individual to discuss feelings openly.**
- Maintain straightforward communication **to avoid reinforcing manipulative behavior.**
- Explain concern for safety and willingness to help client stay safe.
- Encourage expression of feelings and make time to listen to concerns. **Acknowledges reality of feelings and that they are OK. Helps individual sort out thinking and begin to develop understanding of situation and look at other alternatives.**
- Give permission to express angry feelings in acceptable ways and let client know someone will be available to assist in maintaining control. **Promotes acceptance and sense of safety.**
- Acknowledge reality of suicide as an option. Discuss consequences of actions if they follow through on intent. Ask how

---

Information in brackets added by the authors to clarify and enhance the use of nursing diagnoses.

   Cultural   Collaborative   Community/Home Care

it will help individual to resolve problems. **Helps to focus on consequences of actions and possibility of other options.**

- Maintain observation of client and check environment for hazards that could be used to commit suicide **to increase client safety/reduce risk of impulsive behavior.**
- Help client identify more appropriate solutions/behaviors (e.g., motor activities/exercise) **to lessen sense of anxiety and associated physical manifestations.**
- Provide directions for actions client can take, avoiding negative statements, such as "do nots." **Promotes a positive attitude.**
- Discuss use of psychotropic medication, positive and negative aspects. **There has been concern about the increased risk of suicide from these drugs and research is ongoing to determine whether they help or harm.**
- Reevaluate potential for suicide periodically at key times (e.g., mood changes, increasing withdrawal), as well as when client is feeling better and discharge planning becomes active. **The highest risk is when the client has both suicidal ideation and sufficient energy with which to act.**

NURSING PRIORITY NO. 3. To assist client to plan course of action to correct/deal with existing situation:

- Gear interventions to individual involved (e.g., age, relationship, and current situation).
- Negotiate contract with client regarding willingness not to do anything lethal for a stated period of time. Specify what caregiver will be responsible for and what client responsibilities are.
- Specify alternative actions necessary if client is unwilling to negotiate contract. **May need hospitalization to provide safety.**
- Discuss losses client has experienced and meaning of those losses. **Unresolved issues may be contributing to thoughts of hopelessness.**

NURSING PRIORITY NO. 4. To promote wellness (Teaching/Discharge Considerations):

- Promote development of internal control by helping client look at new ways to deal with problems.
- Assist with learning problem solving, assertiveness training, and social skills.
- Engage in physical activity programs. Releases endorphins **promoting feelings of self-worth and improving sense of well-being.**
- Determine nutritional needs and help client to plan for meeting them.

Information in brackets added by the authors to clarify and enhance the use of nursing diagnoses.

- Involve family/SO(s) in planning **to improve understanding and support.**
- Refer to formal resources as indicated (e.g., individual/group/ marital psychotherapy, substance abuse treatment program, and social services).

Documentation Focus

ASSESSMENT/REASSESSMENT

- Individual findings, including nature of concern (e.g., suicidal/behavioral risk factors and level of impulse control, plan of action/means to carry out plan).
- Client's perception of situation, motivation for change.

PLANNING

- Plan of care and who is involved in the planning.
- Details of contract regarding suicidal ideation/plans.
- Teaching plan.

IMPLEMENTATION/EVALUATION

- Actions taken to promote safety.
- Response to interventions/teaching and actions performed.
- Attainment/progress toward desired outcome(s).
- Modifications to plan of care.

DISCHARGE PLANNING

- Long-range needs and who is responsible for actions to be taken.
- Available resources, specific referrals made.

SAMPLE NURSING OUTCOMES & INTERVENTIONS CLASSIFICATIONS (NOC/NIC)

NOC—Suicide Self-Restraint
NIC—Suicide Prevention

---

delayed Surgical Recovery

Taxonomy II: Activity/Rest—Class 2 Activity/Exercise (00100)
[Diagnostic Division: Safety]
Submitted 1998; Revised 2006

Definition: Extension of the number of postoperative days required to initiate and perform activities that maintain life, health, and well-being

---

Information in brackets added by the authors to clarify and enhance the use of nursing diagnoses.

    Cultural   Collaborative   Community/Home Care

Related Factors

Extensive/prolonged surgical procedure
Pain
Obesity
Preoperative expectations
Postoperative surgical site infection

Defining Characteristics

SUBJECTIVE

Perception that more time is needed to recover
Report of pain/discomfort; fatigue
Loss of appetite with or without nausea
Postpones resumption of work/employment activities

OBJECTIVE

Evidence of interrupted healing of surgical area (e.g., red, indurated, draining, immobilized)
Difficulty in moving about; requires help to complete self-care

Desired Outcomes/Evaluation Criteria—Client Will:

* Display complete healing of surgical area.
* Be able to perform desired self-care activities.
* Report increased energy, able to participate in usual (work/employment) activities.

Actions/Interventions

NURSING PRIORITY NO. 1. To assess causative/contributing factors:

* Identify vulnerable client (e.g., low socioeconomic status, lack of resources, challenges related to poverty, lack of insurance or transportation, severe trauma/prolonged hospitalization with multiple complicating factors) **who is at higher risk for adverse outcomes.**
* Determine extent of surgical involvment of organs/tissues, age/developmental level, and general state of health **to provide anticipatory guidance in postoperative care**.
* Identify underlying condition/pathology (e.g., cancers, burns, diabetes, multiple trauma, infections, cardiopulmomary disorders, debilitating illness), **which may affect healing/recovery.**
* Note other factors that may impede recovery (e.g., obesity, cigarette smoking, sedentary lifestyle, steroid use, prolonged preoperative hospital stay, radiation therapy).

Information in brackets added by the authors to clarify and enhance the use of nursing diagnoses.

 Diagnostic Studies   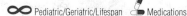 Pediatric/Geriatric/Lifespan   Medications

Side text: delayed SURGICAL RECOVERY

- Ascertain presence/severity of perioperative complications (e.g., lengthy time under anesthesia; trauma/other conditions requiring multiple surgeries) and development of postoperative complications (e.g., surgical site infection, ventilator-associated pneumonia, deep vein thrombosis) **that can prolong recovery.**
- Assess nutritional status and current intake **to determine if nutrition is adequate to support healing.**

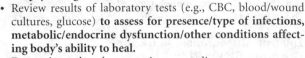

- Review current medication regimen and determine dosages and use of multiple drugs with potential for adverse side effects and interactions **affecting cognition, organ function, and tissue healing.**
- Perform pain assessment **to ascertain whether pain management is adequate to meet client's needs during recovery.**
- Evaluate client's cognitive and emotional state, noting presence of postoperative changes, including confusion, depression, apathy, expressions of helplessness **to determine possible psychological interferences.**
- Review results of laboratory tests (e.g., CBC, blood/wound cultures, glucose) **to assess for presence/type of infections, metabolic/endocrine dysfunction/other conditions affecting body's ability to heal.**
- Determine cultural expectations regarding recovery process and participation of client/others (e.g., client is expected to be inactive and cared for by others).

NURSING PRIORITY NO. 2. To determine impact of delayed recovery:

- Note length of hospitalization and progress in recovery to date and compare with expectations for procedure and situation.
- Determine client's/SO's expectations for recovery and specific stressors related to delay (e.g., return to work/school, home responsibilities/child care, financial difficulties, limited support system).
- Determine energy level and current participation in ADLs. Compare with usual level of function.
- Ascertain whether client usually requires assistance in home setting and who provides it/current availability and capability.
- Obtain psychological assessment of client's emotional status, noting potential problems arising from current situation.

NURSING PRIORITY NO. 3. To promote optimal recovery:

- Inspect incisions/wounds routinely, describing changes (e.g., deepening or healing, wound measurements, presence/type of drainage, development of necrosis).

Information in brackets added by the authors to clarify and enhance the use of nursing diagnoses.

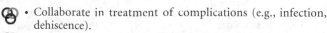

- Collaborate in treatment of complications (e.g., infection, dehiscence).
- Assist with wound care as indicated (e.g., débridement, barrier dressings, wound coverings, skin-protective agents for open/draining wounds).
- Include wound care specialist/stomal therapist as appropriate **to problem solve healing difficulties.**
- Limit/avoid use of plastics or latex materials. **Client may be sensitive.**
- Provide optimal nutrition and adequate protein intake **to provide a positive nitrogen balance, aiding in healing and to achieve general good health.**
- Encourage early ambulation, regular exercise **to promote circulation, improve strength, and reduce risks associated with immobility.**
- Recommend alternating activity with adequate rest periods **to reduce fatigue.**
- Administer medications as indicated (e.g., client may be experiencing stubborn infection requiring IV antibiotics or management of chronic pain).
- Instruct client/SO(s) in necessary self-care of incisions and specific symptom management. **With short hospital stays, client/SO(s) usually provide a great deal of postoperative care and monitoring at home.**
- Encourage client to adhere to medical regimen and follow-up care **to monitor healing process and provide for timely intervention as needed.**
- Refer for outpatient/follow-up care as indicated (e.g., telephone monitoring, home visit, wound care clinic, pain management program).

NURSING PRIORITY NO. 4. To promote wellness (Teaching/Discharge Considerations):

- **Demonstrate self-care skills, provide client/SO(s) with health-related information and psychosocial support** to manage symptoms and pain, enhancing well-being.
- Discuss reality of recovery process in comparison with client's/SO's expectations. **Individuals are often unrealistic regarding energy and time required for healing and own abilities/responsibilities to facilitate process.**
- Involve client/SO(s) in setting incremental goals. **Enhances commitment to plan and reduces likelihood of frustration blocking progress.**
- Refer to physical/occupational therapists, as indicated, **to identify assistive devices to facilitate independence in ADLs.**

Information in brackets added by the authors to clarify and enhance the use of nursing diagnoses.

• Identify suppliers for dressings/wound care items and assistive devices as needed.

• Consult dietitian for individual dietary plan **to meet increased nutritional needs that reflect personal situation/ resources.**

 • Evaluate home situation (e.g., lives alone, bedroom/bathroom on second floor, availability of assistance). **Identifies necessary adjustments, such as moving bedroom to first floor, arranging for commode during recovery, obtaining a Lifeline emergency call system.**

• Discuss alternative placement (e.g., convalescent/rehabilitation center, as appropriate).

• Identify community resources (e.g., visiting nurse, home healthcare agency, Meals on Wheels, respite care). **Facilitates adjustment to home setting.**

 • Recommend support group/self-help program for smoking cessation.

• Refer for counseling/support. **May need additional help to overcome feelings of discouragement, deal with changes in life.**

Documentation Focus

ASSESSMENT/REASSESSMENT

• Assessment findings, including individual concerns, family involvement, and support factors/availability of resources.
• Cultural expectations.
• Assistive device use/need.

PLANNING

• Plan of care and who is involved in planning.
• Teaching plan.

IMPLEMENTATION/EVALUATION

• Responses of client/SO(s) to plan/interventions/teaching and actions performed.
• Attainment/progress toward desired outcome(s).
• Modifications to plan of care.

DISCHARGE PLANNING

• Long-range needs and who is responsible for actions to be taken.
• Specific referrals made.

Information in brackets added by the authors to clarify and enhance the use of nursing diagnoses.

  Cultural Collaborative Community/Home Care

SAMPLE NURSING OUTCOMES & INTERVENTIONS CLASSIFICATIONS (NOC/NIC)

NOC—Self-Care: Activities of Daily Living (ADLs)
NIC—Self-Care Assistance

impaired Swallowing

Taxonomy II: Nutrition—Class 1 Ingestion (00103)
[Diagnostic Division: Food/Fluid]
Submitted 1986; Nursing Diagnosis Extension and
Classification (NDEC) Revision 1998

Definition: Abnormal functioning of the swallowing
mechanism associated with deficits in oral, pharyngeal,
or esophageal structure or function

Related Factors

CONGENITAL DEFICITS

Upper airway anomalies; mechanical obstruction (e.g., edema,
tracheostomy tube, tumor); history of tube feeding
Neuromuscular impairment (e.g., decreased or absent gag
reflex, decreased strength or excursion of muscles involved in
mastication, perceptual impairment, facial paralysis); conditions with significant hypotonia
Respiratory disorders; congenital heart disease
Behavioral feeding problems; self-injurious behavior
Failure to thrive; protein energy malnutrition

NEUROLOGICAL PROBLEMS

Nasal/nasopharyngeal cavity defects; oropharynx/upper airway/
laryngeal anomalies; tracheal/laryngeal/esophageal defects
Gastroesophageal reflux disease; achalasia
Traumas; acquired anatomic defects; cranial nerve involvement;
traumatic head injury; developmental delay; cerebral palsy
Prematurity

Defining Characteristics

SUBJECTIVE

Esophageal Phase Impairment
Complaints [reports] of "something stuck"; odynophagia
Food refusal; volume limiting

Information in brackets added by the authors to clarify and enhance
the use of nursing diagnoses.

 Diagnostic Studies 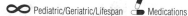 Pediatric/Geriatric/Lifespan Medications **675**

Heartburn; epigastric pain
Nighttime coughing/awakening

OBJECTIVE

Oral Phase Impairment
Weak suck resulting in inefficient nippling
Slow bolus formation; lack of tongue action to form bolus; premature entry of bolus
Incomplete lip closure; food pushed out of/falls from mouth
Lack of chewing
Coughing/choking/gagging before a swallow
Piecemeal deglutition; abnormality in oral phase of swallow study
Inability to clear oral cavity; pooling in lateral sulci; nasal reflux; sialorrhea; drooling
Long meals with little consumption

Pharyngeal Phase Impairment
Food refusal
Altered head positions; delayed/multiple swallows
Inadequate laryngeal elevation; abnormality in pharyngeal phase by swallow study
Choking; coughing; gagging; nasal reflux; gurgly voice quality
Unexplained fevers; recurrent pulmonary infections

Esophageal Phase Impairment
Observed evidence of difficulty in swallowing (e.g., stasis of food in oral cavity, coughing/choking); abnormality in esophageal phase by swallow study
Hyperextension of head (e.g., arching during or after meals)
Repetitive swallowing; bruxism
Unexplained irritability surrounding mealtime
Acidic smelling breath; regurgitation of gastric contents (wet burps); vomitus on pillow; vomiting; hematemesis

Desired Outcomes/Evaluation Criteria—Client Will:

• Pass food and fluid from mouth to stomach safely.
• Maintain adequate hydration as evidenced by good skin turgor, moist mucous membranes, and individually appropriate urine output.
• Achieve and/or maintain desired body weight.

Client/Caregiver Will:

• Verbalize understanding of causative/contributing factors.

Information in brackets added by the authors to clarify and enhance the use of nursing diagnoses.

  Cultural Collaborative Community/Home Care

- Identify individually appropriate interventions/actions to promote intake and prevent aspiration.
- Demonstrate feeding methods appropriate to the individual situation.
- Demonstrate emergency measures in the event of choking.

Actions/Interventions

NURSING PRIORITY NO. 1. To assess causative/contributing factors and degree of impairment:

- Assess sensory-perceptual status (sensory awareness, orientation, concentration, motor coordination).
- Note symmetry of facial structures/muscle tone.
- Assess strength and excursion of muscles involved in mastication and swallowing.
- Inspect oropharyngeal cavity for edema, inflammation, altered integrity of oral mucosa, adequacy of oral hygiene.
- Verify proper fit of dentures if present.
- Ascertain presence and strength of cough and gag reflex.
- Evaluate ability to swallow using small sips of water.
- Determine ability to initiate/sustain effective suck. **Weak suck results in inefficient nippling, suggesting ineffective movement of tongue and mouth muscles, impairing ability to swallow.**
- Note hyperextension of head/arching of neck during/after meals, or repetitive swallowing **suggesting inability to complete swallowing process**.
- Auscultate breath sounds **to evaluate the presence of aspiration.**
- Record current weight/recent changes.
- Prepare for/assist with diagnostic testing of swallowing activity.

NURSING PRIORITY NO. 2. To prevent aspiration and maintain airway patency:

- Identify individual factors that can precipitate aspiration/compromise airway.
- Move client to chair for meals, snacks, and drinks when possible; if client must be in bed, raise head of bed as upright as possible with head in anatomic alignment and slightly flexed forward during feeding. Keep HOB elevated for 30 to 45 minutes after feeding, if possible, **to reduce risk of regurgitation/aspiration**.
- Suction oral cavity prn. Teach client self-suction when appropriate. **Promotes airway safety and independence/sense of control with managing secretions.**

Information in brackets added by the authors to clarify and enhance the use of nursing diagnoses.

 Diagnostic Studies 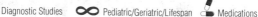 Pediatric/Geriatric/Lifespan Medications

NURSING PRIORITY NO. 3. To enhance swallowing ability to meet fluid and caloric body requirements:

- Refer to gastroenterologist/neurologist as indicated **for treatment/interventions (e.g., reconstructive facial surgery, esophageal dilatation, etc.) that may result in improved swallowing.)**
- Refer to speech therapist **to identify specific techniques to enhance client efforts/safety measures.**
- Encourage a rest period before meals **to minimize fatigue.**
- Provide analgesics prior to feeding, as indicated, **to enhance comfort, being cautious to avoid decreasing awareness/sensory perception.**
- Focus client's attention on feeding/swallowing activity. Decrease environmental stimuli and talking, **which may be distracting or promote choking during feeding.**
- Determine food preferences of client **to incorporate as possible, enhancing intake.** Present foods in an appealing, attractive manner.
- Ensure temperature (hot or cold versus tepid) of foods/fluid, **which will stimulate sensory receptors.**
- Provide a consistency of food/fluid that is most easily swallowed (can be formed into a bolus before swallowing), such as gelatin desserts prepared with less water than usual; pudding and custard; thickened liquids (addition of thickening agent, or yogurt, cream soups prepared with less water); thinned purees (hot cereal with water added); or thick drinks, such as nectars; fruit juices that have been frozen into "slush" consistency (**thin fluids are most difficult to control**); medium-soft boiled or scrambled eggs; canned fruit; soft-cooked vegetables. Avoid milk products and chocolate, **which may thicken oral secretions.**
- Feed one consistency and/or texture of food at a time.
- Place food in unaffected side of client's mouth (**when one side of the mouth is affected by condition, e.g., hemiplegia**), and have client use tongue to assist with moving food bolus to swallowing postion.
- Manage size of bites (e.g., **small bites of 1/2 tsp. or less are usually easier to swallow**). Use a teaspoon/small spoon **to encourage smaller bites**. Cut all solid foods into small pieces.
- Place food midway in oral cavity; provide medium-sized bites (about 15 mL) **to adequately trigger the swallowing reflex.**
- Provide cognitive cues (e.g., remind client to chew/swallow as indicated) **to enhance concentration and performance of swallowing sequence.**

Information in brackets added by the authors to clarify and enhance the use of nursing diagnoses.

       Cultural   Collaborative   Community/Home Care

- Instruct to chew food on unaffected side as appropriate.
- Massage the laryngopharyngeal musculature (sides of trachea and neck) gently **to stimulate swallowing.**
- Observe oral cavity after each bite and have client check around cheeks with tongue for remaining food. Remove food if unable to swallow.
- Incorporate client's eating style and pace when feeding **to avoid fatigue and frustration with process.**
- Allow ample time for eating (feeding).
- Remain with client during meal to reduce anxiety and offer assistance.
- Use a glass with a nose cutout **to avoid posterior head tilting while drinking.** Refrain from pouring liquid into the mouth or "washing food down" with liquid. Note: Some people find drinking from a straw easier than sipping from a cup (if a straw is easier, consider using a flexible one-way straw; if a cup is easier, consider using a "nosey" cup that is double handled and made of durable plastic).
- Monitor intake, output, and body weight to evaluate adequacy of fluid and caloric intake.
- Provide positive feedback for client's efforts.
- Provide oral hygiene following each feeding.
- Consider tube feedings/parenteral solutions, as indicated, **for the client unable to achieve adequate nutritional intake.**
- Consult with dysphagia specialist/rehabilitation team, as indicated.
- Refer to lactation counselor/support group (e.g., La Leche League) **for breastfeeding guidance.**
- Refer to NDs ineffective Breastfeeding; ineffective Infant Feeding Pattern for additional interventions for infants.

NURSING PRIORITY NO. 4. To promote wellness (Teaching/Discharge Considerations):

- Consult with dietitian **to establish optimum dietary plan.**
- Place medication in gelatin, jelly, or puddings. Consult with pharmacist **to determine if pills may be crushed or if liquids/capsules are available.**
- Assist client and/or SO(s) in learning specific feeding techniques and swallowing exercises.
- Encourage continuation of facial exercise program **to maintain/improve muscle strength.**
- Instruct client and/or SO(s) in emergency measures in event of choking.
- Establish routine schedule for monitoring weight.

Information in brackets added by the authors to clarify and enhance the use of nursing diagnoses.

• Refer to ND risk for imbalanced Nutrition: less than body requirements.

Documentation Focus

ASSESSMENT/REASSESSMENT

• Individual findings, including degree/characteristics of impairment, current weight/recent changes.
• Effects on lifestyle/socialization and nutritional status.

PLANNING

• Plan of care and who is involved in planning.
• Teaching plan.

IMPLEMENTATION/EVALUATION

• Response to interventions/teaching and actions performed.
• Attainment/progress toward desired outcome(s).
• Modifications to plan of care.

DISCHARGE PLANNING

• Long-term needs and who is responsible for actions to be taken.
• Available resources and specific referrals made.

SAMPLE NURSING OUTCOMES & INTERVENTIONS CLASSIFICATIONS (NOC/NIC)

NOC—Swallowing Status
NIC—Swallowing Therapy

effective Therapeutic Regimen Management

Taxonomy II: Health Promotion—Class 2 Health Management (00082)
[Diagnostic Division: Teaching/Learning]
Submitted 1994

Definition: Pattern of regulating and integrating into daily living a program for treatment of illness and its sequelae that is satisfactory for meeting specific health goals

Related Factors

To be developed [Complexity of healthcare management; therapeutic regimen]

Information in brackets added by the authors to clarify and enhance the use of nursing diagnoses.

  Cultural Collaborative Community/Home Care

[Added demands made on individual or family]
[Adequate social supports]

Defining Characteristics

SUBJECTIVE

Verbalizes desire to manage the treatment of illness/prevention of sequelae

Verbalizes intent to reduce risk factors for progression of illness and sequelae

OBJECTIVE

Appropriate choices of daily activities for meeting the goals of a treatment/prevention program

Illness symptoms within a normal range of expectation

Desired Outcomes/Evaluation Criteria—Individual Will:

- Develop plan to address individual risk factors for progression of illness/sequelae.
- Demonstrate effective problem solving in integration changes of therapeutic regimen into lifestyle.
- Identify/use available resources.
- Remain free of preventable complications/progression of illness and sequelae.

Actions/Interventions

NURSING PRIORITY NO. 1. To assess situation and individual needs:

- Ascertain client's knowledge/understanding of condition and treatment needs. Note specific health goals.
- Identify individual's perceptions of adaptation to treatment/anticipated changes.
- Note treatments added to present regimen and client's/SO's associated learning needs.
- Discuss present resources used by client **to note whether changes need to be arranged (e.g., increased hours of home care assistance; access to case manager to support complex/long-term program).**

NURSING PRIORITY NO. 2. To assist client/SO(s) in developing strategies to meet increased demands of therapeutic regimen:

- Identify steps necessary to reach desired health goal(s).

Information in brackets added by the authors to clarify and enhance the use of nursing diagnoses.

 Diagnostic Studies   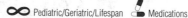 Pediatric/Geriatric/Lifespan   Medications   **681**

effective THERAPEUTIC REGIMEN MANAGEMENT

- Accept client's evaluation of own strengths/limitations while working together to improve abilities. **Promotes sense of self-esteem and confidence to continue efforts.**
- Provide information about individual healthcare needs, using client's/SO's preferred learning style (e.g., pictures, words, video, Internet) **to help client understand own situation and enhance interest/involvement in own health.** Note: When referencing the Internet or nontraditional/unproven resources, the individual must exercise some restraint and determine the reliability of the source/information provided before acting on it.
- Acknowledge individual efforts/capabilities **to reinforce movement toward attainment of desired outcomes.**

NURSING PRIORITY NO. 3. To promote wellness (Teaching/Discharge Considerations):

- Promote client/caregiver choices and involvement in planning and implementing added tasks/responsibilities.
- Provide for follow-up contact/home visit, as appropriate.
- Assist in implementing strategies for monitoring progress/responses to therapeutic regimen. **Promotes proactive problem solving.**
- Refer to family/community support systems, as indicated, **for assistance with lifestyle/relationship issues, finances, housing, or legal concerns (e.g., advance directives, healthcare choices).**

Documentation Focus

ASSESSMENT/REASSESSMENT

- Findings, including dynamics of individual situation.
- Individual strengths/additional needs.

PLANNING

- Plan of care and who is involved in planning.
- Teaching plan.

IMPLEMENTATION/EVALUATION

- Response to interventions/teaching and actions performed.
- Attainment/progress toward desired outcome(s).
- Modifications to plan of care.

DISCHARGE PLANNING

- Short-range and long-range needs and who is responsible for actions.
- Available resources, specific referrals made.

Information in brackets added by the authors to clarify and enhance the use of nursing diagnoses.

     Cultural   Collaborative   🏠 Community/Home Care

SAMPLE NURSING OUTCOMES & INTERVENTIONS CLASSIFICATIONS (NOC/NIC)

NOC—Symptom Control
NIC—Health System Guidance

ineffective Therapeutic Regimen Management

Taxonomy II: Health Promotion—Class 2 Health
 Management (00078)
[Diagnostic Division: Teaching/Learning]
Submitted 1992

Definition: Pattern of regulating and integrating into daily living a program for treatment of illness and the sequelae of illness that is unsatisfactory for meeting specific health goals

Related Factors

Complexity of healthcare system/therapeutic regimen
Decisional conflicts
Economic difficulties
Excessive demands made (e.g., individual or family); family conflict
Family patterns of healthcare
Inadequate number and types of cues to action
Knowledge deficits
Mistrust of regimen/healthcare personnel
Perceived seriousness/susceptibility/barriers/benefits
Powerlessness
Social support deficits

Defining Characteristics

SUBJECTIVE

Verbalizes desire to manage the illness
Verbalizes difficulty with prescribed regimen

OBJECTIVE

Failure to include treatment regimens in daily routines/take action to reduce risk factors
Makes choices in daily living ineffective for meeting the health goals
[Unexpected acceleration of illness symptoms]

Information in brackets added by the authors to clarify and enhance the use of nursing diagnoses.

 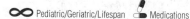

Desired Outcomes/Evaluation Criteria—Client Will:

- Verbalize acceptance of need/desire to change actions to achieve agreed-on health goals.
- Verbalize understanding of factors/blocks involved in individual situation.
- Participate in problem solving of factors interfering with integration of therapeutic regimen.
- Demonstrate behaviors/changes in lifestyle necessary to maintain therapeutic regimen.
- Identify/use available resources.

Actions/Interventions

NURSING PRIORITY NO. 1. To identify causative/contributing factors:

- Ascertain client's knowledge/understanding of condition and treatment needs **so that he or she can make informed decisions about managing self-care**.
- Determine client's/family's health goals and patterns of healthcare.
- Identify cultural values/religious beliefs affecting client's view of situation and willingness to make necessary changes.
- Identify client locus of control: internal (expressions of responsibility for self and ability to control outcomes "I didn't quit smoking") or external (expressions of lack of control over self and environment "Nothing ever works out"; "What bad luck to get lung cancer").
- Identify individual perceptions and expectations of treatment regimen.
- Review complexity of treatment regimen (e.g., number of expected tasks, such as taking medication four times/day or once/day) and evaluate how difficult tasks might be for client (e.g., must stop smoking; or must follow strict dialysis diet even when feeling well, etc.). **These factors are often involved in lack of participation in treatment plan.**
- Note availability/use of resources for assistance, caregiving/respite care.

NURSING PRIORITY NO. 2. To assist client/SO(s) to develop strategies to improve management of therapeutic regimen:

- Use therapeutic communication skills **to assist client to problem solve solution(s).**
- Explore client involvement in or lack of mutual goal setting.

Information in brackets added by the authors to clarify and enhance the use of nursing diagnoses.

    Cultural   Collaborative   Community/Home Care

- Use client's locus of control to develop individual plan to adapt regimen (e.g., for client with internal control, encourage client to take control of own care and for those with external control, begin with small tasks and add, as tolerated).
- Identify steps necessary to reach desired goal(s).
- Contract with the client for participation in care.
- Accept client's evaluation of own strengths/limitations while working together to improve abilities. State belief in client's ability to cope and/or adapt to situation.
- Provide positive reinforcement for efforts **to encourage continuation of desired behaviors.**
- Provide information/encourage client to seek out resources on own. Reinforce previous instructions and rationale, using a variety of learning modalities, including role playing, demonstration, written materials, and so forth.

NURSING PRIORITY NO. 3. To promote wellness (Teaching/Discharge Considerations):

- Emphasize importance of client knowledge and understanding of the need for treatment/medication as well as consequences of actions/choices.
- Promote client/caregiver/SO(s) participation in planning and evaluating process. **Enhances commitment to plan, optimizing outcomes.**
- Assist client to develop strategies for monitoring therapeutic regimen. **Promotes early recognition of changes, allowing proactive response.**
- Mobilize support systems, including family/SO(s), social, financial, and so forth.
- Refer to counseling/therapy (group and individual), as indicated.
- Identify home- and community-based nursing services **for assessment, follow-up care, and education in client's home.**

Documentation Focus

ASSESSMENT/REASSESSMENT

- Findings, including underlying dynamics of individual situation, client's perception of problem/needs, locus of control.
- Cultural values, religious beliefs.
- Family involvement/needs.
- Individual strengths/limitations.
- Availability/use of resources.

Information in brackets added by the authors to clarify and enhance the use of nursing diagnoses.

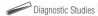
ineffective THERAPEUTIC REGIMEN MANAGEMENT

PLANNING

- Plan of care and who is involved in planning.
- Teaching plan.

IMPLEMENTATION/EVALUATION

- Response to interventions/teaching and actions performed.
- Attainment/progress toward desired outcome(s).
- Modifications to plan of care.

DISCHARGE PLANNING

- Long-range needs and who is responsible for actions to be taken.
- Available resources, specific referrals made.

SAMPLE NURSING OUTCOMES & INTERVENTIONS CLASSIFICATIONS (NOC/NIC)

NOC—Treatment Behavior: Illness or Injury
NIC—Self-Modification Assistance

---

ineffective community Therapeutic Regimen Management

Taxonomy II: Health Promotion—Class 2 Health Management (0081)
[Diagnostic Division: Teaching/Learning]
Submitted 1994

Definition: Pattern of regulating and integrating into community processes programs for treatment of illness and the sequelae of illness that are unsatisfactory for meeting health-related goals

---

Related Factors

To be developed
[Lack of safety for community members]
[Economic insecurity]
[Healthcare not available; unhealthy environment]
[Education not available for all community members]
[Lack of means to meet human needs for recognition, fellowship, security, and membership]

Defining Characteristics

SUBJECTIVE

[Community members/agencies verbalize overburdening of resources/inability to meet therapeutic needs of all members]

Information in brackets added by the authors to clarify and enhance the use of nursing diagnoses.

 Cultural Collaborative Community/Home Care

Deficits in advocates for aggregates

Deficit in community activities for prevention

Illness symptoms above the norm expected for the population; unexpected acceleration of illness

Insufficient healthcare resources (e.g., people, programs); unavailable healthcare resources for illness care

[Deficits in community for collaboration and development of coalitions to address needs]

Desired Outcomes/Evaluation Criteria—Community Will:

- Identify both strengths and limitations affecting community treatment programs for meeting health-related goals.
- Participate in problem solving of factors interfering with regulating and integrating community programs.
- Report unexpected acceleration/illness symptoms near norm expected for the incidence or prevalence of disease(s).

Actions/Interventions

NURSING PRIORITY NO. 1. To identify causative/precipitating factors:

- Evaluate community healthcare resources for illness/sequelae of illness.
- Note reports from members of the community regarding ineffective/inadequate community functioning.
- Investigate unexpected acceleration of illness in the community.
- Identify strengths/limitations of community resources and community commitment to change.
- Ascertain effect of related factors on community activities.
- Determine knowledge/understanding of treatment regimen.
- Note use of resources available to community for developing/funding programs.

NURSING PRIORITY NO. 2. To assist community to develop strategies to improve community functioning/management:

- Foster cooperative spirit of community without negating individuality of members/groups.
- Involve community in determining and prioritizing healthcare goals **to facilitate planning process.**
- Plan together with community health and social agencies **to problem solve solutions to identified and anticipated problems/needs.**
- Identify specific populations at risk or underserved **to actively involve them in process.**

Information in brackets added by the authors to clarify and enhance the use of nursing diagnoses.

ineffective community THERAPEUTIC REGIMEN MANAGEMENT

• Create teaching plan/form speakers' bureau **to disseminate information to community members regarding value of treatment/preventive programs.**

NURSING PRIORITY NO. 3. To promote wellness (Teaching/Discharge Considerations):

 • Assist community to develop a plan for continuing assessment of community needs/functioning and effectiveness of plan. **Promotes proactive approach.**

 • Encourage community to form partnerships within the community and between the community and the larger society **to aid in long-term planning for anticipated/projected needs and concerns.**

Documentation Focus

ASSESSMENT/REASSESSMENT

- Assessment findings, including members' perceptions of community problems, healthcare resources.
- Community use of available resources.

PLANNING

- Plan of care and who is involved in planning.
- Teaching plan.

IMPLEMENTATION/EVALUATION

- Community's response to plan/interventions and actions performed.
- Attainment/progress toward desired outcome(s).
- Modifications to plan of care.

DISCHARGE PLANNING

- Long-range goals and who is responsible for actions to be taken.
- Specific referrals made.

SAMPLE NURSING OUTCOMES & INTERVENTIONS CLASSIFICATIONS (NOC/NIC)

NOC—Community Competence
NIC—Community Health Development

Information in brackets added by the authors to clarify and enhance the use of nursing diagnoses.

  Cultural Collaborative 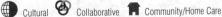 Community/Home Care

ineffective family Therapeutic Regimen Management

Taxonomy II: Health Promotion—Class 2 Health Management (00080)
[Diagnostic Division: Teaching/Learning]
Submitted 1994

Definition: Pattern of regulating and integrating into family processes a program for treatment of illness and the sequelae of illness that is unsatisfactory for meeting specific health goals

Related Factors

Complexity of therapeutic regimen/healthcare system
Decisional conflicts
Economic difficulties
Excessive demands; family conflicts

Defining Characteristics

SUBJECTIVE

Verbalizes difficulty with therapeutic regimen
Verbalizes desire to manage the illness

OBJECTIVE

Inappropriate family activities for meeting health goals
Acceleration of illness symptoms of a family member
Failure to take action to reduce risk factors; lack of attention to illness

Desired Outcomes/Evaluation Criteria—Family Will:

- Identify individual factors affecting regulation/integration of treatment program.
- Participate in problem solving of factors.
- Verbalize acceptance of need/desire to change actions to achieve agreed-on outcomes or health goals.
- Demonstrate behaviors/changes in lifestyle necessary to maintain therapeutic regimen.

Information in brackets added by the authors to clarify and enhance the use of nursing diagnoses.

 Diagnostic Studies   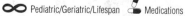 Pediatric/Geriatric/Lifespan   Medications   **689**

Actions/Interventions

NURSING PRIORITY NO. 1. To identify causative/precipitating factors:

 • Ascertain family's perception of efforts to date.

 • Evaluate family functioning/activities as related to appropriateness—looking at frequency/effectiveness of family communication, promotion of autonomy, adaptation to meet changing needs, health of home environment/lifestyle, problem-solving abilities, ties to community.

 • Note family health goals and agreement of individual members. **Presence of conflict interferes with problem solving.**

 • Determine understanding of and value of the treatment regimen to the family.

 • Identify cultural values/religious beliefs affecting view of situation and willingness to make necessary changes.

 • Identify availability and use of resources.

NURSING PRIORITY NO. 2. To assist family to develop strategies to improve management of therapeutic regimen:

 • Provide information to aid family **in understanding the value of the treatment program.**

 • Assist family members to recognize inappropriate family activities. Help the members identify both togetherness and individual needs and behavior **so that effective interactions can be enhanced and perpetuated.**

 • Make a plan jointly with family members to deal with complexity of healthcare regimen/system and other related factors. **Enhances commitment to plan, optimizing outcomes.**

 • Identify community resources, as needed, using the three strategies of education, problem solving, and resource linking **to address specific deficits.**

NURSING PRIORITY NO. 3. To promote wellness as related to future health of family members:

 • Help family identify criteria to promote ongoing self-evaluation of situation/effectiveness and family progress. **Provides opportunity to be proactive in meeting needs.**

 • Make referrals to and/or jointly plan with other health/social and community resources. **Problems often are multifaceted, requiring involvement of numerous providers/agencies.**

 • Provide contact person/case manager for one-to-one assistance, as needed, **to coordinate care, provide support, assist with problem solving, etc.**

• Refer to NDs Caregiver Role Strain; ineffective Therapeutic Regimen Management, as indicated.

Information in brackets added by the authors to clarify and enhance the use of nursing diagnoses.

   Cultural   Collaborative   Community/Home Care

Documentation Focus

ASSESSMENT/REASSESSMENT

- Individual findings, including nature of problem/degree of impairment, family values/health goals, and level of participation and commitment of family members.
- Cultural values, religious beliefs.
- Availability and use of resources.

PLANNING

- Plan of care and who is involved in planning.
- Teaching plan.

IMPLEMENTATION/EVALUATION

- Response to interventions/teaching and actions performed.
- Attainment/progress toward desired outcome(s).
- Modifications of plan of care.

DISCHARGE PLANNING

- Long-term needs, plan for meeting, and who is responsible for actions.
- Specific referrals made.

SAMPLE NURSING OUTCOMES & INTERVENTIONS CLASSIFICATIONS (NOC/NIC)

NOC—Family Participation in Professional Care
NIC—Family Involvement Promotion

readiness for enhanced Therapeutic Regimen Management

Taxonomy II: Health Promotion—Class 2 Health Management (00162)
[Diagnostic Division: Teaching/Learning]
Submitted 2002

Definition: A pattern of regulating and integrating into daily living a program for treatment of illness and its sequelae that is sufficient for meeting health-related goals and can be strengthened

Related Factors

To be developed

Information in brackets added by the authors to clarify and enhance the use of nursing diagnoses.

 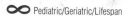

Defining Characteristics

SUBJECTIVE

Expresses desire to manage the illness (e.g., treatment, prevention)
Expresses little difficulty with prescribed regimens
Describes reduction of risk factors

OBJECTIVE

Choices of daily living are appropriate for meeting goals (e.g., treatment, prevention)
No unexpected acceleration of illness symptoms

Desired Outcomes/Evaluation Criteria—Client Will:

- Assume responsibility for managing treatment regimen.
- Demonstrate proactive management by anticipating and planning for eventualities of condition/potential complications.
- Identify/use additional resources as appropriate.
- Remain free of preventable complications/progression of illness and sequelae.

Actions/Interventions

NURSING PRIORITY NO. **1.** To determine motivation for continued growth:

 • Verify client's level of knowledge/understanding of therapeutic regimen. Note specific health goals. **Provides opportunity to assure accuracy and completeness of knowledge base for future learning.**

 • Identify individual's expectations of long-term treatment needs/anticipated changes.

 • Discuss present resources used by client **to note whether changes can be arranged (e.g., increased hours of home care assistance; access to case manager to support complex/long-term program).**

NURSING PRIORITY NO. **2.** To assist client/SO(s) to develop plan to meet individual needs:

 • Identify steps necessary to reach desired health goal(s). **Understanding the process enhances commitment and the likelihood of achieving the goals.**

 • Accept client's evaluation of own strengths/limitations while working together to improve abilities. **Promotes sense of self-esteem and confidence to continue efforts.**

Information in brackets added by the authors to clarify and enhance the use of nursing diagnoses.

  Cultural Collaborative Community/Home Care

- Incorporate client's cultural values/religious beliefs that support attainment of health goals.
- Provide information/bibliotherapy. Help client/SO(s) identify and evaluate resources they can access on their own. **When referencing the Internet or nontraditional/unproven resources, the individual must exercise some restraint and determine the reliability of the source/information provided before acting on it.**
- Acknowledge individual efforts/capabilities to reinforce movement toward attainment of desired outcomes. **Provides positive reinforcement encouraging continued progress toward desired goals.**

NURSING PRIORITY NO. 3. To promote optimum wellness:

- Promote client/caregiver choices and involvement in planning for and implementing added tasks/responsibilities.
- Assist in implementing strategies for monitoring progress/responses to therapeutic regimen. **Promotes proactive problem solving.**
- Identify additional community resources/support groups. **Provides further opportunities for role modeling, skill training, anticipatory problem solving, etc.**

Documentation Focus

ASSESSMENT/REASSESSMENT

- Findings, including dynamics of individual situation.
- Individual strengths/additional needs.
- Cultural values, religious beliefs.

PLANNING

- Plan of care and who is involved in planning.
- Teaching plan.

IMPLEMENTATION/EVALUATION

- Response to interventions/teaching and actions performed.
- Attainment/progress toward desired outcome(s).
- Modifications to plan of care.

DISCHARGE PLANNING

- Short-range and long-range needs and who is responsible for actions.
- Available resources, specific referrals made.

Information in brackets added by the authors to clarify and enhance the use of nursing diagnoses.

SAMPLE NURSING OUTCOMES & INTERVENTIONS CLASSIFICATIONS (NOC/NIC)

NOC—Symptom Control
NIC—Health System Guidance

ineffective Thermoregulation

Taxonomy II: Safety/Protection—Class 6 Thermoregulation (00008)
[Diagnostic Division: Safety]
Submitted 1986

Definition: Temperature fluctuation between hypothermia and hyperthermia

Related Factors

Trauma; illness [e.g., cerebral edema, CVA, intracranial surgery, or head injury]
Immaturity; aging [e.g., loss/absence of brown adipose tissue]
Fluctuating environmental temperature
[Changes in hypothalamic tissue causing alterations in emission of thermosensitive cells and regulation of heat loss/production]
[Changes in metabolic rate/activity; changes in level/action of thyroxine and catecholamines]
[Chemical reactions in contracting muscles]

Defining Characteristics

OBJECTIVE

Fluctuations in body temperature above and below the normal range
Tachycardia
Reduction in body temperature below normal range; cool skin; moderate pallor; mild shivering; piloerection; cyanotic nailbeds; slow capillary refill; hypertension
Warm to touch; flushed skin; increased respiratory rate; seizures

Desired Outcomes/Evaluation Criteria—Client/Caregiver Will:

- Verbalize understanding of individual factors and appropriate interventions.
- Demonstrate techniques/behaviors to correct underlying condition/situation.
- Maintain body temperature within normal limits.

Information in brackets added by the authors to clarify and enhance the use of nursing diagnoses.

 Cultural Collaborative 🏠 Community/Home Care

Actions/Interventions

NURSING PRIORITY NO. 1. To identify causative/contributing factors:
- Identify individual factor(s)/underlying condition (e.g., environmental exposure, infectious process, brain injury, effects of drugs/toxins, salt or water depletion, obesity, confined to bed, drug overdose, etc.). **Influences choice of interventions.**

- Note extremes of age (e.g., premature neonate, young child, or aging adult) **as this can directly impact ability to maintain/regulate body temperature.**
- Monitor laboratory studies (e.g., tests indicative of infection, thyroid/other endocrine tests, organ damage, drug screens).

NURSING PRIORITY NO. 2. To assist with measures to correct/treat underlying cause:

- Initate emergent and/or immediate interventions **to restore/ maintain body temperature within normal range,** as indicated in NDs Hypothermia; Hyperthermia; risk for imbalanced Body Temperature.
- Administer fluids, electrolytes, and medications, as appropriate, **to restore or maintain body/organ function.**
- Prepare client for/assist with procedures (e.g., surgical intervention or administering neoplastic agents, antibiotics) **to treat underlying cause of hypothermia or hyperthermia.**

NURSING PRIORITY NO. 3. To promote wellness (Teaching/Discharge Considerations):

- Review causative/related factors and risk factors, if appropriate, with client/SO(s).
- Provide information concerning disease processes, current therapies, and post-discharge precautions, as appropriate to situation.
- Refer to teaching section in NDs Hypothermia; Hyperthermia.

Documentation Focus

ASSESSMENT/REASSESSMENT

- Individual findings, including nature of problem, degree of impairment/fluctuations in temperature.

PLANNING

- Plan of care and who is involved in planning.
- Teaching plan.

IMPLEMENTATION/EVALUATION

- Responses to interventions/teaching actions performed.

Information in brackets added by the authors to clarify and enhance the use of nursing diagnoses.

 Diagnostic Studies   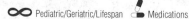 Pediatric/Geriatric/Lifespan   Medications   **695**

ineffective THERMOREGULATION

- Attainment/progress toward desired outcome(s).
- Modifications to plan of care.

DISCHARGE PLANNING

- Long-term needs and who is responsible for actions to be taken.
- Specific referrals made.

SAMPLE NURSING OUTCOMES & INTERVENTIONS CLASSIFICATIONS (NOC/NIC)

NOC—Thermoregulation
NIC—Temperature Regulation

disturbed Thought Processes

Taxonomy II: Perception/Cognition—Class 4 Cognition (00130)
[Diagnostic Division: Neurosensory]
Submitted 1973; Revised 1996

Definition: Disruption in cognitive operations and activities

Related Factors

To be developed
[Physiological changes, aging, hypoxia, head injury, malnutrition, infections]
[Biochemical changes, medications, substance abuse]
[Sleep deprivation]
[Psychological conflicts, emotional changes, mental disorders]

Defining Characteristics

SUBJECTIVE

[Ideas of reference, hallucinations, delusions]

OBJECTIVE

Inaccurate interpretation of environment
Inappropriate thinking; egocentricity
Memory deficit; [confabulation]
Hypervigilance; hypovigilance
Cognitive dissonance [decreased ability to grasp ideas, make decisions, problem solve, use abstract reasoning or conceptualize, calculate; disordered thought sequencing]

Information in brackets added by the authors to clarify and enhance the use of nursing diagnoses.

   Cultural   Collaborative Community/Home Care

Distractibility; [altered attention span]
[Inappropriate social behavior]

Desired Outcomes/Evaluation Criteria—Client Will:

- Recognize changes in thinking/behavior.
- Verbalize understanding of causative factors when known/able.
- Identify interventions to deal effectively with situation.
- Demonstrate behaviors/lifestyle changes to prevent/minimize changes in mentation.
- Maintain usual reality orientation.

Actions/Interventions

NURSING PRIORITY NO. 1. To assess causative/contributing factors:

- Identify factors present; for example, acute/chronic brain syndrome (recent stroke/Alzheimer's disease); brain injury/increased intracranial pressure; anoxic event; acute infections, especially in elderly; malnutrition; sleep or sensory deprivation; chronic mental illness, such as schizophrenia.
- Determine alcohol/other drug use (prescription/OTC/illicit). **Drugs can have direct effects on the brain, or have side effects, dose-related effects, and/or cumulative effects that alter thought patterns and sensory perception.**
- Note schedule of drug administration (**may be significant when evaluating cumulative effects/drug interactions**).
- Assess dietary intake/nutritional status.
- Monitor laboratory values for abnormalities, such as metabolic alkalosis, hypokalemia, anemia, elevated ammonia levels, and signs of infection.

NURSING PRIORITY NO. 2. To assess degree of impairment:

- Assist with testing/review results evaluating mental status according to age and developmental capacity, noting extent of impairment in thinking ability, memory (remote/recent), orientation to person/place/time, insight and judgment.
- Assess attention span/distractibility and ability to make decisions or problem solve. **Determines ability to participate in planning/executing care.**
- Test ability to receive, send, and appropriately interpret communications.
- Note behavior such as untidy personal habits, slowing and/or slurring of speech.

Information in brackets added by the authors to clarify and enhance the use of nursing diagnoses.

disturbed THOUGHT PROCESSES

- Note occurrence of paranoia and delusions, hallucinations.
- Interview SO(s)/caregiver(s) to determine client's usual thinking ability, changes in behavior, length of time problem has existed, and other pertinent information **to provide baseline for comparison.**
- Determine client's anxiety level in relation to situation.
- Assist with in-depth testing of specific cognitive abilities/ executive brain functions, as appropriate.

NURSING PRIORITY NO. 3. To prevent further deterioration, maximize level of function:

- Assist with treatment for underlying problems, such as anorexia, brain injury/increased intracranial pressure, sleep disorders, biochemical imbalances. **Cognition/thinking often improves with treatment/correction of medical/psychiatric problems.**
- Establish alternate means for self-expression if unable to communicate verbally. (Refer to ND impaired verbal Communication for related interventions.)
- Monitor and document vital signs periodically, as appropriate.
- Perform periodic neurological/behavioral assessments, as indicated, and compare with baseline. Note changes in level of consciousness and cognition (e.g., increased lethargy, confusion, drowsiness, irritability; changes in ability to communicate and/or appropriateness of thinking and behavior). **Early recognition of changes promotes proactive modifications to plan of care.**
- Reorient to time/place/person, as needed. **Inability to maintain orientation is a sign of deterioration.**
- Have client write name periodically; keep this record for comparison and report differences.
- Note behavior that may be indicative of potential for violence and take appropriate actions. (Refer to NDs risk for self- or other-directed Violence.)
- Provide safety measures (e.g., side rails, padding, as necessary; close supervision, seizure precautions), as indicated.
- Schedule structured activity and rest periods. **Provides stimulation while reducing fatigue.**
- Monitor medication regimen. Verify that physician is aware of all medications client is taking, noting possible interactions/ cumulative effects.
- Encourage family/SO(s) to participate in reorientation and provide ongoing input (e.g., current news and family happenings).
- Refer to appropriate rehabilitation providers (e.g., cognitive retraining program, speech therapist, psychosocial resources, biofeedback, counselor).

Information in brackets added by the authors to clarify and enhance the use of nursing diagnoses.

  Cultural Collaborative Community/Home Care

NURSING PRIORITY NO. 4. To create therapeutic milieu and assist client/SO(s) to develop coping strategies—especially when condition is irreversible:

- Provide opportunities for SO(s)/caregivers(s) to ask questions and obtain information.
- Maintain a pleasant, quiet environment and approach client in a slow, calm manner. **Client may respond with anxious or aggressive behaviors if startled or overstimulated.**
- Give simple directions, using short words and simple sentences.
- Listen with regard **to convey interest and worth to individual.**
- Allow ample time for client to respond to questions/comments and make simple decisions.
- Maintain reality-oriented relationship and environment (clocks, calendars, personal items, seasonal decorations).
- Present reality concisely and briefly and do not challenge illogical thinking—**defensive reactions may result.**
- Reduce provocative stimuli, negative criticism, arguments, and confrontations **to avoid triggering fight/flight responses.**
- Refrain from forcing activities and communications. **Client may feel threatened and may withdraw or rebel.**
- Respect individuality and personal space.
- Use touch judiciously, respecting personal needs/cultural beliefs, but keeping in mind physical and psychological importance of touch.
- Provide for nutritionally well-balanced diet, incorporating client's preferences as able. Encourage client to eat. Provide pleasant environment and allow sufficient time to eat. **Enhances intake and general well-being.**
- Assist client/SO(s) with grieving process for loss of self/abilities, as in Alzheimer's disease.
- Encourage participation in resocialization activities/groups when available.

NURSING PRIORITY NO. 5. To promote wellness (Teaching/Discharge Considerations):

- Assist in identifying ongoing treatment needs/rehabilitation program for the individual **to maintain gains and continue progress if able.**
- Emphasize importance of cooperation with therapeutic regimen.
- Promote socialization within individual limitations.
- Identify problems related to aging that are remediable and assist client/SO(s) to seek appropriate assistance/access resources. **Encourages problem solving to improve condition rather than accept the status quo.**

Information in brackets added by the authors to clarify and enhance the use of nursing diagnoses.

 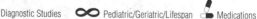

- Help client/SO(s) develop plan of care when problem is progressive/long term. **Advance planning addressing home care, transportation, assistance with care activities, support and respite for caregivers, enhances management of client in home setting.** (Refer to ND Caregiver Role Strain for related interventions.)
- Refer to community resources (e.g., day-care programs, support groups, drug/alcohol rehabilitation, mental health treatment programs).
- Refer to NDs acute Confusion; chronic Confusion; impaired Environmental Interpretation Syndrome; impaired Memory; Self-Care Deficit; Grieving; disturbed Sensory Perception, as appropriate, for additional interventions.

Documentation Focus

ASSESSMENT/REASSESSMENT

- Individual findings, including nature of problem, current and previous level of function, effect on independence and lifestyle.
- Results of tests/diagnostic studies, and mental status/cognitive evaluations.
- SO/family support and participation.
- Availability/use of resources.

PLANNING

- Plan of care and who is involved in planning.
- Teaching plan.

IMPLEMENTATION/EVALUATION

- Response to interventions/teaching and actions performed.
- Attainment/progress toward desired outcome(s).
- Modifications to plan of care.

DISCHARGE PLANNING

- Long-term needs/referrals and who is responsible for actions to be taken.
- Available resources, specific referrals made.

SAMPLE NURSING OUTCOMES & INTERVENTIONS CLASSIFICATIONS (NOC/NIC)

NOC—Distorted Thought Control
NIC—Dementia Management

Information in brackets added by the authors to clarify and enhance the use of nursing diagnoses.

 Cultural Collaborative Community/Home Care

impaired Tissue Integrity

Taxonomy II: Safety/Protection—Class 2 Physical Injury
   (00044)
[Diagnostic Division: Safety]
Submitted 1986; Revised 1998 (by small group work
   1996)

Definition: Damage to mucous membrane, corneal,
integumentary, or subcutaneous tissues

Related Factors

Altered circulation
Nutritional factors (e.g., deficit or excess); [metabolic/endocrine
   dysfunction]
Fluid deficit/excess
Impaired physical mobility
Chemical irritants [including body excretions, secretions,
   medications]; radiation [including therapeutic radiation]
Temperature extremes
Mechanical (e.g., pressure, shear, friction); [surgery]
Knowledge deficit
[Infection]

Defining Characteristics

OBJECTIVE

Damaged tissue (e.g., cornea, mucous membrane, integumentary, subcutaneous)
Destroyed tissue

Desired Outcomes/Evaluation
Criteria—Client Will:

• Verbalize understanding of condition and causative factors.
• Identify interventions appropriate for specific condition.
• Demonstrate behaviors/lifestyle changes to promote healing
  and prevent complications/recurrence.
• Display progressive improvement in wound/lesion healing.

Actions/Interventions

NURSING PRIORITY NO. 1. To identify causative/contributing factors:

• Identify underlying condition/pathology involved in tissue
  injury (e.g., diabetic neuropathies; peripheral arterial disorders;
  sensory/perceptual deficits; cognitively impaired/debilitated

   Information in brackets added by the authors to clarify and enhance
the use of nursing diagnoses.

 Diagnostic Studies   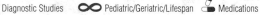 Pediatric/Geriatric/Lifespan   Medications   **701** elderly; emotional/psychological problems; developmental delay; surgery/traumatic injuries; debilitating illness; long-term immobility). **Suggests treatment options, desire/ability to protect self, and potential for recurrence of tissue damage**.

- Identify specific behaviors, such as occupational/sports hazards or toxic exposures; lifestyle choices (e.g., unsafe sex practices); or need for/use of restraints or prosthetic devices (e.g., limbs, artificial eye, contact lenses, dentures, artificial airway, indwelling catheter).

- Note poor hygiene/health practices (e.g., lack of cleanliness, frequent use of enemas, poor dental care) **that may be impacting tissue health.**

- Determine nutritional status/impact of malnutrition on situation (e.g., pressure points on emaciated and/or elderly client, obesity, lack of activity, slow healing/failure to heal).

- Assess environmental location of home/work as well as recent travel. **Some areas of a country or city may be more susceptible to certain disease conditions/environmental pollutants.**

- Note race/ethnic background, familial history for genetic/sociocultural/religious factors **that may make individual vulnerable to particular condition or impact treatment.**

- Note evidence of deep organ/tissue involvement in client with wound **(e.g., draining fistula through the integumentary and subcutaneous tissue may involve a bone infection).**

- Assess blood supply and sensation (nerve damage) of affected area. Evaluate pulses/calculate ankle-brachial index **to evaluate actual/potential for impairment of circulation to lower extremities. Result less than 0.9 indicates need for close monitoring/more aggressive intervention (e.g., tighter blood glucose and weight control in diabetic client).**

- Obtain specimens of exudate/lesions for Gram's stain, culture/sensitivity, etc., when appropriate.

NURSING PRIORITY NO. 2. To assess degree of impairment:

- Obtain a history of condition (e.g., pressure, venous, or diabetic wound; eye or oral lesions, etc.), including whether condition is acute or recurrent; original site/characteristics of wound; duration of problem and changes that have occurred over time.

- Assess skin/tissues, bony prominences, pressure areas and wounds **for comparative baseline**:
  Note color, texture, and turgor.
  Assess areas of least pigmentation for color changes (e.g., sclera, conjunctiva, nailbeds, buccal mucosa, tongue, palms, and soles of feet).
  Note presence, location, and degree of edema (e.g., 4+ pitting).

Information in brackets added by the authors to clarify and enhance the use of nursing diagnoses.

 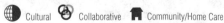

Record size (depth, width), color, location, temperature, texture of wounds/lesions.

Determine degree/depth of injury/damage to integumentary system (involves epidermis, dermis, and/or underlying tissues), extent of tunneling/undermining, if present. Note: Full extent of lesions of mucous membranes or subcutaneous tissue may not be discernible.

Identify stage of ulcers/wound (I-IV) and classify burns using appropriate measuring tool.

Document with drawings and/or photograph wound/lesion(s)/burns, as appropriate.

Observe for other distinguishing characteristics of surrounding tissue (e.g., exudate; granulation; cyanosis/pallor; tight, shiny skin).

Describe wound drainage (e.g., amount, color/odor).

- Assist with diagnostic procedures (e.g., x-rays, imaging scans, biopsies, debridement). **May be necessary to determine extent of impairment.**
- Determine psychological effects of condition on client/SO(s). **Can be devastating for client's body/self-image and esteem, especially if condition is severe/disfiguring or chronic, as well as costly and burdensome for SO(s)/caregiver.**

NURSING PRIORITY NO. 3. To assist client to correct/minimize impairment and to promote healing:

- Modify/eliminate factors contributing to condition, if possible. Assist with treatment of underlying condition(s), as appropriate.
- Inspect lesions/wounds daily, or as appropriate, for changes (e.g., signs of infection/complications or healing). **Promotes timely intervention/revision of plan of care.**
- Promote optimum nutrition with high-quality protein and sufficient calories, vitamins, and mineral supplements **to facilitate healing.**
- Encourage adequate periods of rest and sleep **to limit metabolic demands, maximize energy available for healing, and meet comfort needs.**
- Limit/avoid use of caffeine/alcohol and medications affecting REM sleep.
- Provide/assist with oral care (e.g., teaching oral/dental hygiene, avoiding extremes of hot or cold, changing position of ET/NG tubes, lubricating lips, etc.) **to prevent damage to mucous membranes.**
- Promote early mobility. Assist with/encourage position changes, active/passive and assistive exercises **to promote circulation and prevent excessive tissue pressure.**

Information in brackets added by the authors to clarify and enhance the use of nursing diagnoses.

 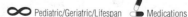

- Provide appropriate protective and healing devices (e.g., eye pads/goggles, heel protectors, padding/cushions, therapeutic beds and mattresses, splints, chronic ulcer dressings, compression wrap, etc.).
- Practice aseptic technique for cleansing/dressing/medicating lesions. **Reduces risk of cross-contamination.**
- Monitor laboratory studies (e.g., CBC, electrolytes, glucose, cultures) **for changes indicative of healing or infection/ complications.**
- Protect client from environmental hazards when vision/ hearing or cognitive deficits impact safety.
- Advise smoking cessation/refer for resources, if indicated. **Smoking causes vasoconstriction/interferes with healing.**

NURSING PRIORITY NO. 4. To promote wellness (Teaching/Discharge Considerations):

- Encourage verbalizations of feelings and expectations regarding condition and potential for recovery of structure and function.
- Help client and family to identify effective successful coping mechanisms and to implement them **to reduce pain/discomfort and to improve quality of life.**
- Discuss importance of early detection and reporting of changes in condition or any unusual physical discomforts/ changes in pain characteristics. **Promotes early intervention/reduces potential for complications.**
- Emphasize need for adequate nutritional/fluid intake **to optimize healing potential.**
- Instruct in dressing changes (technique and frequency) and proper disposal of soiled dressings **to prevent spread of infectious agent.**
- Review medical regimen (e.g., proper use of topical sprays, creams, ointments, soaks, or irrigations).
- Stress importance of follow-up care, as appropriate (e.g., diabetic foot care clinic, wound care specialist/clinic, enterostomal therapist).
- Identify required changes in lifestyle, occupation, or environment **necessitated by limitations imposed by condition or to avoid causative factors.**
- Refer to community/governmental resources, as indicated (e.g., Public Health Department, OSHA, National Association for the Prevention of Blindness).
- Refer to NDs dependent on individual situation (e.g., impaired Skin Integrity; impaired Oral Mucous Membrane; risk for perioperative positioning Injury; impaired physical/bed

---

Information in brackets added by the authors to clarify and enhance the use of nursing diagnoses.

  Cultural Collaborative 🏠 Community/Home Care

Mobility; disturbed visual Sensory Perception; ineffective Tissue Perfusion; risk for Trauma; risk for Infection).

Documentation Focus

ASSESSMENT/REASSESSMENT

- Individual findings, including history of condition, characteristics of wound/lesion, evidence of other organ/tissue involvement.
- Impact on functioning/lifestyle.
- Availability/use of resources.

PLANNING

- Plan of care and who is involved in planning.
- Teaching plan.

IMPLEMENTATION/EVALUATION

- Responses to interventions/teaching, actions performed.
- Attainment/progress toward desired outcome(s).
- Modifications to plan of care.

DISCHARGE PLANNING

- Long-term needs/referrals and who is responsible for actions to be taken.
- Specific referrals made.

SAMPLE NURSING OUTCOMES & INTERVENTIONS CLASSIFICATIONS (NOC/NIC)

NOC—Tissue Integrity: Skin & Mucous Membranes
NIC—Wound Care

ineffective Tissue Perfusion
(Specify Type: Renal, Cerebral, Cardiopulmonary, Gastrointestinal, Peripheral)

Taxonomy II: Activity/Rest—Class 4 Cardiovascular/
   Pulmonary Responses (00024)
[Diagnostic Division: Circulation]
Submitted 1980; Revised 1998 (by small group work
   1996)

Definition: Decrease in oxygen resulting in the failure to nourish the tissues at the capillary level. [Tissue perfusion problems can exist without decreased cardiac output; however, there may be a relationship between cardiac output and tissue perfusion.]

Information in brackets added by the authors to clarify and enhance the use of nursing diagnoses.

 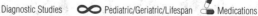

Related Factors

Hypervolemia; hypovolemia

Interruption of blood flow

Decreased hemoglobin concentration in blood; enzyme poisoning

Altered affinity of hemoglobin for oxygen; impaired transport of oxygen

Mismatch of ventilation with blood flow; exchange problems

Hypoventilation

Defining Characteristics

SUBJECTIVE

Cardiopulmonary

Chest pain

Dyspnea

Sense of "impending doom"

Gastrointestinal

Nausea

Abdominal pain or tenderness

Peripheral

Claudication

OBJECTIVE

Renal

Altered blood pressure outside of acceptable parameters

Oliguria; anuria; hematuria

Elevation in BUN/creatine ratio

Cerebral

Altered mental status; speech abnormalities

Behavioral changes; [restlessness]

Changes in motor response; extremity weakness; paralysis

Changes in pupillary reactions

Difficulty in swallowing

Cardiopulmonary

Arrhythmias

Capillary refill >3 sec

Altered respiratory rate outside of acceptable parameters

Use of accessory muscles; chest retraction; nasal flaring

Bronchospasms

Abnormal arterial blood gases

[Hemoptysis]

Information in brackets added by the authors to clarify and enhance the use of nursing diagnoses.

  Cultural Collaborative 🏠 Community/Home Care

Gastrointestinal

Hypoactive/absent bowel sounds
Abdominal distention
[Vomiting]

Peripheral

Altered skin characteristics (e.g., hair, nails, moisture)
Skin temperature changes
Skin discolorations; skin color pales on elevation, color does not return on lowering the leg
Altered sensations
Blood pressure changes in extremities; weak/absent pulses; diminished arterial pulsations; bruits
Edema
Delayed healing
Positive Homans' sign

Desired Outcomes/Evaluation Criteria—Client Will:

- Verbalize understanding of condition, therapy regimen, side effects of medications, and when to contact healthcare provider.
- Demonstrate behaviors/lifestyle changes to improve circulation (e.g., cessation of smoking, relaxation techniques, exercise/dietary program).
- Demonstrate increased perfusion as individually appropriate (e.g., skin warm/dry, peripheral pulses present/strong, vital signs within client's normal range, alert/oriented, balanced intake/output, absence of edema, free of pain/discomfort).

Actions/Interventions

NURSING PRIORITY NO. 1. To assess causative/contributing factors:

- Determine factors related to individual situation; for example, previous history of/at risk for formation of thrombus or emboli, diabetes with hyperinsulinemia, lipid abnormalities, fractures (especially long bone/pelvis), diagnosis of Raynaud's or Buerger's disease, pheochromocytoma/other endocrine imbalances, pancreatitis/intraperitoneal hemorrhage.
- Note presense of conditions/situations that can affect multiple systems (e.g., brain injury, sepsis, systemic lupus, Addison's disease, mycardial infarction/congestive heart failure, history of alcohol abuse, history of penetrating abdominal trauma).
- Identify changes related to systemic and/or peripheral alterations in circulation (e.g., altered mentation, vital sign

---

Information in brackets added by the authors to clarify and enhance the use of nursing diagnoses.

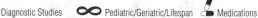

changes, pain, changes in skin/tissue/organ function, signs of metabolic imbalances).
- Evaluate for signs of infection, especially when immune system is compromised.
- Note signs of pulmonary emboli: sudden onset of chest pain, cyanosis, respiratory distress, hemoptysis, diaphoresis, hypoxia, anxiety, restlessness.

NURSING PRIORITY NO. 2. To note degree of impairment/organ involvement:
- Determine duration of problem/frequency of recurrence, precipitating/aggravating factors.
- Note customary baseline data (e.g., usual BP, weight, mentation, ABGs, and other appropriate laboratory study values). **Provides comparison with current findings.**
- Review results of diagnostic studies (e.g., x-rays, ultrsound/CT/other imaging scans, organ/compartment pressure measurements, endoscopy) **to determine location/severity of condition.**
- Ascertain impact of condition on functioning/lifestyle.

Renal
- Determine usual voiding pattern; compare with current situation.
- Note characteristics of urine; measure specific gravity.
- Review laboratory studies (e.g., BUN/Cr levels, proteinuria, specific gravity, serum electrolytes).
- Note mentation (**may be altered by increased BUN/Cr).**
- Auscultate BP, ascertain client's usual range (**decreased glomerular filtration rate—GFR—may increase renin release and raise BP).**
- Note presence, location, intensity, duration of pain.
- Observe for dependent/generalized edema.

Cerebral
- Determine presence of visual, sensory/motor changes, headache, dizziness, altered mental status, personality changes.
- Note history of syncope, brief/intermittent periods of confusion/blackout. **Suggestive of a transient ischemic attack (TIA).**
- Interview SO(s) regarding their perception of situation.
- Review medication regimen for possible adverse side effects/interactions, improper use of antihypertensives, drug overdose.

Cardiopulmonary
- Investigate reports of chest pain/angina; note precipitating factors, changes in characteristics of pain episodes.

Information in brackets added by the authors to clarify and enhance the use of nursing diagnoses.

- Evaluate vital signs, noting changes in BP, heart rate, and respirations.
- Note presence/degree of dyspnea, cyanosis, hemoptysis.
- Determine cardiac rhythm, note presence of dysrhythmias.
- Review baseline ABGs, electrolytes, BUN/Cr, cardiac enzymes.

Gastrointestinal

- Note reports of nausea/vomiting.
- Ascertain location/type/intensity/timing of abdominal pain. **Note: Midepigastric pain following meals and lasting several hours suggests abdominal angina reflecting atherosclerotic occlusive disease.**
- Investigate reports of pain out of proportion to degree of injury. **May reflect developing abdominal compartment syndrome.**
- Auscultate bowel sounds.
- Measure abdominal girth; ascertain client's customary waist size/belt length; investigate reports of difficulty breathing related to abdominal distention.
- Note changes in stool frequency/characteristics, presence of blood.
- Monitor for temperature, especially in presence of bright red blood in stool. **May indicate ischemic colitis.**
- Review laboratory studies (e.g., metabolic panel, CBC, amylase and lipase, clotting studies).

Peripheral

- Ascertain history/characteristics of pain, such as present with activity and/or at rest, cramping accompanied by temperature/color changes, trophic skin changes (e.g., hair loss, thin skin, thick nails), precipitated by heat, presence of paresthesias, etc. **Note: Pain combined with pallor, parasthesia, paralysis, and pulselessness indicates compartment syndrome.**
- Investigate reports of pain out of proportion to degree of injury. **May reflect developing compartment syndrome.**
- Measure circumference of extremities, as indicated. **Useful in identifying edema in involved extremity.**
- Assess lower extremities, noting skin texture; absence of body hair; presence of edema, ulcerations, non-healing wounds.
- Measure capillary refill; palpate for presence/absence and quality of pulses. Calculate ankle-brachial index (ABI), as appropriate (e.g., diabetic clients or others with impaired circulation to lower extremities). **Result less than 0.9 indicates need for more aggressive preventive interventions to manage peripheral vascular disease**.
- Auscultate for systolic/continuous bruits below obstruction in extremities.

Information in brackets added by the authors to clarify and enhance the use of nursing diagnoses.

- Check for calf tenderness (Homans' sign), swelling, and redness, **which may indicate thrombus formation.**
- Review diagnostic studies and laboratory tests (e.g., venogram, angiography, clotting times, Hb/Hct).
- Observe for signs of shock/sepsis. Note presence of bleeding or signs of DIC.

NURSING PRIORITY NO. 3. To maximize tissue perfusion:

- Assist with treatment of underlying conditions (e.g., stent placement, surgical reperfusion procedures, medications, fluid replacement/rehydration, nutrients, treatment of sepsis, etc.), as indicated, **to improve tissue perfusion/organ function.**

Renal
- Monitor vital signs.
- Measure urine output on a regular schedule. (Intake may be calculated against output.)
- Weigh daily.
- Administer medications (e.g., anticoagulants in presence of thrombosis, steroids in membranous nephropathy).
- Provide for diet restrictions, as indicated, while providing adequate calories to meet the body's needs. **Restriction of protein helps limit BUN.**
- Provide psychological support for client/SO(s), especially when progression of disease and resultant treatment (dialysis) may be long term.

Cerebral
- Elevate HOB (e.g., 10 degrees) and maintain head/neck in midline or neutral position **to promote circulation/venous drainage.**
- Administer medications (e.g., antihypertensive agents, steroids/diuretics [**may be used to decrease edema**], anticoagulants).
- Assist with/monitor hypothermia therapy, **which may be used to decrease metabolic and O_2 needs.**
- Prepare client for surgery, as indicated (e.g., carotid endarterectomy, evacuation of hematoma/space-occupying lesion).
- Refer to ND decreased Intracranial Adaptive Capacity.

Cardiopulmonary
- Monitor vital signs, hemodynamics, heart sounds, and cardiac rhythm.
- Encourage quiet, restful atmosphere. **Conserves energy/lowers tissue O_2 demands.**
- Caution client to avoid activities that increase cardiac workload (e.g., straining at stool).

Information in brackets added by the authors to clarify and enhance the use of nursing diagnoses.

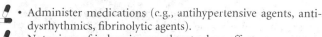

- Administer medications (e.g., antihypertensive agents, anti-dysrhythmics, fibrinolytic agents).
- Note signs of ischemia secondary to drug effects.
- Refer to ND decreased Cardiac Output.

Gastrointestinal

- Maintain gastric/intestinal decompression, when indicated, and measure output periodically.
- Provide small/easily digested food and fluids, when tolerated.
- Encourage rest after meals **to maximize blood flow to stomach, enhancing digestion.**
- Prepare client for emergency surgery (e.g., resection, bypass graft, mesenteric endarterectomy), as indicated.
- Refer to ND imbalanced Nutrition: less than body requirements.

Peripheral

- Perform assistive/active range-of-motion exercises (e.g., Buerger and Buerger-Allen).
- Encourage early ambulation, when possible. **Enhances venous return.**
- Discourage sitting/standing for long periods, wearing constrictive clothing, crossing legs.
- Elevate the legs when sitting, avoiding sharp angulation of the hips or knees.
- Avoid use of knee gatch on bed; elevate entire foot, as indicated.
- Provide air mattress, foam padding, bed/foot cradle **to protect the extremities.**
- Elevate HOB at night **to increase gravitational blood flow.**
- Apply antithromboembolic hose/compression bandages to lower extremities before arising from bed **to prevent venous stasis.**
- Avoid massaging the leg **when at risk for embolus.**
- Exercise caution in use of hot water bottles or heating pads. **Tissues may have decreased sensitivity due to ischemia, and heat also increases the metabolic demands of already compromised tissues.**
- Monitor circulation/movement/sensation above and below casts/traction device. Apply ice and elevate limb, as appropriate, **to reduce edema.**
- Emphasize necessity for smoking cessation.
- Assist with/prepare for surgical procedures (e.g., sympathectomy, vein graft, fasciotomy) **to improve peripheral circulation, relieve excessive tissue pressure.**
- Monitor closely for signs of shock when sympathectomy is done (**result of unmediated vasodilation**).
- Administer medications with caution (e.g., vasodilators, papaverine, antilipemics, anticoagulants). **Drugs used to**

Information in brackets added by the authors to clarify and enhance the use of nursing diagnoses.

 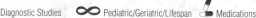

improve tissue perfusion also carry risk of adverse responses (e.g., altered drug response, changes in half-life/drug clearance, problems with interactions).

• Monitor for signs of bleeding during use of fibrinolytic agents.

NURSING PRIORITY NO. 4. To promote wellness (Teaching/Discharge Considerations):

• Discuss individual risk factors (e.g., family history, obesity, age, smoking, hypertension, diabetes, clotting disorders) and potential outcomes of atherosclerosis (e.g., systemic and peripheral vascular disease conditions). **Information necessary for client to make informed choices about remedial risk factors and commitment to lifestyle changes, as appropriate, to prevent onset of complications/manage symptoms when condition is present.**

• Instruct in blood pressure monitoring at home, advise purchase of home monitoring equipment, refer to community resources, as indicated. **Facilitates management of hypertension, which is a major risk factor for damage to blood vessels/organ function.**

• Encourage discussion of feelings regarding prognosis/long-term effects of condition.

• Identify necessary changes in lifestyle and assist client to incorporate disease management into ADLs.

• Encourage smoking cessation, provide information/refer to stop-smoking programs. **Smoking causes vasoconstriction and may further compromise perfusion.**

• Demonstrate/encourage use of relaxation activities, exercises/techniques **to decrease tension level.** Establish/encourage regular exercise program.

• Review specific dietary changes/restrictions with client (e.g., reduction of cholesterol and triglycerides, high or low protein intake, avoidance of rye in Buerger's disease).

• Discuss care of dependent limbs, body hygiene, foot care when circulation is impaired.

• Recommend avoidance of vasoconstricting drugs.

• Discourage massaging calf in presence of varicose veins/thrombophlebitis **to prevent embolization.**

• Emphasize importance of avoiding use of aspirin, some OTC drugs, vitamins containing potassium, mineral oil, or alcohol when taking anticoagulants.

• Review medical regimen and appropriate safety measures (e.g., use of electric razor when taking anticoagulants; foot care if diabetic or prone to venous statis).

• Discuss preventing exposure to cold, dressing warmly, and use of natural fibers to retain heat more efficiently.

Information in brackets added by the authors to clarify and enhance the use of nursing diagnoses.

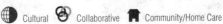

Cultural   Collaborative   Community/Home Care

- Provide preoperative teaching appropriate for the situation.
- Refer to specific support groups, counseling, as appropriate.

Documentation Focus

ASSESSMENT/REASSESSMENT

- Individual findings, noting nature/extent and duration of problem, effect on independence/lifestyle.
- Characteristics of pain, precipitators, and what relieves pain.
- Vital signs, cardiac rhythm/dysrhythmias.
- Pulses/BP, including above/below suspected lesion, as appropriate.
- I/O and weight, as indicated.

PLANNING

- Plan of care and who is involved in planning.
- Teaching plan.

IMPLEMENTATION/EVALUATION

- Response to interventions/teaching and actions performed.
- Attainment/progress toward desired outcome(s).
- Modifications to plan of care.

DISCHARGE PLANNING

- Long-term needs and who is responsible for actions to be taken.
- Available resources, specific referrals made.

SAMPLE NURSING OUTCOMES & INTERVENTIONS CLASSIFICATIONS (NOC/NIC)

RENAL

NOC—Urinary
NIC—Fluid/Electrolyte Management

CEREBRAL

NOC— Tissue Perfusion: Cerebral
NIC—Cerebral Perfusion Promotion

CARDIOPULMONARY

NOC—Tissue Perfusion: Cardiac
NIC—Cardiac Care

GASTROINTESTINAL

NOC—Tissue Perfusion: Abdominal Organ
NIC—Gastrointestinal Intubation

Information in brackets added by the authors to clarify and enhance the use of nursing diagnoses.

 Diagnostic Studies 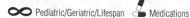 Pediatric/Geriatric/Lifespan Medications **713**

PERIPHERAL

NOC—Tissue Perfusion: Peripheral
NIC—Circulatory Care: Arterial/Venous Insufficiency

impaired Transfer Ability

Taxonomy II: Activity/Rest—Class 2 Activity/Exercise
  (00090)
[Diagnostic Division: Activity/Rest]
Submitted 1998; Revised 2006

Definition: Limitation of independent movement
between two nearby surfaces

Related Factors

Insufficient muscle strength; deconditioning; neuromuscular
  impairment; musculoskeletal impairment (e.g., contractures)
Impaired balance
Pain
Obesity
Impaired vision
Lack of knowledge; cognitive impairment
Environment constraints (e.g., bed height, inadequate space,
  wheelchair type, treatment equipment, restraints)

Defining Characteristics

SUBJECTIVE OR OBJECTIVE

Inability to transfer: from bed to chair/chair to bed; from chair to
  car/car to chair; from chair to floor/floor to chair; on or off a
  toilet/commode; in or out of tub/shower; from bed to stand-
  ing/standing to bed; from chair to standing/standing to chair;
  from standing to floor/floor to standing; between uneven levels
Note: Specify level of independence using a standardized functional scale —[refer to ND impaired physical Mobility, for
  suggested functional level classification]

Desired Outcomes/Evaluation
Criteria—Client/Caregiver Will:

• Verbalize understanding of situation and appropriate safety
  measures.
• Master techniques of transfer successfully.
• Make desired transfer safely.

Information in brackets added by the authors to clarify and enhance
the use of nursing diagnoses.

 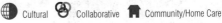

Actions/Interventions

NURSING PRIORITY NO. 1. To assess causative/contributing factors:
- Determine diagnosis that contributes to transfer problems (e.g., MS, fractures, back injuries, quadriplegia/paraplegia, agedness, dementias, brain injury, etc.).
- Note current situations such as surgery, amputation, contractures, traction apparatus, mechanical ventilation, multiple tubings that restrict movement.

NURSING PRIORITY NO. 2. To assess functional ability:
- Evaluate degree of impairment using 0 to 4 functional level classification.
- Note emotional/behavioral responses of client/SO(s) to problems of immobility.
- Determine presence/degree of perceptual/cognitive impairment and ability to follow directions.

NURSING PRIORITY NO. 3. To promote optimal level of movement:

- Assist with treatment of underlying condition causing dysfunction.
- Consult with PT/OT/rehabilitation team **in identifying balance, gait, and mobility aids/adjunctive devices.**
- Demonstrate/assist with use of siderails, overhead trapeze, transfer boards, transfer/sit-to-stand hoist, specialty slings, safety grab bars, cane, walker, wheelchair, crutches, as indicated.
- Position devices (e.g., call light, bed-positioning switch) within easy reach on the bed/chair. **Facilitates transfer/allows client to obtain assistance for transfer, as needed.**
- Provide instruction/reinforce information for client and caregivers regarding positioning **to improve/maintain balance when transferring**.
- Monitor body alignment/posture and balance, and encourage wide base of support when standing to transfer.
- Use full-length mirror, as needed, **to facilitate client's view of own postural alignment.**
- Demonstrate/reinforce safety measures, as indicated, such as transfer board, gait belt, supportive footwear, good lighting, clearing floor of clutter **to avoid possibility of fall and subsequent injury.**

NURSING PRIORITY NO. 4. To promote wellness (Teaching/Discharge Considerations):

- Assist client/caregivers to learn safety measures as individually indicated (e.g., using correct body mechanics for particular

---

Information in brackets added by the authors to clarify and enhance the use of nursing diagnoses.

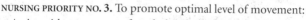

Diagnostic Studies ∞ Pediatric/Geriatric/Lifespan Medications

715

transfer, locking wheelchair before transfer, using properly placed/functioning hoists, ascertaining that floor surface is even and clutter-free).

 • Refer to appropriate community resources for evaluation and modification of environment (e.g., shower/tub, uneven floor surfaces/steps, use of ramps/standing tables/lifts, etc.).

Documentation Focus

ASSESSMENT/REASSESSMENT

• Individual findings, including level of function/ability to participate in desired transfers.
• Mobility aids/transfer devices used.

PLANNING

• Plan of care and who is involved in the planning.
• Teaching plan.

IMPLEMENTATION/EVALUATION

• Responses to interventions/teaching and actions performed.
• Attainment/progress toward desired outcome(s).
• Modifications to plan of care.

DISCHARGE PLANNING

• Discharge/long-range needs, noting who is responsible for each action to be taken.
• Specific referrals made.
• Sources of/maintenance for assistive devices.

SAMPLE NURSING OUTCOMES & INTERVENTIONS CLASSIFICATIONS (NOC/NIC)

NOC—Transfer Performance
NIC—Transport

risk for Trauma

Taxonomy II: Safety/Protection—Class 2 Physical Injury (00038)
[Diagnostic Division: Safety]
Submitted 1980

Definition: Accentuated risk of accidental tissue injury (e.g., wound, burn, fracture)

Information in brackets added by the authors to clarify and enhance the use of nursing diagnoses.

 Cultural Collaborative Community/Home Care

Risk Factors

INTERNAL

Weakness; balancing difficulties; reduced muscle/hand/eye coordination

Poor vision

Reduced sensation

Lack of safety education/precautions

Insufficient finances

Cognitive/emotional difficulties

History of previous trauma

EXTERNAL [INCLUDES BUT IS NOT LIMITED TO]

Slippery floors (e.g., wet or highly waxed); unanchored rugs/electric wires

Bathtub without antislip equipment

Use of unsteady ladder/chairs

Obstructed passageways; entering unlighted rooms

Inadequate stair rails; children playing without gates at top of stairs

High beds; inappropriate call-for-aid mechanisms for bedresting client

Unsafe window protection in homes with young children

Pot handles facing toward front of stove; bathing in very hot water (e.g., unsupervised bathing of young children)

Potential igniting gas leaks; delayed lighting of gas appliances

Wearing flowing clothes around open flames; flammable children's clothing/toys

Smoking in bed/near oxygen; grease waste collected on stoves

Children playing with dangerous objects; accessibility of guns

Playing with explosives; experimenting with chemicals; inadequately stored combustibles (e.g., matches, oily rags)/corrosives (e.g., lye); contact with corrosives

Overloaded fuse boxes; faulty electrical plugs; frayed wires; defective appliances; overloaded electrical outlets

Exposure to dangerous machinery; contact with rapidly moving machinery

Struggling with restraints

Contact with intense cold; lack of protection from heat source; overexposure to radiation

Large icicles hanging from the roof

Use of cracked dishware; knives stored uncovered

High-crime neighborhood

Information in brackets added by the authors to clarify and enhance the use of nursing diagnoses.

Driving a mechanically unsafe vehicle; driving at excessive speeds; driving without necessary visual aids; driving while intoxicated

Children riding in the front seat of car; nonuse/misuse of seat restraints

Unsafe road/walkways; physical proximity to vehicle pathways (e.g., driveways, lanes, railroad tracks)

Misuse [/nonuse] of necessary headgear [e.g., for bicycles, motorcycles, skateboarding, skiing]

> NOTE: A risk diagnosis is not evidenced by signs and symptoms, as the problem has not occurred and nursing interventions are directed at prevention.

Desired Outcomes/Evaluation Criteria—Client/Caregiver Will:

• Identify and correct potential risk factors in the environment.
• Demonstrate appropriate lifestyle changes to reduce risk of injury.
• Identify resources to assist in promoting a safe environment.
• Recognize need for/seek assistance to prevent accidents/injuries.

Actions/Interventions

This ND is a compilation of a number of situations that can result in injury. Refer to specific NDs—risk for imbalanced Body Temperature; risk for Contamination; impaired Environmental Interpretation Syndrome; risk for Falls; impaired Home Maintenance; Hypothermia; Hyperthermia; impaired physical Mobility; risk for Injury; risk for Poisoning; impaired Skin Integrity; risk for impaired Parenting; disturbed Sensory Perception; risk for Suffocation; disturbed Thought Processes; impaired Tissue Integrity; risk for self-/other-directed Violence; impaired Walking, as appropriate, for more specific interventions.

NURSING PRIORITY NO. 1. To assess causative/contributing factors:

• Determine factors related to individual situation, as listed in Risk Factors, and extent of risk. **Influences scope and intensity of interventions to manage threat to safety.**
∞ • Note client's age/gender/developmental stage, decision-making ability, level of cognition/competence. **Affects client's ability to protect self and/or others, and influences choice of interventions and teaching.**

Information in brackets added by the authors to clarify and enhance the use of nursing diagnoses.

 Cultural Collaborative Community/Home Care

• Ascertain knowledge of safety needs/injury prevention and motivation to prevent injury in home, community, and work setting.

• Note socioeconomic status/availability and use of resources.

• Assess influence of client's lifestyle/stress on potential for injury.

 • Review history of accidents noting circumstances (e.g., time of day, activities coinciding with accident, who was present, type of injury sustained).

 • Determine potential for abusive behavior by family members/SO(s)/peers.

• Review diagnostic studies /laboratory tests for impairments/ imbalances **that may result in/exacerbate conditions, such as confusion, tetany, pathological fractures, etc.**

NURSING PRIORITY NO. 2. To promote safety measures required by individual situation:

• Implement interventions regarding safety issues when planning for client care and/or discharge from care. **Failure to accurately assess, intervene, and/or refer these issues can place the client at needless risk and create negligence issues for the healthcare practitioner:**

Orient client to environment.

Make arrangement for call system for bedridden client in home/hospital setting. Demonstrate use and place device within client's reach.

Keep bed in low position or place mattress on floor, as appropriate.

Use and pad side rails, as indicated.

Provide seizure precautions.

Lock wheels on bed/movable furniture. Clear travel paths. Provide adequate area lighting.

Assist with activities and transfers, as needed.

Provide well-fitting, non-skid footwear.

Demonstrate/monitor use of assistive devices, such as cane, walker, crutches, wheelchair, safety bars.

Provide supervision while client is smoking.

Provide for appropriate disposal of potentially injurious items (e.g., needles, scalpel blades).

Follow facility protocol/closely monitor use of restraints, when required (e.g., vest, limb, belt, mitten).

NURSING PRIORITY NO. 3. To treat underlying medical/psychiatric condition:

• Assist with treatments for underlying medical/surgical/psychiatric conditions **to improve cognition/thinking processes,**

Information in brackets added by the authors to clarify and enhance the use of nursing diagnoses.

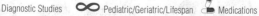

musculoskeletal function, awareness of own safety needs, and general well-being.

- Provide quiet environment and reduced stimulation, as indicated. **Helps limit confusion or overstimulation for clients at risk for such conditions as seizures, tetany, autonomic hyperreflexia.**

 • Refer to counseling/psychotherapy, as need indicates, especially when individual is "accident-prone"/self-destructive behavior is noted. (Refer to NDs risk for other-directed/self-directed Violence.)

NURSING PRIORITY NO. 4. To promote wellness (Teaching/Discharge Considerations):

- Review client's therapeutic regimen on a continual basis when under direct care (e.g., client's vital signs, medications, treatment modalities, infusions, nutrition, physical environment) **to prevent healthcare-related complications**

 • Stress importance of obtaining assistance when weak and when problems of balance, coordination, or postural hypotension are present **to reduce risk of syncope/falls.**

- Encourage use of warm-up/stretching exercises before engaging in athletic activity **to prevent muscle injuries.**

- Recommend use of seat belts; fitted helmets for cyclists, skate/snowboarders, skiers; approved infant seat; avoidance of hitchhiking; substance abuse programs **to promote transportation safety.**

- Refer to accident prevention programs (e.g., medication/drug safety; mobility/transfer device training; driving instruction; parenting classes, firearms safety, workplace erogomics, etc.).

- Develop fire safety program (e.g., family fire drills; use of smoke detectors; yearly chimney cleaning; purchase of fire-retardant clothing, especially children's nightwear; safe use of in-home oxygen; fireworks safety).

- Problem solve with client/parent to provide adequate child supervision after school, during working hours, on school holidays; or day program for frail/confused elder.

- Discuss necessary environmental changes (e.g., decals on glass doors to show when they are closed, lowering temperature on hot water heater, adequate lighting of stairways; tamper-proof medication containers, safe chemical/poisons storage) **to prevent/reduce risk of accidents.**

- Identify community resources (e.g., financial **to assist with necessary corrections/improvements/purchases**).

- Recommend involvement in community self-help programs, such as Neighborhood Watch, Helping Hand.

Information in brackets added by the authors to clarify and enhance the use of nursing diagnoses.

Documentation Focus

ASSESSMENT/REASSESSMENT

- Individual risk factors, past/recent history of injuries, awareness of safety needs.

PLANNING

- Plan of care and who is involved in the planning.
- Teaching plan.

IMPLEMENTATION/EVALUATION

- Responses to interventions/teaching, actions performed.
- Attainment/progress toward desired outcome(s).
- Modifications to plan of care.

DISCHARGE PLANNING

- Long-term needs and who is responsible for actions to be taken.
- Available resources, specific referrals made.

SAMPLE NURSING OUTCOMES & INTERVENTIONS CLASSIFICATIONS (NOC/NIC)

NOC—Safety Status: Physical Injury
NIC—Environmental Management: Safety

impaired Urinary Elimination

Taxonomy II: Elimination—Class 1 Urinary System (00016)
[Diagnostic Division: Elimination]
Submitted 1973; Revised 2006

Definition: Dysfunction in urine elimination

Related Factors

Multiple causality; sensory motor impairment; anatomical obstruction; UTI; [mechanical trauma; fluid/volume states; psychogenic factors; surgical diversion]

Defining Characteristics

SUBJECTIVE

Frequency; urgency
Hesitancy

Information in brackets added by the authors to clarify and enhance the use of nursing diagnoses.

 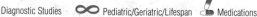

Dysuria
Nocturia [enuresis]

OBJECTIVE

Incontinence
Retention

Desired Outcomes/Evaluation Criteria—Client Will:

- Verbalize understanding of condition.
- Identify specific causative factors.
- Achieve normal elimination pattern or participate in measures to correct/compensate for defects.
- Demonstrate behaviors/techniques to prevent urinary infection.
- Manage care of urinary catheter, or stoma and appliance following urinary diversion.

Actions/Interventions

NURSING PRIORITY NO. **1.** To assess causative/contributing factors:

- Identify conditions that may be present, such as urinary tract infection, interstitial cystitis/painful bladder syndrome; dehydration; surgery (including urinary diversion); neurological involvement (e.g., MS, stroke, Parkinson's disease, paraplegia/tetraplegia); mental/emotional dysfunction (e.g., impaired cognition, delirium/confusion, depression, Alzheimer's disease); prostate disorders; recent/multiple pregnancies; pelvic trauma.
- Determine pathology of bladder dysfunction relative to medical diagnosis identified. **For example, in such neurological/demyelinating diseases as MS, problem may be related to inability to store urine, empty the bladder, or both.**
- Assist with physical examination (e.g., cough test for incontinence, palpation for bladder retention/masses, prostate size, observation for urethral stricture, etc.).
- Note age and gender of client. **Incontinence and urinary tract infections are more prevalent in women and older adults; painful bladder syndrome/interstitial cystitis (PBS/IC) is more common in women.**
- Investigate pain, noting location, duration, intensity; presence of bladder spasms; or back or flank pain **to assist in differentiating between bladder and kidney as cause of dysfunction. Bladder pain located suprapubically, vaginally, in the perineum, low back, or in the medial aspects of the thighs–that is**

Information in brackets added by the authors to clarify and enhance the use of nursing diagnoses.

  Cultural Collaborative 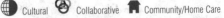 Community/Home Care

relieved by voiding and often recurs with bladder filling–suggests presence of PBS/IC.

- Have client complete Pelvic Pain and Urgency/Frequency (PUF) patient symptom survey, as indicated. **Helps to evaluate the presence and severity of PBS/IC symptoms.**

- Note reports of exacerbations and spontaneous remissions of symptoms of urgency and frequency, which may/may not be accompanied by pain, pressure, or spasm. **Clients with PBS/IC void approximately 16 times per day with voided volumes usually less then normal.**

- Determine client's usual daily fluid intake (both amount and beverage choices/use of caffeine). Note condition of skin and mucous membranes, color of urine **to help determine level of hydration.**

- Review medication regimen **for drugs that can alter bladder or kidney function (e.g., antihypertensive agents [e.g., ACE inhibiotors, beta blockers]; anticholinergics [e.g., antihistamines, anti-parkinsonian drugs]; antidepressants/antipsychotics; sedatives/hypnotics/opioids; caffeine and alcohol).**

- Send urine specimen (midstream clean-voided or catheterized) for culture and sensitivities in presence of signs of urinary tract infection—cloudy, foul odor; bloody urine.

- Rule out gonorrhea in men when urethritis with a penile discharge is present and there are no bacteria in the urine.

- Obtain specimen for antibody-coated bacteria assay **to diagnose bacterial infection of the kidney or prostate.**

- Assist with/perform potassium sensitivity test (instillation of potassium solution into bladder). **Eighty percent of patients with PBS/IC will react positively.**

- Review laboratory tests for hyperglycemia/hyperparathyroidism/other metabolic conditions; changes in renal function; culture for presence of infection/sexually transmitted disease (STD), urine cytology for cancer.

- Strain all urine for calculi and describe stones expelled and/or send to laboratory for analysis.

- Review results of diagnostic studies (e.g., uroflowmetry, cystometogram, post-void residual, pressure flow and leak point pressure measurement, videourodynamics, electromyography, kidneys/ureters/bladder [KUB] imaging, etc.) **to identify presence/type of elimination problem.**

NURSING PRIORITY NO. 2. To assess degree of interference/disability:

- Ascertain client's previous pattern of elimination **for comparison with current situation**. Ask about/note reports of problems (e.g., frequency, urgency, painful urination; leaking/

Information in brackets added by the authors to clarify and enhance the use of nursing diagnoses.

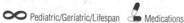

incontinence; changes in size/force of urinary stream; problems emptying bladder completely; nocturia/enuresis).

- Ascertain client's/SO's perception of problem/degree of disability (e.g., client is restricting social/employment/travel activities; having sexual/relationship difficulties; incurring sleep deprivation; experiencing depression).
- Determine cultural factors impacting client's self-image regarding urinary problem (e.g., presence of urostomy and need to empty bag at intervals; painful bladder that interferes with daily activities/employment).
- Have client keep a voiding diary for three days to record fluid intake, voiding times, precise urine output, and dietary intake. **Helps determine baseline symptoms, severity of frequency/urgency, and whether diet is a factor (if symptoms worsen).**

NURSING PRIORITY NO. 3. To assist in treating/preventing urinary alteration:

- Refer to specific NDs Urinary Incontinence (specify); Urinary Retention for additional related interventions.
- Encourage fluid intake up to 3000 or more mL/day (within cardiac tolerance), including cranberry juice, **to help maintain renal function, prevent infection and formation of urinary stones, avoid encrustation around catheter, or to flush urinary diversion appliance.**
- Discuss possible dietary restrictions (e.g., especially coffee, alcohol, carbonated drinks, citrus, tomatoes, and chocolate) based on individual symptoms.
- Assist with developing toileting routines (e.g., timed voiding, bladder training, prompted voiding, habit retraining), as appropriate. Note: Bladder retraining is not recommended for clients with PBS.
- Encourage client to verbalize fears/concerns (e.g., disruption in sexual activity, inability to work). **Open expression allows client to deal with feelings and begin problem solving.**
- Implement/monitor interventions for specific elimination problem (e.g., pelvic floor exercises/other bladder retraining modalities; medication regimen, including antimicrobials [single-dose is frequently being used for UTI], sulfonamides, antispasmodics); and evaluate client's response **to modify treatment, as needed.**
- Discuss possible surgical procedures and medical regimen, as indicated (e.g., client with benign prostatic hypertrophy bladder/prostatic cancer, PBS/IC, and so forth). **For example, cystoscopy with bladder hydrodistention for PBS/IC, or an electrical stimulator may be implanted to treat**

Information in brackets added by the authors to clarify and enhance the use of nursing diagnoses.

 Cultural Collaborative Community/Home Care

chronic urinary urge incontinence, nonobstructive urinary retention, and symptoms of urgency and frequency.

NURSING PRIORITY NO. 4. To assist in management of long-term urinary alterations:

- Keep bladder deflated by use of an indwelling catheter connected to closed drainage. Investigate alternatives when possible (e.g., intermittent catheterization, surgical interventions, urinary drugs, voiding maneuvers, condom catheter).
- Provide latex-free catheter and care supplies **to reduce risk of latex sensitivity.**
- Check frequently for bladder distention and observe for overflow **to reduce risk of infection and/or autonomic hyperreflexia.**
- Maintain acidic environment of the bladder by the use of agents, such as vitamin C, Mandelamine, when appropriate, **to discourage bacterial growth.**
- Adhere to a regular bladder/diversion appliance emptying schedule **to avoid accidents.**
- Provide for routine diversion appliance care, and assist client to recognize and deal with problems, such as alkaline salt encrustation, ill-fitting appliance, malodorous urine, infection, and so forth.

NURSING PRIORITY NO. 5. To promote wellness (Teaching/Discharge Considerations):

- Emphasize importance of keeping area clean and dry **to reduce risk of infection and/or skin breakdown.**
- Instruct female clients with UTI to drink large amounts of fluid, void immediately after intercourse, wipe from front to back, promptly treat vaginal infections, and take showers rather than tub baths **to limit risk/avoid reinfection.**
- Recommend smoking cessation program, as appropriate. **Cigarette smoking can also be a source of bladder irritation.**
- Encourage SO(s) who participate in routine care to recognize complications (including latex allergy) necessitating medical evaluation/intervention.
- Instruct in proper application and care of appliance for urinary diversion. Encourage liberal fluid intake, avoidance of foods/medications that produce strong odor, use of white vinegar or deodorizer in pouch **to promote odor control.**
- Identify sources for supplies, programs/agencies providing financial assistance **to obtain needed equipment.**
- Recommend avoidance of gas-forming foods in presence of ureterosigmoidostomy **as flatus can cause urinary incontinence.**

Information in brackets added by the authors to clarify and enhance the use of nursing diagnoses.

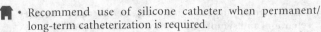

readiness for enhanced URINARY ELIMINATION (side margin)

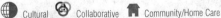

- Recommend use of silicone catheter when permanent/long-term catheterization is required.
- Demonstrate proper positioning of catheter drainage tubing and bag **to facilitate drainage/prevent reflux.**
- Refer client/SO(s) to appropriate community resources, such as ostomy specialist, support group, sex therapist, psychiatric clinical nurse specialist, **to deal with changes in body image/function, when indicated.**

Documentation Focus

ASSESSMENT/REASSESSMENT

- Individual findings, including previous and current pattern of voiding, nature of problem, effect on desired lifestyle.
- Cultural factors/concerns.

PLANNING

- Plan of care and who is involved in planning.
- Teaching plan.

IMPLEMENTATION/EVALUATION

- Response to interventions/teaching and actions performed.
- Attainment/progress toward desired outcome(s).
- Modifications to plan of care.

DISCHARGE PLANNING

- Long-term needs and who is responsible for actions to be taken.
- Available resources/specific referrals made.
- Individual equipment needs and sources.

SAMPLE NURSING OUTCOMES & INTERVENTIONS CLASSIFICATIONS (NOC/NIC)

NOC—Urinary Elimination
NIC—Urinary Elimination Management

readiness for enhanced Urinary Elimination

Taxonomy II: Elimination—Class 1 Urinary System (00166)
[Diagnostic Division: Elimination]
Submitted 2002

Definition: A pattern of urinary functions that is sufficient for meeting eliminatory needs and can be strengthened

---

Information in brackets added by the authors to clarify and enhance the use of nursing diagnoses.

 Cultural  Collaborative Community/Home Care

Related Factors

To be developed

Defining Characteristics

SUBJECTIVE

Expresses willingness to enhance urinary elimination
Positions self for emptying of bladder

OBJECTIVE

Urine is straw colored/odorless
Amount of output/specific gravity is within normal limits
Fluid intake is adequate for daily needs

Desired Outcomes/Evaluation Criteria—Client Will:

- Verbalize understanding of condition that has potential for altering elimination.
- Achieve normal/acceptable elimination pattern emptying bladder/voiding in appropriate amounts.
- Alter lifestyle/environment to accommodate individual needs.

Actions/Interventions

NURSING PRIORITY NO. 1. To assess status and adaptive skills being used by client:

- Identify physical conditions (e.g., surgery, childbirth, recent/multiple pregnancies, pelvic trauma, neurogenic bladder from central nervous system disorders or neuropathies [stroke/spinal cord injury, diabetes], mental/emotional dysfunction, prostate disease/surgery) **that can impact client's elimination patterns.**
- Determine client's usual pattern of elimination and compare with current situation. Review voiding diary, if indicated. **Provides baseline for future comparison.**
- Observe voiding patterns, time, color, and amount voided, if indicated (e.g., postsurgical or postpartum client) **to document normalization of elimination.**
- Ascertain methods of self-management (e.g., limiting or increasing liquid intake, acting on urge in timely manner, established voiding schedule, regularly spaced catherization) **to identify strengths/areas of concern in elimination management**.

Information in brackets added by the authors to clarify and enhance the use of nursing diagnoses.

readiness for enhanced URINARY ELIMINATION

 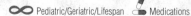

- Determine client's usual daily fluid intake. **Both amount and beverage choices are important in managing elimination.**

NURSING PRIORITY NO. 2. To assist client to improve management of urinary elimination:

- Encourage fluid intake, including water and cranberry juice, **to help maintain renal function, prevent infection.**
- Regulate liquid intake at prescheduled times **to promote predictable voiding pattern.** Restrict fluid intake 2 to 3 hours before bedtime **to reduce voiding during the night.**
- Assist with modifying current routines, as appropriate. **Client may benefit from additional information in enhancing success, such as regarding cues/urge to void; adjusting schedule of voiding/catheterization (shorter or longer); relaxation and/or distraction techniques; standing or sitting upright during voiding to ensure that bladder is completely empty; and/or practicing pelvic muscle strengthening exercises.**
- Provide assistance/devices, as indicated (e.g., providing means of summoning assistance; placing bedside commode, urinal, or bedpan within client's reach; using elevated toilet seats; mobility devices) **when client is frail or mobility impaired.**
- Modify/recommend diet changes, if indicated. **For example, reduction of caffeine, because of its bladder irritant effect; or weight reduction, to reduce overactive bladder symptoms and incontinence by decreasing pressure on the bladder.**
- Modify medication regimens, as appropriate (e.g., administer prescribed diuretics in the morning **to lessen nighttime voiding**). Reduce or eliminate use of hypnotics, if possible, **as client may be too sedated to recognize/respond to urge to void.**
- Refer to appropriate resources (e.g., medical supply company, ostomy nurse, rehabilitation team) **for assistance, as desired/needed to promote self-care.**

NURSING PRIORITY NO. 3. To promote optimum wellness:

- Encourage continuation of successful toileting program and identify possible alterations to meet individual needs (e.g., use of adult briefs for extended outing or travel with limited access to toilet). **Promotes proactive problem solving and supports self-esteem and normalization of social interactions/desired lifestyle activities.**
- Instruct client/SO(s)/caregivers in cues that client needs, such as voiding on routine schedule, showing client location of the bathroom, providing adequate room lighting, signs, color coding of door **to assist client in continued continence, especially when in unfamiliar surroundings.**

Information in brackets added by the authors to clarify and enhance the use of nursing diagnoses.

   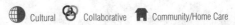 Cultural   Collaborative   Community/Home Care

- Review with client/SO(s) the signs/symptoms of urinary complications and need for expedient medical follow-up care. **Promotes timely intervention to limit or prevent adverse events.**

Documentation Focus

ASSESSMENT/REASSESSMENT

- Findings/adaptive skills being used.

PLANNING

- Plan of care and who is involved in planning.
- Teaching plan.

IMPLEMENTATION/EVALUATION

- Responses to treatment plan/interventions and actions performed.
- Attainment/progress toward desired outcome(s).
- Modifications to plan of care.

DISCHARGE PLANNING

- Available resources, equipment needs/sources.

SAMPLE NURSING OUTCOMES & INTERVENTIONS CLASSIFICATIONS (NOC/NIC)

NOC—Urinary Elimination
NIC—Urinary Elimination Management

functional Urinary Incontinence

Taxonomy II: Elimination—Class 1 Urinary System (00020)
[Diagnostic Division: Elimination]
Submitted 1986; Nursing Diagnosis Extension and Classification (NDEC) Revision 1998

Definition: Inability of usually continent person to reach toilet in time to avoid unintentional loss of urine

Related Factors

Altered environmental factors [e.g., poor lighting or inability to locate bathroom]
Neuromuscular limitations
Weakened supporting pelvic structures
Impaired vision/cognition

Information in brackets added by the authors to clarify and enhance the use of nursing diagnoses.

Psychological factors; [reluctance to call for assistance/use bedpan; fluctuation in mentation]
[Increased urine production]

Defining Characteristics

SUBJECTIVE

Senses need to void
[Voiding in large amounts]

OBJECTIVE

Loss of urine before reaching toilet; amount of time required to
reach toilet exceeds length of time between sensing urge and
uncontrolled voiding
Able to completely empty bladder
May only be incontinent in early morning

Desired Outcomes/Evaluation
Criteria—Client/Caregiver Will:

- Verbalize understanding of condition and identify interven-
tions to prevent incontinence.
- Alter environment to accommodate individual needs.
- Report voiding in individually appropriate amounts.
- Urinate at acceptable times and places.

Actions/Interventions

NURSING PRIORITY NO. 1. To assess causative/contributing factors:

- Identify/differentiate client with functional incontinence
(e.g., bladder and urethra are functioning normally, but client
either cannot get to toilet, or has impaired mental function
that interferes with recognizing need to urinate and getting to
toilet on time) from other forms of incontinence.
- Evaluate cognition. **Disease process/medications can affect
mental status/orientation to place, recognition of urge to
void, and/or its significance.**
- Note presence/type of functional impairments (e.g., poor eye-
sight, mobility problems, dexterity problems/self-care
deficits) **that can hinder ability to get to bathroom.**
- Identify environmental conditions that interfere with timely
access to bathroom/successful toileting process. **Unfamiliar
surroundings, poor lighting, improperly fitted chair walker,
low toilet seat, absence of safety bars, and travel distance to
toilet may affect self-care ability.**

Information in brackets added by the authors to clarify and enhance
the use of nursing diagnoses.

Cultural Collaborative Community/Home Care

- Determine if client is voluntarily postponing urination.
- Review medical history for condition or use of medication/substances known to increase urine output and/or alter bladder tone (e.g., diuretics, alcohol, caffeine).

NURSING PRIORITY NO. 2. To assess degree of interference/disability:

- Determine frequency and timing of continent/incontinent voids. Note time of day/night when incontinence occurs, as well as timing issues (e.g., difference between the time it takes to get to bathroom/remove clothing and involuntary loss of urine).
- Ascertain effect on client's lifestyle (including socialization and sexuality) and self-esteem.

NURSING PRIORITY NO. 3. To assist in treating/preventing incontinence:

- Remind client to void when needed and schedule voiding times **to reduce incontinence episodes/promote comfort for client who ambulates slowly because of physical limitations or who has cognitive decline.**
- Administer prescribed diuretics in the morning **to lessen nighttime voidings.**
- Reduce or eliminate use of hypnotics, if possible, **as client may be too sedated to recognize/respond to urge to void.**
- Provide means of summoning assistance (e.g., call light or bell).
- Use night-lights **to mark bathroom location.**
- Provide cues, such as adequate room lighting, signs, color coding of door, **to assist client who is disoriented to find the bathroom.**
- Remove throw rugs, excess furniture in travel path to bathroom.
- Provide bedside commode, urinal, or bedpan, as indicated.
- Adapt clothes for quick removal: Velcro fasteners, full skirts, crotchless panties or no panties, suspenders or elastic waists instead of belts on pants. **Facilitates toileting once urge to void is noted.**
- Schedule voiding for every 3 hours **to minimize bladder pressure.**
- Restrict fluid intake 2 to 3 hours before bedtime **to reduce nighttime voidings.**
- Include physical/occupational therapist in determining ways to alter environment and identifying appropriate assistive devices to meet client's individual needs.

NURSING PRIORITY NO. 4. To promote wellness (Teaching/Discharge Considerations):

Information in brackets added by the authors to clarify and enhance the use of nursing diagnoses.

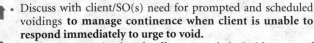

- Discuss with client/SO(s) need for prompted and scheduled voidings **to manage continence when client is unable to respond immediately to urge to void.**
- Suggest limiting intake of coffee, tea, and alcohol **because of diuretic effect and impact on voiding pattern.**
- Maintain positive regard **to reduce embarrassment associated with incontinence, need for assistance, use of bedpan.**
- Promote participation in developing long-term plan of care.
- Refer to NDs reflex Urinary Incontinence; stress Urinary Incontinence; total Urinary Incontinence; urge Urinary Incontinence.

Documentation Focus

ASSESSMENT/REASSESSMENT

- Current elimination pattern/assessment findings and effect on lifestyle and self-esteem.

PLANNING

- Plan of care and who is involved in planning.
- Teaching plan.

IMPLEMENTATION/EVALUATION

- Response to interventions/teaching and actions performed.
- Attainment/progress toward desired outcome(s).
- Modifications to plan of care.

DISCHARGE PLANNING

- Long-term needs and who is responsible for actions to be taken.
- Specific referrals made.

SAMPLE NURSING OUTCOMES & INTERVENTIONS CLASSIFICATIONS (NOC/NIC)

NOC—Urinary Continence
NIC—Prompted Voiding

overflow Urinary Incontinence

Taxonomy II: Elimination—Class 1 Urinary System (00176)
[Diagnostic Division: Elimination]
Submitted 2006

Definition: Involuntary loss of urine associated with overdistention of the bladder

Information in brackets added by the authors to clarify and enhance the use of nursing diagnoses.

 Cultural   Collaborative   Community/Home Care

Related Factors

Bladder outlet obstruction; fecal impaction

Urethral obstruction; severe pelvic prolapse

Detrusor external sphincter dyssynergia; detrusor hypocontractility

Side effects of anticholinergic/decongestant medications; calcium channel blockers

Defining Characteristics

SUBJECTIVE

Reports involuntary leakage of small volumes of urine

Nocturia

OBJECTIVE

Bladder distention

High post-void residual volume

Observed involuntary leakage of small volumes of urine

Desired Outcomes/Evaluation Criteria—Client Will:

- Verbalize understanding of causative factors and appropriate interventions for individual situation.
- Demonstrate techniques/behaviors to alleviate/prevent overflow incontinence.
- Void in sufficient amounts with no palpable bladder distention; experience no post-void residuals greater than 50 mL; have no dribbling/overflow.

Actions/Interventions

NURSING PRIORITY NO. 1. To assess causative/contributing factors:

- Review client's history for 1) bladder outlet obstruction (e.g., prostatic hypertrophy, urethral stricture, urinary stones or tumors); 2) nonfunctioning detrusor muscle (i.e., sensory or motor paralytic bladder due to underlying neurologic disease); or 3) atonic bladder that has lost its muscular tone (i.e., chronic overdistention) **to identify potential for/presence of conditions associated with overflow incontinence.**
- Note client's age and gender. **Urinary incontinence due to overflow bladder is more common in men because of the prevalence of obstructive prostate gland enlargement.**
- Review medication regimen **for drugs that can cause/exacerbate retention and overflow incontinence (e.g., anticholinergic**

Information in brackets added by the authors to clarify and enhance the use of nursing diagnoses.

 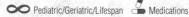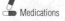

agents, calcium channel blockers, psychotropics, anesthesia, opiates, sedatives, alpha- and beta-blockers, antihistamines, neuroleptics).

NURSING PRIORITY NO. 2. To determine degree of interference/disability:

• Note client reports of symptoms common to overflow incontinence, such as:

    feeling no need to urinate, while simultaneously losing urine

    feeling the urge to urinate, but not being able to

    feeling as though the bladder is never completely empty

    passing a dribbling stream of urine, even after spending a long time at the toilet

    frequently getting up at night to urinate

 • Prepare for/assist with urodynamic testing (e.g., uroflowmetry **to assess urine speed and volume;** cystometrogram **to measure bladder pressure and volume;** bladder scan **to measure retention and/or post-void residual,** leak point pressure, etc.).

NURSING PRIORITY NO. 3. To assist in treating/preventing overflow incontinence:

• Collaborate in treatment of underlying conditions (e.g., medications or surgery for prostatic hypertrophy; use of medication, such as terazosin, to relax urinary sphincter; altering dose/discontinuing medications contributing to retention). **If the underlying cause of the overflow problem can be treated or eliminated, client may be able to return to normal voiding pattern.**

• Demonstrate/instruct client/SO(s) in use of gentle massage over bladder (Credé's maneuver). **May facilitate bladder emptying when cause is detrusor weakness.**

• Implement intermittent or continuous catheterization. **Short-term use may be required while acute conditions are treated (e.g., infection, surgery for enlarged prostate); long-term use is required for permanent conditions (e.g., spinal cord injury/other neuromuscular conditions resulting in permanent bladder dysfunction).**

NURSING PRIORITY NO. 4. To promote wellness (Teaching/Discharge Considerations);

• Establish regular schedule for bladder emptying whether voiding or using catheter.

• Stress need for adequate fluid intake, including use of acidifying fruit juices or ingestion of vitamin C **to discourage bacterial growth and stone formation.**

Information in brackets added by the authors to clarify and enhance the use of nursing diagnoses.

- Instruct client/SO(s) in clean intermittent self-catheterization (CISC) techniques.
- Review signs/symptoms of complications requiring prompt medical evaluation/intervention.

Documentation Focus

ASSESSMENT/REASSESSMENT

- Current elimination pattern/assessment findings and effect on lifestyle/sleep.

PLANNING

- Plan of care and who is involved in planning.
- Teaching plan.

IMPLEMENTATION/EVALUATION

- Response to interventions/teaching and actions performed.
- Attainment/progress toward desired outcome(s).
- Modifications to plan of care.

DISCHARGE PLANNING

- Long-term needs and who is responsible for actions to be taken.
- Specific referrals made.

SAMPLE NURSING OUTCOMES & INTERVENTIONS CLASSIFICATIONS (NOC/NIC)

NOC—Urinary Continence
NIC—Urinary Retention Care

reflex Urinary Incontinence

Taxonomy II: Elimination—Class 1 Urinary System (00018)
[Diagnostic Division: Elimination]
Submitted 1986; Nursing Diagnosis Extension and Classification (NDEC) Revision 1998

Definition: Involuntary loss of urine at somewhat predictable intervals when a specific bladder volume is reached

Related Factors

Tissue damage (e.g., due to radiation cystitis, inflammatory bladder conditions, radical pelvic surgery)

Information in brackets added by the authors to clarify and enhance the use of nursing diagnoses.

 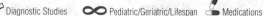
reflex URINARY INCONTINENCE

Neurological impairment above level of sacral/pontine micturition center

Defining Characteristics

SUBJECTIVE

No sensation of bladder fullness/urge to void/voiding

Sensation of urgency without voluntary inhibition of bladder contraction

Sensations associated with full bladder (e.g., sweating, restlessness, abdominal discomfort)

OBJECTIVE

Predictable pattern of voiding

Inability to voluntarily inhibit/initiate voiding

Complete emptying with [brain] lesion above pontine micturition center

Incomplete emptying with [spinal cord] lesion above sacral micturition center

Desired Outcomes/Evaluation Criteria—Client Will:

- Verbalize understanding of condition/contributing factors.
- Establish bladder regimen appropriate for individual situation.
- Demonstrate behaviors/techniques to control condition and prevent complications.
- Urinate at acceptable times and places.

Actions/Interventions

NURSING PRIORITY NO. 1. To assess degree of interference/disability:

- Note condition/disease process as listed in Related Factors (e.g., pelvic cancer/radiation/surgery, central nervous system disorders, stroke, MS, Parkinson's disease, spinal cord injuries, and brain tumors resulting in neurogenic bladder [either hypnotic or spastic]) **affecting bladder storage, emptying, and control.**
- Note whether client experiences any sense of bladder fullness or awareness of incontinence. **Loss of sensation of bladder filling can result in overfilling, inadequate emptying (retention), and dribbling.** (Refer to NDs acute/chronic Urinary Retention; overflow Urinary Incontinence.)
- Review voiding diary, if available, or record frequency and time of urination. Compare timing of voidings, particularly in relation to liquid intake and medications.

Information in brackets added by the authors to clarify and enhance the use of nursing diagnoses.

  Cultural Collaborative 🏠 Community/Home Care

- Measure amount of each voiding **because incontinence often occurs once a specific bladder volume is achieved.**

- Determine actual bladder volume (via bladder scan) in client with incomplete emptying/on scheduled catheterization **when attempting toilet training and to avoid unnecessary catheterizations.**
- Measure/scan post-void residuals/catheterization volumes. **Determines frequency for emptying bladder and reduces incontinence episodes.**
- Evaluate client's ability to manipulate/use urinary collection device or catheter **to determine long-term need for assistance.**
- Refer to urologist/appropriate specialist for testing of bladder capacity and muscle fibers/sphincter control.

NURSING PRIORITY NO. 2. To assist in managing incontinence:

- Collaborate in treatment of underlying cause/management of reflex incontinence.
- Determine availability/use of resources or assistance.
- Involve client/SO/caregiver in developing plan of care to address specific needs.
- Encourage minimum of 1500 to 2000 mL of fluid intake daily. **Regulate liquid intake at prescheduled times (with and between meals) to promote predictable voiding pattern.**
- Restrict fluids 2 to 3 hours before bedtime **to reduce night-time voiding.**
- Instruct client, or take to toilet before the expected time of incontinence, **in an attempt to stimulate the reflex for voiding.**
- Instruct in measures, such as pouring warm water over perineum; running water in sink; stimulating/massaging tissues over bladder, lower abdomen, thighs **to stimulate voiding reflexes.**
- Set alarm to awaken during night to maintain schedule, or use external catheter/external collection device, as appropriate.
- Implement continuous catheterization or intermittent self-catheterization using small-lumen straight catheter, if condition indicates, **to prevent overdistention with consequent infection and detrusor muscle damage.**

NURSING PRIORITY NO. 3. To promote wellness (Teaching/Discharge Considerations):

- Encourage continuation of regular toileting or bladder program **to limit overdistention and related complications.**
- Suggest use of incontinence pads/pants during day and social contact, if appropriate, dependent on client's activity level, amount of urine loss, manual dexterity, and cognitive ability.

Information in brackets added by the authors to clarify and enhance the use of nursing diagnoses.

• Stress importance of perineal care following voiding and fre-quent changing of incontinence pads, if used.

• Encourage limited intake of coffee, tea, and alcohol **because of diuretic effect, which may affect predictability of voiding pattern.**

• Instruct in proper care of catheter and cleaning techniques **to reduce risk of infection.**

• Review signs/symptoms of urinary complications and need for timely medical follow-up care.

Documentation Focus

ASSESSMENT/REASSESSMENT

• Findings/degree of disability and effect on lifestyle.
• Availability of resources/support person.

PLANNING

• Plan of care and who is involved in planning.
• Teaching plan.

IMPLEMENTATION/EVALUATION

• Responses to treatment plan/interventions and actions per-formed.
• Attainment/progress toward desired outcome(s).
• Modifications to plan of care.

DISCHARGE PLANNING

• Long-term needs and who is responsible for actions to be taken.
• Available resources, equipment needs/sources.

SAMPLE NURSING OUTCOMES & INTERVENTIONS CLASSIFICATIONS (NOC/NIC)

NOC—Urinary Continence
NIC—Urinary Bladder Training

---

risk for urge Urinary Incontinence

Taxonomy II: Elimination—Class 1 Urinary System (00022)
[Diagnostic Division: Elimination]
Submitted 1998 (Nursing Diagnosis Extension and Classification [NDEC])

Definition: At risk for an involuntary loss of urine associated with a sudden, strong sensation or urinary urgency

---

Information in brackets added by the authors to clarify and enhance the use of nursing diagnoses.

   Cultural   Collaborative   Community/Home Care

Risk Factors

Effects of medications/caffeine/alcohol

Detrusor hyperreflexia (e.g., from cystitis, urethritis, tumors, renal calculi, CNS disorders above pontine micturition center)

Impaired bladder contractility; involuntary sphincter relaxation

Ineffective toileting habits

Small bladder capacity

> NOTE: A risk diagnosis is not evidenced by signs and symptoms as the problem has not occurred; rather, nursing interventions are directed at prevention.

Desired Outcomes/Evaluation Criteria—Client Will:

- Identify individual risk factors and appropriate interventions.
- Demonstrate behaviors or lifestyle changes to prevent development of problem.

Actions/Interventions

NURSING PRIORITY NO. 1. To assess potential for developing incontinence:

- Identify client with potential for urge incontinence as noted in Risk Factors.
- Note presence of conditions often associated with urgent voiding (e.g., stroke, MS, Parkinson's disease, spinal cord injury, Alzheimer's disease, obesity, pelvic inflammatory disease, abdominal/pelvic surgeries, urinary tract infections) **affecting bladder capacity, pelvic/bladder/urethral musculature tone and/or innervation.**
- Determine use/presence of bladder irritants (e.g., significant intake of alcohol or caffeine, resulting in increased output or concentrated urine).
- Review client's medication regimen (e.g., diuretics, antipsychotic agents, sedatives) **for use of drugs that increase urine production or that may impair client's recognition of/ability to respond to urge to void.**
- Review history for long-standing habits or medical conditions (e.g., frequent voluntary voiding, impaired mobility, use of sedatives) **that may reduce bladder capacity.**
- Note conditions that may affect ability to respond to urge to void (e.g., impaired sensory perception or mobility, cognitive impairment/dementia, central nervous system disorders).

Information in brackets added by the authors to clarify and enhance the use of nursing diagnoses.

• Measure amount of urine voided, especially noting amounts less than 100 mL or greater than 550 mL **to determine bladder capacity and effectiveness of bladder contractions to facilitate emptying.**

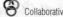 • Prepare for/assist with appropriate testing (e.g., urinalysis, non-invasive bladder scanning, cystometrogram) **to evaluate voiding pattern, identify potential functional concerns.**

NURSING PRIORITY NO. 2. To prevent occurrence of problem:

 • Assist in treatment of underlying conditions that may contribute to urge incontinence.

 • Ascertain client's awareness/concerns about developing problem and whether lifestyle might be affected (e.g., daily living activites, socialization, sexual patterns).

 • Regulate liquid intake at prescheduled times (with and between meals) **to promote predictable voiding pattern.**

 • Establish schedule for voiding (habit training) based on client's usual voiding pattern.

 • Provide assistance/devices, as indicated, for clients who are mobility impaired (e.g., providing means of summoning assistance; placing bedside commode, urinal, or bedpan within client's reach).

 • Encourage regular pelvic floor strengthening exercises/Kegel exercises.

NURSING PRIORITY NO. 3. To promote wellness (Teaching/Discharge Considerations):

 • Provide information to client/SO(s) about potential for urge incontinence and lifestyle measures to prevent/limit incontinence:

Recommend limiting intake of coffee, tea, and alcohol **because of their irritating effect on the bladder.**

Suggest wearing loose-fitting or especially adapted clothing **to facilitate response to voiding urge.**

• Emphasize importance of perineal care after each voiding **to reduce risk of ascending infection.**

Documentation Focus

ASSESSMENT/REASSESSMENT

• Individual findings, including specific risk factors and pattern of voiding.

PLANNING

• Plan of care/interventions and who is involved in planning.
• Teaching plan.

Information in brackets added by the authors to clarify and enhance the use of nursing diagnoses.

 Cultural   Collaborative   Community/Home Care

IMPLEMENTATION/EVALUATION

- Response to interventions/teaching and actions performed.
- Attainment/progress toward desired outcome(s).
- Modifications to plan of care.

DISCHARGE PLANNING

- Discharge needs/referrals and who is responsible for actions to be taken.
- Specific referrals made.

SAMPLE NURSING OUTCOMES & INTERVENTIONS CLASSIFICATIONS (NOC/NIC)

NOC—Urinary Continence
NIC—Urinary Habit Training

stress Urinary Incontinence

Taxonomy II: Elimination—Class 1 Urinary System (00017)
[Diagnostic Division: Elimination]
Submitted 1986; Revised 2006

Definition: Sudden leakage of urine with activities that increase intra-abdominal pressure

Related Factors

Degenerative changes in pelvic muscles; weak pelvic muscles
High intra-abdominal pressure [e.g., obesity, gravid uterus]
Intrinsic urethral sphincter deficiency

Defining Characteristics

SUBJECTIVE

Reported involuntary leakage of small amounts of urine: on exertion [e.g., lifting, impact aerobics]; with sneezing, laughing, or coughing; in the absence of detrusor contraction/an overdistended bladder

OBJECTIVE

Observed involuntary leakage of small amounts of urine: on exertion [e.g., lifting, impact aerobics]; with sneezing, laughing, or coughing; in the absence of detrusor contraction/an overdistended bladder

---

Information in brackets added by the authors to clarify and enhance the use of nursing diagnoses.

 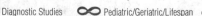

Desired Outcomes/Evaluation Criteria—Client Will:

- Verbalize understanding of condition and interventions for bladder conditioning.
- Demonstrate behaviors/techniques to strengthen pelvic floor musculature.
- Remain continent even with increased intra-abdominal pressure.

Actions/Interventions

NURSING PRIORITY NO. 1. To assess causative/contributing factors:

- Identify physiological causes of increased intra-abdominal pressure (e.g., obesity, gravid uterus) and contributing history such as multiple births; bladder or pelvic trauma/fractures; surgery (e.g., radical prostatectomy, bladder/other pelvic surgeries that may damage sphincter muscles); participation in high-impact athletic activities, repeated heavy lifting. **Note: Female athletes engaged in high-impact sports/soldiers on field exercises are at increased risk for stress incontinence.**
- Assess for urine loss (usually small amount) with coughing/sneezing or sports activities, relaxed pelvic musculature and support, noting inability to start/stop stream while voiding, bulging of perineum when bearing down.
- Review client's medications for those that may cause/exacerbate stress incontinence (e.g., alpha-blockers, angiotension-converting ezyme (ACE) inhibitors, loop diuretics).

NURSING PRIORITY NO. 2. To assess degree of interference/disability:

- Observe voiding patterns, time and amount voided, and stimulus provoking incontinence. Review voiding diary, if available.
- Prepare for/assist with appropriate testing (e.g., urinalysis, non-invasive bladder scanning, cystogram, urodynamics, leak point pressure, etc.) **to evaluate functional concerns.**
- Determine effect on lifestyle (including daily activities, participation in sports/exercise and recreation, socialization, sexuality, and self-esteem).
- Ascertain methods of self-management (e.g., regularly timed voiding, limiting liquid intake, using undergarment protection).
- Assess for concomitant urge or functional incontinence, noting whether bladder irritability, reduced bladder capacity, or voluntary overdistention is present. (Refer to appropriate NDs.)

NURSING PRIORITY NO. 3. To assist in treating/preventing incontinence:

- Suggest/implement self-help techniques:

Information in brackets added by the authors to clarify and enhance the use of nursing diagnoses.

 Cultural　 Collaborative　 Community/Home Care

Practice timed voidings (e.g., every 3 hours during the day) **to keep bladder relatively empty.**

Void before physical exertion, such as exercise/sports activites, heavy lifting, **to reduce potential for incontinence.**

Encourage weight loss, as indicated, **to reduce pressure on pelvic organs.**

Suggest limiting use of coffee, tea, and alcohol **because of diuretic effect.**

Recommend regular pelvic floor strengthening exercises (Kegel exercises).

Suggest starting and stopping stream 2 or 3 times during voiding **to isolate muscles involved in voiding process for exercise training.**

Incorporate "bent-knee sit-ups" into exercise program **to increase abdominal muscle tone.**

Restrict intake 2 to 3 hours prior to bedtime **to decrease incontinence during sleep.**

- Assist with medical treatment of underlying urological condition, as indicated (e.g., surgery to reposition bladder/strengthen pelvic musclulature; use of vaginal cones; electrical stimulation; biofeedback; medications [e.g., tricylic antidepressants, hormone replacement therapy]).

NURSING PRIORITY NO. 4. To promote wellness (Teaching/Discharge Considerations):

- Discuss participation in/incontinence management for activities, such as heavy lifting, impact aerobics, **that increase intra-abdominal pressure.** Substitute swimming, bicycling, or low-impact exercise.

- Refer to weight-loss program/support group **when obesity is a contributing factor.**

- Suggest use of incontinence pads/pants, as needed. Consider client's activity level, amount of urine loss, physical size, manual dexterity, and cognitive ability **to determine specific product choices best suited to individual situation and needs.**

- Stress importance of perineal care following voiding and frequent changing of incontinence pads **to prevent irritation and infection.** Recommend application of oil-based emollient **to protect skin from irritation.**

- Review use of sympathomimetic drugs, if prescribed, **to improve resting tone of the bladder neck and proximal urethra.**

Information in brackets added by the authors to clarify and enhance the use of nursing diagnoses.

Diagnostic Studies   Pediatric/Geriatric/Lifespan   Medications   **743**

Documentation Focus

ASSESSMENT/REASSESSMENT

- Findings/pattern of incontinence and physical factors present.
- Effect on lifestyle and self-esteem.
- Client understanding of condition.

PLANNING

- Plan of care and who is involved in the planning.
- Teaching plan.

IMPLEMENTATION/EVALUATION

- Responses to interventions/teaching, actions performed, and changes that are identified.
- Attainment/progress toward desired outcome(s).
- Modifications to plan of care.

DISCHARGE PLANNING

- Long-term needs/referrals and who is responsible for specific actions.
- Specific referrals made.

SAMPLE NURSING OUTCOMES & INTERVENTIONS CLASSIFICATIONS (NOC/NIC)

NOC—Urinary Continence
NIC—Pelvic Muscle Exercise

total Urinary Incontinence

Taxonomy II: Elimination—Class 1 Urinary System (00021)
[Diagnostic Division: Elimination]
Submitted 1986

Definition: Continuous and unpredictable loss of urine

Related Factors

Neuropathy preventing transmission of reflex [signals to the reflex arc] indicating bladder fullness
Neurological dysfunction [e.g., cerebral lesions]
Independent contraction of detrusor reflex
Trauma/disease affecting spinal cord nerves [destruction of sensory or motor neurons below the injury level]
Anatomic (fistula)

Information in brackets added by the authors to clarify and enhance the use of nursing diagnoses.

 Cultural Collaborative Community/Home Care

Defining Characteristics

SUBJECTIVE

Constant flow of urine at unpredictable times without uninhibited bladder contractions/spasm or distention
Nocturia
Lack of bladder/perineal filling [awareness]
Unawareness of incontinence

OBJECTIVE

Unsuccessful incontinence refractory treatments

Desired Outcomes/Evaluation Criteria—Client/Caregiver Will:

* Verbalize awareness of causative/contributing factors.
* Establish bladder regimen for individual situation.
* Demonstrate behaviors, techniques to manage condition and to prevent complications.
* Manage incontinence so that social functioning is regained/maintained.

Actions/Interventions

NURSING PRIORITY NO. 1. To assess causative/contributing factors:

* Identify client with condition(s) causing actual/potential for total incontinence as listed in Related Factors: High-risk persons include frail elderly; women; those with brain lesions (e.g., stroke, tumors, trauma); spinal cord injury (e.g., quadraplegia, paraplegia, herniated disc, pelvic crush injury); chronic neurologic diseases (e.g., MS, Parkinson's disease); genitourinary surgery/trauma (e.g., childbirth, radical hysterectomy, perineal resection, prostatectomy); peripheral neuropathy (e.g., diabetes, AIDS, poliomyelitis); and lifestyle issues (e.g., certain medications, fluid intake, and mobility limitations).
* Be aware of/note effect of global neurological impairment, neuromuscular trauma from surgery/childbirth/radiation; or presence of fistula. **Conditions causing injury to nerves supplying the bladder are associated with loss of integrity of lower urinary tract function.**
* Determine if client is aware of incontinence. **Cognitive, developmental issues, and/or medical conditions can impair client's awareness and sensory perception of voiding need/process and incontinence.**

Information in brackets added by the authors to clarify and enhance the use of nursing diagnoses.

 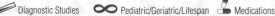

total URINARY INCONTINENCE

- Check for perineal sensation and fecal impaction **to determine whether sensation and reflexes are impaired when neurologic condition is present.**
- Determine concomitant chronic retention (e.g., palpate bladder, scan/catheterize for urine volume and residual). **Retention may be associated with outlet obstruction, urge, and overflow incontinence.**
- Assess for continuous involuntary loss of urine at all times and in all positions. **Usually associated with urinary tract fistula or genital malformation.**
- Carry out/assist with procedures/tests (e.g., post-void residual, urine flowmetry, pressure flow study, cystoscopy, cystogram) **to establish diagnosis/identify needed interventions.**

NURSING PRIORITY NO. 2. To assess degree of interference/disability:

- Determine client's particular symptoms (e.g., continuous dribbling superimposed upon an otherwise normal voiding pattern, or high-volume urine loss that replaces any detectable pattern of bladder filling/storage/voiding). **Influences choice of interventions.**
- Have client/care giver keep an incontinence chart. Note times of voiding and incontinence. **Determines pattern of urination and whether there is any control.**
- 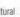 Review history for past interventions regarding alterations in urinary elimination **to ascertain cause for continence failure (e.g., client unable to sustain behavioral management of bladder training program, or medical conditions do not allow for success in voiding efforts).**
- Evaluate client's potential for bladder training/voiding managment program. **Dependent on diagnosed type of incontinence (functional, overflow, reflex, urge).**
- 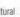 Ascertain effect of condition on lifestyle and self-esteem.

NURSING PRIORITY NO. 3. To assist in preventing/managing incontinence:

- Collaborate in treatment of underlying conditions (e.g., neurologic disorders, prostate problems, chronic urinary tract infections, psychiatric disorders) **that contribute to incontinence.**
- 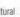 Implement bladder training and/or incontinence management, as indicated:
  Provide ready access to bathroom, commode, bedpan, or urinal.
  Encourage adequate fluid intake and regulate time of intake.
  Establish voiding/bladder emptying schedule.

Information in brackets added by the authors to clarify and enhance the use of nursing diagnoses.

  Cultural   Collaborative   Community/Home Care

Use condom catheter or other external device if tolerated during the day and absorptive pads during the night if external device is not tolerated.

Implement intermittent or continuous catheterization appropriate to client's condition (may be short- or long-term).

Refer to NDs functional, stress, urge, reflex, overflow Urinary Incontinence for related interventions.

Administer medications, as indicated.

• Discuss/prepare for surgical intervention depending on underlying cause (e.g., to treat urethral hypermobility, to suspend bladder, repair vaginal walls, remove obstruction, provide artificial sphinter or bladder reservoir).

NURSING PRIORITY NO. 4. To promote wellness (Teaching/Discharge Considerations):

• Assist client/caregiver to identify regular time for bladder program **to establish a predictable elimination program.**

• Suggest use of incontinence pads/adult briefs, as indicated (e.g., during social contacts), **for extra protection and to enhance confidence.**

• Stress importance of pericare after each voiding (using alcohol-free products) and application of oil-based emollient **to protect the skin from irritation.**

• Instruct in proper care of catheter and cleaning technique **to prevent infection.**

• Recommend use of silicone catheter **when long-term/continuous placement is indicated after other measures/bladder training have failed.**

• Encourage self-monitoring of catheter patency and avoidance of reflux of urine. **Reduces risk of infection.**

• Suggest intake of acidifying juices **to discourage bacterial growth/reduce incidence of infection.**

Documentation Focus

ASSESSMENT/REASSESSMENT

• Current elimination pattern.
• Assessment findings including effect on lifestyle and self-esteem.

PLANNING

• Plan of care/interventions, including who is involved in planning.
• Teaching plan.

Information in brackets added by the authors to clarify and enhance the use of nursing diagnoses.

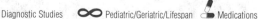

Diagnostic Studies   Pediatric/Geriatric/Lifespan   Medications   **747**

IMPLEMENTATION/EVALUATION

- Response to interventions/teaching and actions performed.
- Attainment/progress toward desired outcome(s).
- Modifications to plan of care.

DISCHARGE PLANNING

- Discharge plan/long-term needs and who is responsible for actions to be taken.
- Specific referrals made.

SAMPLE NURSING OUTCOMES & INTERVENTIONS CLASSIFICATIONS (NOC/NIC)

NOC—Urinary Continence
NIC—Urinary Incontinence Care

urge Urinary Incontinence

Taxonomy II: Elimination—Class 1 Urinary System (00019)
[Diagnostic Division: Elimination]
Submitted 1986; Revised 2006

Definition: Involuntary passage of urine occurring soon after a strong sense of urgency to void

Related Factors

Decreased bladder capacity
Bladder infection; atrophic urethritis/vaginitis
Alcohol/caffeine intake; [increased fluids]
Use of diuretics
Fecal impaction
Detrusor hyperactivity with impaired bladder contractility

Defining Characteristics

SUBJECTIVE

Reports: urinary urgency; involuntary loss of urine with bladder contractions/spasms; inability to reach toilet in time to avoid urine loss

OBJECTIVE

Observed inability to reach toilet in time to avoid urine loss

---

Information in brackets added by the authors to clarify and enhance the use of nursing diagnoses.

  Cultural Collaborative Community/Home Care

Desired Outcomes/Evaluation Criteria—Client Will:

- Verbalize understanding of condition.
- Demonstrate behaviors/techniques to control/correct situation.
- Report increase in interval between urge and involuntary loss of urine.
- Void every 3 to 4 hours in individually appropriate amounts.

Actions/Interventions

NURSING PRIORITY NO. 1. To assess causative/contributing factors:

- Note presence of conditions often associated with urgent voiding (e.g., stroke, MS, Parkinson's disease, spinal cord injury, Alzheimer's disease, obesity; pelvic inflammatory disease, abdominal/pelvic surgeries, recent/lengthy use of indwelling urinary catheter) **affecting bladder capacity, pelvic/ bladder/urethral musculature tone, and/or innervation.**
- Ask client about urgency (more than just normal desire to void). Urgency **(also sometimes called overactive bladder syndrome) is a sudden compelling need to void that is difficult to defer and may be accompanied by leaking/incontinence.**
- Note factors that may affect ability to respond to urge to void in timely manner (e.g., impaired mobility, debilitation, sensory/perceptual impairments).
- Review client's medications/substance use (e.g., diuretics, antipsychotic agents, sedatives, caffeine, alcohol) **for agents that increase urine production or exert a bladder irritant effect.**
- Assess for signs and symptoms of bladder infection (e.g., cloudy, odorous urine; burning pain with voiding; bacteriuria) **associated with acute, painful urgency symptoms.**
- Prepare for/assist with appropriate testing (e.g., pre-/post-void bladder scanning; pelvic examination for strictures; impaired perineal sensation or musculature; urinalysis; uroflometry voiding pressures; cystoscopy; cystometrogram) **to determine anatomic and functional status of bladder and urethra.**
- Assess for concomitant stress or functional incontinence. **Older women often have a mix of stress and urge incontinence, while individuals with dementia or disabling neurologic disorders tend to have urge and functional incontinence.** (Refer to NDs stress/functional Urinary Incontinence for additional interventions.)

Information in brackets added by the authors to clarify and enhance the use of nursing diagnoses.

NURSING PRIORITY NO. 2. To assess degree of interference/disability:

- Record frequency of voiding during a typical 24-hour period.
- Discuss degree of urgency and length of warning time between initial urge and loss of urine.
- Ascertain if client experiences triggers (e.g., sound of running water, putting hands in water, seeing a restroom sign, "key-in-the-lock" syndrome, etc.).
- Measure amount of urine voided, especially noting amounts less than 100 mL or greater than 550 mL. **Bladder capacity may be impaired or bladder contractions facilitating emptying may be ineffective.** (Refer to ND [acute/chronic] Urinary Retention.)
- Ascertain effect on lifestyle (including daily activities, socialization, sexuality) and self-esteem.

NURSING PRIORITY NO. 3. To assist in treating/preventing incontinence:

- Collaborate in treating underlying cause and/or managing urge symptoms.
- Administer medications as indicated (e.g., antibiotic for urinary tract infection, or antimuscarinics [e.g., oxybutynin, tolterodine]) **to reduce voiding frequency and urgency by blocking overactive detrusor contractions.**
- Provide assistance/devices, as indicated, for client who is mobility impaired (e.g., provide means of summoning assistance; place bedside commode, urinal, or bedpan within client's reach).
- Offer assistance to cognitively impaired client (e.g., prompt client/or take to bathroom on regularly timed schedule) **to reduce frequency of incontinence episodes/promote comfort.**
- Recommend lifestyle changes:
  Adjust fluid intake to 1500 to 2000 mL/day. Regulate liquid intake at prescheduled times (with and between meals) and limit fluids 2–3 hours prior to bedtime **to promote predictable voiding pattern and limit nocturia.**
  Modify diet as indicated (e.g., reduce caffeine, citrus juices, spicy foods, etc.) **to reduce bladder irritation.**
  Manage bowel elimination **to prevent urinary problems associated with constipation/fecal impaction.**
- Encourage client to participate in behavioral interventions, if able:
  Establish voiding schedule (habit and bladder training) based on client's usual voiding pattern and gradually increase time interval.

Information in brackets added by the authors to clarify and enhance the use of nursing diagnoses.

  Cultural 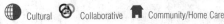 Collaborative Community/Home Care

Recommend consciously delaying voiding by using distraction (e.g., slow deep breaths); self-statements (e.g., "I can wait"); and contracting pelvic muscles when exposed to triggers. **Behavioral techniques for urge suppression.**

Encourage regular pelvic floor strengthening exercises/Kegel exercises as indicated by specific condition.

Instruct client to tighten pelvic floor muscles before arising from bed. **Helps prevent loss of urine as abdominal pressure changes.**

Suggest starting and stopping stream two or more times during voiding **to isolate muscles involved in voiding process for exercise training.**

• Refer to specialists/treament program, as indicated, for additional/specialized interventions (e.g., biofeedback, use of vaginal cones, electronic stimulation therapy, possible surgical interventions).

NURSING PRIORITY NO. 4. To promote wellness (Teaching/Discharge Considerations):

• Encourage comfort measures (e.g., use of incontinence pads/undergarments, wearing loose-fitting or especially adapted clothing) **to prepare for/manage urge incontinence symptoms over the long term, and enhance sense of security/confidence in abilities to be socially active.**

• Emphasize importance of regular perineal care **to prevent skin irritation/incontinence-related dermatitis.**

• Identify signs/symptoms indicating urinary complications and need for timely medical follow-up care.

Documentation Focus

ASSESSMENT/REASSESSMENT

• Individual findings, including pattern of incontinence, effect on lifestyle, and self-esteem.

PLANNING

• Plan of care/interventions and who is involved in planning.
• Teaching plan.

IMPLEMENTATION/EVALUATION

• Response to interventions/teaching and actions performed.
• Attainment/progress toward desired outcome(s).
• Modifications to plan of care.

Information in brackets added by the authors to clarify and enhance the use of nursing diagnoses.

DISCHARGE PLANNING

- Discharge needs/referrals and who is responsible for actions to be taken.
- Specific referrals made.

SAMPLE NURSING OUTCOMES & INTERVENTIONS CLASSIFICATIONS (NOC/NIC)

NOC—Urinary Continence
NIC—Urinary Habit Training

[acute/chronic] Urinary Retention

Taxonomy II: Elimination—Class 1 Urinary System (00023)
[Diagnostic Division: Elimination]
Submitted 1986

Definition: Incomplete emptying of the bladder

Related Factors

High urethral pressure
Inhibition of reflex arc
Strong sphincter; blockage [e.g., benign prostatic hypertrophy–BPH, perineal swelling]
[Habituation of reflex arc]
[Infections; neurological diseases/trauma]
[Use of medications with side effect of retention (e.g., atropine, belladonna, psychotropics, antihistamines, opiates)]

Defining Characteristics

SUBJECTIVE

Sensation of bladder fullness
Dribbling
Dysuria

OBJECTIVE

Bladder distention
Small/frequent voiding; absence of urine output
Residual urine [150 mL or more]
Overflow incontinence
[Reduced stream]

Information in brackets added by the authors to clarify and enhance the use of nursing diagnoses.

Desired Outcomes/Evaluation Criteria—Client Will:

- Verbalize understanding of causative factors and appropriate interventions for individual situation.
- Demonstrate techniques/behaviors to alleviate/prevent retention.
- Void in sufficient amounts with no palpable bladder distention; experience no post-void residuals greater than 50 mL; have no dribbling/overflow.

Actions/Interventions

ACUTE

NURSING PRIORITY NO. 1. To assess causative/contributing factors:

- Note presence of pathological conditions (e.g., urinary tract infection, neurological disorders/trauma, stone formation, prostate hypertrophy).
- Investigate reports of sudden loss of ability to pass urine/great difficulty passing urine, pain with urination, blood in urine. **May indicate urinary tract infection or obstruction.**
- Obtain urine/review results of urinalysis (e.g., presence of red/white blood cells, nitrates, glucose, bacteria) and culture, as indicated, **to determine presence of treatable condition.**
- Review medications, noting those that can cause/exacerbate retention (e.g., psychotropics, anesthesia, opiates, sedatives, alpha- and beta-blockers, anticholinergics, antihistamines, neuroleptics).
- Examine for fecal impaction, surgical site swelling, postpartal edema, vaginal or rectal packing, enlarged prostate, or other factors (e.g., recent removal of indwelling catheter with urethral swelling/spasm) **that may produce a blockage of the urethra.**
- Determine anxiety level (e.g., **client may be too embarrassed to void in presence of others**).

NURSING PRIORITY NO. 2. To determine degree of interference/disability:

- Ascertain whether client has sensation of bladder fullness, and determine level of discomfort. **Sensation and discomfort can vary, depending on underlying cause of retention.**
- Determine if there has been any significant urine output in the last 6 to 8 hours; presence of frequent/small voidings, and whether dribbling (overflow) is occurring.
- Palpate height of the bladder.

Information in brackets added by the authors to clarify and enhance the use of nursing diagnoses.

 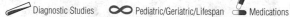

- Note recent amount/type of fluid intake.
- Prepare for/assist with urodynamic testing (e.g., cystometro-gram **to measure bladder pressure and volume,** bladder scan **to measure retention volume and/or post-void residual,** leak point pressure).

NURSING PRIORITY NO. 3. To assist in treating/preventing retention:

- Relieve pain by administering appropriate medications and measures **to reduce swelling/treat underlying cause.**
- Assist client to sit upright on bedpan/commode or stand **to provide functional position of voiding.**
- Provide privacy.
- Use ice techniques, spirits of wintergreen, stroking inner thigh, running water in sink or warm water over perineum **to stimulate reflex arc.**
- Remove blockage if possible (e.g., vaginal packing, bowel impaction). Prepare for more aggressive intervention (e.g., surgery/prostatectomy).
- Catheterize with intermittent or indwelling catheter **to resolve acute retention.**
- Drain bladder with straight catheter per agency protocol. **References are mixed as to need for fractional drainage in increments of 200 mL at a time to prevent possibility of bladder spasm, syncope/hypotension.**
- Reduce recurrences by controlling causative/contributing factors when possible (e.g., ice to perineum **to prevent swelling,** use of stool softeners/laxatives, change of medication/dosage).

NURSING PRIORITY NO. 4. To promote wellness (Teaching/Discharge Considerations):

- Encourage client to report problems immediately **so treatment can be instituted promptly.**
- Emphasize need for adequate fluid intake.

CHRONIC

NURSING PRIORITY NO. 1. To assess causative/contributing factors:

- Review medical history for diagnoses, such as congenital defects; neurological disorders (e.g., MS, polio); prostatic hypertrophy/surgery; birth canal injury/scarring; spinal cord injury with lower motor neuron injury **that may suggest detrusor muscle atrophy/dysfunction; or chronic overdis-tention because of outlet obstruction.**
- Determine presence of weak or absent sensory and/or motor impulses (as with stroke, spinal injury, or diabetes).
- Evaluate customary fluid intake.

Information in brackets added by the authors to clarify and enhance the use of nursing diagnoses.

   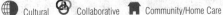 Cultural   Collaborative   Community/Home Care

• Assess for effects of psychotropics, antihistamines, atropine, belladonna, and so forth.

NURSING PRIORITY NO. 2. To determine degree of interference/disability:

• Measure amount voided and post-void residuals.
• Determine frequency and timing of voiding, and/or dribbling.
• Note size and force of urinary stream.
• Palpate height of bladder.
• Determine presence of bladder spasms.
• Ascertain effect of condition on functioning/lifestyle.
 • Prepare for/assist with urodynamic testing (e.g., uroflowmetry **to assess urine speed and volume,** cystometrogram **to measure bladder pressure and volume,** bladder scan **to measure retention and/or post-void residual,** leak point pressure).

NURSING PRIORITY NO. 3. To assist in treating/preventing retention:

• Collaborate in treatment of underlying conditions.
• Recommend client void on frequent, timed schedule **to maintain low bladder pressures.**
• Maintain consistent fluid intake **to wash out bacteria/avoid infections and limit stone formation.**
• Adjust fluid amount and timing, if indicated, **to prevent bladder distention.**
• Demonstrate and instruct client/SO(s) in use of Credé's maneuver **to facilitate emptying of the bladder.**
• Encourage client to use Valsalva's maneuver if appropriate **to increase intra-abdominal pressure.**
• Establish regular voiding/self-catheterization program **to prevent reflux and increased renal pressures.**
• Refer for consideration of advanced/research-based therapies (e.g., implanted sacral/tibial/pelvic electrical stimulating device) **for long-term management of retention.**

NURSING PRIORITY NO. 4. To promote wellness (Teaching/Discharge Considerations):

• Establish regular schedule for bladder emptying whether voiding or using catheter.
• Stress need for adequate fluid intake, including use of acidifying fruit juices or ingestion of vitamin C, **to discourage bacterial growth and stone formation.**
• Instruct client/SO(s) in clean intermittent self-catheterization (CISC) techniques.

Information in brackets added by the authors to clarify and enhance the use of nursing diagnoses.

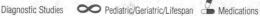

impaired spontaneous VENTILATION

- Review signs/symptoms of complications requiring medical evaluation/intervention.

Documentation Focus

ASSESSMENT/REASSESSMENT

- Individual findings, including nature of problem, degree of impairment, and whether client is incontinent.

PLANNING

- Plan of care and who is involved in planning.
- Teaching plan.

IMPLEMENTATION/EVALUATION

- Response to interventions.
- Attainment/progress toward desired outcome(s).
- Modifications to plan of care.

DISCHARGE PLANNING

- Long-term needs/referrals and who is responsible for actions to be taken.
- Specific referrals made.

SAMPLE NURSING OUTCOMES & INTERVENTIONS CLASSIFICATIONS (NOC/NIC)

NOC—Urinary Elimination
NIC—Urinary Retention Care

impaired spontaneous Ventilation

Taxonomy II: Activity/Rest—Class 2 Cardiovascular/Pulmonary Response (00033)
[Diagnostic Division: Respiration]
Submitted 1992

Definition: Decreased energy reserves results in an individual's inability to maintain breathing adequate to support life

Related Factors

Metabolic factors; [hypermetabolic state (e.g., infection), nutritional deficits/depletion of energy stores]
Respiratory muscle fatigue
[Airway size/resistance; inadequate secretion management]

Information in brackets added by the authors to clarify and enhance the use of nursing diagnoses.

  Cultural Collaborative 🏠 Community/Home Care

Defining Characteristics

SUBJECTIVE

Dyspnea
Apprehension

OBJECTIVE

Increased metabolic rate
Increased heart rate
Increased restlessness; decreased cooperation
Increased use of accessory muscles
Decreased tidal volume
Decreased Po_2/Sao_2; increased Pco_2

Desired Outcomes/Evaluation Criteria—Client Will:

- Reestablish/maintain effective respiratory pattern via ventilator with absence of retractions/use of accessory muscles, cyanosis, or other signs of hypoxia; and with ABGs/SaO_2 within acceptable range.
- Participate in efforts to wean (as appropriate) within individual ability.

Caregiver Will:

- Demonstrate behaviors necessary to maintain respiratory function.

Actions/Interventions

NURSING PRIORITY NO. 1. To determine degree of impairment:

- Identify client with actual or impending respiratory failure (e.g., apnea or slow, shallow breathing; obtudation with need for airway protection; respiratory distress with altered mentation).
- Assess spontaneous respiratory pattern, noting rate, depth, rhythm, symmetry of chest movement, use of accessory muscles **to measure work of breathing.**
- Auscultate breath sounds, noting presence/absence and equality of breath sounds, adventitious breath sounds.
- Evaluate ABGs and/or pulse oximetry and capnograpy **to determine presence/degree of arterial hypoxemia (<55%) and hypercapnea (CO_2 >45%), resulting in impaired ventilation requiring ventilatory support.**
- Obtain/review results of pulmonary function studies (e.g., lung volumes, **inspiratory and expiratory pressures, and**

Information in brackets added by the authors to clarify and enhance the use of nursing diagnoses.

 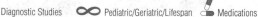

forced vital capacity), as appropriate, to assess presence/degree of respiratory insufficiency.

 • Investigate etiology of respiratory failure **to determine ventilation needs and most appropriate type of ventilatory support.**

• Review serial chest x-rays and imaging MRI/CT scans results **to diagnose disorder and monitor response to treatment.**

 • Note response to respiratory therapy (e.g., bronchodilators, supplemental oxygen, IPPB treatments).

NURSING PRIORITY NO. 2. To provide/maintain ventilatory support:

 • Assist with implementation of ventilatory support, as indicated (e.g., endotracheal/tracheal intubation with mechanical ventilation **to support compromised ventilation.**)

• Observe overall breathing pattern, distinguishing between spontaneous respirations and ventilator breaths.

• Count client's respirations for one full minute and compare to desired/ventilator set rate.

• Verify that client's respirations are in phase with the ventilator. **Decreases work of breathing, maximizes O_2 delivery.**

• Inflate tracheal/endotracheal tube cuff properly using minimal leak/occlusive technique. Check cuff inflation every 4 to 8 hours and whenever cuff is deflated/reinflated **to prevent risk associated with underinflation/overinflation.**

• Check tubing for obstruction (e.g., kinking or accumulation of water). Drain tubing as indicated; avoid draining toward client, or back into the reservoir **resulting in contamination/providing medium for growth of bacteria.**

• Check ventilator alarms for proper functioning. Do not turn off alarms, even for suctioning. Remove from ventilator and ventilate manually if source of ventilator alarm cannot be quickly identified and rectified. Verify that alarms can be heard in the nurses' station by care providers.

• Assess ventilator settings routinely and readjust as indicated according to client's primary disease and results of diagnostic testing.

• Verify that oxygen line is in proper outlet/tank; monitor inline oxygen analyzer or perform periodic oxygen analysis.

• Verify tidal volume set to volume needed for individual situation, and proper functioning of spirometer, bellows, or computer readout of delivered volume. Note alterations from desired volume delivery **to determine alteration in lung compliance or leakage through machine/around tube cuff (if used).**

• Monitor airway pressure **for developing complications/equipment problems.**

• Monitor inspiratory and expiratory (I:E) ratio.

Information in brackets added by the authors to clarify and enhance the use of nursing diagnoses.

      Cultural   Collaborative   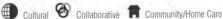 Community/Home Care

- Promote maximal ventilation of alveoli; check sigh rate intervals (usually 11/2 to 2 times tidal volume). **Reduces risk of atelectasis, helps mobilize secretions.**
- Note inspired humidity and temperature; maintain hydration **to liquefy secretions, facilitating removal.**
- Auscultate breath sounds periodically. Investigate frequent crackles or rhonchi that do not clear with coughing/suctioning—**suggestive of developing complications (atelectasis, pneumonia, acute bronchospasm, pulmonary edema).**
- Suction as needed **to clear secretions/maintain airway.**
- Note changes in chest symmetry. **May indicate improper placement of ET tube, development of barotrauma.**
- Keep resuscitation bag at bedside and ventilate manually whenever indicated (e.g., if client is removed from ventilator or troubleshooting equipment problems).
- 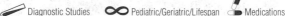 Administer sedation as required **to synchronize respirations and reduce work of breathing/energy expenditure, as indicated.**
- Administer and monitor response to medications that promote airway patency and gas exchange.

NURSING PRIORITY NO. 3. To prepare for/assist with weaning process if appropriate:

- Determine physical/psychological readiness to wean, including specific respiratory parameters, absence of infection/cardiac failure, client alert and/or able to sustain spontaneous respiration, nutritional status sufficient to maintain work of breathing.
- Explain weaning activities/techniques, individual plan, and expectations. **Reduces fear of unknown.**
- Elevate head of bed/place in orthopedic chair, if possible, or position **to alleviate dyspnea and to facilitate oxygenation.**
- Assist client in "taking control" of breathing if weaning is attempted or ventilatory support is interrupted during procedure/activity.
- Coach client to take slower, deeper breaths, practice abdominal/pursed-lip breathing, assume position of comfort, and use relaxation techniques **to maximize respiratory function.**
- Assist client to practice effective coughing, secretion management.
- Provide quiet environment, calm approach, undivided attention of nurse. **Promotes relaxation, decreasing energy/oxygen requirements.**
- Involve family/SO(s) as appropriate. Provide diversional activity. **Helps client focus on something other than breathing.**

Information in brackets added by the authors to clarify and enhance the use of nursing diagnoses.

- Instruct client in use of energy-saving techniques during care activities **to limit oxygen consumption/fatigue.**
- Acknowledge and provide ongoing encouragement for client's efforts. Communicate hope for successful weaning response (even partial). **Enhances commitment to continue activity, maximizing outcomes.**

NURSING PRIORITY NO. 4. To prepare for discharge on ventilator when indicated:

 • Ascertain plan for discharge placement (e.g., return home, short-term/permanent placement in long-term care).

 • Determine specific equipment needs. Identify resources for equipment needs/maintenance and arrange for delivery prior to client discharge.

 • Review layout of home, noting size of rooms, doorways, placement of furniture, number/type of electrical outlets, **to identify specific safety needs.**

 • Obtain no-smoking signs to be posted in home. Encourage family members to refrain from smoking.

 • Have family/SO(s) notify utilities companies and fire department about ventilator in home.

 • Review and provide written or audiovisual materials regarding proper ventilator management, maintenance, and safety **for reference in home setting, enhancing client's/SO's knowledge and level of comfort.**

 • Demonstrate airway management techniques and proper equipment cleaning practices.

 • Instruct SO(s)/caregivers in other pulmonary physiotherapy measures as indicated (e.g., chest physiotherapy).

 • Allow sufficient opportunity for SO(s)/caregivers to practice new skills. Role play potential crisis situations **to enhance confidence in ability to handle client's needs.**

 • Identify signs/symptoms requiring prompt medical evaluation/intervention. **Timely treatment may prevent progression of problem.**

 • Provide positive feedback and encouragement for efforts of SO(s)/caregivers. **Promotes continuation of desired behaviors.**

 • List names and phone numbers for identified contact persons/resources. **Round-the-clock availability reduces sense of isolation and enhances likelihood of obtaining appropriate information/assistance when needed.**

NURSING PRIORITY NO. 5. To promote wellness (Teaching/Discharge Considerations):

Information in brackets added by the authors to clarify and enhance the use of nursing diagnoses.

   Cultural   Collaborative   Community/Home Care

- Discuss impact of specific activities on respiratory status and problem solve solutions to maximize weaning effort.
- Engage client in specialized exercise program **to enhance respiratory muscle strength and general endurance.**
- Protect client from sources of infection (e.g., monitor health of visitors, roommate, caregivers).
- Recommend involvement in support group; introduce to individuals dealing with similar problems **to provide role models, assistance for problem solving.**
- Encourage time-out for caregivers **so that they may attend to personal needs, wellness, and growth.**
- Provide opportunities for client/SO(s) to discuss termination of therapy/end-of-life decisions.
- Refer to individual(s) who are ventilator-dependent/have managed home ventilation successfully **to encourage hope for the future.**
- Refer to additional resources (e.g., spiritual advisor, counselor).

Documentation Focus

ASSESSMENT/REASSESSMENT

- Baseline findings, subsequent alterations in respiratory function.
- Results of diagnostic testing.
- Individual risk factors/concerns.

PLANNING

- Plan of care and who is involved in planning.
- Teaching plan.

IMPLEMENTATION/EVALUATION

- Client's/SO's responses to interventions, teaching, and actions performed.
- Skill level/assistance needs of SO(s)/family.
- Attainment, progress toward desired outcome(s).
- Modifications to plan of care.

DISCHARGE PLANNING

- Discharge plan, including appropriate referrals, action taken, and who is responsible for each action.
- Equipment needs and source.
- Resources for support persons/home care providers.

Information in brackets added by the authors to clarify and enhance the use of nursing diagnoses.

SAMPLE NURSING OUTCOMES & INTERVENTIONS CLASSIFICATIONS (NOC/NIC)

NOC—Respiratory Status: Ventilation
NIC—Mechanical Ventilation

dysfunctional Ventilatory Weaning Response

Taxonomy II: Activity/Rest—Class 4 Cardiovascular/
    Pulmonary Responses (00034)
[Diagnostic Division: Respiration]
Submitted 1992

Definition: Inability to adjust to lowered levels of
mechanical ventilator support that interrupts and
prolongs the weaning process

Related Factors

PHYSIOLOGICAL

Ineffective airway clearance
Sleep pattern disturbance
Inadequate nutrition
Uncontrolled pain
[Muscle weakness/fatigue; inability to control respiratory mus-
    cles; immobility]

PSYCHOLOGICAL

Knowledge deficit of the weaning process
Patient's perceived inefficacy about the ability to wean
Decreased motivation/self-esteem
Anxiety; fear; insufficient trust in the nurse
Hopelessness; powerlessness
[Unprepared for weaning attempt]

SITUATIONAL

Uncontrolled episodic energy demands
Inappropriate pacing of diminished ventilator support
Inadequate social support
Adverse environment (e.g., noisy, active environment; negative
    events in the room; low nurse–patient ratio; unfamiliar nurs-
    ing staff)
History of ventilator dependence >4 days
History of multiple unsuccessful weaning attempts

Information in brackets added by the authors to clarify and enhance
the use of nursing diagnoses.

    Cultural   Collaborative   Community/Home Care

Defining Characteristics

MILD

Subjective
Expressed feelings of increased need for O_2; breathing discomfort; fatigue; warmth
Queries about possible machine malfunction

Objective
Restlessness
Slight increase of respiratory rate from baseline
Increased concentration on breathing

MODERATE

Subjective
Apprehension

Objective
Slight increase from baseline blood pressure (<20 mm Hg)/heart rate <20 beats/min)
Baseline increase in respiratory rate (<5 breaths/min); slight respiratory accessory muscle use; decreased air entry on auscultation
Hypervigilance to activities; wide-eyed look
Inability to respond to coaching/cooperate
Diaphoresis
Color changes; pale; slight cyanosis

SEVERE

Objective
Agitation; decreased level of consciousness
Deterioration in arterial blood gases from current baseline
Increase from baseline blood pressure (20 mm Hg)/heart rate (20 beats/min)
Respiratory rate increases significantly from baseline; full respiratory accessory muscle use; shallow/gasping breaths; paradoxical abdominal breathing
Adventitious breath sounds, audible airway secretions
Asynchronized breathing with the ventilator
Profuse diaphoresis
Cyanosis

Desired Outcomes/Evaluation Criteria—Client Will:

- Actively participate in the weaning process.
- Reestablish independent respiration with ABGs within client's normal range and be free of signs of respiratory failure.

Information in brackets added by the authors to clarify and enhance the use of nursing diagnoses.

 Diagnostic Studies 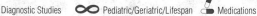 Pediatric/Geriatric/Lifespan   Medications

• Demonstrate increased tolerance for activity/participate in self-care within level of ability.

Actions/Interventions

NURSING PRIORITY NO. 1. To identify contributing factors/degree of dysfunction:

• Determine extent and nature of underlying disorders/factors (e.g., preexisting cardiopulmonary diseases, significant trauma, neuromuscular disorders, complications from surgical procedures) **that contribute to client's reliance on mechanical support and can affect future weaning efforts.**

• Note length of time client has been receiving ventilator support. Review previous episodes of extubation/reintubation. **Previous unsuccessful weaning attempts (e.g., due to inability to protect airway or clear secretions; oxygen saturation less than 50% on room air, etc.) that can influence future weaning interventions.**

• Assess systemic parameters that may affect readiness for weaning using Burns Weaning Assessment Program (BWAP) or similar checklist (e.g., stability of vital signs, factors that increase metabolic rate [e.g., sepsis, fever]; hydration status; need for/recent use of analgesia or sedation; nutritional state; muscle strength; and activity level).

• Ascertain client's alertness and understanding of weaning process, expectations, and concerns. **Client/SO(s) may need specific and repeated instructions during process.**

• Determine psychological readiness, presence/degree of anxiety. Introduce client to individual who has shared similar experiences with successful outcome if desired/indicated **to provide support and encourgement for successful outcome.**

 • Review laboratory studies (e.g., CBC reflecting number/integrity of red blood cells [**affects O_2 transport**], serum albumim and electrolyte levels indicating nutritional status [**to confirm sufficient energy to meet demands of weaning**]).

 • Review chest x-ray, pulse oximetry/capnography, and/or ABGs.

NURSING PRIORITY NO. 2. To support weaning process:

 • Consult with dietitian, nutritional support team for adjustments in composition of diet **to prevent excessive production of CO_2, which could alter respiratory drive.**

 • Implement weaning protocols and mode (e.g., spontaneous breathing trials, partial client suppport [SIMV], or pressure support [PSV] during client's spontaneous breathing); **to**

Information in brackets added by the authors to clarify and enhance the use of nursing diagnoses.

  Cultural Collaborative Community/Home Care

determine if client can assume the full work of breathing and to provide support for spontaneous ventilation.

- Discuss with client/SO(s) individual plan and expectations. Assure client of nurse's presence and assistance during weaning attempts. **May reduce client's anxiety about process and ultimate outcome and enhance willingness to work at spontaneous breathing.**
- Note response to activity/client care during weaning and limit, as indicated. Provide undisturbed rest/sleep periods. Avoid stressful procedures/situations or nonessential activities. **Prevents excessive O_2 consumption/demand with increased possibility of weaning failure.**
- Time medications during weaning efforts **to minimize sedative effects.**
- Provide quiet room, calm approach, undivided attention of nurse. **Enhances relaxation, conserving energy.**
- Involve SO(s)/family, as appropriate (e.g., sitting at bedside, providing encouragement, and helping monitor client status).
- Provide diversional activity (e.g., watching TV, reading aloud) **to focus attention away from breathing when not actively working at breathing exercises.**
- Auscultate breath sounds periodically; suction airway, as indicated.
- Acknowledge and provide ongoing encouragement for client's efforts.
- Minimize setbacks, focus client attention on gains and progress to date **to reduce frustration that may further impair progress.**
- Suspend weaning (take a "holiday") periodically, as individually appropriate (e.g., initially may "rest" 45 or 50 minutes each hour, progressing to a 20-minute rest every 4 hours, then weaning during daytime and resting during night).
- Prepare client/SO(s) for alternative actions when client is unable to resume spontaneous ventilation (e.g., tracheostomy with long-term ventilation support in alternate care setting, palliative care/end-of-life procedures).

NURSING PRIORITY NO. 3. To promote wellness (Teaching/Discharge Considerations):

- Discuss impact of specific activities on respiratory status and problem solve solutions to maximize weaning effort.
- Engage in rehabilitation program **to enhance respiratory muscle strength and general endurance.**
- Teach client/SO(s) how to protect client from sources of infection (e.g., monitor health of visitors, persons involved in care; avoid crowds during flu season).

Information in brackets added by the authors to clarify and enhance the use of nursing diagnoses.

dysfunctional VENTILATORY WEANING RESPONSE

 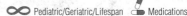

[actual/] risk for other-directed VIOLENCE

• Identify conditions requiring immediate medical intervention **to prevent respiratory failure.**

Documentation Focus

ASSESSMENT/REASSESSMENT

• Baseline findings and subsequent alterations.
• Results of diagnostic testing/procedures.
• Individual risk factors.

PLANNING

• Plan of care/interventions and who is involved in the planning.
• Teaching plan.

IMPLEMENTATION/EVALUATION

• Client response to interventions.
• Attainment of/progress toward desired outcome(s).
• Modifications to plan of care.

DISCHARGE PLANNING

• Status at discharge, long-term needs and referrals, indicating who is to be responsible for each action.
• Equipment needs/supplier.

SAMPLE NURSING OUTCOMES & INTERVENTIONS CLASSIFICATIONS (NOC/NIC)

NOC—Respiratory Status: Ventilation
NIC—Mechanical Ventilatory Weaning

> NOTE: NANDA has separated the diagnosis of Violence into its two elements: "directed at others" and "self-directed." However, the interventions in general address both situations and have been left in one block following the definition and supporting data of the two diagnoses.

[actual/] risk for other-directed Violence

Taxonomy II: Safety/Protection—Class 3 Violence (00138)
[Diagnostic Division: Safety]
Submitted 1980; Revised 1996

Definition: At risk for behaviors in which an individual demonstrates that he or she can be physically, emotionally, and/or sexually harmful to others

Information in brackets added by the authors to clarify and enhance the use of nursing diagnoses.

 Cultural Collaborative Community/Home Care

Risk Factors/[Indicators]*

HISTORY OF:

Violence against others (e.g., hitting, kicking, scratching, biting or spitting, throwing objects at someone; attempted rape, rape, sexual molestation; urinating/defecating on a person)

Threats (e.g., verbal threats against property/person, social threats, cursing, threatening notes/letters, threatening gestures, sexual threats)

Violent antisocial behavior (e.g., stealing, insistent borrowing, insistent demands for privileges, insistent interruption of meetings, refusal to eat/take medication, ignoring instructions)

Indirect violence (e.g., tearing off clothes, urinating/defecating on floor, stamping feet, temper tantrum, running in corridors, yelling, writing on walls, ripping objects off walls, throwing objects, breaking a window, slamming doors, sexual advances)

Childhood abuse/witnessing family violence

Neurological impairment (e.g., positive EEG, CT, or MRI; neurological findings; head trauma; seizure disorders)

Cognitive impairment (e.g., learning disabilities, attention deficit disorder, decreased intellectual functioning); [organic brain syndrome]

Cruelty to animals; firesetting

Prenatal/perinatal complications

History of substance abuse; pathological intoxication; [toxic reaction to medication]

Psychotic symptomatology (e.g., auditory, visual, command hallucinations; paranoid delusions; loose, rambling, or illogical thought processes); [panic states; rage reactions; catatonic/manic excitement]

Motor vehicle offenses (e.g., frequent traffic violations, use of a motor vehicle to release anger)

Suicidal behavior; impulsivity; availability of weapon(s)

Body language (e.g., rigid posture, clenching of fists and jaw, hyperactivity, pacing, breathlessness, threatening stances)

[Hormonal imbalance (e.g., premenstrual syndrome—PMS, postpartal depression/psychosis)]

[Expressed intent/desire to harm others directly or indirectly]

[Almost continuous thoughts of violence]

---

*Although a risk diagnosis does not have defining characteristics (signs and symptoms), the factors identified here can be used to denote an actual diagnosis or as indicators of risk for/escalation of violence.

Information in brackets added by the authors to clarify and enhance the use of nursing diagnoses.

 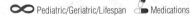

[actual/] risk for self-directed Violence

Taxonomy II: Safety/Protection—Class 3 Violence (00140)
[Diagnostic Division: Safety]
Submitted 1994

Definition: At risk for behaviors in which an individual demonstrates that he or she can be physically, emotionally, and/or sexually harmful to self

Risk Factors/[Indicators]*

Ages 15 to 19/over 45
Marital status (single, widowed, divorced)
Employment problems (e.g., unemployed, recent job loss/failure); occupation (executive, administrator/owner of business, professional, semi-skilled worker)
Conflictual interpersonal relationships
Family background (e.g., chaotic or conflictual, history of suicide)
Sexual orientation (bisexual [active], homosexual [inactive])
Physical health problems (e.g., hypochondriac, chronic or terminal illness)
Mental health problems (e.g., severe depression, [bipolar disorder] psychosis, severe personality disorder, alcoholism or drug abuse)
Emotional problems (e.g., hopelessness, [lifting of depressed mood], despair, increased anxiety, panic, anger, hostility); history of multiple suicide attempts; suicidal ideation; suicidal plan
Lack of personal resources (e.g., poor achievement, poor insight, affect unavailable and poorly controlled)
Lack of social resources (e.g., poor rapport, socially isolated, unresponsive family)
Verbal clues (e.g., talking about death, "better off without me," asking questions about lethal dosages of drugs)
Behavioral clues (e.g., writing forlorn love notes, directing angry messages at a significant other who has rejected the person, giving away personal items, taking out a large life insurance policy)

Desired Outcomes/Evaluation Criteria—[For Other-Directed/Self-Directed] Client Will:

• Acknowledge realities of the situation.
• Verbalize understanding of why behavior occurs.

---

*Although a risk diagnosis does not have defining characteristics (signs and symptoms), the factors identified here can be used to denote an actual diagnosis or as indicators of risk for/escalation of violence.

Information in brackets added by the authors to clarify and enhance the use of nursing diagnoses.

 Cultural Collaborative 🏠 Community/Home Care

- Identify precipitating factors.
- Express realistic self-evaluation and increased sense of self-esteem.
- Participate in care and meet own needs in an assertive manner.
- Demonstrate self-control as evidenced by relaxed posture, nonviolent behavior.
- Use resources and support systems in an effective manner.

Actions/Interventions

(Addresses both "other-directed" and "self-directed")

NURSING PRIORITY NO. 1. To assess causative/contributing factors:

- Determine underlying dynamics as listed in the Risk Factors.
- Ascertain client's perception of self/situation. Note use of defense mechanisms (e.g., denial, projection).
- Observe/listen for early cues of distress/increasing anxiety (e.g., irritability, lack of cooperation, demanding behavior, body posture/expression). **May indicate possibility of loss of control and intervention at this point can prevent a blow-up.**
- Identify conditions such as acute/chronic brain syndrome, panic state, hormonal imbalance (e.g., PMS, postpartal psychosis), drug-induced, postanesthesia/postseizure confusion, traumatic brain injury. **These physical conditions may interfere with ability to control own behavior and will need specific interventions to manage.**
- Review laboratory findings (e.g., blood alcohol, blood glucose, ABGs, electrolytes, renal function tests).
- Observe for signs of suicidal/homicidal intent (e.g., perceived morbid or anxious feeling while with the client; warning from the client, "It doesn't matter," "I'd/They'd be better off dead"; mood swings; "accident-prone"/self-destructive behavior; suicidal attempts; possession of alcohol and/or other drug(s) in known substance abuser). (Refer to ND risk for Suicide.)
- Note family history of suicidal/homicidal behavior. **Children who grow up in homes where violence is accepted tend to grow up to use violence as a means of solving problems.**
- Ask directly if the person is thinking of acting on thoughts/feelings **to determine violent intent.**
- Determine availability of homicidal means.
- Assess client coping behaviors already present. **Note: Client believes there are no alternatives other than violence, especially if they have come from a family background of violence.**

Information in brackets added by the authors to clarify and enhance the use of nursing diagnoses.

[actual/] risk for VIOLENCE

 • Identify risk factors and assess for indicators of child abuse/neglect: unexplained/frequent injuries, failure to thrive, and so forth.

NURSING PRIORITY NO. 2. To assist client to accept responsibility for impulsive behavior and potential for violence:

• Develop therapeutic nurse-client relationship. Provide consistent caregiver when possible. **Promotes sense of trust, allowing client to discuss feelings openly.**

• Maintain straightforward communication **to avoid reinforcing manipulative behavior.**

 • Discuss motivation for change (e.g., failing relationships, job loss, involvement with judicial system). **Crisis situation can provide impetus for change, but requires timely therapeutic intervention to sustain efforts.**

 • Help client recognize that own actions may be in response to own fear (**may be afraid of own behavior, loss of control**), dependency, and feeling of powerlessness.

 • Make time to listen to expressions of feelings. Acknowledge reality of client's feelings and that feelings are OK. (Refer to ND Self-Esteem [specify].)

 • Confront client's tendency to minimize situation/behavior. **In domestic violence situations, individual may be remorseful after incident and will apologize and say that it won't happen again.**

 • Review factors (feelings/events) involved in precipitating violent behavior.

 • Discuss impact of behavior on others/consequences of actions.

 • Acknowledge reality of suicide/homicide as an option. Discuss consequences of actions if they were to follow through on intent. Ask how it will help client to resolve problems. **Provides an opportunity for client to look at reality of choices and potential outcomes.**

• Accept client's anger without reacting on emotional basis. Give permission to express angry feelings in acceptable ways and let client know that staff will be available to assist in maintaining control. **Promotes acceptance and sense of safety.**

 • Help client identify more appropriate solutions/behaviors (e.g., motor activities/exercise) **to lessen sense of anxiety and associated physical manifestations.**

 • Provide directions for actions client can take, avoiding negatives, such as "do nots."

Information in brackets added by the authors to clarify and enhance the use of nursing diagnoses.

  Cultural Collaborative Community/Home Care

NURSING PRIORITY NO. 3. To assist client in controlling behavior:

- Contract with client regarding safety of self/others.
- Give client as much control as possible within constraints of individual situation. **Enhances self-esteem, promotes confidence in ability to change behavior.**
- Be truthful when giving information and dealing with client. **Builds trust, enhancing therapeutic relationship, and prevents manipulative behavior.**
- Identify current/past successes and strengths. Discuss effectiveness of coping techniques used and possible changes. (Refer to ND ineffective Coping.) **Client is often not aware of positive aspects of life, and once recognized, they can be used as a basis for change.**
- Assist client to distinguish between reality and hallucinations/delusions.
- Approach in positive manner, acting as if the client has control and is responsible for own behavior. Be aware, though, that the client may not have control, especially if under the influence of drugs (including alcohol).
- Maintain distance and do not touch client without permission when situation indicates client does not tolerate such closeness (e.g., post-trauma response).
- Remain calm and state limits on inappropriate behavior (including consequences) in a firm manner.
- Direct client to stay in view of staff/caregiver.
- Administer prescribed medications (e.g., anti-anxiety/antipsychotic), taking care not to oversedate client. **The chemistry of the brain is changed by early violence and has been shown to respond to serotonin, as well as related neurotransmitter systems, which play a role in restraining aggressive impulses.**
- Monitor for possible drug interactions, cumulative effects of drug regimen (e.g., anticonvulsants/antidepressants).
- Give positive reinforcement for client's efforts. **Encourages continuation of desired behaviors.**
- Explore death fantasies when expressed (e.g., "I'll look down and watch them suffer; she'll be sorry") or the idea that death is not final (e.g., "I can come back").

NURSING PRIORITY NO. 4. To assist client/SO(s) to correct/deal with existing situation:

- Gear interventions to individual(s) involved, based on age, relationship, and so forth.
- Maintain calm, matter-of-fact, nonjudgmental attitude. **Decreases defensive response.**

Information in brackets added by the authors to clarify and enhance the use of nursing diagnoses.

• Notify potential victims in the presence of serious homicidal threat in accordance with legal/ethical guidelines. **The Tarasoff law requires healthcare providers to report specific threats to the individual named**.

 • Discuss situation with abused/battered person, providing accurate information about choices and effective actions that can be taken.

 • Assist individual to understand that angry, vengeful feelings are appropriate in the situation, but need to be expressed and not acted on. (Refer to ND Post-Trauma Syndrome, as psychological responses may be very similar.)

• Identify resources available for assistance (e.g., battered women's shelter, social services).

NURSING PRIORITY NO. 5. To promote safety in event of violent behavior:

• Provide a safe, quiet environment and remove items from the client's environment that could be used to inflict harm to self/others.
• Maintain distance from client who is striking out/hitting and take evasive/controlling actions, as indicated.
• Call for additional staff/security personnel.
• Approach aggressive/attacking client from the front, just out of reach, in a commanding posture with palms down.
• Tell client to *STOP*. **This may be sufficient enough to help client control own actions**.
• Maintain direct/constant eye contact, when appropriate.
• Speak in a low, commanding voice.
• Provide client with a sense that caregiver is in control of the situation **to provide feeling of safety.**
• Maintain clear route for staff and client and be prepared to move quickly.
• Hold client, using restraints or seclusion, when necessary, until client regains self-control.
• Administer medication, as indicated, **to help client until able to regain self-control.**

NURSING PRIORITY NO. 6. To promote wellness (Teaching/Discharge Considerations):

 • Promote client involvement in planning care within limits of situation, allowing for meeting own needs for enjoyment. **Individuals often believe they are not entitled to pleasure and good things in their lives and need to learn how to meet these needs.**

 • Assist client to learn assertive rather than manipulative, nonassertive, or aggressive behavior. **Promotes behaviors**

Information in brackets added by the authors to clarify and enhance the use of nursing diagnoses.

 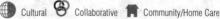

that help client to engage in positive social activities with others.

• Discuss reasons for client's behavior with SO(s). Determine desire/commitment of involved parties to sustain current relationships.

∞ • Develop strategies to help parents learn more effective parenting skills (e.g., parenting classes, appropriate ways of dealing with frustrations). **Mothering has a powerful effect on helping children to learn impulse control.**

🏠 • Identify support systems (e.g., family/friends, clergy). **In addition to the client, those around him or her need to learn how to be positive role models and display a broader array of skills for resolving problems.**

⊘ • Refer to formal resources, as indicated (e.g., individual/group psychotherapy, substance abuse treatment program, social services, safe house facility, parenting classes).

• Refer to NDs impaired Parenting; family Coping [specify]; Post-Trauma Syndrome.

Documentation Focus

ASSESSMENT/REASSESSMENT

• Individual findings, including nature of concern (e.g., suicidal/homicidal), behavioral risk factors and level of impulse control, plan of action/means to carry out plan.
• Client's perception of situation, motivation for change.
• Family history of violence.
• Availability/use of resources.

PLANNING

• Plan of care and who is involved in the planning.
• Details of contract regarding violence to self/others.
• Teaching plan.

IMPLEMENTATION/EVALUATION

• Actions taken to promote safety, including notification of parties at risk.
• Response to interventions/teaching and actions performed.
• Attainment/progress toward desired outcome(s).
• Modifications to plan of care.

DISCHARGE PLANNING

• Long-range needs and who is responsible for actions to be taken.
• Available resources, specific referrals made.

Information in brackets added by the authors to clarify and enhance the use of nursing diagnoses.

[actual/] risk for VIOLENCE

SAMPLE NURSING OUTCOMES & INTERVENTIONS CLASSIFICATIONS (NOC/NIC)

NOC—Aggression Control
NIC—Anger Control Assistance

impaired Walking

Taxonomy II: Activity/Rest—Class 2 Activity/Exercise (00088)
[Diagnostic Division: Activity/Rest]
Submitted 1998

Definition: Limitation of independent movement within the environment on foot

Related Factors

Insufficient muscle strength; neuromuscular impairment; musculoskeletal impairment (e.g., contractures)
Limited endurance; deconditioning
Fear of falling; impaired balance
Impaired vision
Pain
Obesity
Depressed mood; cognitive impairment
Lack of knowledge
Environmental constraints (e.g., stairs, inclines, uneven surfaces, unsafe obstacles, distances, lack of assistive devices or persons, restraints)

Defining Characteristics

SUBJECTIVE OR OBJECTIVE

Impaired ability to walk required distances; walk on an incline/ decline; walk on uneven surfaces; to navigate curbs, climb stairs
[Specify level of independence—refer to ND impaired physical Mobility, for suggested functional level classification]

Desired Outcomes/Evaluation Criteria—Client Will:

• Be able to move about within environment as needed/desired within limits of ability or with appropriate adjuncts.
• Verbalize understanding of situation/risk factors and safety measures.

Information in brackets added by the authors to clarify and enhance the use of nursing diagnoses.

  Cultural Collaborative 🏠 Community/Home Care

Actions/Interventions

NURSING PRIORITY NO. 1. To assess causative/contributing factors:

- Identify condition/diagnoses that contribute to difficulty walking (e.g., advanced age; acute illness; weakness/chronic illness [e.g., cardiopulmonary disorders, cancer, kidney disease]; recent surgery/trauma; osteo/rheumatoid/gouty arthritis; leg/hip/knee trauma/other disorders [e.g., fractures, tendon or ligament injury, amputation]; balance problems [e.g., inner ear infection/brain injury/stroke]; nerve disorders [e.g., MS, Parkinson's disease, cerebral palsy]; spinal abnormalities [disease, trauma, degeneration]; neuropathies [e.g., peripheral, diabetic, alcoholic]; degenerative muscle disorders [e.g., muscular dystrophy, myositis]; vision impairments; foot conditions [e.g., plantar warts, bunions, ingrown toenails, pressure ulcers]; cognitive dysfunction).
- Note client's particular symptoms related to walking (e.g., unable to bear weight, can't walk usual distance, limping, staggering, stiff leg, leg pain, shuffling, asymmetric or unsteady gait).
- Determine ability to follow directions and note emotional/behavioral responses that may be affecting the situation.

NURSING PRIORITY NO. 2. To assess functional ability:

- Determine degree of impairment in relation to suggested functional scale (0 to 4), noting that impairment can be either temporary/permanent or progressive.
- Assist with/review results of mobility testing (e.g., timing of walking over fixed distance, distance walked over set period of time [endurance], limb movement analysis, leg strength and speed of walking, ambulatory activity monitoring) **for differential diagnosis and to guide treatment interventions.**
- Note emotional/behavioral responses of client/SO(s) to problems of mobility.

NURSING PRIORITY NO. 3. To promote safe, optimal level of independence in walking:

- Assist with treatment of underlying condition causing dysfunction, as indicated by individual situation.
- Consult with PT/OT/rehabilitation team **for individualized mobility/walking program, and identify/develop appropriate devices (e.g., shoe insert, leg brace to maintain proper foot alignment for walking, quad cane, hemiwalker).**
- Demonstrate use of/help client become comfortable with adjunctive devices (e.g., cane, crutches, walking cast/boot, walker, limb prosthesis, mobility scooter).

Information in brackets added by the authors to clarify and enhance the use of nursing diagnoses.

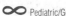 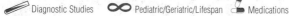

• Provide assistance when indicated (e.g., walking on uneven surfaces; client is weak or has to walk a distance; or vision, coordination, or posture are impaired).

 • Schedule walking/exercise activities interspersed with adequate rest periods **to reduce fatigue.**

 • Provide ample time to perform mobility-related tasks **to reduce risk of falling and manage fatigue or pain.**

 • Encourage active and passive exercises. Advance levels of exercise, as able, **to increase stamina/endurance.**

• Provide safety measures, as indicated, including skin/tissue care, environmental management/fall prevention.

NURSING PRIORITY NO. 4. To promote wellness (Teaching/Discharge Considerations):

 • Involve client/SO(s) in care, assisting them to learn ways of managing deficits **to enhance safety for client and SO(s)/ caregivers.**

 • Identify appropriate resources for obtaining and maintaining appliances, equipment, and environmental modifications **to promote mobility.**

 • Instruct client/SO(s) in safety measures, as individually indicated (e.g., maintaining safe travel pathway, proper lighting/ handrails on stairs, etc.) **to reduce risk of falls.**

Documentation Focus

ASSESSMENT/REASSESSMENT

• Individual findings, including level of function/ability to participate in specific/desired activities.
• Equipment/assistive device needs.

PLANNING

• Plan of care and who is involved in the planning.
• Teaching plan.

IMPLEMENTATION/EVALUATION

• Responses to interventions/teaching and actions performed.
• Attainment/progress toward desired outcome(s).
• Modifications to plan of care.

DISCHARGE PLANNING

• Discharge/long-range needs, noting who is responsible for each action to be taken.
• Specific referrals made.
• Sources of/maintenance for assistive devices.

Information in brackets added by the authors to clarify and enhance the use of nursing diagnoses.

SAMPLE NURSING OUTCOMES & INTERVENTIONS CLASSIFICATIONS (NOC/NIC)

NOC—Ambulation: Walking
NIC—Exercise Therapy: Ambulation

Wandering
[Specify Sporadic or Continuous]

Taxonomy II: Activity/Rest—Class 2 Activity/Exercise (00154)
[Diagnostic Division: Safety]
Submitted 2000

Definition: Meandering, aimless, or repetitive locomotion that exposes the individual to harm; frequently incongruent with boundaries, limits, or obstacles

Related Factors

Cognitive impairment (e.g., memory and recall deficits, disorientation, poor visuoconstructive or visuospatial ability, language defects); sedation

Cortical atrophy

Premorbid behavior (e.g., outgoing, sociable personality; premorbid dementia)

Separation from familiar environment; overstimulating environment

Emotional state (e.g., frustration, anxiety, boredom, depression, agitation)

Physiological state or need (e.g., hunger, thirst, pain, urination, constipation)

Time of day

Defining Characteristics

OBJECTIVE

Frequent/continuous movement from place to place, often revisiting the same destinations

Persistent locomotion in search of something; scanning/searching behaviors

Haphazard locomotion; fretful locomotion; pacing; long periods of locomotion without an apparent destination

Locomotion into unauthorized or private spaces; trespassing

Locomotion resulting in unintended leaving of a premise

Information in brackets added by the authors to clarify and enhance the use of nursing diagnoses.

 Diagnostic Studies ∞ Pediatric/Geriatric/Lifespan 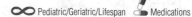 Medications

Inability to locate significant landmarks in a familiar setting; getting lost

Locomotion that cannot be easily dissuaded; shadowing a caregiver's locomotion

Hyperactivity

Periods of locomotion interspersed with periods of non-locomotion (e.g., sitting, standing, sleeping)

Desired Outcomes/Evaluation Criteria—Client Will:

• Be free of injury, or unplanned exits.

CAREGIVER(S) WILL:

• Modify environment, as indicated, to enhance safety.
• Provide for maximal independence of client.

Actions/Interventions

NURSING PRIORITY NO. 1. To assess degree of impairment/stage of disease process:

• Ascertain history of client's memory loss and cognitive changes.
• Note results of diagnostic testing, confirming diagnosis and type of dementia.
• Evaluate client's mental status during daytime and nighttime, noting when client's confusion is most pronounced and when client sleeps.
• Monitor client's use/need for assistive devices, such as glasses, hearing aids, cane.
• Assess frequency and pattern of wandering behavior (e.g., client may be goal-directed or non-goal directed, may start wandering in late afternoon or evening [nocturnal]) **to determine individual risks/safety needs.**
• Determine bowel/bladder elimination pattern, timing of incontinence, presence of constipation **for possible correlation to wandering behavior.**
• Identify client's reason for wandering, if possible (e.g., looking for lost item, desire to go home, boredom, need for activity, hunger, thirst, or discomfort).
• Ascertain if client has delusions due to shadows, lights, and noises.

NURSING PRIORITY NO. 2. To assist client/caregiver to deal with situations:

Information in brackets added by the authors to clarify and enhance the use of nursing diagnoses.

🏠 • Provide a structured daily routine. **Decreases wandering behavior and minimizes caregiver stress.**

🏠 • Encourage participation in family activities and familiar routines, such as folding laundry, listening to music, shared-walking time outdoors. **Activities and exercises may reduce anxiety and restlessness.**

🏠 • Offer drink of water or snack, bring client to bathroom on a regular schedule. **Wandering may at times be expressing a need.**

🏠 • Provide safe place for client to wander, away from safety hazards (e.g., hot water/kitchen stove, open stairway) and other noisy clients. Arrange furniture, remove scatter rugs, electrical cords, and other high-risk items **to accommodate safe wandering.**

🏠 • Make sure that doors or gates have alarms/chimes and that alarms are turned on. Provide door and window locks that are not within line of sight or easily opened **to prevent unsafe exits.**

🏠 • Provide 24-hour supervision/reality orientation. **(Client can be awake at any time and fail to recognize day/night routines.)**

🏠 • Sit with client and visit/reminiscence. Provide TV/radio/music.

• Avoid overstimulation from activities or new partner/roommate during rest periods when client is in a facility.

🏠 • Use pressure-sensitive bed/chair alarms **to alert caregivers of movement.**

🏠 • Avoid using physical or chemical restraints (sedatives) to control wandering behavior. **May increase agitation, sensory deprivation, and falls, and may contribute to wandering behavior.**

• Provide consistent staff as much as possible.

• Provide room near monitoring station; check client location on frequent basis.

NURSING PRIORITY NO. 3. To Promote Wellness (Teaching/Discharge Considerations):

🏠 • Identify problems that are remediable and assist client/SO(s) to seek appropriate assistance and access resources. **Encourages problem solving to improve condition rather than accept the status quo.**]

🏠 • Notify neighbors about client's condition and request that they contact client's family or local police if they see client outside alone. **Community awareness can prevent/reduce risk of client being lost or hurt.**

Information in brackets added by the authors to clarify and enhance the use of nursing diagnoses.

- Register client with community/national resources, such as Alzheimer's Association Safe Return Program, **to assist in identification, location, and safe return of individual with wandering behaviors.**
- Help SO(s) develop plan of care when problem is progressive.
- Refer to community resources, such as day care programs, support groups.
- Refer to NDs acute Confusion; chronic Confusion; impaired Environmental Interpretation Syndrome; disturbed Sensory Perception (specify); risk for Injury; risk for Falls.

Documentation Focus

ASSESSMENT/REASSESSMENT

- Assessment findings, including individual concerns, family involvement, and support factors/availability of resources.

PLANNING

- Plan of care and who is involved in planning.
- Teaching plan.

IMPLEMENTATION/EVALUATION

- Responses of client/SO(s) to plan interventions and actions performed.
- Attainment/progress toward desired outcome(s).
- Modifications to plan of care.

DISCHARGE PLANNING

- Long-range needs and who is responsible for actions to be taken.
- Specific referrals made.

SAMPLE NURSING OUTCOMES & INTERVENTIONS CLASSIFICATIONS (NOC/NIC)

NOC—Risk Control
NIC—Elopement Precautions

Information in brackets added by the authors to clarify and enhance the use of nursing diagnoses.

 Cultural   Collaborative   Community/Home Care

CHAPTER 5

Health Conditions and Client Concerns with Associated Nursing Diagnoses

This chapter presents over 400 disorders/health conditions/life situations reflecting all specialty areas, with associated nursing diagnoses written as client problem/need statements that include the "related to" and "evidenced by" components.

This section will facilitate and help validate the assessment and diagnosis steps of the nursing process. Because the nursing process is perpetual and ongoing, other nursing diagnoses may be appropriate based on changing individual situations. Therefore, the nurse must continually assess, identify, and validate new client needs and evaluate subsequent care. Once the appropriate nursing diagnoses have been selected from this chapter, the reader may refer to Chapter 4, which lists the 187 NANDA diagnoses, and review the diagnostic definition, defining characteristics, and related or risk factors for further validation. This step is necessary to determine if the nursing diagnosis is an accurate match, if more data are required, or if another diagnosis needs to be investigated.

To facilitate access to the health conditions/concerns and nursing diagnoses, the client needs have been listed alphabetically and coded to identify nursing specialty areas.

MS: Medical-Surgical
PED: Pediatric
OB: Obstetric
CH: Community/Home
PSY: Psychiatric/Behavioral
GYN: Gynecological

A separate category for geriatric has not been made because geriatric concerns/conditions actually are subsumed under the other specialty areas, because elderly persons are susceptible to the majority of these problems.

Abdominal hysterectomy   **MS**
(Refer to Hysterectomy)

Abdominal perineal resection   MS
(Also refer to Surgery, general)

disturbed Body Image may be related to presence of surgical wounds, possibly evidenced by verbalizations of feelings/perceptions, fear of reaction by others, preoccupation with change.

risk for Constipation: risk factors may include decreased physical activity/gastric motility, abdominal muscle weakness, insufficient fluid intake, change in usual foods/eating pattern.*

risk for Sexual Dysfunction: risk factors may include altered body structure/function, radical resection/treatment procedures, vulnerability/psychological concern about response of significant other(s) [SO(s)], and disruption of sexual response pattern (e.g., erection difficulty).*

Abortion, elective termination   OB

risk for decisional Conflict: risk factors may include unclear personal values/beliefs, lack of experience or interference with decision making, information from divergent sources, deficient support system.*

deficient Knowledge [Learning Need] regarding reproduction, contraception, self-care, Rh factor may be related to lack of exposure/recall or misinterpretation of information, possibly evidenced by request for information, statement of misconception, inaccurate follow-through of instructions, development of preventable events/complications.

risk for Spiritual Distress/moral Distress: risk factors may include perception of moral/ethical implications of therapeutic procedure, time constraints for decision making.*

Anxiety [specify level] may be related to situational/maturational crises, unmet needs, unconscious conflict about essential values/beliefs, possibly evidenced by increased tension, apprehension, fear of unspecific consequences, sympathetic stimulation, focus on self.

acute Pain/[Discomfort] may be related to aftereffects of procedure/drug effect, possibly evidenced by verbal report, distraction behaviors, changes in muscle tone, autonomic responses/changes in vital signs.

risk for maternal Injury: risk factors may include surgical procedure, effects of anesthesia/medications.*

Abortion, spontaneous termination   OB

deficient Fluid Volume [isotonic] may be related to excessive blood loss, possibly evidenced by decreased pulse volume and pressure, delayed capillary refill, or changes in sensorium.

risk for Spiritual Distress: risk factors may include need to adhere to personal religious beliefs/practices, blame for loss directed at self or God.*

deficient Knowledge [Learning Need] regarding cause of abortion, self-care, contraception/future pregnancy may be related to lack of familiarity with new self/healthcare needs, sources for support, possibly evidenced by requests for information and statement of concern/misconceptions, development of preventable complications.

Grieving related to perinatal loss, possibly evidenced by crying, expressions of sorrow, or changes in eating habits/sleep patterns.

---

*A risk diagnosis is not evidenced by signs and symptoms, as the problem has not occurred and nursing interventions are directed at prevention.

risk for ineffective Sexuality Pattern: risk factors may include increasing fear of pregnancy and/or repeat loss, impaired relationship with SO(s), self-doubt regarding own femininity.*

Abruptio placentae OB

deficient Fluid Volume [isotonic] may be related to excessive blood loss, possibly evidenced by hypotension, increased heart rate, decreased pulse volume and pressure, delayed capillary refill, or changes in sensorium.

Fear related to threat of death (perceived or actual) to fetus/self, possibly evidenced by verbalization of specific concerns, increased tension, sympathetic stimulation.

acute Pain may be related to collection of blood between uterine wall and placenta, uterine contractions, possibly evidenced by verbal reports, abdominal guarding, muscle tension, or alterations in vital signs.

impaired fetal Gas Exchange may be related to altered uteroplacental O_2 transfer, possibly evidenced by alterations in fetal heart rate and movement.

Abscess, brain (acute) MS

acute Pain may be related to inflammation, edema of tissues, possibly evidenced by reports of headache, restlessness, irritability, and moaning.

risk for Hyperthermia: risk factors may include inflammatory process/hypermetabolic state and dehydration.*

acute Confusion may be related to physiological changes (e.g., cerebral edema/altered perfusion, fever), possibly evidenced by fluctuation in cognition/level of consciousness, increased agitation/restlessness, hallucinations.

risk for Suffocation/Trauma: risk factors may include development of clonic/tonic muscle activity and changes in consciousness (seizure activity).*

Abscess, skin/tissue CH/MS

impaired Skin/Tissue Integrity may be related to immunological deficit/infection, possibly evidenced by disruption of skin, destruction of skin layers/tissues, invasion of body structures.

risk for Infection [spread]: risk factors may include broken skin/traumatized tissues, chronic disease, malnutrition, insufficient knowledge.*

Abuse CM

(Also refer to Battered child syndrome)

risk for Trauma: risk factors may include vulnerable client, recipient of verbal threats, history of physical abuse.*

Powerlessness may be related to abusive relationship, lifestyle of helplessness as evidenced by verbal expressions of having no control, reluctance to express true feelings, apathy, passivity.

chronic low Self-Esteem may be related to continual negative evaluation of self/capabilities, personal vulnerability, willingness to tolerate possible life-threatening domestic violence as evidenced by self-negative verbalization, evaluates self as unable to deal with events, rationalizes away/rejects positive feedback.

---

*A risk diagnosis is not evidenced by signs and symptoms, as the problem has not occurred and nursing interventions are directed at prevention.

Achalasia (cardiac sphincter)   MS

impaired Swallowing may be related to neuromuscular impairment, possibly evidenced by observed difficulty in swallowing or regurgitation.

imbalanced Nutrition: less than body requirements may be related to inability and/or reluctance to ingest adequate nutrients to meet metabolic demands/nutritional needs, possibly evidenced by reported/observed inadequate intake, weight loss, and pale conjunctiva and mucous membranes.

acute Pain may be related to spasm of the lower esophageal sphincter, possibly evidenced by reports of substernal pressure, recurrent heartburn, or gastric fullness (gas pains).

Anxiety [specify level]/Fear may be related to recurrent pain, choking sensation, altered health status, possibly evidenced by verbalizations of distress, apprehension, restlessness, or insomnia.

risk for Aspiration: risk factors may include regurgitation/spillover of esophageal contents.*

deficient Knowledge [Learning Need] regarding condition, prognosis, self-care, and treatment needs may be related to lack of familiarity with pathology and treatment of condition, possibly evidenced by requests for information, statement of concern, or development of preventable complications.

Acidosis, metabolic   MS
(Refer to Diabetic ketoacidosis)

Acidosis, respiratory   MS
(Also refer to underlying cause/condition)

impaired Gas Exchange may be related to ventilation perfusion imbalance (decreased O_2-carrying capacity of blood, altered O_2 supply, alveolar-capillary membrane changes), possibly evidenced by dyspnea with exertion, tachypnea, changes in mentation, irritability, tachycardia, hypoxia, hypercapnia.

Acne   CH/PED

impaired Skin Integrity may be related to secretions, infectious process as evidenced by disruptions of skin surface.

disturbed Body Image may be related to change in visual appearance as evidenced by fear of rejection of others, focus on past appearance, negative feelings about body, change in social involvement.

situational low Self-Esteem may be related to adolescence, negative perception of appearance as evidenced by self-negating verbalizations, expressions of helplessness.

Acquired immune deficiency syndrome   CH
(Refer to AIDS)

Acromegaly   CH

chronic Pain may be related to soft tissue swelling, joint degeneration, peripheral nerve compression possibly evidenced by verbal reports, altered ability to continue previous activities, changes in sleep pattern, fatigue.

---

*A risk diagnosis is not evidenced by signs and symptoms, as the problem has not occurred and nursing interventions are directed at prevention.

disturbed Body Image may be related to biophysical illness/changes, possibly evidenced by verbalization of feelings/concerns, fear of rejection or of reaction of others, negative comments about body, actual change in structure/appearance, change in social involvement.

risk for Sexual Dysfunction: risk factors may include altered body structure, changes in libido.*

Acute respiratory distress syndrome (ARDS)   MS

ineffective Airway Clearance may be related to loss of ciliary action, increased amount and viscosity of secretions, and increased airway resistance, possibly evidenced by presence of dyspnea, changes in depth/rate of respiration, use of accessory muscles for breathing, wheezes/crackles, cough with or without sputum production.

impaired Gas Exchange may be related to changes in pulmonary capillary permeability with edema formation, alveolar hypoventilation and collapse, with intrapulmonary shunting; possibly evidenced by tachypnea, use of accessory muscles, cyanosis, hypoxia per arterial blood gases (ABGs)/oximetry, anxiety, and changes in mentation.

risk for deficient Fluid Volume: risk factors may include active loss from diuretic use and restricted intake.*

risk for decreased Cardiac Output: risk factors may include alteration in preload (hypovolemia, vascular pooling, diuretic therapy, and increased intrathoracic pressure/use of ventilator/positive end expiratory pressure–PEEP).*

Anxiety [specify level]/Fear may be related to physiological factors (effects of hypoxemia), situational crisis, change in health status/threat of death possibly evidenced by increased tension, apprehension, restlessness, focus on self, and sympathetic stimulation.

risk for barotrauma Injury: risk factors may include increased airway pressure associated with mechanical ventilation (PEEP).*

Adams-Stokes syndrome   CH
(Refer to Dysrhythmia)

ADD   PED/PSY
(Refer to Attention deficit disorder)

Addiction   CH/PSY
(Refer to specific substances; Substance dependence/abuse rehabilitation)

Addison's disease   MS

deficient Fluid Volume [hypotonic] may be related to vomiting, diarrhea, increased renal losses, possibly evidenced by delayed capillary refill, poor skin turgor, dry mucous membranes, report of thirst.

decreased Cardiac Output may be related to hypovolemia and altered electrical conduction (dysrhythmias) and/or diminished cardiac muscle mass, possibly evidenced by alterations in vital signs, changes in mentation, and irregular pulse or pulse deficit.

---

*A risk diagnosis is not evidenced by signs and symptoms, as the problem has not occurred and nursing interventions are directed at prevention.

Fatigue may be related to decreased metabolic energy production, altered body chemistry (fluid, electrolyte, and glucose imbalance), possibly evidenced by unremitting overwhelming lack of energy, inability to maintain usual routines, decreased performance, impaired ability to concentrate, lethargy, and disinterest in surroundings.

disturbed Body Image may be related to changes in skin pigmentation, mucous membranes, loss of axillary/pubic hair, possibly evidenced by verbalization of negative feelings about body and decreased social involvement.

risk for impaired physical Mobility: risk factors may include neuromuscular impairment (muscle wasting/weakness) and dizziness/syncope.*

imbalanced Nutrition: less than body requirements may be related to glucocorticoid deficiency; abnormal fat, protein, and carbohydrate metabolism; nausea, vomiting, anorexia, possibly evidenced by weight loss, muscle wasting, abdominal cramps, diarrhea, and severe hypoglycemia.

risk for impaired Home Maintenance: risk factors may include effects of disease process, impaired cognitive functioning, and inadequate support systems.*

Adenoidectomy   PED/MS

Anxiety [specify level]/Fear may be related to separation from supportive others, unfamiliar surroundings, and perceived threat of injury/abandonment, possibly evidenced by crying, apprehension, trembling, and sympathetic stimulation (pupil dilation, increased heart rate).

risk for ineffective Airway Clearance: risk factors may include sedation, collection of secretions/blood in oropharynx, and vomiting.*

risk for deficient Fluid Volume: risk factors may include operative trauma to highly vascular site/hemorrhage.*

acute Pain may be related to physical trauma to oronasopharynx, presence of packing, possibly evidenced by restlessness, crying, and facial mask of pain.

Adjustment disorder   PSY

moderate to severe Anxiety may be related to situational/maturational crisis, threat to self-concept, unmet needs, fear of failure, dysfunctional family system, fixation in earlier level of development, possibly evidenced by overexcitement/restlessness, increased tension, insomnia, feelings of inadequacy, focus on self, difficulty concentrating, continuous attention-seeking behaviors, numerous physical complaints.

risk for self-/other-directed Violence: risk factors may include depressed mood, hopelessness, powerlessness, inability to tolerate frustration, rage reactions, unmet needs, negative role modeling, substance use/abuse, history of suicide attempt.*

ineffective Coping may be related to situational/maturational crisis, dysfunctional family system, negative role modeling, unmet dependency needs, retarded ego development, possibly evidenced by inability to problem solve, chronic worry, depressed/anxious mood, manipulation

---

*A risk diagnosis is not evidenced by signs and symptoms, as the problem has not occurred and nursing interventions are directed at prevention.

of others, destructive behaviors, increased dependency, refusal to follow rules.

complicated Grieving may be related to real or perceived loss of any concept of value to individual, bereavement overload/cumulative grief, thwarted grieving response, feelings of guilt generated by ambivalent relationship with the lost concept/person, possibly evidenced by difficulty in expressing/denial of loss, excessive/inappropriately expressed anger, labile affect, developmental regression, changes in concentration/pursuit of tasks.

Hopelessness may be related to lifestyle of helplessness (repeated failures, dependency), incomplete grief work of losses in life, lost belief in transcendent values/God possibly evidenced by verbal cues/despondent content, apathy/passivity, decreased response to stimuli, lack of initiative, nonparticipation in care or decision making.

Adoption/loss of child custody   PSY

risk for complicated Grieving: risk factors may include actual loss of child, expectations for future of child/self, thwarted grieving response to loss.*

risk for Powerlessness: risk factors may include perceived lack of options, no input into decision process, no control over outcome.*

Adrenal crisis, acute   MS

(Also refer to Addison's disease; Shock)

deficient Fluid Volume [hypotonic] may be related to failure of regulatory mechanism (damage to/suppression of adrenal gland), inability to concentrate urine, possibly evidenced by decreased venous filling/pulse volume and pressure, hypotension, dry mucous membranes, changes in mentation, decreased serum sodium.

acute Pain may be related to effects of disease process/metabolic imbalances, decreased tissue perfusion, possibly evidenced by reports of severe pain in abdomen, lower back, or legs.

impaired physical Mobility may be related to neuromuscular impairment, decreased muscle strength/control, possibly evidenced by generalized weakness, inability to perform desired activities/movements.

risk for Hyperthermia: risk factors may include presence of illness/infectious process, dehydration.*

risk for ineffective Protection: risk factors may include hormone deficiency, drug therapy, nutritional/metabolic deficiencies.*

Adrenalectomy   MS

ineffective Tissue Perfusion (specify) may be related to hypovolemia and vascular pooling (vasodilation), possibly evidenced by diminished pulse, pallor/cyanosis, hypotension, and changes in mentation.

risk for Infection: risk factors may include inadequate primary defenses (incision, traumatized tissues), suppressed inflammatory response, invasive procedures.*

deficient Knowledge [Learning Need] regarding condition, prognosis, self-care and treatment needs may be related to unfamiliarity with long-term therapy requirements, possibly evidenced by request for information and statement of concern/misconceptions.

---

*A risk diagnosis is not evidenced by signs and symptoms, as the problem has not occurred and nursing interventions are directed at prevention.

Adrenal insufficiency   CH
(Refer to Addison's disease)

Affective disorder   PSY
(Refer to Bipolar disorder; Depressive disorders, major)

Affective disorder, seasonal   PSY
(Also refer to Depressive disorders, major)
intermittent ineffective Coping may be related to situational crisis
    (fall/winter season), disturbance in pattern of tension release, and
    inadequate resources available, possibly evidenced by verbalizations
    of inability to cope, changes in sleep pattern (too little or too much),
    reports of lack of energy/fatigue, lack of resolution of problem,
    behavioral changes (irritability, discouragement).
risk for imbalanced Nutrition: more/less than body requirements:
    risk factors may include eating in response to internal cues other
    than hunger, alteration in usual coping patterns, change in usual
    activity level, decreased appetite, lack of energy/interest to prepare
    food.*

Agoraphobia   PSY
(Also refer to Phobia)
Anxiety [panic] may be related to contact with feared situation (public
    place/crowds), possibly evidenced by tachycardia, chest pain, dysp-
    nea, gastrointestinal distress, faintness, sense of impending doom.

Agranulocytosis   MS
risk for infection: risk factors may include suppressed inflammatory
    response.*
risk for impaired Oral Mucous Membrane: risk factors may include
    infection.*
risk for imbalanced Nutrition: less than body requirements: risk factors
    may include inability to ingest food/fluids (lesions of oral cavity).*

AIDS (acquired immunodeficiency syndrome)   MS
(Also refer to HIV positive)
risk for Infection [progression to sepsis/onset of new opportunistic
    infection]: risk factors may include depressed immune system, use of
    antimicrobial agents, inadequate primary defenses, broken skin, trau-
    matized tissue, malnutrition, and chronic disease processes.*
risk for deficient Fluid Volume: risk factors may include excessive losses:
    copious diarrhea, profuse sweating, vomiting, hypermetabolic state
    or fever, and restricted intake (nausea, anorexia, lethargy).*
acute/chronic Pain may be related to tissue inflammation/destruction:
    infections, internal/external cutaneous lesions, rectal excoriation,
    malignancies, necrosis, peripheral neuropathies, myalgias and arthral-
    gias, possibly evidenced by verbal reports, self-focusing/narrowed

---

*A risk diagnosis is not evidenced by signs and symptoms, as the
problem has not occurred and nursing interventions are directed at
prevention.

focus, alteration in muscle tone, paresthesias, paralysis, guarding behaviors, changes in vital signs (acute), autonomic responses, and restlessness.

CH

imbalanced Nutrition: less than body requirements may be related to altered ability to ingest, digest, and/or absorb nutrients (nausea/vomiting, hyperactive gag reflex, intestinal disturbances); increased metabolic activity/nutritional needs (fever, infection); possibly evidenced by weight loss, decreased subcutaneous fat/muscle mass, lack of interest in food/aversion to eating, altered taste sensation, abdominal cramping, hyperactive bowel sounds, diarrhea, sore and inflamed buccal cavity.

Fatigue may be related to decreased metabolic energy production, increased energy requirements (hypermetabolic state), overwhelming psychological/emotional demands, altered body chemistry (side effects of medication, chemotherapy), possibly evidenced by unremitting/overwhelming lack of energy, inability to maintain usual routines, decreased performance, impaired ability to concentrate, lethargy/restlessness, and disinterest in surroundings.

ineffective Protection may be related to chronic disease affecting immune and neurological systems, inadequate nutrition, drug therapies, possibly evidenced by deficient immunity, impaired healing, neurosensory alterations, maladaptive stress response, fatigue, anorexia, disorientation.

PSY

Social Isolation may be related to changes in physical appearance/mental status, state of wellness, perceptions of unacceptable social or sexual behavior/values, physical isolation, phobic fear of others (transmission of disease), possibly evidenced by expressed feelings of aloneness/rejection, absence of supportive SO(s), and withdrawal from usual activities.

disturbed Thought Processes/chronic Confusion may be related to physiological changes (hypoxemia, central nervous system—CNS—infection by HIV, brain malignancies, and/or disseminated systemic opportunistic infection), altered drug metabolism/excretion, accumulation of toxic elements (renal failure, severe electrolyte imbalance, hepatic insufficiency), possibly evidenced by clinical evidence of organic impairment, altered attention span, distractibility, memory deficit, disorientation, cognitive dissonance, delusional thinking, impaired ability to make decisions/problem solve, inability to follow complex commands/mental tasks, loss of impulse control, and altered personality.

AIDS dementia   CH
(Also refer to Dementia, presenile/senile)

impaired Environmental Interpretation Syndrome may be related to dementia, depression, possibly evidenced by consistent disorientation, inability to follow simple directions/instructions, loss of social functioning from memory decline.

ineffective Protection may be related to chronic disease affecting immune and neurological systems, inadequate nutrition, drug therapies, possibly evidenced by deficient immunity, impaired healing, neurosensory alterations, maladaptive stress response, fatigue, anorexia, disorientation.

Alcohol abuse/withdrawal   CH/MS/PSY
(Refer to Drug overdose, acute [depressants]; Delirium tremens; Substance dependency/abuse rehabilitation)

Alcohol intoxication, acute   MS
(Also refer to Delirium tremens)
acute Confusion may be related to substance abuse, hypoxemia, possibly evidenced by hallucinations, exaggerated emotional response, fluctuation in cognition/level of consciousness, increased agitation.
risk for ineffective Breathing Pattern: risk factors may include neuromuscular impairment/CNS depression.*
risk for Aspiration: risk factors may include reduced level of consciousness, depressed cough/gag reflexes, delayed gastric emptying.*

Aldosteronism, primary   MS
deficient Fluid Volume [isotonic] may be related to increased urinary losses, possibly evidenced by dry mucous membranes, poor skin turgor, dilute urine, excessive thirst, weight loss.
impaired physical Mobility may be related to neuromuscular impairment, weakness, and pain, possibly evidenced by impaired coordination, decreased muscle strength, paralysis, and positive Chvostek's and Trousseau's signs.
risk for decreased Cardiac Output: risk factors may include hypovolemia and altered electrical conduction/dysrhythmias.*

Alkalosis, respiratory   MS
(Also refer to underlying cause/condition)
impaired Gas Exchange may be related to ventilation-perfusion imbalance (decreased O_2 carrying capacity of blood, altered O_2 supply, alveolar-capillary membrane changes), possibly evidenced by dyspnea, tachypnea, changes in mentation, tachycardia, hypoxia, hypocapnia.

Allergies, seasonal   CH
(Refer to Hay fever)

Alopecia   CH
disturbed Body Image may be related to effects of illness/therapy or aging process, change in appearance, possibly evidenced by verbalization of feelings/concerns, fear of rejection/reaction of others, focus on past appearance, preoccupation with change, feelings of helplessness.

ALS   CH
(Refer to Amyotrophic lateral sclerosis)

Alzheimer's disease   CH
(Also refer to Dementia, presenile/senile)

---

*A risk diagnosis is not evidenced by signs and symptoms, as the problem has not occurred and nursing interventions are directed at prevention.

<u>risk for Injury/Trauma:</u> risk factors may include inability to recognize/identify danger in environment, disorientation, confusion, impaired judgment, weakness, muscular incoordination, balancing difficulties, and altered perception.*

<u>chronic Confusion</u> related to physiological changes (neuronal degeneration), possibly evidenced by inaccurate interpretation of/response to stimuli, progressive/long-standing cognitive impairment, short-term memory deficit, impaired socialization, altered personality, and clinical evidence of organic impairment.

<u>disturbed Sensory Perception (specify)</u> may be related to altered sensory reception, transmission, and/or integration (neurological disease/deficit), socially restricted environment (homebound/institutionalized), sleep deprivation, possibly evidenced by changes in usual response to stimuli, change in problem-solving abilities, exaggerated emotional responses (anxiety, paranoia, hallucinations), inability to tell position of body parts, diminished/altered sense of taste.

<u>Insomnia</u> may be related to sensory impairment, changes in activity patterns, psychological stress (neurological impairment), possibly evidenced by wakefulness, disorientation (day/night reversal), increased aimless wandering, inability to identify need/time for sleeping, changes in behavior/performance, lethargy; dark circles under eyes, and frequent yawning.

<u>ineffective Health Maintenance</u> may be related to deterioration affecting ability in all areas, including coordination/communication, cognitive impairment, ineffective individual/family coping, possibly evidenced by reported or observed inability to take responsibility for meeting basic health practices, lack of equipment/financial or other resources, and impairment of personal support system.

PSY

<u>risk for Stress Overload:</u> risk factors may include inadequate resources, chronic illness, physical demands, threats of violence.*

<u>compromised family Coping/Caregiver Role Strain</u> may be related to family disorganization, role changes, family/caregiver isolation, long-term illness/complexity and amount of homecare needs exhausting supportive/financial capabilities of family member(s), lack of respite, possibly evidenced by verbalizations of frustrations in dealing with day-to-day care, reports of conflict, feelings of depression, expressed anger/guilt directed toward client, and withdrawal from interaction with client/social contacts.

<u>risk for Relocation Stress Syndrome:</u> risk factors may include little or no preparation for transfer to a new setting, changes in daily routine, sensory impairment, physical deterioration, separation from support systems.*

Amphetamine abuse   PSY
(Refer to Stimulant abuse)

---

*A risk diagnosis is not evidenced by signs and symptoms, as the problem has not occurred and nursing interventions are directed at prevention.

Amputation   MS

risk for ineffective peripheral Tissue Perfusion: risk factors may include reduced arterial/venous blood flow, tissue edema, hematoma formation, hypovolemia.*

acute Pain may be related to tissue and nerve trauma, psychological impact of loss of body part, possibly evidenced by reports of incisional/phantom pain, guarding/protective behavior, narrowed/self-focus, and autonomic responses.

impaired physical Mobility may be related to loss of limb (primarily lower extremity), altered sense of balance, pain/discomfort, possibly evidenced by reluctance to attempt movement; impaired coordination; decreased muscle strength, control, and mass.

disturbed Body Image may be related to loss of a body part, possibly evidenced by verbalization of feelings of powerlessness, grief, preoccupation with loss, and unwillingness to look at/touch stump.

Amyotrophic lateral sclerosis (ALS)   MS

impaired physical Mobility may be related to muscle wasting/weakness, possibly evidenced by impaired coordination, limited range of motion, and impaired purposeful movement.

ineffective Breathing Pattern/impaired spontaneous Ventilation may be related to neuromuscular impairment, decreased energy, fatigue, tracheobronchial obstruction, possibly evidenced by shortness of breath, fremitus, respiratory depth changes, and reduced vital capacity.

impaired Swallowing may be related to muscle wasting and fatigue, possibly evidenced by recurrent coughing/choking and signs of aspiration.

PSY

Powerlessness [specify level] may be related to chronic/debilitating nature of illness, lack of control over outcome, possibly evidenced by expressions of frustration about inability to care for self and depression over physical deterioration.

Grieving may be related to perceived potential loss of self/physiopsychosocial well-being, possibly evidenced by sorrow, choked feelings, expression of distress, changes in eating habits, sleeping patterns, and altered communication patterns/libido.

CH

impaired verbal Communication may be related to physical barrier (neuromuscular impairment), possibly evidenced by impaired articulation, inability to speak in sentences, and use of nonverbal cues (changes in facial expression).

risk for Caregiver Role Strain: risk factors may include illness severity of care receiver, complexity and amount of home-care needs, duration of caregiving required, caregiver is spouse, family/caregiver isolation, lack of respite/recreation for caregiver.*

---

*A risk diagnosis is not evidenced by signs and symptoms, as the problem has not occurred and nursing interventions are directed at prevention.

Anaphylaxis
(Also refer to Shock)

CH

A

ineffective Airway Clearance may be related to airway spasm (bronchial), laryngeal edema, possibly evidenced by diminished/adventitious breath sounds, cough ineffective or absent, difficulty vocalizing, wide-eyed.

decreased Cardiac Output may be related to decreased preload, increased capillary permeability (third spacing) and vasodilation, possibly evidenced by tachycardia/palpitations, changes in blood pressure (BP), anxiety, restlessness.

Anemia

CH

Activity Intolerance may be related to imbalance between O_2 supply (delivery) and demand, possibly evidenced by reports of fatigue and weakness, abnormal heart rate or BP response, decreased exercise/activity level, and exertional discomfort or dyspnea.

imbalanced Nutrition: less than body requirements may be related to failure to ingest/inability to digest food or absorb nutrients necessary for formation of normal red blood cells (RBCs), possibly evidenced by weight loss/weight below normal for age, height, body build, decreased triceps skinfold measurement, changes in gums/oral mucous membranes, decreased tolerance for activity, weakness, and loss of muscle tone.

deficient Knowledge [Learning Need] regarding condition, prognosis, self-care and treatment needs may be related to inadequate understanding or misinterpretation of dietary/physiological needs, possibly evidenced by inadequate dietary intake, request for information, and development of preventable complications.

Anemia, sickle cell

MS

impaired Gas Exchange may be related to decreased O_2-carrying capacity of blood, reduced RBC life span, abnormal RBC structure, increased blood viscosity, predisposition to bacterial pneumonia/pulmonary infarcts, possibly evidenced by dyspnea, use of accessory muscles, cyanosis/signs of hypoxia, tachycardia, changes in mentation, and restlessness.

ineffective Tissue Perfusion: (specify) may be related to stasis, vaso-occlusive nature of sickling, inflammatory response, atrioventricular (AV) shunts in pulmonary and peripheral circulation, myocardial damage (small infarcts, iron deposits, fibrosis), possibly evidenced by signs and symptoms dependent on system involved, for example: renal: decreased specific gravity and pale urine in face of dehydration; cerebral: paralysis and visual disturbances; peripheral: distal ischemia, tissue infarctions, ulcerations, bone pain; cardiopulmonary: angina, palpitations.

CH

acute/chronic Pain may be related to intravascular sickling with localized vascular stasis, occlusion, infarction/necrosis and deprivation of O_2 and nutrients, accumulation of noxious metabolites, possibly evidenced by reports of localized, generalized, or migratory joint and/or abdominal/back pain, guarding and distraction behaviors (moaning, crying, restlessness), facial grimacing, narrowed focus, and autonomic responses.

deficient Knowledge [Learning Need] regarding disease process, genetic factors, prognosis, self-care and treatment needs may be related to lack of exposure/recall, misinterpretation of information, unfamiliarity with resources, possibly evidenced by questions, statement of concern/misconceptions, exacerbation of condition, inadequate follow-through of therapy instructions, and development of preventable complications.

delayed Growth and Development may be related to effects/limitations of physical condition, possibly evidenced by altered physical growth and delay/difficulty performing skills typical of age group.

risk for sedentary Lifestyle: risk factors may include lack of interest/motivation, lack of resources, lack of training or knowledge of specific exercise needs, safety concerns/fear of injury.

compromised family Coping may be related to chronic nature of disease/disability, family disorganization, presence of other crises/situations impacting significant person/parent, lifestyle restrictions, possibly evidenced by significant person/parent expressing preoccupation with own reaction and displaying protective behavior disproportionate to client's ability or need for autonomy.

Aneurysm, abdominal aortic (AAA)   MS
(Refer to Aortic aneurysm, abdominal)

Angina pectoris   MS
acute Pain may be related to decreased myocardial blood flow, increased cardiac workload/O_2 consumption, possibly evidenced by verbal reports, narrowed focus, distraction behaviors (restlessness, moaning), and autonomic responses (diaphoresis, changes in vital signs).

decreased Cardiac Output may be related to inotropic changes (transient/prolonged myocardial ischemia, effects of medications), alterations in rate/rhythm and electrical conduction, possibly evidenced by changes in hemodynamic readings, dyspnea, restlessness, decreased tolerance for activity, fatigue, diminished peripheral pulses, cool/pale skin, changes in mental status, and continued chest pain.

Anxiety [specify level] may be related to situational crises, change in health status and/or threat of death, negative self-talk, possibly evidenced by verbalized apprehension, facial tension, extraneous movements, and focus on self.

CH

Activity Intolerance may be related to imbalance between O_2 supply and demand, possibly evidenced by exertional dyspnea, abnormal pulse/BP response to activity, and electrocardiogram (ECG) changes.

deficient Knowledge [Learning Need] regarding condition, prognosis, self-care and treatment needs may be related to lack of exposure, inaccurate/misinterpretation of information, possibly evidenced by questions, request for information, statement of concern, and inaccurate follow-through of instructions.

risk for sedentary Lifestyle: risk factors may include lack of training or knowledge of specific exercise needs, safety concerns/fear of myocardial injury.

risk for risk-prone health Behavior: risk factors may include condition requiring long-term therapy/change in lifestyle, multiple stressors, assault to self-concept, and altered locus of control.*

Anorexia nervosa   MS

imbalanced Nutrition: less than body requirements may be related to psychological restrictions of food intake and/or excessive activity, self-induced vomiting, laxative abuse, possibly evidenced by weight loss, poor skin turgor/muscle tone, denial of hunger, unusual hoarding or handling of food, amenorrhea, electrolyte imbalance, cardiac irregularities, hypotension.

risk for deficient Fluid Volume: risk factors may include inadequate intake of food and liquids, chronic/excessive laxative or diuretic use, self-induced vomiting.*

PSY

disturbed Thought Processes may be related to severe malnutrition/electrolyte imbalance, psychological conflicts, possibly evidenced by impaired ability to make decisions, problem solve, nonreality-based verbalizations, ideas of reference, altered sleep patterns, altered attention span/distractibility, perceptual disturbances with failure to recognize hunger, fatigue, anxiety, and depression.

disturbed Body Image/chronic low Self-Esteem may be related to altered perception of body, perceived loss of control in some aspect of life, unmet dependency needs, personal vulnerability, dysfunctional family system, possibly evidenced by negative feelings, distorted view of body, use of denial, feeling powerless to prevent/make changes, expressions of shame/guilt, overly conforming, dependent on others' opinions.

interrupted Family Processes may be related to ambivalent family relationships and ways of transacting issues of control, situational/maturational crises, possibly evidenced by enmeshed family, dissonance among family members, family developmental tasks not being met, family members acting as enablers.

Antisocial personality disorder   PSY

risk for other-directed Violence: risk factors may include contempt for authority/rights of others, inability to tolerate frustration, need for immediate gratification, easy agitation, vulnerable self-concept, inability to verbalize feelings, use of maladjusted coping mechanisms including substance use.*

ineffective Coping may be related to very low tolerance for external stress, lack of experience of internal anxiety (e.g., guilt/shame), personal vulnerability, unmet expectations, multiple life changes, possibly evidenced by choice of aggression and manipulation to handle

---

*A risk diagnosis is not evidenced by signs and symptoms, as the problem has not occurred and nursing interventions are directed at prevention.

A

problems/conflicts, inappropriate use of defense mechanisms (e.g., denial, projection), chronic worry, anxiety, destructive behaviors, high rate of accidents.

chronic low Self-Esteem may be related to lack of positive and/or repeated negative feedback, unmet dependency needs, retarded ego development, dysfunctional family system, possibly evidenced by acting-out behaviors (e.g., substance abuse, sexual promiscuity, feelings of inadequacy, nonparticipation in therapy).

compromised/disabled family Coping may be related to family disorganization/role changes, highly ambivalent family relationships, client providing little support in turn for the primary person(s), history of abuse/neglect in the home, possibly evidenced by expressions of concern or complaints, preoccupation of primary person with own reactions to situation, display of protective behaviors disproportionate to client's abilities, or need for autonomy.

impaired Social Interaction may be related to inadequate personal resources (shallow feelings), immature interests, underdeveloped conscious, unaccepted social values, possibly evidenced by difficulty meeting expectations of others, lack of belief that rules pertain to self, sense of emptiness/inadequacy covered by expressions of self-conceit/arrogance/contempt, behavior unaccepted by dominant cultural group.

Anxiety disorder, generalized   PSY

Anxiety [specify level]/Powerlessness may be related to real or perceived threat to physical integrity or self-concept (may or may not be able to identify the threat), unconscious conflict about essential values/beliefs and goals of life, unmet needs, negative self-talk, possibly evidenced by sympathetic stimulation, extraneous movements (foot shuffling, hand/arm fidgeting, rocking movements, restlessness), persistent feelings of apprehension and uneasiness, a general anxious feeling that client has difficulty alleviating, poor eye contact, focus on self, impaired functioning, free-floating anxiety, and nonparticipation in decision making.

ineffective Coping may be related to level of anxiety being experienced by the client, personal vulnerability, unmet expectations/unrealistic perceptions, inadequate coping methods and/or support systems, possibly evidenced by verbalization of inability to cope/problem solve, excessive compulsive behaviors (e.g., smoking, drinking), and emotional/muscle tension, alteration in societal participation, high rate of accidents.

Insomnia may be related to psychological stress, repetitive thoughts, possibly evidenced by reports of difficulty in falling asleep/awakening earlier or later than desired, reports of not feeling rested, dark circles under eyes, and frequent yawning.

risk for compromised family Coping: risk factors may include inadequate/incorrect information or understanding by a primary person, temporary family disorganization and role changes, prolonged disability that exhausts the supportive capacity of SO(s).*

*A risk diagnosis is not evidenced by signs and symptoms, as the problem has not occurred and nursing interventions are directed at prevention.

impaired Social Interaction/Social Isolation may be related to low self-concept, inadequate personal resources, misinterpretation of internal/external stimuli, hypervigilance, possibly evidenced by discomfort in social situations, withdrawal from or reported change in pattern of interactions, dysfunctional interactions, expressed feelings of difference from others, sad, dull affect.

Anxiolytic abuse   PSY
(Refer to Depressant abuse)

Aortic aneurysm, abdominal (AAA)   MS
risk for ineffective peripheral Tissue Perfusion: risk factors may include interruption of arterial blood flow [embolus formation, spontaneous blockage of aorta].*
risk for Infection: risk factors may include turbulent blood flow through arteriosclerotic lesion.*
acute Pain may be related to vascular enlargement-dissection/rupture, possibly evidenced by verbal coded reports, guarding behavior, facial mask, change in abdominal muscle tone.

Aortic aneurysm repair, abdominal   MS
(Also refer to Surgery, general)
Fear related to threat of injury/death, surgical intervention, possibly evidenced by verbal reports, apprehension, decreased self-assurance, increased tension, changes in vital signs.
risk for deficient Fluid Volume: risk factors may include weakening of vascular wall, failure of vascular repair.*
risk for ineffective renal/peripheral Tissue Perfusion: risk factors may include interruption of arterial blood flow, hypovolemia.*

Aortic stenosis   MS
decreased Cardiac Output may be related to structural changes of heart valve, left ventricular outflow obstruction, alteration of afterload (increased left ventricular end-diastolic pressure and systemic vascular resistance—SVR), alteration in preload/increased atrial pressure and venous congestion, alteration in electrical conduction, possibly evidenced by fatigue, dyspnea, changes in vital signs/hemodynamic parameters, and syncope.
risk for impaired Gas Exchange: risk factors may include alveolar-capillary membrane changes/congestion.*

                                                                 CH
risk for acute Pain: risk factors may include episodic ischemia of myocardial tissues and stretching of left atrium.*
Activity Intolerance may be related to imbalance between O_2 supply and demand (decreased/fixed cardiac output), possibly evidenced by exertional dyspnea, reported fatigue/weakness, and abnormal blood pressure or ECG changes/dysrhythmias in response to activity.

---

*A risk diagnosis is not evidenced by signs and symptoms, as the problem has not occurred and nursing interventions are directed at prevention.

Aplastic anemia   CH
(Also refer to Anemia)

risk for ineffective Protection: risk factors may include abnormal blood profile (leukopenia, thrombocytopenia), drug therapies (antineoplastics, antibiotics, NSAIDs [nonsteroidal anti-inflammatory drugs], anticonvulsants).*

Fatigue may be related to anemia, disease states, malnutrition, possibly evidenced by verbalization of overwhelming lack of energy, inability to maintain usual routines/level of physical activity, tired, decreased libido, lethargy, increase in physical complaints.

Appendicitis   MS

acute Pain may be related to distention of intestinal tissues by inflammation, possibly evidenced by verbal reports, guarding behavior, narrowed focus, and autonomic responses (diaphoresis, changes in vital signs).

risk for deficient Fluid Volume: risk factors may include nausea, vomiting, anorexia, and hypermetabolic state.*

risk for Infection: risk factors may include release of pathogenic organisms into peritoneal cavity.*

ARDS   MS
(Refer to Acute respiratory distress syndrome)

Arrhythmia, cardiac   MS/CH
(Refer to Dysrhythmia, cardiac)

Arterial occlusive disease, peripheral   CH

ineffective peripheral Tissue Perfusion may be related to decreased arterial blood flow, possibly evidenced by skin discolorations, temperature changes, altered sensation, claudication, delayed healing.

risk for impaired Walking: risk factors may include presence of circulatory problems, pain with activity.*

risk for impaired Skin/Tissue Integrity risk factors may include altered circulation/sensation.*

Arthritis, juvenile rheumatoid   PED/CH
(Also refer to Arthritis, rheumatoid)

risk for delayed Development: risk factors may include effects of physical disability and required therapy.*

risk for Social Isolation: risk factors may include delay in accomplishing developmental task, altered state of wellness, and changes in physical appearance.*

Arthritis, rheumatoid   CH

acute/chronic Pain may be related to accumulation of fluid/inflammatory process, degeneration of joint, and deformity, possibly evidenced by verbal reports, narrowed focus, guarding/protective behaviors, and physical and social withdrawal.

impaired physical Mobility may be related to musculoskeletal deformity, pain/discomfort, decreased muscle strength, possibly evidenced

---

*A risk diagnosis is not evidenced by signs and symptoms, as the problem has not occurred and nursing interventions are directed at prevention.

by limited range of motion, impaired coordination, reluctance to attempt movement, and decreased muscle strength/control and mass.

Self-Care Deficit [specify] may be related to musculoskeletal impairment, decreased strength/endurance and range of motion, pain on movement, possibly evidenced by inability to manage activities of daily living (ADLs).

disturbed Body Image/ineffective Role Performance may be related to change in body structure/function, impaired mobility/ability to perform usual tasks, focus on past strength/function/appearance, possibly evidenced by negative self-talk, feelings of helplessness, change in lifestyle/physical abilities, dependence on others for assistance, decreased social involvement.

Arthritis, septic   CH

acute Pain may be related to joint inflammation, possibly evidenced by verbal/coded reports, guarding behaviors, restlessness, narrowed focus.

impaired physical Mobility may be related to joint stiffness, pain/discomfort, reluctance to initiate movement, possibly evidenced by limited range of motion, slowed movement.

Self-Care Deficit [specify] may be related to musculoskeletal impairment, pain/discomfort, decreased strength, impaired coordination, possibly evidenced by inability to perform desired ADLs.

risk for Infection [spread]: risk factors may include presence of infectious process, chronic disease states, invasive procedures.*

Arthroplasty   MS

risk for Infection: risk factors may include breach of primary defenses (surgical incision), stasis of body fluids at operative site, and altered inflammatory response.*

risk for deficient Fluid Volume [isotonic]: risk factors may include surgical procedure/trauma to vascular area.*

impaired physical Mobility may be related to decreased strength, pain, musculoskeletal changes, possibly evidenced by impaired coordination and reluctance to attempt movement.

acute Pain may be related to tissue trauma, local edema, possibly evidenced by verbal reports, narrowed focus, guarded movement, and autonomic responses (diaphoresis, changes in vital signs).

Arthroscopy, knee   MS

deficient Knowledge [Learning Need] regarding procedure/outcomes and self-care needs may be related to unfamiliarity with information/resources, misinterpretations, possibly evidenced by questions and requests for information, misconceptions.

risk for impaired Walking: risk factors may include joint stiffness, discomfort, prescribed movement restrictions, use of assistive devices/crutches for ambulation.*

Asthma   MS
(Also refer to Emphysema)

---

*A risk diagnosis is not evidenced by signs and symptoms, as the problem has not occurred and nursing interventions are directed at prevention.

ineffective Airway Clearance may be related to increased production/ retained pulmonary secretions, bronchospasm, decreased energy/ fatigue, possibly evidenced by wheezing, difficulty breathing, changes in depth/rate of respirations, use of accessory muscles, and persistent ineffective cough with or without sputum production.

impaired Gas Exchange may be related to altered delivery of inspired O_2/air trapping, possibly evidenced by dyspnea, restlessness, reduced tolerance for activity, cyanosis, and changes in ABGs and vital signs.

Anxiety [specify level] may be related to perceived threat of death, possibly evidenced by apprehension, fearful expression, and extraneous movements.

CH

Activity Intolerance may be related to imbalance between O_2 supply and demand, possibly evidenced by fatigue and exertional dyspnea.

risk for Contamination: risk factors may include presence of atmospheric pollutants, environmental contaminants in the home (e.g., smoking/second-hand tobacco smoke).

Athlete's foot   CH

impaired Skin Integrity may be related to fungal invasion, humidity, secretions, possibly evidenced by disruption of skin surface, reports of painful itching.

risk for Infection [spread]: risk factors may include multiple breaks in skin, exposure to moist/warm environment.*

Atrial fibrillation   CH
(Refer to Dysrhythmias)

Atrial flutter   CH
(Refer to Dysrhythmias)

Atrial tachycardia   CH
(Refer to Dysrhythmias)

Attention deficit disorder (ADD)   PED/PSY

ineffective Coping may be related to situational/maturational crisis, retarded ego development, low self-concept, possibly evidenced by easy distraction by extraneous stimuli, shifting between uncompleted activities.

chronic low Self-Esteem may be related to retarded ego development, lack of positive/repeated negative feedback, negative role models, possibly evidenced by lack of eye contact, derogatory self comments, hesitance to try new tasks, inadequate level of confidence.

deficient Knowledge [Learning Need] regarding condition, prognosis, therapy may be related to misinformation/misinterpretations, unfamiliarity with resources, possibly evidenced by verbalization of problems/misconceptions, poor school performance, unrealistic expectations of medication regimen.

---

*A risk diagnosis is not evidenced by signs and symptoms, as the problem has not occurred and nursing interventions are directed at prevention.

Autistic disorder   PED/PSY

impaired Social Interaction may be related to abnormal response to sensory input/inadequate sensory stimulation, organic brain dysfunction, delayed development of secure attachment/trust, lack of intuitive skills to comprehend and accurately respond to social cues, disturbance in self-concept, possibly evidenced by lack of responsiveness to others, lack of eye contact or facial responsiveness, treating persons as objects, lack of awareness of feelings in others, indifference/aversion to comfort, affection, or physical contact, failure to develop cooperative social play and peer friendships in childhood.

impaired verbal Communication may be related to inability to trust others, withdrawal into self, organic brain dysfunction, abnormal interpretation/response to and/or inadequate sensory stimulation, possibly evidenced by lack of interactive communication mode, no use of gestures or spoken language, absent or abnormal nonverbal communication, lack of eye contact or facial expression, peculiar patterns of speech (form, content, or speech production), and impaired ability to initiate or sustain conversation despite adequate speech.

risk for Self-Mutilation: risk factors may include organic brain dysfunction, inability to trust others, disturbance in self-concept, inadequate sensory stimulation or abnormal response to sensory input (sensory overload), history of physical, emotional, or sexual abuse, and response to demands of therapy, realization of severity of condition.*

disturbed Personal Identity may be related to organic brain dysfunction, lack of development of trust, maternal deprivation, fixation at presymbiotic phase of development, possibly evidenced by lack of awareness of the feelings or existence of others, increased anxiety resulting from physical contact with others, absent or impaired imitation of others, repeating what others say, persistent preoccupation with parts of objects, obsessive attachment to objects, marked distress over changes in environment, autoerotic/ritualistic behaviors, self-touching, rocking, swaying.

compromised/disabled family Coping may be related to family members unable to express feelings, excessive guilt, anger, or blaming among family members regarding child's condition, ambivalent or dissonant family relationships, prolonged coping with problem exhausting supportive ability of family members, possibly evidenced by denial of existence or severity of disturbed behaviors, preoccupation with personal emotional reaction to situation, rationalization that problem will be outgrown, attempts to intervene with child are achieving increasingly ineffective results, family withdraws from or becomes overly protective of child.

Barbiturate abuse   CH/PSY
(Refer to Depressant abuse)

Battered child syndrome   PED/CH
(Also refer to Abuse)

---

*A risk diagnosis is not evidenced by signs and symptoms, as the problem has not occurred and nursing interventions are directed at prevention.

risk for Trauma: risk factors may include dependent position in rela-
tionship(s), vulnerability (e.g., congenital problems/chronic illness),
history of previous abuse/neglect, lack/nonuse of support systems by
caregiver(s).*

interrupted Family Processes/impaired Parenting may be related to
poor role model/identity, unrealistic expectations, presence of stressors, and lack of support, possibly evidenced by verbalization of negative feelings, inappropriate caretaking behaviors, and evidence of
physical/psychological trauma to child.

PSY

chronic low Self-Esteem may be related to deprivation and negative
feedback of family members, personal vulnerability, feelings of abandonment, possibly evidenced by lack of eye contact, withdrawal from
social contacts, discounting own needs, nonassertive/passive, indecisive, or overly conforming behaviors.

Post-Trauma Syndrome may be related to sustained/recurrent physical
or emotional abuse; possibly evidenced by acting-out behavior, development of phobias, poor impulse control, and emotional numbness.

ineffective Coping may be related to situational or maturational crisis,
overwhelming threat to self, personal vulnerability, inadequate support systems, possibly evidenced by verbalized concern about ability
to deal with current situation, chronic worry, anxiety, depression,
poor self-esteem, inability to problem solve, high illness rate, destructive behavior toward self/others.

Benign prostatic hyperplasia   CH/MS

[acute/chronic] Urinary Retention/overflow Urinary Incontinence may
be related to mechanical obstruction (enlarged prostate), decompensation of detrusor musculature, inability of bladder to contract adequately, possibly evidenced by frequency, hesitancy, inability to empty
bladder completely, incontinence/dribbling, nocturia, bladder distention, residual urine.

acute Pain may be related to mucosal irritation, bladder distention, colic,
urinary infection, and radiation therapy, possibly evidenced by verbal
reports (bladder/rectal spasm), narrowed focus, altered muscle tone, grimacing, distraction behaviors, restlessness, and autonomic responses.

risk for deficient Fluid Volume: risk factors may include postobstructive
diuresis, endocrine/electrolyte imbalances.*

Fear/Anxiety [specify level] may be related to change in health status
(possibility of surgical procedure/malignancy); embarrassment/loss
of dignity associated with genital exposure before, during, and after
treatment, and concern about sexual ability, possibly evidenced by
increased tension, apprehension, worry, expressed concerns regarding
perceived changes, and fear of unspecific consequences.

Bipolar disorder   PSY

risk for other-directed Violence: risk factors may include irritability,
impulsive behavior, delusional thinking, angry response when ideas

---

*A risk diagnosis is not evidenced by signs and symptoms, as the
problem has not occurred and nursing interventions are directed at
prevention.

are refuted or wishes denied, manic excitement, with possible indicators of threatening body language/verbalizations, increased motor activity, overt and aggressive acts, hostility.*

imbalanced Nutrition: less than body requirements may be related to inadequate intake in relation to metabolic expenditures, possibly evidenced by body weight 20% or more below ideal weight, observed inadequate intake, inattention to mealtimes, and distraction from task of eating, laboratory evidence of nutritional deficits/imbalances.

risk for Poisoning [lithium toxicity]: risk factors may include narrow therapeutic range of drug, client's ability (or lack of) to follow-through with medication regimen and monitoring, and denial of need for information/therapy.*

Insomnia may be related to psychological stress, lack of recognition of fatigue/need to sleep, hyperactivity, possibly evidenced by denial of need to sleep, interrupted nighttime sleep, one or more nights without sleep, changes in behavior and performance, increasing irritability/restlessness, and dark circles under eyes.

disturbed Sensory Perception (specify) [overload] may be related to decrease in sensory threshold, endogenous chemical alteration, psychological stress, sleep deprivation, possibly evidenced by increased distractibility and agitation, anxiety, disorientation, poor concentration, auditory/visual hallucination, bizarre thinking, and motor incoordination.

interrupted Family Processes may be related to situational crises (illness, economics, change in roles), euphoric mood and grandiose ideas/actions of client, manipulative behavior and limit testing, client's refusal to accept responsibility for own actions, possibly evidenced by statements of difficulty coping with situation, lack of adaptation to change, or not dealing constructively with illness, ineffective family decision-making process, failure to send and to receive clear messages, and inappropriate boundary maintenance.

Bone cancer   MS/CH
(Also refer to Myeloma, multiple; Amputation)

acute Pain may be related to bone destruction, pressure on nerves, possibly evidenced by verbal or coded report, protective behavior, autonomic responses.

risk for Trauma: risk factors may include increased bone fragility, general weakness, balancing difficulties.*

Borderline personality disorder   PSY

risk for self-/other-directed Violence/Self-Mutilation: risk factors may include use of projection as a major defense mechanism, pervasive problems with negative transference, feelings of guilt/need to "punish" self, distorted sense of self, inability to cope with increased psychological/physiological tension in a healthy manner.*

Anxiety [severe to panic] may be related to unconscious conflicts (experience of extreme stress), perceived threat to self-concept, unmet needs, possibly evidenced by easy frustration and feelings of hurt,

---

*A risk diagnosis is not evidenced by signs and symptoms, as the problem has not occurred and nursing interventions are directed at prevention.

abuse of alcohol/other drugs, transient psychotic symptoms, and performance of self-mutilating acts.

chronic low Self-Esteem/disturbed personal Identity may be related to lack of positive feedback, unmet dependency needs, retarded ego development/fixation at an earlier level of development, possibly evidenced by difficulty identifying self or defining self-boundaries, feelings of depersonalization, extreme mood changes, lack of tolerance of rejection or of being alone, unhappiness with self, striking out at others, performance of ritualistic self-damaging acts, and belief that punishing self is necessary.

Social Isolation may be related to immature interests, unaccepted social behavior, inadequate personal resources, and inability to engage in satisfying personal relationships, possibly evidenced by alternating clinging and distancing behaviors, difficulty meeting expectations of others, experiencing feelings of difference from others, expressing interests inappropriate to developmental age, and exhibiting behavior unaccepted by dominant cultural group.

Botulism (food-borne)   MS

deficient Fluid Volume [isotonic] may be related to active losses—vomiting, diarrhea, decreased intake—nausea, dysphagia, possibly evidenced by reports of thirst, dry skin/mucous membranes, decreased BP and urine output, change in mental state, increased hematocrit (Hct).

impaired physical Mobility may be related to neuromuscular impairment, possibly evidenced by limited ability to perform gross/fine motor skills.

Anxiety [specify level]/Fear may be related to threat of death, interpersonal transmission, possibly evidenced by expressed concerns, apprehension, awareness of physiological symptoms, focus on self.

risk for impaired spontaneous Ventilation: risk factors may include neuromuscular impairment, presence of infectious process.*

                                                        CH

Contamination may be related to lack of proper precautions in food storage/preparation as evidenced by gastointestinal and neurological effects of exposure to biological agent.*

Brain tumor   MS

acute Pain may be related to pressure on brain tissues, possibly evidenced by reports of headache, facial mask of pain, narrowed focus, and autonomic responses (changes in vital signs).

disturbed Thought Processes may be related to altered circulation to and/or destruction of brain tissue, possibly evidenced by memory loss, personality changes, impaired ability to make decisions/conceptualize, and inaccurate interpretation of environment.

disturbed Sensory Perception (specify) may be related to compression/displacement of brain tissue, disruption of neuronal conduction, possibly evidenced by changes in visual acuity, alterations in sense of balance/gait disturbance, and paresthesia.

---

*A risk diagnosis is not evidenced by signs and symptoms, as the problem has not occurred and nursing interventions are directed at prevention.

risk for deficient Fluid Volume: risk factors may include recurrent vomiting from irritation of vagal center in medulla and decreased intake.*

Self-Care Deficit [specify] may be related to sensory/neuromuscular impairment interfering with ability to perform tasks, possibly evidenced by unkempt/disheveled appearance, body odor, and verbalization/observation of inability to perform ADLs.

Breast cancer   MS/CH
(Also refer to Cancer)

Anxiety [specify level] may be related to change in health status, threat of death, stress, interpersonal transmission, possibly evidenced by expressed concerns, apprehension, uncertainty, focus on self, diminished productivity.

deficient Knowledge [Learning Need] regarding diagnosis, prognosis, and treatment options may be related to lack of exposure/unfamiliarity with information resources, information misinterpretation, cognitive limitation/anxiety, possibly evidenced by verbalizations, statements of misconceptions, inappropriate behaviors.

risk for disturbed Body Image: risk factors may include significance of body part with regard to sexual perceptions.*

risk for ineffective Sexuality Pattern: risk factors may include health-related changes, medical treatments, concern about relationship with SO.*

Bronchitis   CH
ineffective Airway Clearance may be related to excessive, thickened mucus secretions, possibly evidenced by presence of rhonchi, tachypnea, and ineffective cough.

Activity Intolerance [specify level] may be related to imbalance between O_2 supply and demand, possibly evidenced by reports of fatigue, dyspnea, and abnormal vital sign response to activity.

acute Pain may be related to localized inflammation, persistent cough, aching associated with fever, possibly evidenced by reports of discomfort, distraction behavior, and facial mask of pain.

Bronchopneumonia   MS/CH
(Also refer to Bronchitis)

ineffective Airway Clearance may be related to tracheal bronchial inflammation, edema formation, increased sputum production, pleuritic pain, decreased energy, fatigue, possibly evidenced by changes in rate/depth of respirations, abnormal breath sounds, use of accessory muscles, dyspnea, cyanosis, effective/ineffective cough—with or without sputum production.

impaired Gas Exchange may be related to inflammatory process, collection of secretions affecting O_2 exchange across alveolar membrane, and hypoventilation, possibly evidenced by restlessness/changes in mentation, dyspnea, tachycardia, pallor, cyanosis, and ABGs/oximetry evidence of hypoxia.

risk for Infection [spread]: risk factors may include decreased ciliary action, stasis of secretions, presence of existing infection.*

*A risk diagnosis is not evidenced by signs and symptoms, as the problem has not occurred and nursing interventions are directed at prevention.

Bulimia nervosa   PSY/MS
(Also refer to Anorexia nervosa)

impaired Dentition may be related to dietary habits, poor oral hygiene, chronic vomiting, possibly evidenced by erosion of tooth enamel, multiple caries, abraded teeth.

impaired Oral Mucous Membrane may be related to malnutrition or vitamin deficiency, poor oral hygiene, chronic vomiting, possibly evidenced by sore, inflamed buccal mucosa, swollen salivary glands, ulcerations of mucosa, reports of constant sore mouth/throat.

risk for deficient Fluid Volume: risk factors may include consistent self-induced vomiting, chronic/excessive laxative/diuretic use, esophageal erosion or tear (Mallory-Weiss syndrome).*

deficient Knowledge [Learning Need] regarding condition, prognosis, complication, treatment may be related to lack of exposure to/unfamiliarity with information about condition, learned maladaptive coping skills, possibly evidenced by verbalization of misconception of relationship of current situation and behaviors, distortion of body image, binging and purging behaviors, verbalized need for information/desire to change behaviors.

Burn (dependent on type, degree,   MS/CH
and severity of the injury)

risk for deficient Fluid Volume: risk factors may include loss of fluids through wounds, capillary damage and evaporation, hypermetabolic state, insufficient intake, hemorrhagic losses.*

risk for ineffective Airway Clearance: risk factors may include mucosal edema and loss of ciliary action (smoke inhalation), direct upper airway injury by flame, steam, chemicals.*

risk for Infection: risk factors may include loss of protective dermal barrier, traumatized/necrotic tissue, decreased hemoglobin, suppressed inflammatory response, environmental exposure/invasive procedures.*

acute/chronic Pain may be related to destruction of/trauma to tissue and nerves, edema formation, and manipulation of impaired tissues, possibly evidenced by verbal reports, narrowed focus, distraction and guarding behaviors, facial mask of pain, and autonomic responses (changes in vital signs).

risk for imbalanced Nutrition: less than body requirements: risk factors may include hypermetabolic state in response to burn injury/stress, inadequate intake, protein catabolism.*

Post-Trauma Syndrome may be related to life-threatening event, possibly evidenced by reexperiencing the event, repetitive dreams/nightmares, psychic/emotional numbness, and sleep disturbance.

ineffective Protection may be related to extremes of age, inadequate nutrition, anemia, impaired immune system, possibly evidenced by impaired healing, deficient immunity, fatigue, anorexia.

                                                              PED

deficient Diversional Activity may be related to long-term hospitalization, frequent lengthy treatments, and physical limitations, possibly

---

*A risk diagnosis is not evidenced by signs and symptoms, as the problem has not occurred and nursing interventions are directed at prevention.

evidenced by expressions of boredom, restlessness, withdrawal, and requests for something to do.

risk for delayed Development: risk factors may include effects of physical disability, separation from SO(s), and environmental deficiencies.*

Bursitis CH
acute/chronic Pain may be related to inflammation of affected joint, possibly evidenced by verbal reports, guarding behavior, and narrowed focus.

impaired physical Mobility may be related to inflammation and swelling of joint, and pain, possibly evidenced by diminished range of motion, reluctance to attempt movement, and imposed restriction of movement by medical treatment.

Calculi, urinary CH/MS
acute Pain may be related to increased frequency/force of ureteral contractions, tissue distention/trauma and edema formation, cellular ischemia, possibly evidenced by reports of sudden, severe, colicky pains, guarding and distraction behaviors, self-focus, and autonomic responses.

impaired Urinary Elimination may be related to stimulation of the bladder by calculi, renal or ureteral irritation, mechanical obstruction of urinary flow, edema formation, inflammation, possibly evidenced by urgency and frequency, oliguria (retention), hematuria.

risk for deficient Fluid Volume: risk factors may include stimulation of renal-intestinal reflexes causing nausea, vomiting, and diarrhea, changes in urinary output, postoperative diuresis, and decreased intake.*

risk for Infection: risk factors may include stasis of urine.*

deficient Knowledge [Learning Need] regarding condition, prognosis, self-care, and treatment needs may be related to lack of exposure/recall and information misinterpretation, possibly evidenced by requests for information, statements of concern, and recurrence/development of preventable complications.

Cancer MS
(Also refer to Chemotherapy)

Fear/death Anxiety may be related to situational crises, threat to/change in health/socioeconomic status, role functioning, interaction patterns, threat of death, separation from family, interpersonal transmission of feelings, possibly evidenced by expressed concerns, feelings of inadequacy/helplessness, insomnia, increased tension, restlessness, focus on self, sympathetic stimulation.

Grieving may be related to potential loss of physiological well-being (body part/function), perceived separation from SO(s)/lifestyle (death), possibly evidenced by anger, sadness, withdrawal, choked feelings, changes in eating/sleep patterns, activity level, libido, and communication patterns.

---

*A risk diagnosis is not evidenced by signs and symptoms, as the problem has not occurred and nursing interventions are directed at prevention.

acute/chronic Pain may be related to the disease process (compression of nerve tissue, infiltration of nerves or their vascular supply, obstruction of a nerve pathway, inflammation), or side effects of therapeutic agents, possibly evidenced by verbal reports, self-focusing/narrowed focus, alteration in muscle tone, facial mask of pain, distraction/guarding behaviors, autonomic responses, and restlessness.

Fatigue may be related to decreased metabolic energy production, increased energy requirements (hypermetabolic state), overwhelming psychological/emotional demands, and altered body chemistry (side effects of medications, chemotherapy), possibly evidenced by unremitting/overwhelming lack of energy, inability to maintain usual routines, decreased performance, impaired ability to concentrate, lethargy/listlessness, and disinterest in surroundings.

impaired Home Maintenance may be related to debilitation, lack of resources, and/or inadequate support systems, possibly evidenced by verbalization of problem, request for assistance, and lack of necessary equipment or aids.

PSY/PED

compromised/disabled family Coping may be related to chronic nature of disease and disability, ongoing treatment needs, parental supervision, and lifestyle restrictions, possibly evidenced by expression of denial/despair, depression, and protective behavior disproportionate to client's abilities or need for autonomy.

readiness for enhanced family Coping may be related to the fact that the individual's needs are being sufficiently gratified and adaptive tasks effectively addressed, enabling goals of self-actualization to surface, possibly evidenced by verbalizations of impact of crisis on own values, priorities, goals, or relationships.

Candidiasis   CH

(Also refer to Thrush)

impaired Skin/Tissue Integrity may be related to infectious lesions, possibly evidenced by disruption of skin surfaces/mucous membranes.

acute Pain/[Discomfort] may be related to exposure of irritated skin/mucous membranes to excretions (urine/feces), possibly evidenced by verbal/coded reports, restlessness, guarding behaviors.

risk for Sexual Dysfunction: risk factors include presence of infectious process/vaginal discomfort.*

Cannabis abuse   CH

(Refer to Stimulant abuse)

Cardiac surgery   MS/PED

Anxiety [specify level]/Fear may be related to change in health status and threat to self-concept/of death, possibly evidenced by sympathetic stimulation, increased tension, and apprehension.

risk for decreased Cardiac Output: risk factors may include decreased preload (hypovolemia), depressed myocardial contractility, changes in SVR (afterload), and alterations in electrical conduction (dysrhythmias).*

---

*A risk diagnosis is not evidenced by signs and symptoms, as the problem has not occurred and nursing interventions are directed at prevention.

deficient Fluid Volume [isotonic] may be related to intraoperative bleeding with inadequate blood replacement; bleeding related to insufficient heparin reversal, fibrinolysis, or platelet destruction; or volume depletion effects of intraoperative/postoperative diuretic therapy, possibly evidenced by increased pulse rate, decreased pulse volume/pressure, decreased urine output, hemoconcentration.

risk for impaired Gas Exchange: risk factors may include alveolar-capillary membrane changes (atelectasis), intestinal edema, inadequate function or premature discontinuation of chest tubes, and diminished O_2-carrying capacity of the blood.*

acute Pain/[Discomfort] may be related to tissue inflammation/trauma, edema formation, intraoperative nerve trauma, and myocardial ischemia, possibly evidenced by reports of incisional discomfort/pain in chest and donor site; paresthesia/pain in hand, arm, shoulder; anxiety, restlessness, irritability; distraction behaviors; and autonomic responses.

impaired Skin/Tissue Integrity related to mechanical trauma (surgical incisions, puncture wounds) and edema evidenced by disruption of skin surface/tissues.

Cardiogenic shock   MS
(Refer to Shock, cardiogenic)

Cardiomyopathy   CH/MS
decreased Cardiac Output may be related to altered contractility, possibly evidenced by dyspnea, fatigue, chest pain, dizziness, syncope.

Activity Intolerance may be related to imbalance between O_2 supply and demand, possibly evidenced by weakness/fatigue, dyspnea, abnormal heart rate/BP response to activity, ECG changes.

ineffective Role Performance may be related to changes in physical health, stress, demands of job/life, possibly evidenced by change in usual patterns of responsibility, role strain, change in capacity to resume role.

Carpal tunnel syndrome   CH/MS
acute/chronic Pain may be related to pressure on median nerve, possibly evidenced by verbal reports, reluctance to use affected extremity, guarding behaviors, expressed fear of reinjury, altered ability to continue previous activities.

impaired physical Mobility may be related to neuromuscular impairment and pain, possibly evidenced by decreased hand strength, weakness, limited range of motion, and reluctance to attempt movement.

risk for Peripheral Neurovascular Dysfunction: risk factors may include mechanical compression (e.g., brace, repetitive tasks/motions), immobilization.*

deficient Knowledge [Learning Need] regarding condition, prognosis, and treatment/safety needs may be related to lack of exposure/recall, information misinterpretation, possibly evidenced by questions, statements of concern, request for information, inaccurate follow-through of instructions/development of preventable complications.

---

*A risk diagnosis is not evidenced by signs and symptoms, as the problem has not occurred and nursing interventions are directed at prevention.

C

Casts CH/MS

(Also refer to Fractures)

risk for Peripheral Neurovascular Dysfunction: risk factors may include presence of fracture(s), mechanical compression (cast), tissue trauma, immobilization, vascular obstruction.*

risk for impaired Skin Integrity: risk factors may include pressure of cast, moisture/debris under cast, objects inserted under cast to relieve itching, and/or altered sensation/circulation.*

Self-Care Deficit [specify] may be related to impaired ability to perform self-care tasks, possibly evidenced by statements of need for assistance and observed difficulty in performing ADLs.

Cataract CH

disturbed visual Sensory Perception may be related to altered sensory reception/status of sense organs, and therapeutically restricted environment (surgical procedure, patching), possibly evidenced by diminished acuity, visual distortions, and change in usual response to stimuli.

risk for Trauma: risk factors may include poor vision, reduced hand/eye coordination.*

Anxiety [specify level]/Fear may be related to alteration in visual acuity, threat of permanent loss of vision/independence, possibly evidenced by expressed concerns, apprehension, and feelings of uncertainty.

deficient Knowledge [Learning Need] regarding ways of coping with altered abilities, therapy choices, lifestyle changes may be related to lack of exposure/recall, misinterpretation, or cognitive limitations, possibly evidenced by requests for information, statement of concern, inaccurate follow-through of instructions/development of preventable complications.

Cat scratch disease CH

acute Pain may be related to effects of circulating toxins (fever, headache, and lymphadenitis), possibly evidenced by verbal reports, guarding behavior, and autonomic response (changes in vital signs).

Hyperthermia may be related to inflammatory process, possibly evidenced by increased body temperature, flushed warm skin, tachypnea, and tachycardia.

Cerebrovascular accident (CVA) MS

ineffective cerebral Tissue Perfusion may be related to interruption of blood flow (occlusive disorder, hemorrhage, cerebral vasospasm/edema), possibly evidenced by altered level of consciousness, changes in vital signs, changes in motor/sensory responses, restlessness, memory loss, as well as sensory, language, intellectual, and emotional deficits.

impaired physical Mobility may be related to neuromuscular involvement (weakness, paresthesia, flaccid/hypotonic paralysis, spastic paralysis), perceptual/cognitive impairment, possibly evidenced by inability to purposefully move involved body parts/limited range of motion, impaired coordination, and/or decreased muscle strength/control.

---

*A risk diagnosis is not evidenced by signs and symptoms, as the problem has not occurred and nursing interventions are directed at prevention.

impaired verbal [and/or written] Communication may be related to impaired cerebral circulation, neuromuscular impairment, loss of facial/oral muscle tone and control, generalized weakness/fatigue, possibly evidenced by impaired articulation, does not/cannot speak (dysarthria), inability to modulate speech, find and/or name words, identify objects and/or inability to comprehend written/spoken language, inability to produce written communication.

Self-Care Deficit [specify] may be related to neuromuscular impairment, decreased strength/endurance, loss of muscle control/coordination, perceptual/cognitive impairment, pain/discomfort, and depression, possibly evidenced by stated/observed inability to perform ADLs, requests for assistance, disheveled appearance, and incontinence.

risk for impaired Swallowing: risk factors may include muscle paralysis and perceptual impairment.*

risk for unilateral Neglect: risk factors may include sensory loss of part of visual field with perceptual loss of corresponding body segment.*

CH

impaired Home Maintenance may be related to condition of individual family member, insufficient finances/family organization or planning, unfamiliarity with resources, and inadequate support systems, possibly evidenced by members expressing difficulty in managing home in a comfortable manner/requesting assistance with home maintenance, disorderly surroundings, and overtaxed family members.

situational low Self-Esteem/disturbed Body Image/ineffective Role Performance may be related to biophysical, psychosocial, and cognitive/perceptual changes, possibly evidenced by actual change in structure and/or function, change in usual patterns of responsibility/physical capacity to resume role, and verbal/nonverbal response to actual or perceived change.

risk for complicated Grieving: risk factors may include preloss psychological symptoms, predisposition for anxiety and feelings of inadequacy, frequency of major life events.*

Cervix, dysfunctional OB
(Refer to Dilation of cervix, premature)

Cesarean birth, postpartal OB
(Also refer to Postpartal period)

risk for impaired parent/infant Attachment: risk factors may include developmental transition/gain of a family member, situational crisis (e.g., surgical intervention, physical complications interfering with initial acquaintance/interaction, negative self-appraisal).*

acute Pain/[Discomfort] may be related to surgical trauma, effects of anesthesia, hormonal effects, bladder/abdominal distention, possibly evidenced by verbal reports (e.g., incisional pain, cramping/afterpains, spinal headache), guarding/distraction behaviors, irritability, facial mask of pain.

---

*A risk diagnosis is not evidenced by signs and symptoms, as the problem has not occurred and nursing interventions are directed at prevention.

risk for situational low Self-Esteem: risk factors may include perceived "failure" at life event, maturational transition, perceived loss of control in unplanned delivery.*

risk for Injury: risk factors may include biochemical or regulatory functions (e.g., orthostatic hypotension, development of PIH or eclampsia), effects of anesthesia, thromboembolism, abnormal blood profile (anemia/excessive blood loss, rubella sensitivity, Rh incompatibility), tissue trauma.*

risk for Infection: risk factors may include tissue trauma/broken skin, decreased Hb, invasive procedures and/or increased environmental exposure, prolonged rupture of amniotic membranes, malnutrition.*

Self-Care Deficit (specify) may be related to effects of anesthesia, decreased strength and endurance, physical discomfort, possibly evidenced by verbalization of inability to perform desired ADL(s).

Cesarean birth, unplanned   OB
(Also refer to Cesarean birth, postpartal)

deficient Knowledge [Learning Need] regarding underlying procedure, pathophysiology, and self-care needs may be related to incomplete/inadequate information, possibly evidenced by request for information, verbalization of concerns/misconceptions, and inappropriate/exaggerated behavior.

Anxiety [specify level] may be related to actual/perceived threat to mother/fetus, emotional threat to self-esteem, unmet needs/expectations, interpersonal transmission, possibly evidenced by increased tension, apprehension, feelings of inadequacy, sympathetic stimulation, and narrowed focus, restlessness.

Powerlessness may be related to interpersonal interaction, perception of illness-related regimen, lifestyle of helplessness, possibly evidenced by verbalization of lack of control, lack of participation in care or decision making, passivity.

risk for impaired fetal Gas Exchange: risk factors may include altered blood flow to placenta and/or through umbilical cord.*

risk for acute Pain: risk factors may include increased/prolonged contractions, psychological reaction.*

risk for Infection: risk factors may include invasive procedures, rupture of amniotic membranes, break in skin, decreased hemoglobin, exposure to pathogens.*

Chemotherapy   MS/CH
(Also refer to Cancer)

risk for deficient Fluid Volume: risk factors may include gastrointestinal losses (vomiting), interference with adequate intake (stomatitis/anorexia), losses through abnormal routes (indwelling tubes, wounds, fistulas), hypermetabolic state.*

imbalanced Nutrition: less than body requirements may be related to inability to ingest adequate nutrients (nausea, stomatitis, and fatigue), hypermetabolic state, possibly evidenced by weight loss

---

*A risk diagnosis is not evidenced by signs and symptoms, as the problem has not occurred and nursing interventions are directed at prevention.

(wasting), aversion to eating, reported altered taste sensation, sore and inflamed buccal cavity, diarrhea and/or constipation.

impaired Oral Mucous Membrane may be related to side effects of therapeutic agents/radiation, dehydration, and malnutrition, possibly evidenced by ulcerations, leukoplakia, decreased salivation, and reports of pain.

disturbed Body Image may be related to anatomical/structural changes, loss of hair and weight, possibly evidenced by negative feelings about body, preoccupation with change, feelings of helplessness/hopelessness, and change in social environment.

ineffective Protection may be related to inadequate nutrition, drug therapy/radiation, abnormal blood profile, disease state (cancer), possibly evidenced by impaired healing, deficient immunity, anorexia, fatigue.

readiness for enhanced Hope may be related to expectations of therapeutic interventions, results of diagnostic procedures as evidenced by expressed desire to enhance belief in possibilities/sense of meaning to life.

Cholecystectomy   MS

acute Pain may be related to interruption in skin/tissue layers with mechanical closure (sutures/staples) and invasive procedures (including T-tube/nasogastric—NG—tube), possibly evidenced by verbal reports, guarding/distraction behaviors, and autonomic responses (changes in vital signs).

ineffective Breathing Pattern may be related to decreased lung expansion (pain and muscle weakness), decreased energy/fatigue, ineffective cough, possibly evidenced by fremitus, tachypnea, and decreased respiratory depth/vital capacity.

risk for deficient Fluid Volume: risk factors may include vomiting/NG aspiration, medically restricted intake, altered coagulation.*

Cholelithiasis   CH

acute Pain may be related to inflammation and distortion of tissues, ductal spasm, possibly evidenced by verbal reports, guarding/distraction behaviors, and autonomic responses (changes in vital signs).

imbalanced Nutrition: less than body requirements may be related to inability to ingest/absorb adequate nutrients (food intolerance/pain, nausea/vomiting, anorexia), possibly evidenced by aversion to food/ decreased intake and weight loss.

deficient Knowledge [Learning Need] regarding pathophysiology, therapy choices, and self-care needs may be related to lack of information, misinterpretation, possibly evidenced by verbalization of concerns, questions, and recurrence of condition.

Chronic obstructive lung disease   CH/MS

impaired Gas Exchange may be related to altered O_2 delivery (obstruction of airways by secretions/bronchospasm, air trapping) and alveoli destruction, possibly evidenced by dyspnea, restlessness, confusion, abnormal ABG values, and reduced tolerance for activity.

*A risk diagnosis is not evidenced by signs and symptoms, as the problem has not occurred and nursing interventions are directed at prevention.

ineffective Airway Clearance may be related to bronchospasm, increased production of tenacious secretions, retained secretions, and decreased energy/fatigue, possibly evidenced by presence of wheezes, crackles, tachypnea, dyspnea, changes in depth of respirations, use of accessory muscles, cough (persistent), and chest x-ray findings.

Activity Intolerance may be related to imbalance between O_2 supply and demand, and generalized weakness, possibly evidenced by verbal reports of fatigue, exertional dyspnea, and abnormal vital sign response.

imbalanced Nutrition: less than body requirements may be related to inability to ingest adequate nutrients (dyspnea, fatigue, medication side effects, sputum production, anorexia), possibly evidenced by weight loss, reported altered taste sensation, decreased muscle mass/subcutaneous fat, poor muscle tone, and aversion to eating/lack of interest in food.

risk for Infection: risk factors may include decreased ciliary action, stasis of secretions, and debilitated state/malnutrition.*

Circumcision   PED

deficient Knowledge [Learning Need] regarding surgical procedure, prognosis, and treatment may be related to lack of exposure, misinterpretation, unfamiliarity with information resources, possibly evidenced by request for information, verbalization of concern/misconceptions, inaccurate follow-through of instructions.

acute Pain may be related to trauma to/edema of tender tissues, possibly evidenced by crying, changes in sleep pattern, refusal to eat.

impaired urinary Elimination may be related to tissue injury/inflammation or development of urethral fistula, possibly evidenced by edema, difficulty voiding.

risk for Injury [hemorrhage]: risk factors may include decreased clotting factors immediately after birth, previously undiagnosed problems with bleeding/clotting.*

risk for Infection: risk factors may include immature immune system, invasive procedure/tissue trauma, environmental exposure.*

Cirrhosis   MS/CH

(Also refer to Substance dependence/abuse rehabilitation; Hepatitis, acute viral)

risk for impaired Liver Function: risk factors may include viral infection, alcohol abuse.*

imbalanced Nutrition: less than body requirements may be related to inability to ingest/absorb nutrients (anorexia, nausea, indigestion, early satiety), abnormal bowel function, impaired storage of vitamins, possibly evidenced by aversion to eating, observed lack of intake, muscle wasting, weight loss, and imbalances in nutritional studies.

excess Fluid Volume may be related to compromised regulatory mechanism (e.g., syndrome of inappropriate antidiuretic hormone—SIADH, decreased plasma proteins/malnutrition) and excess sodium/

---

*A risk diagnosis is not evidenced by signs and symptoms, as the problem has not occurred and nursing interventions are directed at prevention.

fluid intake, possibly evidenced by generalized or abdominal edema, weight gain, dyspnea, BP changes, positive hepatojugular reflex, change in mentation, altered electrolytes, changes in urine specific gravity, and pleural effusion.

risk for impaired Skin Integrity: risk factors may include altered circulation/metabolic state, poor skin turgor, skeletal prominence, presence of edema/ascites, and accumulation of bile salts in skin.*

risk for acute Confusion: risk factors may include alcohol abuse, increased serum ammonia level, and inability of liver to detoxify certain enzymes/drugs.*

situational low Self-Esteem/disturbed Body Image may be related to biophysical changes/altered physical appearance, uncertainty of prognosis, changes in role function, personal vulnerability, self-destructive behavior (alcohol-induced disease), possibly evidenced by verbalization of changes in lifestyle, fear of rejection/reaction of others, negative feelings about body/abilities, and feelings of helplessness/hopelessness/powerlessness.

risk for ineffective Protection: risk factors may include abnormal blood profile (altered clotting factors), portal hypertension/development of esophageal varices.*

Cocaine hydrochloride poisoning, acute   MS
(Also refer to Stimulant abuse; Substance dependence/abuse rehabilitation)

ineffective Breathing Pattern may be related to pharmacological effects on respiratory center of the brain, possibly evidenced by tachypnea, altered depth of respiration, shortness of breath, and abnormal ABGs.

risk for decreased Cardiac Output: risk factors may include drug effect on myocardium (degree dependent on drug purity/quality used), alterations in electrical rate/rhythm/conduction, preexisting myocardiopathy.*

CH

risk for impaired Liver Function: risk factors may include cocaine abuse.*

imbalanced Nutrition: less than body requirements may be related to anorexia, insufficient/inappropriate use of financial resources, possibly evidenced by reported inadequate intake, weight loss/less than normal weight gain, lack of interest in food, poor muscle tone, signs/laboratory evidence of vitamin deficiencies.

risk for Infection: risk factors may include injection techniques, impurities of drugs, localized trauma/nasal septum damage, malnutrition, altered immune state.*

PSY

ineffective Coping may be related to personal vulnerability, negative role modeling, inadequate support systems, ineffective/inadequate coping skills with substitution of drug, possibly evidenced by use of harmful substance despite evidence of undesirable consequences.

---

*A risk diagnosis is not evidenced by signs and symptoms, as the problem has not occurred and nursing interventions are directed at prevention.

disturbed Sensory Perception (specify) may be related to exogenous chemical, altered sensory reception/transmission/integration (hallucination), altered status of sense organs, possibly evidenced by responding to internal stimuli from hallucinatory experiences, bizarre thinking, anxiety/panic, changes in sensory acuity (sense of smell/taste).

Coccidioidomycosis (San Joaquin/Valley Fever)   CH

acute Pain may be related to inflammation, possibly evidenced by verbal reports, distraction behaviors, and narrowed focus.

Fatigue may be related to decreased energy production, states of discomfort, possibly evidenced by reports of overwhelming lack of energy, inability to maintain usual routine, emotional lability/irritability, impaired ability to concentrate, and decreased endurance/libido.

deficient Knowledge [Learning Need] regarding nature/course of disease, therapy and self-care needs may be related to lack of information, possibly evidenced by statements of concern and questions.

Colitis, ulcerative   MS

Diarrhea may be related to inflammation or malabsorption of the bowel, presence of toxins and/or segmental narrowing of the lumen, possibly evidenced by increased bowel sounds/peristalsis, urgency, frequency/watery stools (acute phase), changes in stool color, and abdominal pain/cramping.

acute/chronic Pain may be related to inflammation of the intestines/hyperperistalsis and anal/rectal irritation, possibly evidenced by verbal reports, guarding/distraction behaviors.

risk for deficient Fluid Volume: risk factors may include continued GI losses (diarrhea, vomiting, capillary plasma loss), altered intake, hypermetabolic state.*

    CH

imbalanced Nutrition: less than body requirements may be related to altered intake/absorption of nutrients (medically restricted intake, fear that eating may cause diarrhea) and hypermetabolic state, possibly evidenced by weight loss, decreased subcutaneous fat/muscle mass, poor muscle tone, hyperactive bowel sounds, steatorrhea, pale conjunctiva and mucous membranes, and aversion to eating.

ineffective Coping may be related to chronic nature and indefinite outcome of disease, multiple stressors (repeated over time), personal vulnerability, severe pain, inadequate sleep, lack of/ineffective support systems, possibly evidenced by verbalization of inability to cope, discouragement, anxiety, preoccupation with physical self, chronic worry, emotional tension, depression, and recurrent exacerbation of symptoms.

risk for Powerlessness: risk factors may include unresolved dependency conflicts, feelings of insecurity/resentment, repression of anger and

---

*A risk diagnosis is not evidenced by signs and symptoms, as the problem has not occurred and nursing interventions are directed at prevention.

aggressive feelings, lacking a sense of control in stressful situations, sacrificing own wishes for others, and retreat from aggression or frustration.*

Colostomy   MS

risk for impaired Skin Integrity: risk factors may include absence of sphincter at stoma and chemical irritation from caustic bowel contents, reaction to product/removal of adhesive, and improperly fitting appliance.*

risk for Diarrhea/Constipation: risk factors may include interruption/alteration of normal bowel function (placement of ostomy), changes in dietary/fluid intake, and effects of medication.*

                                                                CH

deficient Knowledge [Learning Need] regarding changes in physiological function and self-care/treatment needs may be related to lack of exposure/recall, information misinterpretation, possibly evidenced by questions, statement of concern, and inaccurate follow-through of instruction/development of preventable complications.

disturbed Body Image may be related to biophysical changes (presence of stoma, loss of control of bowel elimination) and psychosocial factors (altered body structure, disease process/associated treatment regimen, e.g., cancer, colitis), possibly evidenced by verbalization of change in perception of self, negative feelings about body, fear of rejection/reaction of others, not touching/looking at stoma, and refusal to participate in care.

impaired Social Interaction may be related to fear of embarrassing situation secondary to altered bowel control with loss of contents, odor, possibly evidenced by reduced participation and verbalized/observed discomfort in social situations.

risk for Sexual Dysfunction: risk factors may include altered body structure/function, radical resection/treatment procedures, vulnerability/psychological concern about response of SO(s), and disruption of sexual response pattern (e.g., erection difficulty).*

Coma, diabetic   MS
(Refer to Diabetic ketoacidosis; Unconsciousness)

Concussion, brain   CH
acute Pain may be related to trauma to/edema of cerebral tissue, possibly evidenced by reports of headache, guarding/distraction behaviors, and narrowed focus.

risk for deficient Fluid Volume: risk factors may include vomiting, decreased intake, and hypermetabolic state (fever).*

risk for disturbed Thought Processes: risk factors may include trauma to/edema of cerebral tissue.*

deficient Knowledge [Learning Need] regarding condition, treatment/safety needs, and potential complications may be related to lack of recall, misinterpretation, cognitive limitation, possibly evidenced by questions/statement of concerns, development of preventable complications.

---

*A risk diagnosis is not evidenced by signs and symptoms, as the problem has not occurred and nursing interventions are directed at prevention.

Conduct disorder (childhood, adolescence) PSY/PED

risk for self-/other-directed Violence: risk factors may include retarded ego development, antisocial character, poor impulse control, dysfunctional family system, loss of significant relationships, history of suicidal/acting-out behaviors.*

defensive Coping may be related to inadequate coping strategies, maturational crisis, multiple life changes/losses, lack of control of impulsive actions, and personal vulnerability, possibly evidenced by inappropriate use of defense mechanisms, inability to meet role expectations, poor self-esteem, failure to assume responsibility for own actions, hypersensitivity to slight or criticism, and excessive smoking/drinking/drug use.

disturbed Thought Processes may be related to physiological changes, lack of appropriate psychological conflict, biochemical changes, as evidenced by tendency to interpret the intentions/actions of others as blaming and hostile, deficits in problem-solving skills, with physical aggression the solution most often chosen.

chronic low Self-Esteem may be related to life choices perpetuating failure, personal vulnerability, possibly evidenced by self-negating verbalizations, anger, rejection of positive feedback, frequent lack of success in life events.

CH

compromised/disabled family Coping may be related to excessive guilt, anger, or blaming among family members regarding child's behavior; parental inconsistencies; disagreements regarding discipline, limit setting, and approaches; and exhaustion of parental resources (prolonged coping with disruptive child), possibly evidenced by unrealistic parental expectations, rejection or overprotection of child; and exaggerated expressions of anger, disappointment, or despair regarding child's behavior or ability to improve or change.

impaired Social Interaction may be related to retarded ego development, developmental state (adolescence), lack of social skills, low self-concept, dysfunctional family system, and neurological impairment, possibly evidenced by dysfunctional interaction with others (difficulty waiting turn in games or group situations, not seeming to listen to what is being said), difficulty playing quietly and maintaining attention to task or play activity, often shifting from one activity to another and interrupting or intruding on others.

Congestive heart failure MS
(Refer to Heart failure, chronic)

Conn's syndrome MS/CH
(Refer to Aldosteronism, primary)

Constipation CH
Constipation may be related to weak abdominal musculature, GI obstructive lesions, pain on defecation, diagnostic procedures, pregnancy, possibly evidenced by change in character/frequency of stools,

---

*A risk diagnosis is not evidenced by signs and symptoms, as the problem has not occurred and nursing interventions are directed at prevention.

feeling of abdominal/rectal fullness or pressure, changes in bowel sounds, abdominal distention.

acute Pain may be related to abdominal fullness/pressure, straining to defecate, and trauma to delicate tissues, possibly evidenced by verbal reports, reluctance to defecate, and distraction behaviors.

deficient Knowledge [Learning Need] regarding dietary needs, bowel function, and medication effect may be related to lack of information/misconceptions, possibly evidenced by development of problem and verbalization of concerns/questions.

Coronary artery bypass surgery   **MS**

risk for decreased Cardiac Output: risk factors may include decreased myocardial contractility, diminished circulating volume (preload), alterations in electrical conduction, and increased SVR (afterload).*

acute Pain may be related to direct chest tissue/bone trauma, invasive tubes/lines, donor site incision, tissue inflammation/edema formation, intraoperative nerve trauma, possibly evidenced by verbal reports, autonomic responses (changes in vital signs), and distraction behaviors/(restlessness), irritability.

disturbed Sensory Perception (specify) may be related to restricted environment (postoperative/acute), sleep deprivation, effects of medications, continuous environmental sounds/activities, and psychological stress of procedure, possibly evidenced by disorientation, alterations in behavior, exaggerated emotional responses, and visual/auditory distortions.

CH

ineffective Role Performance may be related to situational crises (dependent role)/recuperative process, uncertainty about future, possibly evidenced by delay/alteration in physical capacity to resume role, change in usual role or responsibility, change in self/others' perception of role.

Crohn's disease   **MS/CH**
(Also refer to Colitis, ulcerative)

imbalanced Nutrition: less than body requirements may be related to intestinal pain after eating, decreased transit time through bowel, possibly evidenced by weight loss, aversion to eating, and observed lack of intake.

Diarrhea may be related to inflammation of small intestine, presence of toxins, particular dietary intake, possibly evidenced by hyperactive bowel sounds, cramping, and frequent loose liquid stools.

deficient Knowledge [Learning Need] regarding condition, nutritional needs, and prevention of recurrence may be related to insufficient information/misinterpretation, unfamiliarity with resources, possibly evidenced by statements of concern/questions, inaccurate follow-through of instructions, and development of preventable complications/exacerbation of condition.

---

*A risk diagnosis is not evidenced by signs and symptoms, as the problem has not occurred and nursing interventions are directed at prevention.

Croup   PED/CH

ineffective Airway Clearance may be related to presence of thick, tenacious mucus and swelling/spasms of the epiglottis, possibly evidenced by harsh/brassy cough, tachypnea, use of accessory breathing muscles, and presence of wheezes.

deficient Fluid Volume [isotonic] may be related to decreased ability/aversion to swallowing, presence of fever, and increased respiratory losses, possibly evidenced by dry mucous membranes, poor skin turgor, and scanty/concentrated urine.

Croup, membranous   PED/CH

(Also refer to Croup)

risk for Suffocation: risk factors may include inflammation of larynx with formation of false membrane.*

Anxiety [specify level]/Fear may be related to change in environment, perceived threat to self (difficulty breathing), and transmission of anxiety of adults, possibly evidenced by restlessness, facial tension, glancing about, and sympathetic stimulation.

C-Section   OB

(Refer to Cesarean birth, unplanned)

Cushing's syndrome   CH/MS

risk for excess Fluid Volume: risk factors may include compromised regulatory mechanism (fluid/sodium retention).*

risk for Infection: risk factors may include immunosuppressed inflammatory response, skin and capillary fragility, and negative nitrogen balance.*

imbalanced Nutrition: less than body requirements may be related to inability to utilize nutrients (disturbance of carbohydrate metabolism), possibly evidenced by decreased muscle mass and increased resistance to insulin.

Self-Care Deficit [specify] may be related to muscle wasting, generalized weakness, fatigue, and demineralization of bones, possibly evidenced by statements of/observed inability to complete or perform ADLs.

disturbed Body Image may be related to change in structure/appearance (effects of disease process, drug therapy), possibly evidenced by negative feelings about body, feelings of helplessness, and changes in social involvement.

Sexual Dysfunction may be related to loss of libido, impotence, and cessation of menses, possibly evidenced by verbalization of concerns and/or dissatisfaction with and alteration in relationship with SO.

risk for Trauma [fractures]: risk factors may include increased protein breakdown, negative protein balance, demineralization of bones.*

CVA   MS/CH

(Refer to Cerebrovascular accident)

Cystic fibrosis   CH/PED

ineffective Airway Clearance may be related to excessive production of thick mucus and decreased ciliary action, possibly evidenced by

---

*A risk diagnosis is not evidenced by signs and symptoms, as the problem has not occurred and nursing interventions are directed at prevention.

abnormal breath sounds, ineffective cough, cyanosis, and altered respiratory rate/depth.

risk for Infection: risk factors may include stasis of respiratory secretions and development of atelectasis.*

imbalanced Nutrition: less than body requirements may be related to impaired digestive process and absorption of nutrients, possibly evidenced by failure to gain weight, muscle wasting, and retarded physical growth.

deficient Knowledge [Learning Need] regarding pathophysiology of condition, medical management, and available community resources may be related to insufficient information/misconceptions, possibly evidenced by statements of concern and questions, inaccurate follow-through of instructions, development of preventable complications.

compromised family Coping may be related to chronic nature of disease and disability, inadequate/incorrect information or understanding by a primary person, possibly evidenced by significant person attempting assistive or supportive behaviors with less than satisfactory results, protective behavior disproportionate to client's abilities, or need for autonomy.

Cystitis CH

acute Pain may be related to inflammation and bladder spasms, possibly evidenced by verbal reports, distraction behaviors, and narrowed focus.

impaired Urinary Elimination may be related to inflammation/irritation of bladder, possibly evidenced by frequency, nocturia, and dysuria.

deficient Knowledge [Learning Need] regarding condition, treatment, and prevention of recurrence may be related to inadequate information/misconceptions, possibly evidenced by statements of concern and questions, recurrent infections.

Cytomegalic inclusion disease CH
(Refer to Cytomegalovirus infection)

Cytomegalovirus (CMV) infection CH

risk for disturbed visual Sensory Perception: risk factors may include inflammation of the retina.*

risk for fetal Infection: risk factors may include transplacental exposure, contact with blood/body fluids.*

Deep Vein Thrombosis (DVT) CH/MS
(Refer to Thrombophlebitis)

Degenerative joint disease CH
(Refer to Arthritis, rheumatoid)

Dehiscence (abdominal) MS

impaired Skin Integrity may be related to altered circulation, altered nutritional state (obesity/malnutrition), and physical stress on incision,

---

*A risk diagnosis is not evidenced by signs and symptoms, as the problem has not occurred and nursing interventions are directed at prevention.

possibly evidenced by poor/delayed wound healing and disruption of skin surface/wound closure.

risk for Infection: risk factors may include inadequate primary defenses (separation of incision, traumatized intestines, environmental exposure).*

risk for impaired Tissue Integrity: risk factors may include exposure of abdominal contents to external environment.*

Fear/[severe] Anxiety may be related to crises, perceived threat of death, possibly evidenced by fearfulness, restless behaviors, and sympathetic stimulation.

deficient Knowledge [Learning Need] regarding condition/prognosis and treatment needs may be related to lack of information/recall and misinterpretation of information, possibly evidenced by development of preventable complication, requests for information, and statement of concern.

Dehydration   PED/CH

deficient Fluid Volume [specify] may be related to etiology as defined by specific situation, possibly evidenced by dry mucous membranes, poor skin turgor, decreased pulse volume/pressure, and thirst.

risk for impaired Oral Mucous Membrane: risk factors may include dehydration and decreased salivation.*

deficient Knowledge [Learning Need] regarding fluid needs may be related to lack of information/misinterpretation, possibly evidenced by questions, statement of concern, and inadequate follow-through of instructions/development of preventable complications.

Delirium tremens (acute alcohol   MS/PSY
withdrawal)

Anxiety [severe/panic]/Fear may be related to cessation of alcohol intake/physiological withdrawal, threat to self-concept, perceived threat of death, possibly evidenced by increased tension, apprehension, fear of unspecified consequences, identifies object of fear.

disturbed Sensory Perception (specify) may be related to exogenous (alcohol consumption/sudden cessation)/endogenous (electrolyte imbalance, elevated ammonia and blood urea nitrogen—BUN) chemical alterations, sleep deprivation, and psychological stress, possibly evidenced by disorientation, restlessness, irritability, exaggerated emotional responses, bizarre thinking, and visual and auditory distortions/hallucinations.

risk for decreased Cardiac Output: risk factors may include direct effect of alcohol on heart muscle, altered SVR, presence of dysrhythmias.*

risk for Trauma: risk factors may include alterations in balance, reduced muscle coordination, cognitive impairment, and involuntary clonic/tonic muscle activity.*

imbalanced Nutrition: less than body requirements may be related to poor dietary intake, effects of alcohol on organs involved in digestion, interference with absorption/metabolism of nutrients and amino acids, possibly evidenced by reports of inadequate food intake, altered

---

*A risk diagnosis is not evidenced by signs and symptoms, as the problem has not occurred and nursing interventions are directed at prevention.

taste sensation, lack of interest in food, debilitated state, decreased subcutaneous fat/muscle mass, signs of mineral/electrolyte deficiency including abnormal laboratory findings.

Delivery, precipitous/out of hospital   OB
(Also refer to Labor, precipitous; Labor stages I–II)
risk for deficient Fluid Volume: risk factors may include presence of nausea/vomiting, lack of intake, excessive vascular loss.*
risk for Infection: risk factors may include broken/traumatized tissue, increased environmental exposure, rupture of amniotic membranes.*
risk for fetal Injury: risk factors may include rapid descent/pressure changes, compromised circulation, environmental exposure.*

Delusional disorder   PSY
risk for self-/other-directed Violence: risk factors may include perceived threats of danger, increased feelings of anxiety, acting out in an irrational manner.*
[severe] Anxiety may be related to inability to trust, possibly evidenced by rigid delusional system, frightened of other people and own hostility.
Powerlessness may be related to lifestyle of helplessness, feelings of inadequacy, interpersonal interaction, possibly evidenced by verbal expressions of no control/influence over situation(s), use of paranoid delusions, aggressive behavior to compensate for lack of control.
disturbed Thought Processes may be related to psychological conflicts, increasing anxiety/fear, possibly evidenced by interference with ability to think clearly/logically, fragmentation and autistic thinking, delusions, beliefs and behaviors of suspicion/violence.
impaired Social Interaction may be related to mistrust of others/delusional thinking, lack of knowledge/skills to enhance mutuality, possibly evidenced by discomfort in social situations, difficulty in establishing relationships with others, expression of feelings of rejection, no sense of belonging.

Dementia, presenile/senile   CH/PSY
(Also refer to Alzheimer's disease)
impaired Memory may be related to neurological disturbances, possibly evidenced by observed experiences of forgetting, inability to determine if a behavior was performed, inability to perform previously learned skills, inability to recall factual information or recent/past events.
Fear may be related to decreases in functional abilities, public disclosure of disabilities, further mental/physical deterioration, possibly evidenced by social isolation, apprehension, irritability, defensiveness, suspiciousness, aggressive behavior.
Self-Care Deficit [specify] may be related to cognitive decline, physical limitations, frustration over loss of independence, depression, possibly evidenced by impaired ability to perform ADLs.
risk for Trauma: risk factors may include changes in muscle coordination/balance, impaired judgment, seizure activity.*

---

*A risk diagnosis is not evidenced by signs and symptoms, as the problem has not occurred and nursing interventions are directed at prevention.

risk for sedentary Lifestyle: risk factors may include lack of interest/ motivation, lack of resources, lack of training or knowledge of specific exercise needs, safety concerns/fear of injury. *

risk for Caregiver Role Strain: risk factors may include illness severity of care receiver, duration of caregiving required, care receiver exhibiting deviant/bizarre behavior; family/caregiver isolation, lack of respite/recreation, spouse is caregiver.*

risk for complicated Grieving: risk factors may include preloss psychological symptoms, predisposition for anxiety and feelings of inadequacy, frequency of major life events.*

Depressant abuse   CH/PSY
(Also refer to Drug overdose, acute [depressants])

ineffective Denial may be related to weak underdeveloped ego, unmet self-needs, possibly evidenced by inability to admit impact of condition on life, minimizes symptoms/problem, refuses healthcare attention.

ineffective Coping may be related to weak ego, possibly evidenced by abuse of chemical agents, lack of goal-directed behavior, inadequate problem solving, destructive behavior toward self.

imbalanced Nutrition: less than body requirements may be related to use of substance in place of nutritional food, possibly evidenced by loss of weight, pale conjunctiva and mucous membranes, electrolyte imbalances, anemias.

risk for Injury: risk factors may include changes in sleep, decreased concentration, loss of inhibitions.*

Depressive disorders, major   PSY
depression, dysthymia

risk for self-directed Violence: risk factors may include depressed mood and feeling of worthlessness and hopelessness.*

[moderate to severe] Anxiety/disturbed Thought Processes may be related to psychological conflicts, unconscious conflict about essential values/goals of life, unmet needs, threat to self-concept, sleep deprivation, interpersonal transmission/contagion, possibly evidenced by reports of nervousness or fearfulness, feelings of inadequacy; agitation, angry/tearful outbursts, rambling/discoordinated speech, restlessness, hand rubbing or wringing, tremulousness, poor memory/concentration, decreased ability to grasp ideas, inability to follow/impaired ability to make decisions, numerous/repetitious physical complaints without organic cause, ideas of reference, hallucinations/delusions.

Insomnia may be related to biochemical alterations (decreased serotonin), unresolved fears and anxieties, and inactivity, possibly evidenced by difficulty in falling/remaining asleep, early morning awakening/awakening later than desired, reports of not feeling rested, physical signs (e.g., dark circles under eyes, excessive yawning).

Social Isolation/impaired Social Interaction may be related to alterations in mental status/thought processes (depressed mood), inadequate

---

*A risk diagnosis is not evidenced by signs and symptoms, as the problem has not occurred and nursing interventions are directed at prevention.

personal resources, decreased energy/inertia, difficulty engaging in satisfying personal relationships, feelings of worthlessness/low self-concept, inadequacy or absence of significant purpose in life, and knowledge/skill deficit about social interactions, possibly evidenced by decreased involvement with others, expressed feelings of difference from others, remaining in home/room/bed, refusing invitations/suggestions of social involvement, and dysfunctional interaction with peers, family, and/or others.

interrupted Family Processes may be related to situational crises of illness of family member with change in roles/responsibilities, developmental crises (e.g., loss of family member/relationship), possibly evidenced by statements of difficulty coping with situation, family system not meeting needs of its members, difficulty accepting or receiving help appropriately, ineffective family decision-making process, and failure to send and to receive clear messages.

risk for impaired Religiosity: risk factors may include ineffective support/coping, lack of social interaction, depression.*

risk for Injury [effects of electroconvulsive therapy (ECT)]: risk factors may include effects of therapy on the cardiovascular, respiratory, musculoskeletal, and nervous systems; and pharmacological effects of anesthesia.*

Dermatitis, seborrheic   CH

impaired Skin Integrity may be related to chronic inflammatory condition of the skin, possibly evidenced by disruption of skin surface with dry or moist scales, yellowish crusts, erythema, and fissures.

Diabetes mellitus   CH/PED

deficient Knowledge [Learning Need] regarding disease process/treatment and individual care needs may be related to unfamiliarity with information/lack of recall, misinterpretation, possibly evidenced by requests for information, statements of concern/misconceptions, inadequate follow-through of instructions, and development of preventable complications.

risk for unstable blood Glucose: risk factors may include lack of adherence to diabetes management, medication management, inadequate blood glucose monitoring, physical activity level, health status, stress, rapid growth periods.

imbalanced Nutrition: less than body requirements may be related to inability to utilize nutrients (imbalance between intake and utilization of glucose) to meet metabolic needs, possibly evidenced by change in weight, muscle weakness, increased thirst/urination, and hyperglycemia.

risk for risk-prone health Behavior: risk factors may include all-encompassing change in lifestyle, self-concept requiring lifelong adherence to therapeutic regimen and internal/altered locus of control.*

risk for Infection: risk factors may include decreased leukocyte function, circulatory changes, and delayed healing.*

---

*A risk diagnosis is not evidenced by signs and symptoms, as the problem has not occurred and nursing interventions are directed at prevention.

risk for disturbed Sensory Perception (specify): risk factors may include endogenous chemical alteration (glucose/insulin and/or electrolyte imbalance).*

compromised family Coping may be related to inadequate or incorrect information or understanding by primary person(s), other situational/developmental crises or situations the significant person(s) may be facing, lifelong condition requiring behavioral changes impacting family, possibly evidenced by family expressions of confusion about what to do, verbalizations that they are having difficulty coping with situation, family does not meet physical/emotional needs of its members; SO(s) preoccupied with personal reaction (e.g., guilt, fear), display protective behavior disproportionate (too little/too much) to client's abilities or need for autonomy.

Diabetic ketoacidosis   CH/MS

deficient Fluid Volume [specify] may be related to hyperosmolar urinary losses, gastric losses and inadequate intake, possibly evidenced by increased urinary output/dilute urine; reports of weakness, thirst, sudden weight loss, hypotension, tachycardia, delayed capillary refill, dry mucous membranes, poor skin turgor.

unstable blood Glucose may be related to medication management, lack of diabetes management, indequate blood glucose moitoring, presence of infection, possibly evidenced by elevated serum glucose level, presence of ketones in urine, nausea, weight loss, blurred vision, irritability.

imbalanced Nutrition: less than body requirements that may be related to inadequate utilization of nutrients (insulin deficiency), decreased oral intake, hypermetabolic state, possibly evidenced by recent weight loss, reports of weakness, lack of interest in food, gastric fullness/abdominal pain,

Fatigue may be related to decreased metabolic energy production, altered body chemistry (insufficient insulin), increased energy demands (hypermetabolic state/infection), possibly evidenced by overwhelming lack of energy, inability to maintain usual routines, decreased performance, impaired ability to concentrate, listlessness.

risk for Infection: risk factors may include high glucose levels, decreased leukocyte function, stasis of body fluids, invasive procedures, alteration in circulation/perfusion.*

Dialysis, general   CH

(Also refer to Dialysis, peritoneal; Hemodialysis)

imbalanced Nutrition: less than body requirements may be related to inadequate ingestion of nutrients (dietary restrictions, anorexia, nausea/vomiting, stomatitis), loss of peptides and amino acids (building blocks for proteins) during procedure, possibly evidenced by reported inadequate intake, aversion to eating, altered taste sensation, poor muscle tone/weakness, sore/inflamed buccal cavity, pale conjunctiva/mucous membranes.

Grieving may be related to actual or perceived loss, chronic and/or fatal illness, and thwarted grieving response to a loss, possibly evidenced

---

*A risk diagnosis is not evidenced by signs and symptoms, as the problem has not occurred and nursing interventions are directed at prevention.

by verbal expression of distress/unresolved issues, denial of loss, altered eating habits, sleep and dream patterns, activity levels, libido, crying, labile affect; feelings of sorrow, guilt, and anger.

disturbed Body Image/situational low Self-Esteem may be related to situational crisis and chronic illness with changes in usual roles/body image, possibly evidenced by verbalization of changes in lifestyle, focus on past function, negative feelings about body, feelings of helplessness/powerlessness, extension of body boundary to incorporate environmental objects (e.g., dialysis setup), change in social involvement, overdependence on others for care, not taking responsibility for self-care/lack of follow-through, and self-destructive behavior.

Self-Care Deficit [specify] may be related to perceptual/cognitive impairment (accumulated toxins), intolerance to activity, decreased strength and endurance, pain/discomfort, possibly evidenced by reported inability to perform ADLs, disheveled/unkempt appearance, strong body odor.

Powerlessness may be related to illness-related regimen and healthcare environment, possibly evidenced by verbal expression of having no control, depression over physical deterioration, nonparticipation in care, anger, and passivity.

compromised/disabled family Coping may be related to inadequate or incorrect information or understanding by a primary person, temporary family disorganization and role changes, client providing little support in turn for the primary person, and prolonged disease/disability progression that exhausts the supportive capacity of significant persons, possibly evidenced by expressions of concern or reports about response of SO(s)/family to client's health problem, preoccupation of SO(s) with own personal reactions, display of intolerance/rejection, and protective behavior disproportionate (too little or too much) to client's abilities or need for autonomy.

Dialysis, peritoneal   MS/CH
(Also refer to Dialysis, general)

risk for excess Fluid Volume: risk factors may include inadequate osmotic gradient of dialysate, fluid retention (dialysate drainage problems/inappropriate osmotic gradient of solution, bowel distention), excessive PO/IV intake.*

risk for Trauma: risk factors may include improper placement during insertion or manipulation of catheter.*

acute Pain may be related to procedural factors (catheter irritation, improper catheter placement), presence of edema/abdominal distention, inflammation or infection, rapid infusion/infusion of cold or acidic dialysate, possibly evidenced by verbal reports, guarding/distraction behaviors, and self-focus.

risk for Infection [peritoneal]: risk factors may include contamination of catheter/infusion system, skin contaminants, sterile peritonitis (response to composition of dialysate).*

---

*A risk diagnosis is not evidenced by signs and symptoms, as the problem has not occurred and nursing interventions are directed at prevention.

risk for ineffective Breathing Pattern: risk factors may include increased abdominal pressure with restricted diaphragmatic excursion, rapid infusion of dialysate, pain/discomfort, inflammatory process (e.g., atelectasis/pneumonia).*

Diaper rash   PED
(Refer to Candidiasis)

Diarrhea   PED/CH
deficient Knowledge [Learning Need] regarding causative/contributing factors and therapeutic needs may be related to lack of information/misconceptions, possibly evidenced by statements of concern, questions, and development of preventable complications.
risk for deficient Fluid Volume: risk factors may include excessive losses through GI tract, altered intake.*
acute Pain may be related to abdominal cramping and irritation/excoriation of skin, possibly evidenced by verbal reports, facial grimacing, and autonomic responses.
impaired Skin Integrity may be related to effects of excretions on delicate tissues, possibly evidenced by reports of discomfort and disruption of skin surface/destruction of skin layers.

Digitalis toxicity   MS/CH
decreased Cardiac Output may be related to altered myocardial contractility/electrical conduction, properties of digitalis (long half-life and narrow therapeutic range), concurrent medications, age/general health status and electrolyte/acid-base balance, possibly evidenced by changes in rate/rhythm/conduction (development/worsening of dysrhythmias), changes in mentation, worsening of heart failure, elevated serum drug levels.
risk for imbalanced Fluid Volume: risk factors may include excessive losses from vomiting/diarrhea, decreased intake/nausea, decreased plasma proteins, malnutrition, continued use of diuretics; excess sodium/fluid retention.*
deficient Knowledge [Learning Need] regarding condition/therapy and self-care needs may be related to information misinterpretation and lack of recall, possibly evidenced by inaccurate follow-through of instructions and development of preventable complications.
risk for disturbed Thought Processes: risk factors may include physiological effects of toxicity/reduced cerebral perfusion.*

Dilation and curettage (D and C)   OB/GYN
(Also refer to Abortion, elective or spontaneous termination)
deficient Knowledge [Learning Need] regarding surgical procedure, possible postprocedural complications, and therapeutic needs may be related to lack of exposure/unfamiliarity with information, possibly evidenced by requests for information and statements of concern/misconceptions.

Dilation of cervix, premature   OB
(Also refer to Labor, preterm)

---

*A risk diagnosis is not evidenced by signs and symptoms, as the problem has not occurred and nursing interventions are directed at prevention.

<u>Anxiety [specify level]</u> may be related to situational crisis, threat of death/fetal loss, possibly evidenced by increased tension, apprehension, feelings of inadequacy, sympathic stimulation, and repetitive questioning.

<u>risk for maternal Injury</u>: risk factors may include surgical intervention, use of tocolytic drugs.*

<u>risk for fetal Injury</u>: risk factors may include premature delivery, surgical procedure.*

<u>Grieving</u> may be related to perceived potential fetal loss, possibly evidenced by expression of distress, guilt, anger, choked feelings.

Dislocation/subluxation of joint CH

<u>acute Pain</u> may be related to lack of continuity of bone/joint, muscle spasms, edema, possibly evidenced by verbal or coded reports, guarded/protective behaviors, narrowed focus, autonomic responses.

<u>risk for Injury</u>: risk factors may include nerve impingement, improper fitting of splint device.*

<u>impaired physical Mobility</u> may be related to immobilization device/ activity restrictions, pain, edema, decreased muscle strength, possibly evidenced by limited range of motion, limited ability to perform motor skills, gait changes.

Disseminated intravascular coagulation (DIC) MS

<u>risk for deficient Fluid Volume:</u> risk factors may include failure of regulatory mechanism (coagulation process) and active loss/hemorrhage.*

<u>ineffective Tissue Perfusion (specify)</u> may be related to alteration of arterial/venous flow (microemboli throughout circulatory system, and hypovolemia), possibly evidenced by changes in respiratory rate and depth, changes in mentation, decreased urinary output, and development of acral cyanosis/focal gangrene.

<u>Anxiety [specify level]/Fear</u> may be related to sudden change in health status/threat of death, interpersonal transmission/contagion, possibly evidenced by sympathetic stimulation, restlessness, focus on self, and apprehension.

<u>risk for impaired Gas Exchange:</u> risk factors may include reduced O_2-carrying capacity, development of acidosis, fibrin deposition in microcirculation, and ischemic damage of lung parenchyma.*

<u>acute Pain</u> may be related to bleeding into joints/muscles, with hematoma formation, and ischemic tissues with areas of acral cyanosis/focal gangrene, possibly evidenced by verbal reports, narrowed focus, alteration in muscle tone, guarding/distraction behaviors, restlessness, autonomic responses.

Dissociative disorders PSY

<u>Anxiety [severe/panic]/Fear</u> may be related to a maladaptation or ineffective coping continuing from early life, unconscious conflict(s), threat to self-concept, unmet needs, or phobic stimulus, possibly evidenced by maladaptive response to stress (e.g., dissociating self/

---

*A risk diagnosis is not evidenced by signs and symptoms, as the problem has not occurred and nursing interventions are directed at prevention.

fragmentation of the personality), increased tension, feelings of inadequacy, and focus on self, projection of personal perceptions onto the
environment.

risk for self-/other-directed Violence: risk factors may include dissociative state/conflicting personalities, depressed mood, panic states, and
suicidal/homicidal behaviors.*

disturbed Personal Identity may be related to psychological conflicts
(dissociative state), childhood trauma/abuse, threat to physical
integrity/self-concept, and underdeveloped ego, possibly evidenced
by alteration in perception or experience of the self, loss of one's own
sense of reality/the external world, poorly differentiated ego boundaries, confusion about sense of self, confusion regarding purpose or
direction in life, memory loss, presence of more than one personality
within the individual.

compromised family Coping may be related to multiple stressors repeated
over time, prolonged progression of disorder that exhausts the supportive capacity of significant person(s), family disorganization and role
changes, high-risk family situation, possibly evidenced by family/SO(s)
describing inadequate understanding or knowledge that interferes with
assistive or supportive behaviors, relationship and marital conflict.

Diverticulitis   CH

acute Pain may be related to inflammation of intestinal mucosa,
abdominal cramping, and presence of fever/chills, possibly evidenced
by verbal reports, guarding/distraction behaviors, autonomic
responses, and narrowed focus.

Diarrhea/Constipation may be related to altered structure/function and
presence of inflammation, possibly evidenced by signs and symptoms
dependent on specific problem (e.g., increase/decrease in frequency
of stools and change in consistency).

deficient Knowledge [Learning Need] regarding disease process, potential complications, therapeutic and self-care needs may be related to
lack of information/misconceptions, possibly evidenced by statements of concern, request for information, and development of preventable complications.

risk for Powerlessness: risk factors may include chronic nature of disease
process and recurrent episodes despite cooperation with medical regimen.*

Down syndrome   PED/CH
(Also refer to Mental retardation)

delayed Growth and Development may be related to effects of physi-
cal/mental disability, possibly evidenced by altered physical growth,
delay/inability in performing skills and self-care/self-control activities appropriate for age.

risk for Trauma: risk factors may include cognitive difficulties and poor
muscle tone/coordination, weakness.*

imbalanced Nutrition: less than body requirements may be related to
poor muscle tone and protruding tongue, possibly evidenced by weak

---

*A risk diagnosis is not evidenced by signs and symptoms, as the
problem has not occurred and nursing interventions are directed at
prevention.

and ineffective sucking/swallowing and observed lack of adequate intake with weight loss/failure to gain.

interrupted Family Processes may be related to situational/maturational crises requiring incorporation of new skills into family dynamics, possibly evidenced by confusion about what to do, verbalized difficulty coping with situation, unexamined family myths.

risk for complicated Grieving: risk factors may include loss of "the perfect child," chronic condition requiring long-term care, and unresolved feelings.*

risk for impaired parent/infant/child Attachment: risk factors may include ill infant/child who is unable to effectively initiate parental contact due to altered behavioral organization, inability of parents to meet personal needs.*

risk for Social Isolation: risk factors may include withdrawal from usual social interactions and activities, assumption of total childcare, and becoming overindulgent/overprotective.*

Drug overdose, acute (depressants)   MS/PSY
(Also refer to Substance dependence/abuse rehabilitation)

ineffective Breathing Pattern/impaired Gas Exchange may be related to neuromuscular impairment/CNS depression, decreased lung expansion, possibly evidenced by changes in respirations, cyanosis, and abnormal ABGs.

risk for Trauma/Suffocation/Poisoning: risk factors may include CNS depression/agitation, hypersensitivity to the drug(s), psychological stress.*

risk for self-/other-directed Violence: risk factors may include suicidal behaviors, toxic reactions to drug(s).*

risk for Infection: risk factors may include drug injection techniques, impurities in injected drugs, localized trauma; malnutrition, altered immune state.*

Duchenne's muscular dystrophy   PED/CH
(Refer to Muscular dystrophy [Duchenne's])

DVT   CH/MS
(Refer to Thrombophlebitis)

Dysmenorrhea   GYN

acute Pain may be related to exaggerated uterine contractility, possibly evidenced by verbal reports, guarding/distraction behaviors, narrowed focus, and autonomic responses (changes in vital signs).

risk for Activity Intolerance: risk factors may include severity of pain and presence of secondary symptoms (nausea, vomiting, syncope, chills), depression.*

ineffective Coping may be related to chronic, recurrent nature of problem, anticipatory anxiety, and inadequate coping methods, possibly evidenced by muscular tension, headaches, general irritability, chronic depression, and verbalization of inability to cope, report of poor self-concept.

---

*A risk diagnosis is not evidenced by signs and symptoms, as the problem has not occurred and nursing interventions are directed at prevention.

Dysrhythmia, cardiac   MS

risk for decreased Cardiac Output: risk factors may include altered electrical conduction and reduced myocardial contractility.*

Anxiety [specify level] may be related to perceived threat of death, possibly evidenced by increased tension, apprehension, and expressed
concerns.

deficient Knowledge [Learning Need] regarding medical condition/
therapy needs may be related to lack of information/misinterpreta-
tion and unfamiliarity with information resources, possibly evidenced by questions, statement of misconception, failure to improve
on previous regimen, and development of preventable complications.

risk for Activity Intolerance: risk factors may include imbalance
between myocardial O_2 supply and demand, and cardiac depressant
effects of certain drugs (β-blockers, antidysrhythmics).*

risk for Poisoning, [digitalis toxicity]: risk factors may include limited
range of therapeutic effectiveness, lack of education/proper precautions, reduced vision/cognitive limitations.*

Eating disorders   CH/PSY

(Refer to Anorexia nervosa; Bulimia nervosa; Obesity)

Eclampsia   OB

(Refer to Pregnancy-induced hypertension)

Ectopic pregnancy (tubal)   OB

(Also refer to Abortion, spontaneous termination)

acute Pain may be related to distention/rupture of fallopian tube, possibly
evidenced by verbal reports, guarding/distraction behaviors, facial mask
of pain, and autonomic responses (diaphoresis, changes in vital signs).

risk for deficient Fluid Volume [isotonic]: risk factors may include hemorrhagic losses and decreased/restricted intake.*

Anxiety [specify level]/Fear may be related to threat of death and possible loss of ability to conceive, possibly evidenced by increased tension,
apprehension, sympathetic stimulation, restlessness, and focus on self.

Eczema (dermatitis)   CH

Pain/[Discomfort] may be related to cutaneous inflammation and irritation, possibly evidenced by verbal reports, irritability, and scratching.

risk for Infection: risk factors may include broken skin and tissue
trauma.*

Social Isolation may be related to alterations in physical appearance,
possibly evidenced by expressed feelings of rejection and decreased
interaction with peers.

Edema, pulmonary   MS

excess Fluid Volume may be related to decreased cardiac functioning,
excessive fluid/sodium intake, possibly evidenced by dyspnea, presence of crackles (rales), pulmonary congestion on x-ray, restlessness,
anxiety, and increased central venous pressure (CVP)/pulmonary
pressures.

---

*A risk diagnosis is not evidenced by signs and symptoms, as the
problem has not occurred and nursing interventions are directed at
prevention.

impaired Gas Exchange may be related to altered blood flow and decreased alveolar/capillary exchange (fluid collection/shifts into interstitial space/alveoli), possibly evidenced by hypoxia, restlessness, and confusion.

Anxiety [specify level]/Fear may be related to perceived threat of death (inability to breathe), possibly evidenced by responses ranging from apprehension to panic state, restlessness, and focus on self.

Emphysema   CH/MS

impaired Gas Exchange may be related to alveolar capillary membrane changes/destruction, possibly evidenced by dyspnea, restlessness, changes in mentation, abnormal ABG values.

ineffective Airway Clearance may be related to increased production/ retained tenacious secretions, decreased energy level, and muscle wasting, possibly evidenced by abnormal breath sounds (rhonchi), ineffective cough, changes in rate/depth of respirations, and dyspnea.

Activity Intolerance may be related to imbalance between O_2 supply and demand, possibly evidenced by reports of fatigue/weakness, exertional dyspnea, and abnormal vital sign response to activity.

imbalanced Nutrition: less than body requirements may be related to inability to ingest food (shortness of breath, anorexia, generalized weakness, medication side effects), possibly evidenced by lack of interest in food, reported altered taste, loss of muscle mass and tone, fatigue, and weight loss.

risk for Infection: risk factors may include inadequate primary defenses (stasis of body fluids, decreased ciliary action), chronic disease process, and malnutrition.*

Powerlessness may be related to illness-related regimen and healthcare environment, possibly evidenced by verbal expression of having no control, depression over physical deterioration, nonparticipation in therapeutic regimen, anger, and passivity.

Encephalitis   MS

risk for ineffective cerebral Tissue Perfusion: risk factors may include cerebral edema altering/interrupting cerebral arterial/venous blood flow, hypovolemia, exchange problems at cellular level (acidosis).*

Hyperthermia may be related to increased metabolic rate, illness, and dehydration, possibly evidenced by increased body temperature, flushed/warm skin, and increased pulse and respiratory rates.

acute Pain may be related to inflammation/irritation of the brain and cerebral edema, possibly evidenced by verbal reports of headache, photophobia, distraction behaviors, restlessness, and autonomic response (changes in vital signs).

risk for Trauma/Suffocation: risk factors may include restlessness, clonic/tonic activity, altered sensorium, cognitive impairment, generalized weakness, ataxia, vertigo.*

Endocarditis   MS

risk for decreased Cardiac Output: risk factors may include inflammation of lining of heart and structural change in valve leaflets.*

---

*A risk diagnosis is not evidenced by signs and symptoms, as the problem has not occurred and nursing interventions are directed at prevention.

Anxiety [specify level] may be related to change in health status and threat of death, possibly evidenced by apprehension, expressed concerns, and focus on self.

acute Pain may be related to generalized inflammatory process and effects of embolic phenomena, possibly evidenced by verbal reports, narrowed focus, distraction behaviors, and autonomic responses (changes in vital signs).

risk for Activity Intolerance: risk factors may include imbalance between O_2 supply and demand, debilitating condition.*

risk for ineffective Tissue Perfusion (specify): risk factors may include embolic interruption of arterial flow (embolization of thrombi/valvular vegetations).*

Endometriosis   GYN

acute/chronic Pain may be related to pressure of concealed bleeding/formation of adhesions, possibly evidenced by verbal reports (pain between/with menstruation), guarding/distraction behaviors, and narrowed focus.

Sexual Dysfunction may be related to pain secondary to presence of adhesions, possibly evidenced by verbalization of problem, and altered relationship with partner.

deficient Knowledge [Learning Need] regarding pathophysiology of condition and therapy needs may be related to lack of information/misinterpretations, possibly evidenced by statements of concern and misconceptions.

Enteritis   MS/CH
(Refer to Colitis, ulcerative; Crohn's disease)

Epididymitis   MS

acute Pain may be related to inflammation, edema formation, and tension on the spermatic cord, possibly evidenced by verbal reports, guarding/distraction behaviors (restlessness), and autonomic responses (changes in vital signs).

risk for Infection, [spread]: risk factors may include presence of inflammation/infectious process, insufficient knowledge to avoid spread of infection.*

deficient Knowledge [Learning Need] regarding pathophysiology, outcome, and self-care needs may be related to lack of information/misinterpretations, possibly evidenced by statements of concern, misconceptions, and questions.

Epilepsy   CH
(Refer to Seizure disorder)

Erectile dysfunction   CH

Sexual Dysfunction may be related to altered body function possibly evidenced by reports of disruption of sexual response pattern, inability to achieve desired satisfaction.

---

*A risk diagnosis is not evidenced by signs and symptoms, as the problem has not occurred and nursing interventions are directed at prevention.

<u>situational low Self-Esteem</u> may be related to functional impairment; rejection of other(s).

Failure to thrive, infant/child   PED

<u>imbalanced Nutrition: less than body requirements</u> may be related to inability to ingest/digest/absorb nutrients (defects in organ function/metabolism, genetic factors), physical deprivation/psychosocial factors, possibly evidenced by lack of appropriate weight gain/weight loss, poor muscle tone, pale conjunctiva, and laboratory tests reflecting nutritional deficiency.

<u>delayed Growth and Development</u> may be related to inadequate caretaking (physical/emotional neglect or abuse), indifference, inconsistent responsiveness, multiple caretakers, environmental and stimulation deficiencies, possibly evidenced by altered physical growth, flat affect, listlessness, decreased response, delay or difficulty in performing skills or self-control activities appropriate for age group.

<u>risk for impaired Parenting</u>: risk factors may include lack of knowledge, inadequate bonding, unrealistic expectations for self/infant, and lack of appropriate response of child to relationship.*

<u>deficient Knowledge [Learning Need] regarding pathophysiology of condition, nutritional needs, growth/development expectations, and parenting skills</u> may be related to lack of information/misinformation or misinterpretation, possibly evidenced by verbalization of concerns, questions, and misconceptions, or development of preventable complications.

Fatigue syndrome, chronic   CH

<u>Fatigue</u> may be related to disease state, inadequate sleep, possibly evidenced by verbalization of unremitting/overwhelming lack of energy, inability to maintain usual routines, listless, compromised concentration.

<u>chronic Pain</u> may be related to chronic physical disability, possibly evidenced by verbal reports of headache, sore throat, arthralgias, abdominal pain, muscle aches, altered ability to continue previous activities, changes in sleep pattern.

<u>Self-Care Deficit [specify]</u> may be related to tiredness, pain/discomfort, possibly evidenced by reports of inability to perform desired ADLs.

<u>risk for ineffective Role Performance</u>: risk factors may include health alterations, stress.*

Fetal alcohol syndrome   PED

<u>risk for Injury [CNS damage]</u>: risk factors may include external chemical factors (alcohol intake by mother), placental insufficiency, fetal drug withdrawal in utero/postpartum and prematurity.*

<u>disorganized Infant Behavior</u> may be related to prematurity, environmental overstimulation, lack of containment/boundaries, possibly evidenced by change from baseline physiological measures, tremors, startles, twitches, hyperextension of arms/legs, deficient self-regulatory behaviors, deficient response to visual/auditory stimuli.

---

*A risk diagnosis is not evidenced by signs and symptoms, as the problem has not occurred and nursing interventions are directed at prevention.

<u>risk for impaired Parenting</u>: risk factors may include mental and/or physical illness, inability of mother to assume the overwhelming task of unselfish giving and nurturing, presence of stressors (financial/legal problems), lack of available or ineffective role model, interruption of bonding process, lack of appropriate response of child to relationship.*

PSY

<u>ineffective [maternal] Coping</u> may be related to personal vulnerability, low self-esteem, inadequate coping skills, and multiple stressors (repeated over period of time), possibly evidenced by inability to meet basic needs/fulfill role expectations/problem solve, and excessive use of drug(s).

<u>dysfunctional Family Processes: alcoholism</u> may be related to lack of/insufficient support from others, mother's drug problem and treatment status, together with poor coping skills, lack of family stability/overinvolvement of parents with children and multigenerational addictive behaviors, possibly evidenced by abandonment, rejection, neglectful relationships with family members, and decisions and actions by family that are detrimental.

Fetal demise OB

<u>Grieving</u> may be related to death of fetus/infant (wanted or unwanted), possibly evidenced by verbal expressions of distress, anger, loss, crying, alteration in eating habits or sleep pattern.

<u>situational low Self-Esteem</u> may be related to perceived "failure" at a life event, possibly evidenced by negative self-appraisal in response to life event in a person with a previous positive self-evaluation, verbalization of negative feelings about the self (helplessness, uselessness), difficulty making decisions.

<u>risk for Spiritual Distress</u>: risk factors may include loss of loved one, low self-esteem, poor relationships, challenged belief and value system (birth is supposed to be the beginning of life, not of death) and intense suffering.*

Fractures MS/CH

(Also refer to Casts; Traction)

<u>risk for Trauma [additional injury]</u>: risk factors may include loss of skeletal integrity/movement of skeletal fragments, use of traction apparatus, and so on.*

<u>acute Pain</u> may be related to muscle spasms, movement of bone fragments, tissue trauma/edema, traction/immobility device, stress, and anxiety, possibly evidenced by verbal reports, distraction behaviors, self-focusing/narrowed focus, facial mask of pain, guarding/protective behavior, alteration in muscle tone, and autonomic responses (changes in vital signs).

<u>risk for Peripheral Neurovascular Dysfunction</u>: risk factors may include reduction/interruption of blood flow (direct vascular injury, tissue trauma, excessive edema, thrombus formation, hypovolemia).*

---

*A risk diagnosis is not evidenced by signs and symptoms, as the problem has not occurred and nursing interventions are directed at prevention.

impaired physical Mobility may be related to neuromuscular/skeletal impairment, pain/discomfort, restrictive therapies (bedrest, extremity immobilization), and psychological immobility, possibly evidenced by inability to purposefully move within the physical environment, imposed restrictions, reluctance to attempt movement, limited range of motion, and decreased muscle strength/control.

risk for impaired Gas Exchange: risk factors may include altered blood flow, blood/fat emboli, alveolar/capillary membrane changes (interstitial/pulmonary edema, congestion).*

deficient Knowledge [Learning Need] regarding healing process, therapy requirements, potential complications, and self-care needs may be related to lack of exposure, misinterpretation of information, possibly evidenced by statements of concern, questions, and misconceptions.

Frostbite   MS/CH

impaired Tissue Integrity may be related to altered circulation and thermal injury, possibly evidenced by damaged/destroyed tissue.

acute Pain may be related to diminished circulation with tissue ischemia/necrosis and edema formation, possibly evidenced by verbal reports, guarding/distraction behaviors, narrowed focus, and autonomic responses (changes in vital signs).

risk for Infection: risk factors may include traumatized tissue/tissue destruction, altered circulation, and compromised immune response in affected area.*

Gallstones   CH
(Refer to Cholelithiasis)

Gangrene, dry   MS

ineffective peripheral Tissue Perfusion may be related to interruption in arterial flow, possibly evidenced by cool skin temperature, change in color (black), atrophy of affected part, and presence of pain.

acute Pain may be related to tissue hypoxia and necrotic process, possibly evidenced by verbal reports, guarding/distraction behaviors, narrowed focus, and autonomic responses (changes in vital signs).

Gas, lung irritant   MS/CH

ineffective Airway Clearance may be related to irritation/inflammation of airway, possibly evidenced by marked cough, abnormal breath sounds (wheezes), dyspnea, and tachypnea.

risk for impaired Gas Exchange: risk factors may include irritation/inflammation of alveolar membrane (dependent on type of agent and length of exposure).*

Anxiety [specify level] may be related to change in health status and threat of death, possibly evidenced by verbalizations, increased tension, apprehension, and sympathetic stimulation.

Gastritis, acute   MS

acute Pain may be related to irritation/inflammation of gastric mucosa, possibly evidenced by verbal reports, guarding/distraction behaviors, and autonomic responses (changes in vital signs).

---

*A risk diagnosis is not evidenced by signs and symptoms, as the problem has not occurred and nursing interventions are directed at prevention.

risk for deficient Fluid Volume [isotonic]: risk factors may include excessive losses through vomiting and diarrhea, continued bleeding, reluctance to ingest/restrictions of oral intake.*

Gastritis, chronic   CH
risk for imbalanced Nutrition: less than body requirements: risk factors may include inability to ingest adequate nutrients (prolonged nausea/vomiting, anorexia, epigastric pain).*

deficient Knowledge [Learning Need] regarding pathophysiology, psychological factors, therapy needs, and potential complications may be related to lack of information/misinterpretation, possibly evidenced by verbalization of concerns, questions, misconceptions, and continuation of problem.

Gastroenteritis   MS
(Refer to Enteritis; Gastritis, chronic)

Gender identity disorder   PSY
(For individuals experiencing persistent and marked distress regarding uncertainty about issues relating to personal identity, e.g., sexual orientation and behavior.)

Anxiety [specify level] may be related to unconscious/conscious conflicts about essential values/beliefs (ego-dystonic gender identification), threat to self-concept, unmet needs, possibly evidenced by increased tension, helplessness, hopelessness, feelings of inadequacy, uncertainty, insomnia and focus on self, and impaired daily functioning.

ineffective Role Performance/disturbed personal Identity may be related to crisis in development in which person has difficulty knowing/accepting to which sex he or she belongs or is attracted, sense of discomfort and inappropriateness about anatomic sex characteristics, possibly evidenced by confusion about sense of self, purpose or direction in life, sexual identification/preference, verbalization of desire to be/insistence that person is the opposite sex, change in self-perception of role, and conflict in roles.

ineffective Sexuality Pattern may be related to ineffective or absent role models and conflict with sexual orientation and/or preferences, lack of/impaired relationship with an SO, possibly evidenced by verbalizations of discomfort with sexual orientation/role, and lack of information about human sexuality.

risk for compromised/disabled family Coping: risk factors may include inadequate/incorrect information or understanding, SO unable to perceive or to act effectively in regard to client's needs, temporary family disorganization and role changes, and client providing little support in turn for primary person.*

readiness for enhanced family Coping may be related to individual's basic needs being sufficiently gratified and adaptive tasks effectively addressed to enable goals of self-actualization to surface, possibly evidenced by family member's attempts to describe growth/impact of crisis on own values, priorities, goals, or relationships, family member is

---

*A risk diagnosis is not evidenced by signs and symptoms, as the problem has not occurred and nursing interventions are directed at prevention.

moving in direction of health-promoting and enriching lifestyle that supports client's search for self and choosing experiences that optimize wellness.

Genetic disorder   CH/OB

Anxiety may be related to presence of specific risk factors (e.g., exposure to teratogens), situational crisis, threat to self-concept, conscious or unconscious conflict about essential values and life goals, possibly evidenced by increased tension, apprehension, uncertainty, feelings of inadequacy, expressed concerns.

deficient Knowledge [Learning Need] regarding purpose/process of genetic counseling may be related to lack of awareness of ramifications of diagnosis, process necessary for analyzing available options, and information misinterpretation, possibly evidenced by verbalization of concerns, statement of misconceptions, request for information.

risk for interrupted Family Processes: risk factors may include situational crisis, individual/family vulnerability, difficulty reaching agreement regarding options.*

Spiritual Distress may be related to intense inner conflict about the outcome, normal grieving for the loss of the perfect child, anger that is often directed at God/greater power, religious beliefs/moral convictions, possibly evidenced by verbalization of inner conflict about beliefs, questioning of the moral and ethical implications of therapeutic choices, viewing situation as punishment, anger, hostility, and crying.

risk for complicated Grieving: risk factors may include preloss psychological symptoms, predisposition for anxiety and feelings of inadequacy, frequency of major life events.*

Gigantism   CH
(Refer to Acromegaly)

Glaucoma   CH

disturbed visual Sensory Perception may be related to altered sensory reception and altered status of sense organ (increased intraocular pressure/atrophy of optic nerve head), possibly evidenced by progressive loss of visual field.

Anxiety [specify level] may be related to change in health status, presence of pain, possibility/reality of loss of vision, unmet needs, and negative self-talk, possibly evidenced by apprehension, uncertainty, and expressed concern regarding changes in life event.

Glomerulonephritis   PED

excess Fluid Volume may be related to failure of regulatory mechanism (inflammation of glomerular membrane inhibiting filtration), possibly evidenced by weight gain, edema/anasarca, intake greater than output, and blood pressure changes.

acute Pain may be related to effects of circulating toxins and edema/distention of renal capsule, possibly evidenced by verbal reports, guarding/

---

*A risk diagnosis is not evidenced by signs and symptoms, as the problem has not occurred and nursing interventions are directed at prevention.

distraction behaviors, and autonomic responses (changes in vital signs).

imbalanced Nutrition: less than body requirements may be related to anorexia and dietary restrictions, possibly evidenced by aversion to eating, reported altered taste, weight loss, and decreased intake.

deficient Diversional Activity may be related to treatment modality/restrictions, fatigue, and malaise, possibly evidenced by statements of boredom, restlessness, and irritability.

risk for disproportionate Growth: risk factors may include infection, malnutrition, chronic illness.*

Goiter   CH

disturbed Body Image may be related to visible swelling in neck, possibly evidenced by verbalization of feelings, fear of reaction of others, actual change in structure, change in social involvement.

Anxiety may be related to change in health status/progressive growth of mass, perceived threat of death.

risk for imbalanced Nutrition: less than body requirements: risk factors may include decreased ability to ingest/difficulty swallowing.*

risk for ineffective Airway Clearance: risk factors may include tracheal compression/obstruction.*

Gonorrhea   CH

(Also refer to Sexually transmitted disease—STD)

risk for Infection [dissemination/bacteremia]: risk factors may include presence of infectious process in highly vascular area and lack of recognition of disease process.*

acute Pain may be related to irritation/inflammation of mucosa and effects of circulating toxins, possibly evidenced by verbal reports of genital or pharyngeal irritation, perineal/pelvic pain, guarding/distraction behaviors.

deficient Knowledge [Learning Need] regarding disease cause/transmission, therapy, and self-care needs may be related to lack of information/misinterpretation, denial of exposure, possibly evidenced by statements of concern, questions, misconceptions, and inaccurate follow-through of instructions/development of preventable complications.

Gout   CH

acute Pain may be related to inflammation of joint(s), possibly evidenced by verbal reports, guarding/distraction behaviors, and autonomic responses (changes in vital signs).

impaired physical Mobility may be related to joint pain/edema, possibly evidenced by reluctance to attempt movement, limited range of motion, and therapeutic restriction of movement.

deficient Knowledge [Learning Need] regarding cause, treatment, and prevention of condition may be related to lack of information/misinterpretation, possibly evidenced by statements of concern, questions, misconceptions, and inaccurate follow-through of instructions.

---

*A risk diagnosis is not evidenced by signs and symptoms, as the problem has not occurred and nursing interventions are directed at prevention.

Guillain-Barré syndrome (acute polyneuritis) MS

risk for ineffective Breathing Pattern/Airway Clearance: risk factors may include weakness/paralysis of respiratory muscles, impaired gag/ swallow reflexes, decreased energy/fatigue.*

disturbed Sensory Perceptual: (specify) may be related to altered sensory reception/transmission/integration (altered status of sense organs, sleep deprivation), therapeutically restricted environment, endogenous chemical alterations (electrolyte imbalance, hypoxia), and psychological stress, possibly evidenced by reported or observed change in usual response to stimuli, altered communication patterns, and measured change in sensory acuity and motor coordination.

impaired physical Mobility may be related to neuromuscular impairment, pain/discomfort, possibly evidenced by impaired coordination, partial/complete paralysis, decreased muscle strength/control.

Anxiety [specify level]/Fear may be related to situational crisis, change in health status/threat of death, possibly evidenced by increased tension, restlessness, helplessness, apprehension, uncertainty, fearfulness, focus on self, and sympathetic stimulation.

risk for Disuse Syndrome: risk factors include paralysis and pain.*

Hay fever CH

Pain[/Discomfort] may be related to irritation/inflammation of upper airway mucous membranes and conjunctiva, possibly evidenced by verbal reports, irritability, and restlessness.

deficient Knowledge [Learning Need] regarding underlying cause, appropriate therapy, and required lifestyle changes may be related to lack of information, possibly evidenced by statements of concern, questions, and misconceptions.

Heart failure, chronic MS

decreased Cardiac Output may be related to altered myocardial contractility/inotropic changes; alterations in rate, rhythm, and electrical conduction; and structural changes (valvular defects, ventricular aneurysm), possibly evidenced by tachycardia/dysrhythmias, changes in blood pressure, extra heart sounds, decreased urine output, diminished peripheral pulses, cool/ashen skin, orthopnea, crackles; dependent/generalized edema and chest pain.

excess Fluid Volume may be related to reduced glomerular filtration rate/increased ADH production, and sodium/water retention, possibly evidenced by orthopnea and abnormal breath sounds, S_3 heart sound, jugular vein distention, positive hepatojugular reflex, weight gain, hypertension, oliguria, generalized edema.

risk for impaired Gas Exchange: risk factors may include alveolar capillary membrane changes (fluid collection/shifts into interstitial space/alveoli).*

CH

Activity Intolerance may be related to imbalance between O_2 supply/ demand, generalized weakness, and prolonged bedrest/sedentary

---

*A risk diagnosis is not evidenced by signs and symptoms, as the problem has not occurred and nursing interventions are directed at prevention.

lifestyle, possibly evidenced by reported/observed weakness, fatigue, changes in vital signs, presence of dysrhythmias, dyspnea, pallor, and diaphoresis.

deficient Knowledge [Learning Need] regarding cardiac function/disease process, therapy and self-care needs may be related to lack of information/misinterpretation, possibly evidenced by questions, statements of concern/misconceptions; development of preventable complications or exacerbations of condition.

Heatstroke   MS

Hyperthermia may be related to prolonged exposure to hot environment/vigorous activity with failure of regulating mechanism of the body, possibly evidenced by high body temperature (greater than 105°F/40.6°C), flushed/hot skin, tachycardia, and seizure activity.

decreased Cardiac Output may be related to functional stress of hypermetabolic state, altered circulating volume/venous return, and direct myocardial damage secondary to hyperthermia, possibly evidenced by decreased peripheral pulses, dysrhythmias/tachycardia, and changes in mentation.

Hemodialysis   MS/CH
(Also refer to Dialysis, general)

risk for Injury, [loss of vascular access]: risk factors may include clotting/thrombosis, infection, disconnection/hemorrhage.*

risk for deficient Fluid Volume: risk factors may include excessive fluid losses/shifts via ultrafiltration, hemorrhage (altered coagulation/disconnection of shunt), and fluid restrictions.*

risk for excess Fluid Volume: risk factors may include excessive fluid intake, rapid IV, blood/plasma expanders/saline given to support BP during procedure.*

ineffective Protection may be related to chronic disease state, drug therapy, abnormal blood profile, inadequate nutrition, possibly evidenced by altered clotting, impaired healing, deficient immunity, fatigue, anorexia.

Hemophilia   PED

risk for deficient Fluid Volume [isotonic]: risk factors may include impaired coagulation/hemorrhagic losses.*

risk for acute/chronic Pain: risk factors may include nerve compression from hematomas, nerve damage, or hemorrhage into joint space.*

risk for impaired physical Mobility: risk factors may include joint hemorrhage, swelling, degenerative changes, and muscle atrophy.*

ineffective Protection may be related to abnormal blood profile, possibly evidenced by altered clotting.

compromised family Coping may be related to prolonged nature of condition that exhausts the supportive capacity of significant person(s), possibly evidenced by protective behaviors disproportionate to client's abilities/need for autonomy.

---

*A risk diagnosis is not evidenced by signs and symptoms, as the problem has not occurred and nursing interventions are directed at prevention.

Hemorrhoidectomy   MS/CH

acute Pain may be related to edema/swelling and tissue trauma, possibly
    evidenced by verbal reports, guarding/distraction behaviors, focus on
    self, and autonomic responses (changes in vital signs).

risk for Urinary Retention: risk factors may include perineal trauma,
    edema/swelling, and pain.*

deficient Knowledge [Learning Need] regarding therapeutic treatment
    and potential complications may be related to lack of informa-
    tion/misconceptions, possibly evidenced by statements of concern
    and questions.

Hemorrhoids   CH/OB

acute Pain may be related to inflammation and edema of prolapsed
    varices, possibly evidenced by verbal reports, and guarding/distrac-
    tion behaviors.

Constipation may be related to pain on defecation and reluctance to
    defecate, possibly evidenced by frequency less than usual pattern, and
    hard/formed stools.

Hemothorax   MS
(Also refer to Pneumothorax)

risk for Trauma/Suffocation: risk factors may include concurrent dis-
    ease/injury process, dependence on external device (chest drainage
    system), and lack of safety education/precautions.*

Anxiety [specify level] may be related to change in health status and
    threat of death, possibly evidenced by increased tension, restlessness,
    expressed concern, sympathetic stimulation, and focus on self.

Hepatitis, acute viral   MS/CH

impaired Liver Function related to viral infection as evidenced by jaun-
    dice, hepatic enlargement, abdominal pain, marked elevations in
    serum liver function tests.

Fatigue may be related to decreased metabolic energy production and
    altered body chemistry, possibly evidenced by reports of lack of
    energy/inability to maintain usual routines, decreased performance,
    and increased physical complaints.

imbalanced Nutrition: less than body requirements may be related to
    inability to ingest adequate nutrients (nausea, vomiting, anorexia),
    hypermetabolic state, altered absorption and metabolism, possibly
    evidenced by aversion to eating/lack of interest in food, altered taste
    sensation, observed lack of intake, and weight loss.

acute Pain/[Discomfort] may be related to inflammation and swelling
    of the liver, arthralgias, urticarial eruptions, and pruritus, possibly
    evidenced by verbal reports, guarding/distraction behaviors, focus on
    self, and autonomic responses (changes in vital signs).

risk for Infection: risk factors may include inadequate secondary
    defenses and immunosuppression, malnutrition, insufficient knowl-
    edge to avoid exposure to pathogens/spread to others.*

risk for impaired Tissue Integrity: risk factors may include bile salt accu-
    mulation in the tissues.*

---

*A risk diagnosis is not evidenced by signs and symptoms, as the
problem has not occurred and nursing interventions are directed at
prevention.

risk for impaired Home Management: risk factors may include debilitating effects of disease process and inadequate support systems (family, financial, role model).*

deficient Knowledge [Learning Need] regarding disease process/transmission, treatment needs, and future expectations may be related to lack of information/recall, misinterpretation, unfamiliarity with resources, possibly evidenced by questions, statement of concerns/misconceptions, inaccurate follow-through of instructions, and development of preventable complications.

Hernia, hiatal   CH

chronic Pain may be related to regurgitation of acidic gastric contents, possibly evidenced by verbal reports, facial grimacing, and focus on self.

deficient Knowledge [Learning Need] regarding pathophysiology, prevention of complications and self-care needs may be related to lack of information/misconceptions, possibly evidenced by statements of concern, questions, and recurrence of condition.

Herniated nucleus pulposus   CH/MS
(ruptured intervertebral disk)

acute/chronic Pain may be related to nerve compression/irritation and muscle spasms, possibly evidenced by verbal reports, guarding/distraction behaviors, preoccupation with pain, self/narrowed focus, and autonomic responses (changes in vital signs when pain is acute), altered muscle tone/function, changes in eating/sleeping patterns and libido, physical/social withdrawal.

impaired physical Mobility may be related to pain (muscle spasms), therapeutic restrictions (e.g., bedrest, traction/braces), muscular impairment, and depression, possibly evidenced by reports of pain on movement, reluctance to attempt/difficulty with purposeful movement, decreased muscle strength, impaired coordination, and limited range of motion.

deficient Diversional Activity may be related to length of recuperation period and therapy restrictions, physical limitations, pain, and depression, possibly evidenced by statements of boredom, disinterest, "nothing to do," and restlessness, irritability, withdrawal.

Herpes, herpes simplex   CH

acute Pain may be related to presence of localized inflammation and open lesions, possibly evidenced by verbal reports, distraction behaviors, and restlessness.

risk for [secondary] Infection: risk factors may include broken/traumatized tissue, altered immune response, and untreated infection/treatment failure.*

risk for ineffective Sexuality Pattern: risk factors may include lack of knowledge, values conflict, and/or fear of transmitting the disease.*

Herpes zoster (shingles)   CH

acute Pain may be related to inflammation/local lesions along sensory nerve(s), possibly evidenced by verbal reports, guarding/distraction

---

*A risk diagnosis is not evidenced by signs and symptoms, as the problem has not occurred and nursing interventions are directed at prevention.

behaviors, narrowed focus, and autonomic responses (changes in vital signs).

deficient Knowledge [Learning Need] regarding pathophysiology, therapeutic needs, and potential complications may be related to lack of information/misinterpretation, possibly evidenced by statements of concern, questions, and misconceptions.

High altitude pulmonary edema (HAPE)   MS
(Also refer to Mountain sickness, acute)

impaired Gas Exchange may be related to ventilation perfusion imbalance, alveolar-capillary membrane changes, altered O_2 supply, possibly evidenced by dyspnea, confusion, cyanosis, tachycardia, abnormal ABGs.

excess Fluid Volume may be related to compromised regulatory mechanism, possibly evidenced by shortness of breath, anxiety, edema, abnormal breath sounds, pulmonary congestion.

High altitude sickness   MS
(Refer to Mountain sickness, acute; High altitude pulmonary edema)

HIV positive   CH
(Also refer to AIDS)

risk-prone health Behavior may be related to life-threatening, stigmatizing condition/disease, assault to self-esteem, altered locus of control, inadequate support systems, incomplete grieving, medication side effects (fatigue/depression), possibly evidenced by verbalization of nonacceptance/denial of diagnosis, nonexistent or unsuccessful involvement in problem solving/goal setting, extended period of shock and disbelief or anger; lack of future-oriented thinking.

deficient Knowledge [Learning Need] regarding disease, prognosis, and treatment needs may be related to lack of exposure/recall, information misinterpretation, unfamiliarity with information resources, or cognitive limitation, possibly evidenced by statement of misconception/request for information, inappropriate/exaggerated behaviors (hostile, agitated, hysterical, apathetic), inaccurate follow-through of instructions/development of preventable complications.

risk for complicated Grieving: risk factors may include preloss psychological symptoms, predisposition for anxiety and feelings of inadequacy, frequency of major life events.*

Hodgkin's disease   CH/MS
(Also refer to Cancer; Chemotherapy)

Anxiety [specify level]/Fear may be related to threat of self-concept and threat of death, possibly evidenced by apprehension, insomnia, focus on self, and increased tension.

deficient Knowledge [Learning Need] regarding diagnosis, pathophysiology, treatment, and prognosis may be related to lack of information/misinterpretation, possibly evidenced by statements of concern, questions, and misconceptions.

---

*A risk diagnosis is not evidenced by signs and symptoms, as the problem has not occurred and nursing interventions are directed at prevention.

acute Pain/[Discomfort] may be related to manifestations of inflammatory response (fever, chills, night sweats) and pruritus, possibly evidenced by verbal reports, distraction behaviors, and focus on self.
risk for ineffective Breathing Pattern/Airway Clearance: risk factors may
include tracheobronchial obstruction (enlarged mediastinal nodes
and/or airway edema).*

Hospice/End-of-life care   CH

acute/chronic Pain may be related to biological, physical, psychological
agent, possibly evidenced by verbal/coded report, changes in
appetite/eating, sleep pattern, protective behavior, restlessness, irritability.
Activity Intolerance/Fatigue may be related to generalized weakness,
bedrest/immobility, pain, imbalance between O_2 supply and demand,
possibly evidenced by inability to maintain usual routine, verbalized
lack of desire/interest in activity, decreased performance, lethargy.
Grieving/death Anxiety may be related to anticipated loss of physiological well-being, perceived threat of death.
compromised/disabled family Coping/Caregiver Role Strain may be
related to prolonged disease/disability progression, temporary family
disorganization and role changes, unrealistic expectations, inadequate or incorrect information or understanding by primary person.
risk for moral Distress: risk factors may include conflict among decision
makers, cultural conflicts, end-of-life decisions, loss of autonomy,
physical distance of decision makers.*

Hydrocephalus   PED/MS

ineffective cerebral Tissue Perfusion may be related to decreased arte-
rial/venous blood flow (compression of brain tissue), possibly evidenced by changes in mentation, restlessness, irritability, reports of
headache, pupillary changes, and changes in vital signs.
disturbed visual Sensory Perception may be related to pressure on sen-
sory/motor nerves, possibly evidenced by reports of double vision,
development of strabismus, nystagmus, pupillary changes, and optic
atrophy.
risk for impaired physical Mobility: risk factors may include neuromuscular impairment, decreased muscle strength, and impaired coordination.*
risk for decreased Intracranial Adaptive Capacity: risk factors may include
brain injury, changes in perfusion pressure/intracranial pressure.*

                                                          CH
risk for Infection: risk factors may include invasive procedure/presence
of shunt.*
deficient Knowledge [Learning Need] regarding condition, prognosis,
and long-term therapy needs/medical follow-up may be related to
lack of information/misperceptions, possibly evidenced by questions,
statement of concern, request for information, and inaccurate follow-
through of instruction/development of preventable complications.

---

*A risk diagnosis is not evidenced by signs and symptoms, as the
problem has not occurred and nursing interventions are directed at
prevention.

Hyperactivity disorder   PED/PSY

defensive Coping may be related to mild neurological deficits, dysfunctional family system, abuse/neglect, possibly evidenced by denial of obvious problems, projection of blame/responsibility, grandiosity, difficulty in reality testing perceptions.

impaired Social Interaction may be related to retarded ego development, negative role models, neurological impairment, possibly evidenced by discomfort in social situations, interrupts/intrudes on others, difficulty waiting turn in games/group activities, difficulty maintaining attention to task.

disabled family Coping may be related to excessive guilt, anger, or blaming among family members, parental inconsistencies, disagreements regarding discipline/limit-setting/approaches, exhaustion of parental expectations, possibly evidenced by unrealistic parental expectations, rejection or overprotection of child, exaggerated expression of feelings, despair regarding child's behavior.

Hyperbilirubinemia   PED

risk for Injury [CNS involvement]: risk factors may include prematurity, hemolytic disease, asphyxia, acidosis, hyponatremia, and hypoglycemia.*

risk for Injury [effects of treatment]: risk factors may include physical properties of phototherapy and effects on body regulatory mechanisms, invasive procedure (exchange transfusion), abnormal blood profile, chemical imbalances.*

deficient Knowledge [Learning Need] regarding condition prognosis, treatment/safety needs may be related to lack of exposure/recall and information misinterpretation, possibly evidenced by questions, statement of concern, and inaccurate follow-through of instructions/development of preventable complications.

Hyperemesis gravidarum   OB

deficient Fluid Volume [isotonic] may be related to excessive gastric losses and reduced intake, possibly evidenced by dry mucous membranes, decreased/concentrated urine, decreased pulse volume and pressure, thirst, and hemoconcentration.

imbalanced Nutrition: less than body requirements may be related to inability to ingest/digest/absorb nutrients (prolonged vomiting), possibly evidenced by reported inadequate food intake, lack of interest in food/aversion to eating, and weight loss.

risk for ineffective Coping: risk factors may include situational/maturational crisis (pregnancy, change in health status, projected role changes, concern about outcome).*

Hypertension   CH

deficient Knowledge [Learning Need] regarding condition, therapeutic regimen, and potential complications may be related to lack of information/recall, misinterpretation, cognitive limitations, and/or denial of diagnosis, possibly evidenced by statements of concern/questions,

---

*A risk diagnosis is not evidenced by signs and symptoms, as the problem has not occurred and nursing interventions are directed at prevention.

and misconceptions, inaccurate follow-through of instructions, and lack of BP control.

risk-prone health Behavior may be related to condition requiring change in lifestyle, altered locus of control, and absence of feelings/denial of illness, possibly evidenced by verbalization of nonacceptance of health status change and lack of movement toward independence.

risk for Sexual Dysfunction: risk factors may include side effects of medication.*

MS

risk for decreased Cardiac Output: risk factors may include increased afterload (vasoconstriction), fluid shifts/hypovolemia, myocardial ischemia, ventricular hypertrophy/rigidity.*

acute Pain may be related to increased cerebrovascular pressure, possibly evidenced by verbal reports (throbbing pain located in suboccipital region, present on awakening and disappearing spontaneously after being up and about), reluctance to move head, avoidance of bright lights and noise, increased muscle tension.

Hypertension, pulmonary
CH/MS
(Refer to Pulmonary hypertension)

Hyperthyroidism
CH
(Also refer to Thyrotoxicosis)

Fatigue may be related to hypermetabolic imbalance with increased energy requirements, irritability of CNS, and altered body chemistry, possibly evidenced by verbalization of overwhelming lack of energy to maintain usual routine, decreased performance, emotional lability/irritability, and impaired ability to concentrate.

Anxiety [specify level] may be related to increased stimulation of the CNS (hypermetabolic state, pseudocatecholamine effect of thyroid hormones), possibly evidenced by increased feelings of apprehension, overexcitement/distress, irritability/emotional lability, shakiness, restless movements, tremors.

risk for imbalanced Nutrition: less than body requirements: risk factors may include inability to ingest adequate nutrients for hypermetabolic rate/constant activity, impaired absorption of nutrients (vomiting/diarrhea), hyperglycemia/relative insulin insufficiency.*

risk for impaired Tissue Integrity: risk factors may include altered protective mechanisms of eye related to periorbital edema, reduced ability to blink, eye discomfort/dryness, and development of corneal abrasion/ulceration.*

Hypoglycemia
CH
disturbed Thought Processes may be related to inadequate glucose for cellular brain function and effects of endogenous hormone activity, possibly evidenced by irritability, changes in mentation, memory loss, altered attention span, and emotional lability.

---

*A risk diagnosis is not evidenced by signs and symptoms, as the problem has not occurred and nursing interventions are directed at prevention.

risk for unstable blood Glucose: risk factors may include dietary intake, lack of adherence to diabetes management, inadequate blood glucose monitoring, medication management.*

deficient Knowledge [Learning Need] regarding pathophysiology of condition and therapy/self-care needs may be related to lack of information/recall, misinterpretations, possibly evidenced by development of hypoglycemia and statements of questions/misconceptions.

Hypoparathyroidism (acute)   MS
risk for Injury: risk factors may include neuromuscular excitability/tetany and formation of renal stones.*

acute Pain may be related to recurrent muscle spasms and alteration in reflexes, possibly evidenced by verbal reports, distraction behaviors, and narrowed focus.

risk for ineffective Airway Clearance: risk factors may include spasm of the laryngeal muscles.*

Anxiety [specify level] may be related to threat to, or change in, health status, physiological responses.

Hypothermia (systemic)   CH
(Also refer to Frostbite)

Hypothermia may be related to exposure to cold environment, inadequate clothing, age extremes (very young/elderly), damage to hypothalamus, consumption of alcohol/medications causing vasodilation, possibly evidenced by reduction in body temperature below normal range, shivering, cool skin, pallor.

deficient Knowledge [Learning Need] regarding risk factors, treatment needs, and prognosis may be related to lack of information/recall, misinterpretation, possibly evidenced by statement of concerns/misconceptions, occurrence of problem, and development of complications.

Hypothyroidism   CH
(Also refer to Myxedema)

impaired physical Mobility may be related to weakness, fatigue, muscle aches, altered reflexes, and mucin deposits in joints and interstitial spaces, possibly evidenced by decreased muscle strength/control and impaired coordination.

Fatigue may be related to decreased metabolic energy production, possibly evidenced by verbalization of unremitting/overwhelming lack of energy, inability to maintain usual routines, impaired ability to concentrate, decreased libido, irritability, listlessness, decreased performance, increase in physical complaints.

disturbed Sensory Perception (specify) may be related to mucin deposits and nerve compression, possibly evidenced by paresthesias of hands and feet or decreased hearing.

Constipation may be related to decreased peristalsis/physical activity, possibly evidenced by frequency less than usual pattern, decreased bowel sounds, hard dry stools, and development of fecal impaction.

---

*A risk diagnosis is not evidenced by signs and symptoms, as the problem has not occurred and nursing interventions are directed at prevention.

Hysterectomy   GYN/MS

acute Pain may be related to tissue trauma/abdominal incision,
edema/hematoma formation, possibly evidenced by verbal reports,
guarding/distraction behaviors, and autonomic responses (changes
in vital signs).

risk for impaired Urinary Elimination/[acute] Urinary Retention: risk
factors may include mechanical trauma, surgical manipulation, presence of localized edema/hematoma, or nerve trauma with temporary
bladder atony.*

risk for ineffective Sexuality Pattern/Sexual Dysfunction: risk factors
may include concerns regarding altered body function/structure, perceived changes in femininity, changes in hormone levels, loss of
libido, and changes in sexual response pattern.*

risk for complicated Grieving: risk factors may include preloss psychological symptoms, predisposition for anxiety and feelings of inadequacy, frequency of major life events.*

Ileocolitis   MS/CH
(Refer to Crohn's disease)

Ileostomy   MS/CH
(Refer to Colostomy)

Ileus   MS

acute Pain may be related to distention/edema and ischemia of intestinal
tissue, possibly evidenced by verbal reports, guarding/distraction behaviors, narrowed focus, and autonomic responses (changes in vital signs).

Diarrhea/Constipation may be related to presence of obstruction/
changes in peristalsis, possibly evidenced by changes in frequency and
consistency or absence of stool, alterations in bowel sounds, presence
of pain, and cramping.

risk for deficient Fluid Volume: risk factors may include increased intestinal losses (vomiting and diarrhea), and decreased intake.*

Impetigo   PED/CH

impaired Skin Integrity may be related to presence of infectious process
and pruritus, possibly evidenced by open/crusted lesions.

acute Pain may be related to inflammation and pruritus, possibly evidenced by verbal reports, distraction behaviors, and self-focusing.

risk for [secondary] Infection: risk factors may include broken skin,
traumatized tissue, altered immune response, and virulence/conta-
gious nature of causative organism.*

risk for Infection [transmission]: risk factors may include virulent
nature of causative organism, insufficient knowledge to prevent
infection of others.*

Infection, prenatal   OB
(Also refer to AIDS)

risk for maternal/fetal Infection: risk factors may include inadequate
primary defenses (e.g., broken skin, stasis of body fluids), inadequate

---

*A risk diagnosis is not evidenced by signs and symptoms, as the
problem has not occurred and nursing interventions are directed at
prevention.

secondary defenses (e.g., decreased hemoglobin, immunosuppression), inadequate acquired immunity, environmental exposure, malnutrition, rupture of amniotic membranes.*

deficient Knowledge regarding treatment/prevention, prognosis of condition may be related to lack of exposure to information and/or unfamiliarity with resources, misinterpretation possibly evidenced by verbalization of problem, inaccurate follow-through of instructions, development of preventable complications/continuation of infectious process.

[Discomfort] may be related to body response to infective agent, properties of infection (e.g., skin/tissue irritation, development of lesions), possibly evidenced by verbal reports, restlessness, withdrawal from social contacts.

Inflammatory bowel disease   CH
(Refer to Colitis, ulcerative; Crohn's disease)

Influenza   CH
Pain[/Discomfort] may be related to inflammation and effects of circulating toxins, possibly evidenced by verbal reports, distraction behaviors, and narrowed focus.

risk for deficient Fluid Volume: risk factors may include excessive gastric losses, hypermetabolic state, and altered intake.*

Hyperthermia may be related to effects of circulating toxins and dehydration, possibly evidenced by increased body temperature, warm/flushed skin, and tachycardia.

risk for ineffective Breathing: risk factors may include response to infectious process, decreased energy/fatigue.*

Insulin shock   MS/CH
(Refer to Hypoglycemia)

Intestinal obstruction   MS
(Refer to Ileus)

Irritable bowel syndrome   CH
acute Pain may be related to abnormally strong intestinal contractions, increased sensitivity of intestine to distention, hypersensitivity to hormones gastrin and cholecystokinin, skin/tissue irritation/perirectal excoriation, possibly evidenced by verbal reports, guarding behavior, expressive behavior (restlessness, moaning, irritability).

Constipation may be related to motor abnormalities of longitudinal muscles/changes in frequency and amplitude of contractions, dietary restrictions, stress, possibly evidenced by change in bowel pattern/decreased frequency, sensation of incomplete evacuation, abdominal pain/distention.

Diarrhea may be related to motor abnormalities of longitudinal muscles/changes in frequency and amplitude of contractions, possibly evidenced by precipitous passing of liquid stool on rising or immediately after eating, rectal urgency/incontinence, bloating.

---

*A risk diagnosis is not evidenced by signs and symptoms, as the problem has not occurred and nursing interventions are directed at prevention.

Kawasaki disease PED

Hyperthermia may be related to increased metabolic rate and dehydration, possibly evidenced by increased body temperature greater than normal range, flushed skin, increased respiratory rate, and tachycardia.

acute Pain may be related to inflammation and edema/swelling of tissues, possibly evidenced by verbal reports, restlessness, guarding behaviors, and narrowed focus.

impaired Skin Integrity may be related to inflammatory process, altered circulation, and edema formation, possibly evidenced by disruption of skin surface, including macular rash and desquamation.

impaired Oral Mucous Membrane may be related to inflammatory process, dehydration, and mouth breathing, possibly evidenced by pain, hyperemia, and fissures of lips.

risk for decreased Cardiac Output: risk factors may include structural changes/inflammation of coronary arteries and alterations in rate/rhythm or conduction.*

Kidney stone(s) CH
(Refer to Calculi, urinary)

Labor, induced/augmented OB

deficient Knowledge [Learning Need] regarding procedure, treatment needs, and possible outcomes may be related to lack of exposure/recall, information misinterpretation, and unfamiliarity with information resources, possibly evidenced by questions, statement of concern/misconception, and exaggerated behaviors.

risk for maternal Injury: risk factors may include adverse effects/response to therapeutic interventions.*

risk for impaired fetal Gas Exchange: risk factors may include altered placental perfusion/cord prolapse.*

acute Pain may be related to altered characteristics of chemically stimulated contractions, psychological concerns, possibly evidenced by verbal reports, increased muscle tone, distraction/guarding behaviors, and narrowed focus.

Labor, precipitous OB

Anxiety [specify level] may be related to situational crisis, threat to self/fetus, interpersonal transmission, possibly evidenced by increased tension; scared, fearful, restless/jittery; sympathetic stimulation.

risk for impaired Skin/Tissue Integrity: risk factors may include rapid progress of labor, lack of necessary equipment.*

acute Pain may be related to occurrence of rapid, strong muscle contractions; psychological issues, possibly evidenced by verbalizations of inability to use learned pain-management techniques, sympathetic stimulation, distraction behaviors (e.g., moaning, restlessness).

Labor, preterm OB/CH

Activity Intolerance may be related to muscle/cellular hypersensitivity, possibly evidenced by continued uterine contractions/irritability.

---

*A risk diagnosis is not evidenced by signs and symptoms, as the problem has not occurred and nursing interventions are directed at prevention.

risk for Poisoning: risk factors may include dose-related toxic/side effects of tocolytics.*

risk for fetal Injury: risk factors may include delivery of premature/immature infant.*

Anxiety [specify level] may be related to situational crisis, perceived or actual threats to self/fetus, and inadequate time to prepare for labor, possibly evidenced by increased tension, restlessness, expressions of concern, and autonomic responses (changes in vital signs).

deficient Knowledge [Learning Need] regarding preterm labor treatment needs and prognosis may be related to lack of information and misinterpretation, possibly evidenced by questions, statements of concern, misconceptions, inaccurate follow-through of instruction, and development of preventable complications.

Labor, stage I (active phase) OB

acute Pain[/Discomfort] may be related to contraction-related hypoxia, dilation of tissues, and pressure on adjacent structures combined with stimulation of both parasympathetic and sympathetic nerve endings, possibly evidenced by verbal reports, guarding/distraction behaviors (restlessness), muscle tension, and narrowed focus.

impaired Urinary Elimination may be related to altered intake/dehydration, fluid shifts, hormonal changes, hemorrhage, severe intrapartal hypertension, mechanical compression of bladder, and effects of regional anesthesia, possibly evidenced by changes in amount/frequency of voiding, urinary retention, slowed progression of labor, and reduced sensation.

risk for ineffective Coping [Individual/Couple]: risk factors may include situational crises, personal vulnerability, use of ineffective coping mechanisms, inadequate support systems, and pain.*

Labor, stage II (expulsion) OB

acute Pain may be related to strong uterine contractions, tissue stretching/dilation and compression of nerves by presenting part of the fetus, and bladder distention, possibly evidenced by verbalizations, facial grimacing, guarding/distraction behaviors (restlessness), narrowed focus, and autonomic responses (diaphoresis).

Cardiac Output [fluctuation] may be related to changes in SVR, fluctuations in venous return (repeated/prolonged Valsalva's maneuvers, effects of anesthesia/medications, dorsal recumbent position occluding the inferior vena cava and partially obstructing the aorta), possibly evidenced by decreased venous return, changes in vital signs (BP, pulse), urinary output, fetal bradycardia.

risk for impaired fetal Gas Exchange: risk factors may include mechanical compression of head/cord, maternal position/prolonged labor affecting placental perfusion, and effects of maternal anesthesia, hyperventilation.*

risk for impaired Skin/Tissue Integrity: risk factors may include untoward stretching/lacerations of delicate tissues (precipitous labor, hypertonic contractile pattern, adolescence, large fetus) and application of forceps.*

---

*A risk diagnosis is not evidenced by signs and symptoms, as the problem has not occurred and nursing interventions are directed at prevention.

risk for Fatigue: risk factors may include pregnancy, stress, anxiety, sleep deprivation, increased physical exertion, anemia, humidity/temperature, lights.*

Laminectomy (lumbar)   MS

ineffective Tissue Perfusion (specify) may be related to diminished/ interrupted blood flow (dressing, edema/hematoma formation), hypovolemia, possibly evidenced by paresthesia, numbness, decreased range of motion, muscle strength.

risk for [spinal] Trauma: risk factors may include temporary weakness of spinal column, balancing difficulties, changes in muscle tone/coordination.*

acute Pain may be related to traumatized tissues, localized inflammation, and edema, possibly evidenced by altered muscle tone, verbal reports, and distraction/guarding behaviors, autonomic changes.

impaired physical Mobility may be related to imposed therapeutic restrictions, neuromuscular impairment, and pain, possibly evidenced by limited range of motion, decreased muscle strength/control, impaired coordination, and reluctance to attempt movement.

risk for [acute] Urinary Retention: risk factors may include pain and swelling in operative area and reduced mobility/restrictions of position.*

Laryngectomy   MS
(Also refer to Cancer; Chemotherapy)

ineffective Airway Clearance may be related to partial/total removal of the glottis, temporary or permanent change to neck breathing, edema formation, and copious/thick secretions, possibly evidenced by dyspnea/difficulty breathing, changes in rate/depth of respiration, use of accessory respiratory muscles, weak/ineffective cough, abnormal breath sounds, and cyanosis.

impaired Skin/Tissue Integrity may be related to surgical removal of tissues/grafting, effects of radiation or chemotherapeutic agents, altered circulation/reduced blood supply, compromised nutritional status, edema formation, and pooling/continuous drainage of secretions, possibly evidenced by disruption of skin/tissue surface and destruction of skin/tissue layers.

impaired Oral Mucous Membrane may be related to dehydration/ absence of oral intake, poor/inadequate oral hygiene, pathological condition (oral cancer), mechanical trauma (oral surgery), decreased saliva production, difficulty swallowing and pooling/drooling of secretions, and nutritional deficits, possibly evidenced by xerostomia (dry mouth), oral discomfort, thick/mucoid saliva, decreased saliva production, dry and crusted/coated tongue, inflamed lips, absent teeth/gums, poor dental health and halitosis.

                                                           CH

impaired verbal Communication may be related to anatomic deficit (removal of vocal cords), physical barrier (tracheostomy tube), and

*A risk diagnosis is not evidenced by signs and symptoms, as the problem has not occurred and nursing interventions are directed at prevention.

required voice rest, possibly evidenced by inability to speak, change in vocal characteristics, and impaired articulation.

risk for Aspiration: risk factors may include impaired swallowing, facial/neck surgery, presence of tracheostomy/feeding tube.*

Laryngitis   CH/PED
(Refer to Croup)

Latex allergy   CH
latex Allergy Response may be related to no immune mechanism response, possibly evidenced by contact dermatitis—erythema, blisters, delayed hypersensitivity—eczema, irritation, hypersensitivity—generalized edema, wheezing/bronchospasm, hypotension, cardiac arrest.

Anxiety [specify level]/Fear may be related to threat of death, possibly evidenced by expressed concerns, hypervigilance, restlessness, focus on self.

risk for risk-prone health Behavior: risk factors may include health status requiring change in occupation.*

Lead poisoning, acute   PED/CH
(Also refer to Lead poisoning, chronic)
Contamination may be related to flaking/peeling paint (young children), improperly lead-glazed ceramic pottery, unprotected contact with lead (e.g., battery manufacture/recycling, bronzing, soldering/welding), imported herbal products/medicinals, possibly evidenced by abdominal cramping, headache, irritability, decreased attentiveness, constipation, tremors.

risk for Trauma: risk factors may include loss of coordination, altered level of consciousness, clonic or tonic muscle activity, neurological damage.*

risk for deficient Fluid Volume: risk factors may include excessive vomiting, diarrhea, or decreased intake.*

deficient Knowledge [Learning Need] regarding sources of lead and prevention of poisoning may be related to lack of information/misinterpretation, possibly evidenced by statements of concern, questions, and misconceptions.

Lead poisoning, chronic   CH
(Also refer to Lead poisoning, acute)
Contamination may be related to flaking/peeling paint (young children), improperly lead-glazed ceramic pottery, unprotected contact with lead (e.g., battery manufacture/recycling, bronzing, soldering/welding), imported herbal products/medicinals, possibly evidenced by chronic abdominal pain, headache, personality changes, cognitive deficits, seizures, neuropathy.

imbalanced Nutrition: less than body requirements may be related to decreased intake (chemically induced changes in the GI tract), possibly evidenced by anorexia, abdominal discomfort, reported metallic taste, and weight loss.

---

*A risk diagnosis is not evidenced by signs and symptoms, as the problem has not occurred and nursing interventions are directed at prevention.

<u>disturbed Thought Processes</u> may be related to deposition of lead in CNS and brain tissue, possibly evidenced by personality changes, learning disabilities, and impaired ability to conceptualize and reason.

<u>chronic Pain</u> may be related to deposition of lead in soft tissues and bone, possibly evidenced by verbal reports, distraction behaviors, and focus on self.

Leukemia, acute   MS
(Also refer to Chemotherapy)

<u>risk for Infection:</u> risk factors may include inadequate secondary defenses (alterations in mature white blood cells, increased number of immature lymphocytes, immunosuppression and bone marrow suppression), invasive procedures, and malnutrition.*

<u>Anxiety [specify level]/Fear</u> may be related to change in health status, threat of death, and situational crisis, possibly evidenced by sympathetic stimulation, apprehension, feelings of helplessness, focus on self, and insomnia.

<u>Activity Intolerance [specify level]</u> may be related to reduced energy stores, increased metabolic rate, imbalance between O_2 supply and demand, therapeutic restrictions (bedrest)/effect of drug therapy, possibly evidenced by generalized weakness, reports of fatigue and exertional dyspnea, abnormal heart rate or BP response.

<u>acute Pain</u> may be related to physical agents (infiltration of tissues/organs/CNS, expanding bone marrow) and chemical agents (antileukemic treatments), possibly evidenced by verbal reports (abdominal discomfort, arthralgia, bone pain, headache), distraction behaviors, narrowed focus, and autonomic responses (changes in vital signs).

<u>risk for deficient Fluid Volume:</u> risk factors may include excessive losses (vomiting, hemorrhage, diarrhea), decreased intake (nausea, anorexia), increased fluid need (hypermetabolic state/fever), predisposition for kidney stone formation/tumor lysis syndrome.*

Long-term care   CH
(Also refer to condition requiring/contributing to need for facility placement)

<u>Anxiety [specify level]/Fear</u> may be related to change in health status, role functioning, interaction patterns, socioeconomic status, environment; unmet needs, recent life changes, and loss of friends/SO(s), possibly evidenced by apprehension, restlessness, insomnia, repetitive questioning, pacing, purposeless activity, expressed concern regarding changes in life events, and focus on self.

<u>Grieving</u> may be related to perceived/actual or potential loss of physiopsychosocial well-being, personal possessions, and SO(s), as well as cultural beliefs about aging/debilitation, possibly evidenced by denial of feelings, depression, sorrow, guilt, alterations in activity level, sleep patterns, eating habits, and libido.

<u>risk for Poisoning [drug toxicity]:</u> risk factors may include effects of aging (reduced metabolism, impaired circulation, precarious physiological

---

*A risk diagnosis is not evidenced by signs and symptoms, as the problem has not occurred and nursing interventions are directed at prevention.

balance, presence of multiple diseases/organ involvement), and use of multiple prescribed/OTC drugs.*

disturbed Thought Processes may be related to physiological changes of aging (loss of cells and brain atrophy, decreased blood supply), altered sensory input, pain, effects of medications, and psychological conflicts (disrupted life pattern), possibly evidenced by slower reaction times, memory loss, altered attention span, disorientation, inability to follow, altered sleep patterns, and personality changes.

Insomnia may be related to internal factors (illness, psychological stress, inactivity) and external factors (environmental changes, facility routines), possibly evidenced by reports of difficulty in falling asleep/not feeling rested, interrupted sleep/awakening earlier than desired, change in behavior/performance, increasing irritability, and listlessness.

risk for ineffective Sexuality Pattern: risk factors may include biopsychosocial alteration of sexuality, interference in psychological/physical well-being, self-image, and lack of privacy/SO(s).*

risk for Relocation Stress Syndrome: risk factors may include multiple losses, feeling of powerlessness, lack of/inappropriate use of support system, changes in psychosocial/physical health status.*

risk for impaired Religiosity: risk factors may include ineffective support/coping, lack of social interaction, depression. *

Lupus erythematosus, systemic (SLE)　　　　CH

Fatigue may be related to inadequate energy production/increased energy requirements (chronic inflammation), overwhelming psychological or emotional demands, states of discomfort, and altered body chemistry (including effects of drug therapy), possibly evidenced by reports of unremitting and overwhelming lack of energy/inability to maintain usual routines, decreased performance, lethargy, and decreased libido.

acute Pain may be related to widespread inflammatory process affecting connective tissues, blood vessels, serosal surfaces and mucous membranes, possibly evidenced by verbal reports, guarding/distraction behaviors, self-focusing, and autonomic responses (changes in vital signs).

impaired Skin/Tissue Integrity may be related to chronic inflammation, edema formation, and altered circulation, possibly evidenced by presence of skin rash/lesions, ulcerations of mucous membranes, and photosensitivity.

disturbed Body Image may be related to presence of chronic condition with rash, lesions, ulcers, purpura, mottled erythema of hands, alopecia, loss of strength, and altered body function, possibly evidenced by hiding body parts, negative feelings about body, feelings of helplessness, and change in social involvement.

Lyme disease　　　　CH/MS

acute/chronic Pain[/Discomfort] may be related to systemic effects of toxins, presence of rash, urticaria, and joint swelling/inflammation, possibly evidenced by verbal reports, guarding behaviors, autonomic responses, and narrowed focus.

---

*A risk diagnosis is not evidenced by signs and symptoms, as the problem has not occurred and nursing interventions are directed at prevention.

Fatigue may be related to increased energy requirements, altered body chemistry, and states of discomfort evidenced by reports of overwhelming lack of energy/inability to maintain usual routines, decreased performance, lethargy, and malaise.

risk for decreased Cardiac Output: risk factors may include alteration in cardiac rate/rhythm/conduction.*

Macular degeneration   CH

disturbed visual Sensory Perception may be related to altered sensory reception, possibly evidenced by reported/measured change in sensory acuity, change in usual response to stimuli.

Anxiety [specify level]/Fear may be related to situational crisis, threat to or change in health status and role function, possibly evidenced by expressed concerns, apprehension, feelings of inadequacy, diminished productivity, impaired attention.

risk for impaired Home Maintenance: risk factors may include impaired cognitive functioning, inadequate support systems.*

risk for impaired Social Interaction: risk factors may include limited physical mobility, environmental barriers.*

Mallory-Weiss syndrome   MS
(Also refer to Achalasia)

risk for deficient Fluid Volume [isotonic]: risk factors may include excessive vascular losses, presence of vomiting, and reduced intake.*

deficient Knowledge [Learning Need] regarding causes, treatment, and prevention of condition may be related to lack of information/misinterpretation, possibly evidenced by statements of concern, questions, and recurrence of problem.

Mastectomy   MS

impaired Skin/Tissue Integrity may be related to surgical removal of skin/tissue, altered circulation, drainage, presence of edema, changes in skin elasticity/sensation, and tissue destruction (radiation), possibly evidenced by disruption of skin surface and destruction of skin layers/subcutaneous tissues.

impaired physical Mobility may be related to neuromuscular impairment, pain, and edema formation, possibly evidenced by reluctance to attempt movement, limited range of motion, and decreased muscle mass/strength.

bathing/dressing Self-Care Deficit may be related to temporary loss/altered action of one or both arms, possibly evidenced by statements of inability to perform/complete self-care tasks.

disturbed Body Image may be related to loss of body part denoting femininity, possibly evidenced by not looking at/touching area, negative feelings about body, preoccupation with loss, and change in social involvement/relationship.

risk for complicated Grieving: risk factors may include preloss psychological symptoms, predisposition for anxiety and feelings of inadequacy, frequency of major life events. *

---

*A risk diagnosis is not evidenced by signs and symptoms, as the problem has not occurred and nursing interventions are directed at prevention.

Mastitis   OB/GYN

acute Pain may be related to erythema and edema of breast tissues, possibly evidenced by verbal reports, guarding/distraction behaviors,
self-focusing, autonomic responses (changes in vital signs).

risk for Infection [spread/abscess formation]: risk factors may include
traumatized tissues, stasis of fluids, and insufficient knowledge to
prevent complications.*

deficient Knowledge [Learning Need] regarding pathophysiology, treatment, and prevention may be related to lack of information/misin-
terpretation, possibly evidenced by statements of concern, questions,
and misconceptions.

risk for ineffective Breastfeeding: risk factors may include inability to
feed on affected side/interruption in breastfeeding.*

Mastoidectomy   PED/MS

risk for Infection [spread]: risk factors may include preexisting infection, surgical trauma, and stasis of body fluids in close proximity to
brain.*

acute Pain may be related to inflammation, tissue trauma, and edema
formation, possibly evidenced by verbal reports, distraction behaviors, restlessness, self-focusing, and autonomic responses (changes in
vital signs).

disturbed auditory Sensory Perception may be related to presence of
surgical packing, edema, and surgical disturbance of middle ear
structures, possibly evidenced by reported/tested hearing loss in
affected ear.

Measles   CH/PED

acute Pain[/Discomfort] may be related to inflammation of mucous
membranes, conjunctiva, and presence of extensive skin rash with
pruritus, possibly evidenced by verbal reports, distraction behaviors,
self-focusing, and autonomic responses (changes in vital signs).

Hyperthermia may be related to presence of viral toxins and inflammatory response, possibly evidenced by increased body temperature,
flushed/warm skin, and tachycardia.

risk for [secondary] Infection: risk factors may include altered immune
response and traumatized dermal tissues.*

deficient Knowledge [Learning Need] regarding condition, transmission,
and possible complications may be related to lack of information/mis-
interpretation, possibly evidenced by statements of concern, questions,
misconceptions, and development of preventable complications.

Melanoma, malignant   MS/CH
(Refer to Cancer; Chemotherapy)

Meningitis, acute meningococcal   MS

risk for Infection [spread]: risk factors may include hematogenous dissemination of pathogen, stasis of body fluids, suppressed inflammatory
response (medication-induced), and exposure of others to pathogens.*

---

*A risk diagnosis is not evidenced by signs and symptoms, as the
problem has not occurred and nursing interventions are directed at
prevention.

risk for ineffective cerebral Tissue Perfusion: risk factors may include cerebral edema altering/interrupting cerebral arterial/venous blood flow, hypovolemia, exchange problems at cellular level (acidosis).*

Hyperthermia may be related to infectious process (increased metabolic rate) and dehydration, possibly evidenced by increased body temperature, warm/flushed skin, and tachycardia.

acute Pain may be related to inflammation/irritation of the meninges with spasm of extensor muscles (neck, shoulders, and back), possibly evidenced by verbal reports, guarding/distraction behaviors, narrowed focus, photophobia, and autonomic responses (changes in vital signs).

risk for Trauma/Suffocation: risk factors may include alterations in level of consciousness, possible development of clonic/tonic muscle activity (seizures), and generalized weakness/prostration, ataxia, vertigo.*

Meniscectomy   MS/CH

impaired Walking may be related to pain, joint instability, and imposed medical restrictions of movement, possibly evidenced by impaired ability to move about environment as needed/desired.

deficient Knowledge [Learning Need] regarding postoperative expectations, prevention of complications, and self-care needs may be related to lack of information, possibly evidenced by statements of concern, questions, and misconceptions.

Menopause   GYN

ineffective Thermoregulation may be related to fluctuation of hormonal levels, possibly evidenced by skin flushed/warm to touch, diaphoresis, night sweats, cold hands/feet.

Fatigue may be related to change in body chemistry, lack of sleep, depression, possibly evidenced by reports of lack of energy, tired, inability to maintain usual routines, decreased performance.

risk for ineffective Sexuality Pattern: risk factors may include perceived altered body function, changes in physical response, myths/inaccurate information, impaired relationship with SO.*

risk for stress Urinary Incontinence: risk factors may include degenerative changes in pelvic muscles and structural support.*

Health-Seeking Behaviors: management of life cycle changes may be related to maturational change, possibly evidenced by expressed desire for increased control of health practice, demonstrated lack of knowledge in health promotion.

Mental retardation   CH

(Also refer to Down syndrome)

impaired verbal Communication may be related to developmental delay/impairment of cognitive and motor abilities, possibly evidenced by impaired articulation, difficulty with phonation, and inability to modulate speech/find appropriate words (dependent on degree of retardation).

risk for Self-Care Deficit [specify]: risk factors may include impaired cognitive ability and motor skills.*

---

*A risk diagnosis is not evidenced by signs and symptoms, as the problem has not occurred and nursing interventions are directed at prevention.

imbalanced Nutrition: risk for more than body requirements: risk factors may include decreased metabolic rate coupled with impaired cognitive development, dysfunctional eating patterns, and sedentary activity level.*

risk for sedentary Lifestyle: risk factors may include lack of interest/motivation, lack of resources, lack of training or knowledge of specific exercise needs, safety concerns/fear of injury. *

impaired Social Interaction may be related to impaired thought processes, communication barriers, and knowledge/skill deficit about ways to enhance mutuality, possibly evidenced by dysfunctional interactions with peers, family, and/or SO(s), and verbalized/observed discomfort in social situation.

compromised family Coping may be related to chronic nature of condition and degree of disability that exhausts supportive capacity of SO(s), other situational or developmental crises or situations SO(s) may be facing, unrealistic expectations of SO(s), possibly evidenced by preoccupation of SO with personal reaction, SO(s) withdraw(s) or enter(s) into limited interaction with individual, protective behavior disproportionate (too much or too little) to client's abilities or need for autonomy.

impaired Home Maintenance may be related to impaired cognitive functioning, insufficient finances/family organization or planning, lack of knowledge, and inadequate support systems, possibly evidenced by requests for assistance, expression of difficulty in maintaining home, disorderly surroundings, and overtaxed family members.

risk for Sexual Dysfunction: risk factors may include biopsychosocial alteration of sexuality, ineffectual/absent role models, misinformation/lack of knowledge, lack of SO(s), and lack of appropriate behavior control.*

Miscarriage   OB
(Refer to Abortion, spontaneous termination)

Mitral stenosis   MS/CH
Activity Intolerance may be related to imbalance between O_2 supply and demand, possibly evidenced by reports of fatigue, weakness, exertional dyspnea, and tachycardia.

impaired Gas Exchange may be related to altered blood flow, possibly evidenced by restlessness, hypoxia, and cyanosis (orthopnea/paroxysmal nocturnal dyspnea).

decreased Cardiac Output may be related to impeded blood flow as evidenced by jugular vein distention, peripheral/dependent edema, orthopnea/paroxysmal nocturnal dyspnea.

deficient Knowledge [Learning Need] regarding pathophysiology, therapeutic needs, and potential complications may be related to lack of information/recall, misinterpretation, possibly evidenced by statements of concern, questions, inaccurate follow-through of instructions, and development of preventable complications.

---

*A risk diagnosis is not evidenced by signs and symptoms, as the problem has not occurred and nursing interventions are directed at prevention.

Mononucleosis, infectious   CH

Fatigue may be related to decreased energy production, states of discomfort, and increased energy requirements (inflammatory process), possibly evidenced by reports of overwhelming lack of energy, inability to maintain usual routines, lethargy, and malaise.

acute Pain[/Discomfort] may be related to inflammation of lymphoid and organ tissues, irritation of oropharyngeal mucous membranes, and effects of circulating toxins, possibly evidenced by verbal reports, distraction behaviors, and self-focusing.

Hyperthermia may be related to inflammatory process, possibly evidenced by increased body temperature, warm/flushed skin, and tachycardia.

deficient Knowledge [Learning Need] regarding disease transmission, self-care needs, medical therapy, and potential complications may be related to lack of information/misinterpretation, possibly evidenced by statements of concern, misconceptions, and inaccurate follow-through of instructions.

Mood disorders   PSY
(Refer to Depressive disorders)

Mountain sickness, acute (AMS)   CH/MS

acute Pain may be related to reduced O_2 tension, possibly evidenced by reports of headache.

Fatigue may be related to stress, increased physical exertion, sleep deprivation, possibly evidenced by overwhelming lack of energy, inability to restore energy even after sleep, compromised concentration, decreased performance.

risk for deficient Fluid Volume: risk factors may include increased water loss (e.g., overbreathing dry air), exertion, altered fluid intake (nausea).*

Multiple personality   PSY
(Refer to Dissociative disorders)

Multiple sclerosis   CH

Fatigue may be related to decreased energy production/increased energy requirements to perform activities, psychological/emotional demands, pain/discomfort, medication side effects, possibly evidenced by verbalization of overwhelming lack of energy, inability to maintain usual routine, decreased performance, impaired ability to concentrate, increase in physical complaints.

disturbed visual, kinesthetic, tactile Sensory Perception may be related to delayed/interrupted neuronal transmission, possibly evidenced by impaired vision, diplopia, disturbance of vibratory or position sense, paresthesias, numbness, and blunting of sensation.

impaired physical Mobility may be related to neuromuscular impairment; discomfort/pain; sensoriperceptual impairments;, decreased muscle strength, control and/or mass; deconditioning, as evidenced by limited ability to perform motor skills; limited range of motion; gait changes/postural instability.

---

*A risk diagnosis is not evidenced by signs and symptoms, as the problem has not occurred and nursing interventions are directed at prevention.

Powerlessness/Hopelessness may be related to illness-related regimen and lifestyle of helplessness, possibly evidenced by verbal expressions of having no control or influence over the situation, depression over physical deterioration that occurs despite client compliance with regimen, nonparticipation in care or decision making when opportunities are provided, passivity, decreased verbalization/affect.

impaired Home Maintenance may be related to effects of debilitating disease, impaired cognitive and/or emotional functioning, insufficient finances, and inadequate support systems, possibly evidenced by reported difficulty, observed disorderly surroundings, and poor hygienic conditions.

compromised/disabled family Coping may be related to situational crises/temporary family disorganization and role changes, client providing little support in turn for SO(s), prolonged disease/disability progression that exhausts the supportive capacity of SO(s), feelings of guilt, anxiety, hostility, despair, and highly ambivalent family relationships, possibly evidenced by client expressing/confirming concern or report about SO's response to client's illness, SO(s) preoccupied with own personal reactions, intolerance, abandonment, neglectful care of the client, and distortion of reality regarding client's illness.

Mumps PED/CH

acute Pain may be related to presence of inflammation, circulating toxins, and enlargement of salivary glands, possibly evidenced by verbal reports, guarding/distraction behaviors, self-focusing, and autonomic responses (changes in vital signs).

Hyperthermia may be related to inflammatory process (increased metabolic rate) and dehydration, possibly evidenced by increased body temperature, warm/flushed skin, and tachycardia.

risk for deficient Fluid Volume: risk factors may include hypermetabolic state and painful swallowing, with decreased intake.*

Muscular dystrophy (Duchenne's) PED/CH

impaired physical Mobility may be related to musculoskeletal impairment/weakness, possibly evidenced by decreased muscle strength, control, and mass, limited range of motion, and impaired coordination.

delayed Growth and Development may be related to effects of physical disability, possibly evidenced by altered physical growth and altered ability to perform self-care/self-control activities appropriate to age.

risk for imbalanced Nutrition: more than body requirements: risk factors may include sedentary lifestyle and dysfunctional eating patterns.*

compromised family Coping may be related to situational crisis/emotional conflicts around issues about hereditary nature of condition and prolonged disease/disability that exhausts supportive capacity of family members, possibly evidenced by preoccupation with personal reactions regarding disability and displaying protective behavior disproportionate (too little/too much) to client's abilities/need for autonomy.

---

*A risk diagnosis is not evidenced by signs and symptoms, as the problem has not occurred and nursing interventions are directed at prevention.

Myasthenia gravis MS

ineffective Breathing Pattern/Airway Clearance may be related to neuromuscular weakness and decreased energy/fatigue, possibly evidenced by dyspnea, changes in rate/depth of respiration, ineffective cough, and adventitious breath sounds.

impaired verbal Communication may be related to neuromuscular weakness, fatigue, and physical barrier (intubation), possibly evidenced by facial weakness, impaired articulation, hoarseness, and inability to speak.

impaired Swallowing may be related to neuromuscular impairment of laryngeal/pharyngeal muscles and muscular fatigue, possibly evidenced by reported/observed difficulty swallowing, coughing/choking, and evidence of aspiration.

Anxiety [specify level]/Fear may be related to situational crisis, threat to self-concept, change in health/socioeconomic status or role function, separation from support systems, lack of knowledge, and inability to communicate, possibly evidenced by expressed concerns, increased tension, restlessness, apprehension, sympathetic stimulation, crying, focus on self, uncooperative behavior, withdrawal, anger, and noncommunication.

CH

deficient Knowledge [Learning Need] regarding drug therapy, potential for crisis (myasthenic or cholinergic), and self-care management may be related to inadequate information/misinterpretation, possibly evidenced by statements of concern, questions, and misconceptions; development of preventable complications.

impaired physical Mobility may be related to neuromuscular impairment, possibly evidenced by reports of progressive fatigability with repetitive/prolonged muscle use, impaired coordination, and decreased muscle strength/control.

disturbed visual Sensory Perception may be related to neuromuscular impairment, possibly evidenced by visual distortions (diplopia) and motor incoordination.

Myeloma, multiple MS/CH
(Also refer to Cancer)

acute/chronic Pain may be related to destruction of tissues/bone, side effects of therapy, possibly evidenced by verbal or coded reports, guarding/protective behaviors, changes in appetite/weight, sleep; reduced interaction with others.

impaired physical Mobility may be related to loss of integrity of bone structure, pain, deconditioning, depressed mood, possibly evidenced by verbalizations, limited range of motion, slowed movement, gait changes.

risk for ineffective Protection: risk factors may include presence of cancer, drug therapies, radiation treatments, inadequate nutrition.*

Myocardial infarction MS
(Also refer to Myocarditis)

---

*A risk diagnosis is not evidenced by signs and symptoms, as the problem has not occurred and nursing interventions are directed at prevention.

acute Pain may be related to ischemia of myocardial tissue, possibly evidenced by verbal reports, guarding/distraction behaviors (restlessness), facial mask of pain, self-focusing, and autonomic responses (diaphoresis, changes in vital signs).

Anxiety [specify level]/Fear may be related to threat of death, threat of change of health status/role functioning and lifestyle, interpersonal transmission/contagion, possibly evidenced by increased tension, fearful attitude, apprehension, expressed concerns/uncertainty, restlessness, sympathetic stimulation, and somatic complaints.

risk for decreased Cardiac Output: risk factors may include changes in rate and electrical conduction, reduced preload/increased SVR, and altered muscle contractility/depressant effects of some medications, infarcted/dyskinetic muscle, structural defects.*

CH

risk for sedentary Lifestyle: risk factors may include lack of resources, lack of training or knowledge of specific exercise needs, safety concerns/fear of injury.*

Myocarditis   MS
(Also refer to Myocardial infarction)

Activity Intolerance may be related to imbalance in O_2 supply and demand (myocardial inflammation/damage), cardiac depressant effects of certain drugs, and enforced bedrest, possibly evidenced by reports of fatigue, exertional dyspnea, tachycardia/palpitations in response to activity, ECG changes/dysrhythmias, and generalized weakness.

risk for decreased Cardiac Output: risk factors may include degeneration of cardiac muscle.*

deficient Knowledge [Learning Need] regarding pathophysiology of condition/outcomes, treatment, and self-care needs/lifestyle changes may be related to lack of information/misinterpretation, possibly evidenced by statements of concern, misconceptions, inaccurate follow-through of instructions, and development of preventable complications.

Myringotomy   PED/MS
(Refer to Mastoidectomy)

Myxedema   CH
(Also refer to Hypothyroidism)

disturbed Body Image may be related to change in structure/function (loss of hair/thickening of skin, masklike facial expression, enlarged tongue, menstrual and reproductive disturbances), possibly evidenced by negative feelings about body, feelings of helplessness, and change in social involvement.

imbalanced Nutrition: more than body requirements may be related to decreased metabolic rate and activity level, possibly evidenced by weight gain greater than ideal for height and frame.

risk for decreased Cardiac Output: risk factors may include altered electrical conduction and myocardial contractility.*

---

*A risk diagnosis is not evidenced by signs and symptoms, as the problem has not occurred and nursing interventions are directed at prevention.

Neglect/Abuse CH/PSY
(Refer to Abuse; Battered child syndrome)

Neonatal, normal newborn PED
risk for impaired Gas Exchange: risk factors may include prenatal or intrapartal stressors, excess production of mucus, or cold stress.*

risk for imbalanced Body Temperature: risk factors may include large body surface in relation to mass, limited amounts of insulating subcutaneous fat, nonrenewable sources of brown fat and few white fat stores, thin epidermis with close proximity of blood vessels to the skin, inability to shiver, and movement from a warm uterine environment to a much cooler environment.*

risk for impaired parent/infant Attachment: risk factors may include developmental transition (gain of a family member), anxiety associated with the parent role, lack of privacy (intrusive family/visitors).*

risk for imbalanced Nutrition: less than body requirements: risk factors may include rapid metabolic rate, high-caloric requirement, increased insensible water losses through pulmonary and cutaneous routes, fatigue, and a potential for inadequate or depleted glucose stores.*

risk for Infection: risk factors may include inadequate secondary defenses (inadequate acquired immunity, e.g., deficiency of neutrophils and specific immunoglobulins), and inadequate primary defenses (e.g., environmental exposure, broken skin, traumatized tissues, decreased ciliary action).*

Neonatal, premature newborn PED
impaired Gas Exchange may be related to alveolar-capillary membrane changes (inadequate surfactant levels), altered blood flow (immaturity of pulmonary arteriole musculature), altered O_2 supply (immaturity of central nervous system and neuromuscular system, tracheobronchial obstruction), altered O_2-carrying capacity of blood (anemia), and cold stress, possibly evidenced by respiratory difficulties, inadequate oxygenation of tissues, and acidemia.

ineffective Breathing Pattern/Infant Feeding Pattern may be related to immaturity of the respiratory center, poor positioning, drug-related depression and metabolic imbalances, decreased energy/fatigue, possibly evidenced by dyspnea, tachypnea, periods of apnea, nasal flaring/use of accessory muscles, cyanosis, abnormal ABGs, and tachycardia.

risk for ineffective Thermoregulation: risk factors may include immature CNS development (temperature regulation center), decreased ratio of body mass to surface area, decreased subcutaneous fat, limited brown fat stores, inability to shiver or sweat, poor metabolic reserves, muted response to hypothermia, and frequent medical/nursing manipulations and interventions.*

risk for deficit Fluid Volume: risk factors may include extremes of age and weight, excessive fluid losses (thin skin, lack of insulating fat, increased environmental temperature, immature kidney/failure to concentrate urine).*

---

*A risk diagnosis is not evidenced by signs and symptoms, as the problem has not occurred and nursing interventions are directed at prevention.

risk for disorganized Infant Behavior: risk factors may include prematurity (immaturity of CNS system, hypoxia), lack of containment/boundaries, pain, overstimulation, separation from parents.*

Nephrectomy   MS

acute Pain may be related to surgical tissue trauma with mechanical closure (suture), possibly evidenced by verbal reports, guarding/distraction behaviors, self-focusing, and autonomic responses (changes in vital signs).

risk for deficient Fluid Volume: risk factors may include excessive vascular losses and restricted intake.*

ineffective Breathing Pattern may be related to incisional pain with decreased lung expansion, possibly evidenced by tachypnea, fremitus, changes in respiratory depth/chest expansion, and changes in ABGs.

Constipation may be related to reduced dietary intake, decreased mobility, GI obstruction (paralytic ileus), and incisional pain with defecation, possibly evidenced by decreased bowel sounds, reduced frequency/amount of stool, and hard/formed stool.

Nephrolithiasis   MS/CH
(Refer to Calculi, urinary)

Nephrotic syndrome   MS/CH

excess Fluid Volume may be related to compromised regulatory mechanism with changes in hydrostatic/oncotic vascular pressure and increased activation of the renin-angiotensin-aldosterone system, possibly evidenced by edema/anasarca, effusions/ascites, weight gain, intake greater than output, and BP changes.

imbalanced Nutrition: less than body requirements may be related to excessive protein losses and inability to ingest adequate nutrients (anorexia), possibly evidenced by weight loss/muscle wasting (may be difficult to assess due to edema), lack of interest in food, and observed inadequate intake.

risk for Infection: risk factors may include chronic disease and steroidal suppression of inflammatory responses.*

risk for impaired Skin Integrity: risk factors may include presence of edema and activity restrictions.*

Neuralgia, trigeminal   CH

acute Pain may be related to neuromuscular impairment with sudden violent muscle spasm, possibly evidenced by verbal reports, guarding/distraction behaviors, self-focusing, and autonomic responses (changes in vital signs).

deficient Knowledge [Learning Need] regarding control of recurrent episodes, medical therapies, and self-care needs may be related to lack of information/recall and misinterpretation, possibly evidenced by statements of concern, questions, and exacerbation of condition.

---

*A risk diagnosis is not evidenced by signs and symptoms, as the problem has not occurred and nursing interventions are directed at prevention.

Neuritis   CH

acute/chronic Pain may be related to nerve damage usually associated
   with a degenerative process, possibly evidenced by verbal reports,
   guarding/distraction behaviors, self-focusing, and autonomic
   responses (changes in vital signs).

deficient Knowledge [Learning Need] regarding underlying causative
   factors, treatment, and prevention may be related to lack of informa-
   tion/misinterpretation, possibly evidenced by statements of concern,
   questions, and misconceptions.

Obesity   CH/PSY

imbalanced Nutrition: more than body requirements may be related to
   food intake that exceeds body needs, psychosocial factors, socioeconomic status, possibly evidenced by weight of 20% or more over optimum body weight, excess body fat by skinfold/other measurements,
   reported/observed dysfunctional eating patterns, intake more than
   body requirements.

sedentary Lifestyle may be related to lack of interest/motivation, lack of
   resources, lack of training or knowledge of specific exercise needs,
   safety concerns/fear of injury, possibly evidenced by demonstration
   of physical deconditioning, choice of a daily routine lacking physical
   exercise.

disturbed Body Image/chronic low Self-Esteem may be related to view
   of self in contrast to societal values; family/subcultural encouragement of overeating; control, sex, and love issues, possibly evidenced
   by negative feelings about body; fear of rejection/reaction of others;
   feeling of hopelessness/powerlessness; and lack of follow-through
   with treatment plan.

Activity Intolerance may be related to imbalance between O_2 supply and
   demand, and sedentary lifestyle, possibly evidenced by fatigue or
   weakness, exertional discomfort, and abnormal heart rate/BP
   response.

impaired Social Interaction may be related to verbalized/observed discomfort in social situations, self-concept disturbance, possibly evidenced by reluctance to participate in social gatherings, verbalization
   of a sense of discomfort with others, feelings of rejection, absence
   of/ineffective supportive SO(s).

Opioid abuse   CH/PSY
(Refer to Depressant abuse)

Organic brain syndrome   CH
(Refer to Alzheimer's disease)

Osteoarthritis (degenerative joint disease)   CH
(Refer to Arthritis, rheumatoid)
(Although this is a degenerative process versus the inflammatory
   process of rheumatoid arthritis, nursing concerns are the same.)

Osteomyelitis   MS/CH
acute Pain may be related to inflammation and tissue necrosis, possibly
   evidenced by verbal reports, guarding/distraction behaviors, self-
   focus, and autonomic responses (changes in vital signs).

Hyperthermia may be related to increased metabolic rate and infectious process, possibly evidenced by increased body temperature and warm/flushed skin.

ineffective bone Tissue Perfusion may be related to inflammatory reaction with thrombosis of vessels, destruction of tissue, edema, and abscess formation, possibly evidenced by bone necrosis, continuation of infectious process, and delayed healing.

risk for impaired Walking: risk factors may include inflammation and tissue necrosis, pain, joint instability.*

deficient Knowledge [Learning Need] regarding pathophysiology of condition, long-term therapy needs, activity restriction, and prevention of complications may be related to lack of information/misinterpretation, possibly evidenced by statements of concern, questions, and misconceptions, and inaccurate follow-through of instructions.

Osteoporosis CH

risk for Trauma: risk factors may include loss of bone density/integrity increasing risk of fracture with minimal or no stress.*

acute/chronic Pain may be related to vertebral compression on spinal nerve/muscles/ligaments, spontaneous fractures, possibly evidenced by verbal reports, guarding/distraction behaviors, self-focus, and changes in sleep pattern.

impaired physical Mobility may be related to pain and musculoskeletal impairment, possibly evidenced by limited range of motion, reluctance to attempt movement/expressed fear of reinjury, and imposed restrictions/limitations.

Palsy, cerebral (spastic hemiplegia) PED/CH

impaired physical Mobility may be related to muscular weakness/hypertonicity, increased deep tendon reflexes, tendency to contractures, and underdevelopment of affected limbs, possibly evidenced by decreased muscle strength, control, mass; limited range of motion; and impaired coordination.

compromised family Coping may be related to permanent nature of condition, situational crisis, emotional conflicts/temporary family disorganization, and incomplete information/understanding of client's needs, possibly evidenced by verbalized anxiety/guilt regarding client's disability, inadequate understanding and knowledge base, and displaying protective behaviors disproportionate (too little/too much) to client's abilities or need for autonomy.

delayed Growth and Development may be related to effects of physical disability, possibly evidenced by altered physical growth, delay or difficulty in performing skills (motor, social, expressive), and altered ability to perform self-care/self-control activities appropriate to age.

Pancreatitis MS

acute Pain may be related to obstruction of pancreatic/biliary ducts, chemical contamination of peritoneal surfaces by pancreatic exudate/autodigestion, extension of inflammation to the retroperitoneal

---

*A risk diagnosis is not evidenced by signs and symptoms, as the problem has not occurred and nursing interventions are directed at prevention.

nerve plexus, possibly evidenced by verbal reports, guarding/distraction behaviors, self-focusing, grimacing, autonomic responses (changes in vital signs), and alteration in muscle tone.

risk for deficient Fluid Volume: risk factors may include excessive gastric losses (vomiting, nasogastric suctioning), increase in size of vascular bed (vasodilation, effects of kinins), third-space fluid transudation, ascites formation, alteration of clotting process, hemorrhage.*

imbalanced Nutrition: less than body requirements may be related to vomiting, decreased oral intake, as well as altered ability to digest nutrients (loss of digestive enzymes/insulin), possibly evidenced by reported inadequate food intake, aversion to eating, reported altered taste sensation, weight loss, and reduced muscle mass.

risk for Infection: risk factors may include inadequate primary defenses (stasis of body fluids, altered peristalsis, change in pH secretions), immunosuppression, nutritional deficiencies, tissue destruction, and chronic disease.*

Paranoid personality disorder   PSY

risk for self-/other-directed Violence: risk factors may include perceived threats of danger, paranoid delusions, and increased feelings of anxiety.*

[severe] Anxiety may be related to inability to trust (has not mastered task of trust versus mistrust), possibly evidenced by rigid delusional system (serves to provide relief from stress that justifies the delusion), frightened of other people and own hostility.

Powerlessness may be related to feelings of inadequacy, lifestyle of helplessness, maladaptive interpersonal interactions (e.g., misuse of power, force, abusive relationships), sense of severely impaired self-concept, and belief that individual has no control over situation(s), possibly evidenced by paranoid delusions, use of aggressive behavior to compensate, and expressions of recognition of damage paranoia has caused self and others.

disturbed Thought Processes may be related to psychological conflicts, increased anxiety and fear, possibly evidenced by difficulties in the process and character of thought, interference with the ability to think clearly and logically, delusions, fragmentation, and autistic thinking.

compromised family Coping may be related to temporary or sustained family disorganization/role changes, prolonged progression of condition that exhausts the supportive capacity of SO(s), possibly evidenced by family system not meeting physical/emotional/spiritual needs of its members, inability to express or to accept wide range of feelings, inappropriate boundary maintenance, SO(s) describe(s) preoccupation with personal reactions.

Paraplegia   MS/CH
(Also refer to Quadriplegia)

impaired Transfer Ability may be related to loss of muscle function/control, injury to upper extremity joints (overuse).

---

*A risk diagnosis is not evidenced by signs and symptoms, as the problem has not occurred and nursing interventions are directed at prevention.

disturbed kinesthetic/tactile Sensory Perception: may be related to neurological deficit with loss of sensory reception and transmission, psychological stress, possibly evidenced by reported/measured change in sensory acuity and loss of usual response to stimuli.

reflex Urinary Incontinence/impaired Urinary Elimination may be related to loss of nerve conduction above the level of the reflex arc, possibly evidenced by lack of awareness of bladder filling/fullness, absence of urge to void, uninhibited bladder contraction, urinary tract infections (UTIs), kidney stone formation.

disturbed Body Image/ineffective Role Performance may be related to loss of body functions, change in physical ability to resume role, perceived loss of self/identity, possibly evidenced by negative feelings about body/self, feelings of helplessness/powerlessness, delay in taking responsibility for self-care/participation in therapy, and change in social involvement.

Sexual Dysfunction may be related to loss of sensation, altered function, and vulnerability, possibly evidenced by seeking of confirmation of desirability, verbalization of concern, alteration in relationship with SO, and change in interest in self/others.

Parathyroidectomy   MS

acute Pain may be related to presence of surgical incision and effects of calcium imbalance (bone pain, tetany), possibly evidenced by verbal reports, guarding/distraction behaviors, self-focus, and autonomic responses (changes in vital signs).

risk for excess Fluid Volume: risk factors may include preoperative renal involvement, stress-induced release of ADH, and changing calcium/electrolyte levels.*

risk for ineffective Airway Clearance: risk factors may include edema formation and laryngeal nerve damage.*

deficient Knowledge [Learning Need] regarding postoperative care/complications and long-term needs may be related to lack of information/recall, misinterpretation, possibly evidenced by statements of concern, questions, and misconceptions.

Parkinson's disease   CH

impaired Walking may be related to neuromuscular impairment (muscle weakness, tremors, bradykinesia) and musculoskeletal impairment (joint rigidity), possibly evidenced by inability to move about the environment as desired, increased occurrence of falls.

impaired Swallowing may be related to neuromuscular impairment/muscle weakness, possibly evidenced by reported/observed difficulty in swallowing, drooling, evidence of aspiration (choking, coughing).

impaired verbal Communication may be related to muscle weakness and incoordination, possibly evidenced by impaired articulation, difficulty with phonation, and changes in rhythm and intonation.

risk for Stress Overload: risk factors may include inadequate resources, chronic illness, physical demands.*

P

---

*A risk diagnosis is not evidenced by signs and symptoms, as the problem has not occurred and nursing interventions are directed at prevention.

Caregiver Role Strain may be related to illness, severity of care receiver, psychological/cognitive problems in care receiver, caregiver is spouse, duration of caregiving required, lack of respite/recreation for caregiver, possibly evidenced by feeling stressed, depressed, worried; lack of resources/support, family conflict.

Pelvic inflammatory disease   OB/GYN/CH

risk for Infection [spread]: risk factors may include presence of infectious process in highly vascular pelvic structures, delay in seeking treatment.*

acute Pain may be related to inflammation, edema, and congestion of reproductive/pelvic tissues, possibly evidenced by verbal reports, guarding/distraction behaviors, self-focus, and autonomic responses (changes in vital signs).

Hyperthermia may be related to inflammatory process/hypermetabolic state, possibly evidenced by increased body temperature, warm/flushed skin, and tachycardia.

risk for situational low Self-Esteem: risk factors may include perceived stigma of physical condition (infection of reproductive system).*

deficient Knowledge [Learning Need] regarding cause/complications of condition, therapy needs, and transmission of disease to others may be related to lack of information/misinterpretation, possibly evidenced by statements of concern, questions, misconceptions, and development of preventable complications.

Periarteritis nodosa   MS/CH
(Refer to Polyarteritis [nodosa])

Pericarditis   MS

acute Pain may be related to tissue inflammation and presence of effusion, possibly evidenced by verbal reports of pain affected by movement/position, guarding/distraction behaviors, self-focus, and autonomic responses (changes in vital signs).

Activity Intolerance may be related to imbalance between O_2 supply and demand (restriction of cardiac filling/ventricular contraction, reduced cardiac output), possibly evidenced by reports of weakness/fatigue, exertional dyspnea, abnormal heart rate or BP response, and signs of heart failure.

risk for decreased Cardiac Output: risk factors may include accumulation of fluid (effusion) restricted cardiac filling/contractility.*

Anxiety [specify level] may be related to change in health status and perceived threat of death, possibly evidenced by increased tension, apprehension, restlessness, and expressed concerns.

Perinatal loss/death of child   OB/CH

Grieving may be related to death of fetus/infant, possibly evidenced by verbal expressions of distress, anger, loss, guilt; crying, change in eating habits/sleep.

situational low Self-Esteem may be related to perceived failure at a life event, inability to meet personal expectations, possibly evidenced by

---

*A risk diagnosis is not evidenced by signs and symptoms, as the problem has not occurred and nursing interventions are directed at prevention.

negative self-appraisal in response to situation/personal actions, expressions of helplessness/hopelessness, evaluation of self as unable to deal with situation.

risk for ineffective Role Performance: risk factors may include stress, family conflict, inadequate support system.*

risk for interrupted Family Processes: risk factors may include situational crisis, developmental transition [loss of child], family roles shift.*

risk for Spiritual Distress: risk factors may include blame for loss directed at self/God, intense suffering, alienation from other/support systems.*

Peripheral arterial occlusive disease   CH
(Refer to Arterial occlusive disease)

Peripheral vascular disease (atherosclerosis)   CH
ineffective peripheral Tissue Perfusion may be related to reduction or interruption of arterial/venous blood flow, possibly evidenced by changes in skin temperature/color, lack of hair growth, BP/pulse changes in extremity, presence of bruits, and reports of claudication.

Activity Intolerance may be related to imbalance between O_2 supply and demand, possibly evidenced by reports of muscle fatigue/weakness and exertional discomfort (claudication).

risk for impaired Skin/Tissue Integrity: risk factors may include altered circulation with decreased sensation and impaired healing.*

Peritonitis   MS
risk for Infection [spread/septicemia]: risk factors may include inadequate primary defenses (broken skin, traumatized tissue, altered peristalsis), inadequate secondary defenses (immunosuppression), and invasive procedures.*

deficient Fluid Volume [mixed] may be related to fluid shifts from extracellular, intravascular, and interstitial compartments into intestines and/or peritoneal space, excessive gastric losses (vomiting, diarrhea, NG suction), hypermetabolic state, and restricted intake, possibly evidenced by dry mucous membranes, poor skin turgor, delayed capillary refill, weak peripheral pulses, diminished urinary output, dark/concentrated urine, hypotension, and tachycardia.

acute Pain may be related to chemical irritation of parietal peritoneum, trauma to tissues, accumulation of fluid in abdominal/peritoneal cavity, possibly evidenced by verbal reports, muscle guarding/rebound tenderness, distraction behaviors, facial mask of pain, self-focus, autonomic responses (changes in vital signs).

risk for imbalanced Nutrition: less than body requirements: risk factors may include nausea/vomiting, intestinal dysfunction, metabolic abnormalities, increased metabolic needs.*

Pheochromocytoma   MS
Anxiety [specify level] may be related to excessive physiological (hormonal) stimulation of the sympathetic nervous system, situational crises, threat to/change in health status, possibly evidenced by

P

---

*A risk diagnosis is not evidenced by signs and symptoms, as the problem has not occurred and nursing interventions are directed at prevention.

apprehension, shakiness, restlessness, focus on self, fearfulness, diaphoresis, and sense of impending doom.

deficient Fluid Volume [mixed] may be related to excessive gastric losses (vomiting/diarrhea), hypermetabolic state, diaphoresis, and hyperosmolar diuresis, possibly evidenced by hemoconcentration, dry mucous membranes, poor skin turgor, thirst, and weight loss.

decreased Cardiac Output/ineffective Tissue Perfusion (specify) may be related to altered preload/decreased blood volume, altered SVR, and increased sympathetic activity (excessive secretion of catecholamines), possibly evidenced by cool/clammy skin, change in BP (hypertension/postural hypotension), visual disturbances, severe headache, and angina.

deficient Knowledge [Learning Need] regarding pathophysiology of condition, outcome, preoperative and postoperative care needs may be related to lack of information/recall, possibly evidenced by statements of concern, questions, and misconceptions.

Phlebitis   CH
(Refer to Thrombophlebitis)

Phobia   PSY
(Also refer to Anxiety disorder, generalized)

Fear may be related to learned irrational response to natural or innate origins (phobic stimulus), unfounded morbid dread of a seemingly harmless object/situation, possibly evidenced by sympathetic stimulation and reactions ranging from apprehension to panic, withdrawal from/total avoidance of situations that place individual in contact with feared object.

impaired Social Interaction may be related to intense fear of encountering feared object/activity or situation and anticipated loss of control, possibly evidenced by reported change of style/pattern of interaction, discomfort in social situations, and avoidance of phobic stimulus.

Placenta previa   OB
risk for deficient Fluid Volume: risk factors may include excessive vascular losses (vessel damage and inadequate vasoconstriction).*

impaired fetal Gas Exchange: may be related to altered blood flow, altered O_2-carrying capacity of blood (maternal anemia), and decreased surface area of gas exchange at site of placental attachment, possibly evidenced by changes in fetal heart rate/activity and release of meconium.

Fear may be related to threat of death (perceived or actual) to self or fetus, possibly evidenced by verbalization of specific concerns, increased tension, sympathetic stimulation.

risk for deficient Diversional Activity: risk factors may include imposed activity restrictions/bedrest.*

Pleurisy   CH
acute Pain may be related to inflammation/irritation of the parietal pleura, possibly evidenced by verbal reports, guarding/distraction

---

*A risk diagnosis is not evidenced by signs and symptoms, as the problem has not occurred and nursing interventions are directed at prevention.

behaviors, self-focus, and autonomic responses (changes in vital signs).

ineffective Breathing Pattern may be related to pain on inspiration, possibly evidenced by decreased respiratory depth, tachypnea, and dyspnea.

risk for Infection [pneumonia]: risk factors may include stasis of pulmonary secretions, decreased lung expansion, and ineffective cough.*

Pneumonia   CH/MS
(Refer to Bronchitis; Bronchopneumonia)

Pneumothorax   MS
(Also refer to Hemothorax)

ineffective Breathing Pattern may be related to decreased lung expansion (fluid/air accumulation), musculoskeletal impairment, pain, inflammatory process, possibly evidenced by dyspnea, tachypnea, altered chest excursion, respiratory depth changes, use of accessory muscles/nasal flaring, cough, cyanosis, and abnormal ABGs.

risk for decreased Cardiac Output: risk factors may include compression/displacement of cardiac structures.*

acute Pain may be related to irritation of nerve endings within pleural space by foreign object (chest tube), possibly evidenced by verbal reports, guarding/distraction behaviors, self-focus, and autonomic responses (changes in vital signs).

Polyarteritis (nodosa)   MS/CH

ineffective Tissue Perfusion (specify) may be related to reduction/interruption of blood flow, possibly evidenced by organ tissue infarctions, changes in organ function, and development of organic psychosis.

Hyperthermia may be related to widespread inflammatory process, possibly evidenced by increased body temperature and warm/flushed skin.

acute Pain may be related to inflammation, tissue ischemia, and necrosis of affected area, possibly evidenced by verbal reports, guarding/distraction behaviors, self-focus, and autonomic responses (changes in vital signs).

Grieving may be related to perceived loss of self, possibly evidenced by expressions of sorrow and anger, altered sleep and/or eating patterns, changes in activity level, and libido.

Polycythemia vera   CH

Activity Intolerance may be related to imbalance between O_2 supply and demand, possibly evidenced by reports of fatigue/weakness.

ineffective Tissue Perfusion (specify) may be related to reduction/interruption of arterial/venous blood flow (insufficiency, thrombosis, or hemorrhage), possibly evidenced by pain in affected area, impaired mental ability, visual disturbances, and color changes of skin/mucous membranes.

Polyradiculitis   MS
(Refer to Guillain-Barré syndrome)

P

---

*A risk diagnosis is not evidenced by signs and symptoms, as the problem has not occurred and nursing interventions are directed at prevention.

Postoperative recovery period MS

ineffective Breathing Pattern may be related to neuromuscular and perceptual/cognitive impairment, decreased lung expansion/energy, and tracheobronchial obstruction, possibly evidenced by changes in respiratory rate and depth, reduced vital capacity, apnea, cyanosis, and noisy respirations.

risk for imbalanced Body Temperature: risk factors may include exposure to cool environment, effect of medications/anesthetic agents, extremes of age/weight, and dehydration.*

disturbed Sensory Perception (specify)/disturbed Thought Processes may be related to chemical alteration (use of pharmaceutical agents, hypoxia), therapeutically restricted environment, excessive sensory stimuli and physiological stress, possibly evidenced by changes in usual response to stimuli, motor incoordination; impaired ability to concentrate, reason, and make decisions; and disorientation to person, place, and time.

risk for deficit Fluid Volume: risk factors may include restriction of oral intake, loss of fluid through abnormal routes (indwelling tubes, drains) and normal routes (vomiting, loss of vascular integrity, changes in clotting ability), extremes of age and weight.*

acute Pain may be related to disruption of skin, tissue, and muscle integrity; musculoskeletal/bone trauma; and presence of tubes and drains, possibly evidenced by verbal reports, alteration in muscle tone, facial mask of pain, distraction/guarding behaviors, narrowed focus, and autonomic responses.

impaired Skin/Tissue Integrity may be related to mechanical interruption of skin/tissues, altered circulation, effects of medication, accumulation of drainage, and altered metabolic state, possibly evidenced by disruption of skin surface/layers and tissues.

risk for Infection: risk factors may include broken skin, traumatized tissues, stasis of body fluids, presence of pathogens/contaminants, environmental exposure, and invasive procedures.*

Postpartal period OB/CH

risk for impaired parent/infant Attachment/Parenting: risk factors may include lack of support between/from SO(s), ineffective or no role model, anxiety associated with the parental role, unrealistic expectations, presence of stressors (e.g., financial, housing, employment).*

risk for deficient Fluid Volume: risk factors may include excessive blood loss during delivery, reduced intake/inadequate replacement, nausea/vomiting, increased urine output, and insensible losses.*

acute Pain[/Discomfort] may be related to tissue trauma/edema, muscle contractions, bladder fullness, and physical/psychological exhaustion, possibly evidenced by reports of cramping (afterpains), self-focusing, alteration in muscle tone, distraction behaviors, and autonomic responses (changes in vital signs).

impaired Urinary Elimination may be related to hormonal effects (fluid shifts/continued elevation in renal plasma flow), mechanical trauma/tissue edema, and effects of medication/anesthesia, possibly

---

*A risk diagnosis is not evidenced by signs and symptoms, as the problem has not occurred and nursing interventions are directed at prevention.

evidenced by frequency, dysuria, urgency, incontinence, or retention.

Constipation may be related to decreased muscle tone associated with diastasis recti, prenatal effects of progesterone, dehydration, excess analgesia or anesthesia, pain (hemorrhoids, episiotomy, or perineal tenderness), prelabor diarrhea and lack of intake, possibly evidenced by frequency less than usual pattern, hard-formed stool, straining at stool, decreased bowel sounds, and abdominal distention.

Insomnia may be related to pain/discomfort, intense exhilaration/ excitement, anxiety, exhausting process of labor/delivery, and needs/demands of family members, possibly evidenced by verbal reports of difficulty in falling or staying asleep/dissatisfaction with sleep, lack of energy, nonrestorative sleep.

Post-traumatic stress disorder   PSY

Post-Trauma Syndrome related to having experienced a traumatic life event, possibly evidenced by reexperiencing the event, somatic reactions, psychic/emotional numbness, altered lifestyle, impaired sleep, self-destructive behaviors, difficulty with interpersonal relationships, development of phobia, poor impulse control/irritability, and explosiveness.

risk for other-directed Violence: risk factors may include startle reaction, an intrusive memory causing a sudden acting out of a feeling as if the event were occurring, use of alcohol/other drugs to ward off painful effects and produce psychic numbing, breaking through the rage that has been walled off, response to intense anxiety or panic state, and loss of control.*

ineffective Coping may be related to personal vulnerability, inadequate support systems, unrealistic perceptions, unmet expectations, overwhelming threat to self, and multiple stressors repeated over a period of time, possibly evidenced by verbalization of inability to cope or difficulty asking for help, muscular tension/headaches, chronic worry, and emotional tension.

complicated Grieving may be related to actual/perceived object loss (loss of self as seen before the traumatic incident occurred, as well as other losses incurred in/after the incident), loss of physiopsychosocial well-being, thwarted grieving response to a loss, and lack of resolution of previous grieving responses, possibly evidenced by verbal expression of distress at loss, anger, sadness, labile affect; alterations in eating habits, sleep/dream patterns, libido; reliving of past experiences, expression of guilt, and alterations in concentration.

interrupted Family Processes may be related to situational crisis, failure to master developmental transitions, possibly evidenced by expressions of confusion about what to do and that family is having difficulty coping, family system not meeting physical/emotional/spiritual needs of its members, not adapting to change or dealing with traumatic experience constructively, and ineffective family decision-making process.

---

*A risk diagnosis is not evidenced by signs and symptoms, as the problem has not occurred and nursing interventions are directed at prevention.

risk for imbalanced Nutrition: less than body requirements: risk factors may include changes in appetite, insufficient intake (nausea/vomiting, inadequate financial resources and nutritional knowledge), meeting increased metabolic demands (increased thyroid activity associated with the growth of fetal and maternal tissues).*

[Discomfort]/acute Pain may be related to hormonal influences, physical changes, possibly evidenced by verbal reports (nausea, breast changes, leg cramps, hemorrhoids, nasal stuffiness), alteration in muscle tone, restlessness, and autonomic responses (changes in vital signs).

risk for fetal Injury: risk factors may include environmental/hereditary factors and problems of maternal well-being that directly affect the developing fetus (e.g., malnutrition, substance use).*

[maximally compensated] Cardiac Output may be related to increased fluid volume/maximal cardiac effort and hormonal effects of progesterone and relaxin (places the client at risk for hypertension and/or circulatory failure), and changes in peripheral resistance (afterload), possibly evidenced by variations in BP and pulse, syncopal episodes, presence of pathological edema.

readiness for enhanced family Coping may be related to situational/maturational crisis with anticipated changes in family structure/roles, needs sufficiently met and adaptive tasks effectively addressed to enable goals of self-actualization to surface, as evidenced by movement toward health-promoting and enriching lifestyle, choosing experiences that optimize pregnancy experience/wellness.

risk for Constipation: risk factors may include changes in dietary/fluid intake, smooth muscle relaxation, decreased peristalsis, and effects of medications (e.g., iron).*

Fatigue/Insomnia may be related to increased carbohydrate metabolism, altered body chemistry, increased energy requirements to perform ADLs, discomfort, anxiety, inactivity, possibly evidenced by reports of overwhelming lack of energy/inability to maintain usual routines, difficulty falling asleep/dissatisfaction with sleep, decreased quality of life.

risk for ineffective Role Performance: risk factors may include maturational crisis, developmental level, history of maladaptive coping, absence of support systems.*

deficient Knowledge [Learning Need] regarding normal physiological/psychological changes and self-care needs may be related to lack of information/recall and misinterpretation of normal physiological/psychological changes and their impact on the client/family, possibly evidenced by questions, statements of concern, misconceptions, and inaccurate follow-through of instructions/development of preventable complications.

Pregnancy (prenatal period) 2nd trimester　　OB/CH
(Also refer to Pregnancy 1st trimester)

risk for disturbed Body Image: risk factors may include perception of biophysical changes, response of others.*

---

*A risk diagnosis is not evidenced by signs and symptoms, as the problem has not occurred and nursing interventions are directed at prevention.

P

ineffective Breathing Pattern may be related to impingement of the diaphragm by enlarging uterus, possibly evidenced by reports of shortness of breath, dyspnea, and changes in respiratory depth.

risk for [decompensated] Cardiac Output: risk factors may include increased circulatory demand, changes in preload (decreased venous return) and afterload (increased peripheral vascular resistance), and ventricular hypertrophy.*

risk for excess Fluid Volume: risk factors may include changes in regulatory mechanisms, sodium/water retention.

ineffective Sexuality Pattern may be related to conflict regarding changes in sexual desire and expectations, fear of physical injury to woman/fetus, possibly evidenced by reported difficulties, limitations, or changes in sexual behaviors/activities.

Pregnancy (prenatal period) 3rd trimester OB/CH
(Also refer to Pregnancy 1st and 2nd trimester)

deficient Knowledge [Learning Need] regarding preparation for labor/delivery, infant care may be related to lack of exposure/experience, misinterpretations of information, possibly evidenced by request for information, statement of concerns/misconceptions.

impaired Urinary Elimination may be related to uterine enlargement, increased abdominal pressure, fluctuation of renal blood flow, and glomerular filtration rate (GFR), possibly evidenced by urinary frequency, urgency, dependent edema.

risk for ineffective [individual/] family Coping: risk factors may include situational/maturational crisis, personal vulnerability, unrealistic perceptions, absent/insufficient support systems.*

risk for maternal Injury: risk factors may include presence of hypertension, infection, substance use/abuse, altered immune system, abnormal blood profile, tissue hypoxia, premature rupture of membranes.*

Pregnancy, adolescent OB/CH P
(Also refer to Pregnancy, prenatal period)

interrupted Family Processes may be related to situational/developmental transition (economic, change in roles/gain of a family member), possibly evidenced by family expressing confusion about what to do, unable to meet physical/emotional/spiritual needs of the members, family inability to adapt to change or to deal with traumatic experience constructively, does not demonstrate respect for individuality and autonomy of its members, ineffective family decision-making process, and inappropriate boundary maintenance.

Social Isolation may be related to alterations in physical appearance, perceived unacceptable social behavior, restricted social sphere, stage of adolescence, and interference with accomplishing developmental tasks, possibly evidenced by expressions of feelings of aloneness/rejection/difference from others, uncommunicative, withdrawn, no eye contact, seeking to be alone, unacceptable behavior, and absence of supportive SO(s).

---

*A risk diagnosis is not evidenced by signs and symptoms, as the problem has not occurred and nursing interventions are directed at prevention.

disturbed Body Image/situational/chronic low Self-Esteem may be related to situational/maturational crisis, biophysical changes, and fear of failure at life events, absence of support systems, possibly evidenced by self-negating verbalizations, expressions of shame/guilt, fear of rejection/reaction of other, hypersensitivity to criticism, and lack of follow-through/nonparticipation in prenatal care.

deficient Knowledge [Learning Need] regarding pregnancy, developmental/individual needs, future expectations may be related to lack of exposure, information misinterpretation, unfamiliarity with information resources, lack of interest in learning, possibly evidenced by questions, statement of concern/misconception, sense of vulnerability/denial of reality, inaccurate follow-through of instruction, and development of preventable complications.

risk for impaired Parenting: may be related to chronological age/developmental stage, unmet social/emotional/maturational needs of parenting figures, unrealistic expectation of self/infant/partner, ineffective role model/social support, lack of role identity, and presence of stressors (e.g., financial, social).*

Pregnancy, high-risk   OB/CH
(Also refer to Pregnancy 1st, 2nd, 3rd trimester)

Anxiety [specify level] may be related to situational crisis, threat of maternal/fetal death (perceived or actual), interpersonal transmission/contagion, possibly evidenced by increased tension, apprehension, feelings of inadequacy, somatic complaints, difficulty sleeping.

deficient Knowledge [Learning Need] regarding high-risk situation/preterm labor may be related to lack of exposure to/misinterpretation of information, unfamiliarity with individual risks and own role in risk prevention/management, possibly evidenced by request for information, statement of concerns/misconceptions, inaccurate follow-through of instructions.

risk of maternal Injury: risk factors may include preexisting medical conditions, complications of pregnancy.*

risk for Activity Intolerance: risk factors may include presence of circulatory/respiratory problems, uterine irritability.*

risk for ineffective Therapeutic Regimen Management: risk factors may include client value system, health beliefs/cultural influences, issues of control, presence of anxiety, complexity of therapeutic regimen, economic difficulties, perceived susceptibility.*

Pregnancy-induced hypertension   OB/CH
(preeclampsia)

deficient Fluid Volume [isotonic] may be related to a plasma protein loss, decreasing plasma colloid osmotic pressure allowing fluid shifts out of vascular compartment, possibly evidenced by edema formation, sudden weight gain, hemoconcentration, nausea/vomiting, epigastric pain, headaches, visual changes, decreased urine output.

---

*A risk diagnosis is not evidenced by signs and symptoms, as the problem has not occurred and nursing interventions are directed at prevention.

decreased Cardiac Output may be related to hypovolemia/decreased venous return, increased SVR, possibly evidenced by variations in BP/hemodynamic readings, edema, shortness of breath, change in mental status.

ineffective [uteroplacental] Tissue Perfusion: may be related to vasospasm of spiral arteries and relative hypovolemia, possibly evidenced by changes in fetal heart rate/activity, reduced weight gain, and premature delivery/fetal demise.

deficient Knowledge [Learning Need] regarding pathophysiology of condition, therapy, self-care/nutritional needs, and potential complications may be related to lack of information/recall, misinterpretation, possibly evidenced by statements of concern, questions, misconceptions, inaccurate follow-through of instructions/development of preventable complications.

Premenstrual tension syndrome (PMS)   GYN/CH/PSY

chronic/acute Pain may be related to cyclic changes in female hormones affecting other systems (e.g., vascular congestion/spasms), vitamin deficiency, fluid retention, possibly evidenced by increased tension, apprehension, jitteriness, verbal reports, distraction behaviors, somatic complaints, self-focusing, physical and social withdrawal.

excess Fluid Volume may be related to abnormal alterations of hormonal levels, possibly evidenced by edema formation, weight gain, and periodic changes in emotional status/irritability.

Anxiety [specify level] may be related to cyclic changes in female hormones affecting other systems, possibly evidenced by feelings of inability to cope/loss of control, depersonalization, increased tension, apprehension, jitteriness, somatic complaints, and impaired functioning.

deficient Knowledge [Learning Need] regarding pathophysiology of condition and self-care/treatment needs may be related to lack of information/misinterpretation, possibly evidenced by statements of concern, questions, misconceptions, and continuation of condition, exacerbating symptoms.

Pressure ulcer or sore   CH
(Also refer to Ulcer, decubitus)

ineffective peripheral Tissue Perfusion may be related to reduced/interrupted blood flow, possibly evidenced by presence of inflamed, necrotic lesion.

deficient Knowledge [Learning Need] regarding cause/prevention of condition and potential complications may be related to lack of information/misinterpretation, possibly evidenced by statements of concern, questions, misconceptions, and inaccurate follow-through of instructions.

Preterm labor   OB/CH
(Refer to Labor, preterm)

Prostatectomy   MS

impaired Urinary Elimination may be related to mechanical obstruction (blood clots, edema, trauma, surgical procedure, pressure/irritation of catheter/balloon) and loss of bladder tone, possibly evidenced by dysuria, frequency, dribbling, incontinence, retention, bladder fullness, suprapubic discomfort.

risk for deficient Fluid Volume: risk factors may include trauma to highly vascular area with excessive vascular losses, restricted intake, postobstructive diuresis.*

acute Pain may be related to irritation of bladder mucosa and tissue trauma/edema, possibly evidenced by verbal reports (bladder spasms), distraction behaviors, self-focus, and autonomic responses (changes in vital signs).

disturbed Body Image may be related to perceived threat of altered body/sexual function, possibly evidenced by preoccupation with change/loss, negative feelings about body, and statements of concern regarding functioning.

CH

risk for Sexual Dysfunction: risk factors may include situational crisis (incontinence, leakage of urine after catheter removal, involvement of genital area) and threat to self-concept/change in health status.*

Pruritus   **CH**

acute Pain [/Discomfort] may be related to cutaneous hyperesthesia and inflammation, possibly evidenced by verbal reports, distraction behaviors, and self-focus.

risk for impaired Skin Integrity: risk factors may include mechanical trauma (scratching) and development of vesicles/bullae that may rupture.*

Psoriasis   **CH**

impaired Skin Integrity may be related to increased epidermal cell proliferation and absence of normal protective skin layers, possibly evidenced by scaling papules and plaques.

disturbed Body Image may be related to cosmetically unsightly skin lesions, possibly evidenced by hiding affected body part, negative feelings about body, feelings of helplessness, and change in social involvement.

Pulmonary edema, high altitude   **MS**
(Refer to High altitude pulmonary edema)

Pulmonary embolus   **MS**

ineffective Breathing Pattern may be related to tracheobronchial obstruction (inflammation, copious secretions, or active bleeding), decreased lung expansion, inflammatory process, possibly evidenced by changes in depth and/or rate of respiration, dyspnea/use of accessory muscles, altered chest excursion, abnormal breath sounds (crackles, wheezes), and cough (with or without sputum production).

impaired Gas Exchange may be related to altered blood flow to alveoli or to major portions of the lung, alveolar–capillary membrane

---

*A risk diagnosis is not evidenced by signs and symptoms, as the problem has not occurred and nursing interventions are directed at prevention.

changes (atelectasis, airway/alveolar collapse, pulmonary edema/effusion, excessive secretions/active bleeding), possibly evidenced by profound dyspnea, restlessness, apprehension, somnolence, cyanosis, and changes in ABGs/pulse oximetry (hypoxemia and hypercapnia).

ineffective cardiopulmonary Tissue Perfusion may be related to interruption of blood flow (arterial/venous), exchange problems at alveolar level or at tissue level (acidotic shifting of the oxyhemoglobin curve), possibly evidenced by radiology/laboratory evidence of ventilation/perfusion mismatch, dyspnea, and central cyanosis.

Fear/Anxiety [specify level] may be related to severe dyspnea/inability to breathe normally, perceived threat of death, threat to/change in health status, physiological response to hypoxemia/acidosis, and concern regarding unknown outcome of situation, possibly evidenced by restlessness, irritability, withdrawal or attack behavior, sympathetic stimulation (cardiovascular excitation, pupil dilation, sweating, vomiting, diarrhea), crying, voice quivering, and impending sense of doom.

Pulmonary hypertension CH/MS

impaired Gas Exchange may be related to changes in alveolar membrane, increased pulmonary vascular resistance, possibly evidenced by dyspnea, irritability, decreased mental acuity, somnolence, abnormal ABGs.

decreased Cardiac Output may be related to increased pulmonary vascular resistance, decreased blood return to left side of heart, possibly evidenced by increased heart rate, dyspnea, fatigue.

Activity Intolerance may be related to imbalance between O_2 supply and demand, possibly evidenced by reports of weakness/fatigue, abnormal vital signs with activity.

Anxiety may be related to change in health status, stress, threat to self-concept, possibly evidenced by expressed concerns, uncertainty, awareness of physiological symptoms, diminished productivity/ability to problem solve.

Purpura, idiopathic thrombocytopenic CH

ineffective Protection may be related to abnormal blood profile, drug therapy (corticosteroids or immunosuppressive agents), possibly evidenced by altered clotting, fatigue, deficient immunity.

Activity Intolerance may be related to decreased O_2-carrying capacity/imbalance between O_2 supply and demand, possibly evidenced by reports of fatigue/weakness.

deficient Knowledge [Learning Need] regarding therapy choices, outcomes, and self-care needs may be related to lack of information/misinterpretation, possibly evidenced by statements of concern, questions, and misconceptions.

Pyelonephritis MS

acute Pain may be related to acute inflammation of renal tissues, possibly evidenced by verbal reports, guarding/distraction behaviors, self-focus, and autonomic responses (changes in vital signs).

Hyperthermia may be related to inflammatory process/increased metabolic rate, possibly evidenced by increase in body temperature, warm/flushed skin, tachycardia, and chills.

impaired Urinary Elimination may be related to inflammation/
irritation of bladder mucosa, possibly evidenced by dysuria, urgency,
and frequency.
deficient Knowledge [Learning Need] regarding therapy needs and prevention may be related to lack of information/misinterpretation, possibly evidenced by statements of concern, questions, misconceptions,
and recurrence of condition.

Quadriplegia   MS/CH
(Also refer to Paraplegia)
ineffective Breathing Pattern may be related to neuromuscular impairment (diaphragm and intercostal muscle function), reflex abdominal
spasms, gastric distention, possibly evidenced by decreased respiratory depth, dyspnea, cyanosis, and abnormal ABGs.
risk for Trauma [additional spinal injury]: risk factors may include temporary weakness/instability of spinal column.*
Grieving may be related to perceived loss of self, anticipated alterations
in lifestyle and expectations, and limitation of future options/choices,
possibly evidenced by expressions of distress, anger, sorrow, choked
feelings, and changes in eating habits, sleep, communication patterns.
total Self-Care Deficit related to neuromuscular impairment, evidenced
by inability to perform self-care tasks.
impaired bed/wheelchair Mobility may be related to loss of muscle
function/control.
risk for Autonomic Dysreflexia: risk factors may include altered nerve
function (spinal cord injury at T6 or above), bladder/bowel/skin
stimulation (tactile, pain, thermal).*
impaired Home Maintenance may be related to permanent effects of
injury, inadequate/absent support systems and finances, and lack of
familiarity with resources, possibly evidenced by expressions of difficulties, requests for information and assistance, outstanding debts/
financial crisis, and lack of necessary aids and equipment.

Rape   CH
deficient Knowledge [Learning Need] regarding required medical/legal
procedures, prophylactic treatment for individual concerns (STDs,
pregnancy), community resources/supports may be related to lack of
information, possibly evidenced by statements of concern, questions,
misconceptions, and exacerbation of symptoms.
Rape-Trauma Syndrome (acute phase) related to actual or attempted
sexual penetration without consent, possibly evidenced by wide range
of emotional reactions, including anxiety, fear, anger, embarrassment,
and multisystem physical complaints.
risk for impaired Tissue Integrity: risk factors may include forceful sexual penetration and trauma to fragile tissues.*

                                                             PSY
ineffective Coping may be related to personal vulnerability, unmet
expectations, unrealistic perceptions, inadequate support systems/

---

*A risk diagnosis is not evidenced by signs and symptoms, as the
problem has not occurred and nursing interventions are directed at
prevention.

coping methods, multiple stressors repeated over time, overwhelming threat to self, possibly evidenced by verbalizations of inability to cope or difficulty asking for help, muscular tension/headaches, emotional tension, chronic worry.

Sexual Dysfunction may be related to biopsychosocial alteration of sexuality (stress of post-trauma response), vulnerability, loss of sexual desire, impaired relationship with SO, possibly evidenced by alteration in achieving sexual satisfaction, change in interest in self/others, preoccupation with self.

Raynaud's phenomenon CH

acute/chronic Pain may be related to vasospasm/altered perfusion of affected tissues and ischemia/destruction of tissues, possibly evidenced by verbal reports, guarding of affected parts, self-focusing, and restlessness.

ineffective peripheral Tissue Perfusion may be related to periodic reduction of arterial blood flow to affected areas, possibly evidenced by pallor, cyanosis, coolness, numbness, paresthesia, slow healing of lesions.

deficient Knowledge [Learning Need] regarding pathophysiology of condition, potential for complications, therapy/self-care needs may be related to lack of information/misinterpretation, possibly evidenced by statements of concern, questions, and misconceptions; development of preventable complications.

Reflex sympathetic dystrophy (RSD) CH

acute/chronic Pain may be related to continued nerve stimulation, possibly evidenced by verbal reports, distraction/guarding behaviors, narrowed focus, changes in sleep patterns, and altered ability to continue previous activities.

ineffective peripheral Tissue Perfusion may be related to reduction of arterial blood flow (arteriole vasoconstriction), possibly evidenced by reports of pain, decreased skin temperature and pallor, diminished arterial pulsations, and tissue swelling.

disturbed tactile Sensory Perception may be related to altered sensory reception (neurological deficit, pain), possibly evidenced by change in usual response to stimuli/abnormal sensitivity of touch, physiologic anxiety, and irritability.

risk for ineffective Role Performance: risk factors may include situational crisis, chronic disability, debilitating pain.*

risk for compromised family Coping: risk factors may include temporary family disorganization and role changes and prolonged disability that exhausts the supportive capacity of SO(s).*

Regional enteritis CH
(Refer to Crohn's disease)

Renal failure, acute MS

excess Fluid Volume may be related to compromised regulatory mechanisms (decreased kidney function), possibly evidenced by weight

---

*A risk diagnosis is not evidenced by signs and symptoms, as the problem has not occurred and nursing interventions are directed at prevention.

gain, edema/anasarca, intake greater than output, venous congestion, changes in BP/CVP, and altered electrolyte levels.

imbalanced Nutrition: less than body requirements may be related to inability to ingest/digest adequate nutrients (anorexia, nausea/vomiting, ulcerations of oral mucosa, and increased metabolic needs) in addition to therapeutic dietary restrictions, possibly evidenced by lack of interest in food/aversion to eating, observed inadequate intake, weight loss, loss of muscle mass.

risk for Infection: risk factors may include depression of immunological defenses, invasive procedures/devices, and changes in dietary intake/malnutrition.*

disturbed Thought Processes may be related to accumulation of toxic waste products and altered cerebral perfusion, possibly evidenced by disorientation, changes in recent memory, apathy, and episodic obtundation.

Renal transplantation · MS

risk for excess Fluid Volume: risk factors may include compromised regulatory mechanism (implantation of new kidney requiring adjustment period for optimal functioning).*

disturbed Body Image may be related to failure and subsequent replacement of body part and medication-induced changes in appearance, possibly evidenced by preoccupation with loss/change, negative feelings about body, and focus on past strength/function.

Fear may be related to potential for transplant rejection/failure and threat of death, possibly evidenced by increased tension, apprehension, concentration on source, and verbalizations of concern.

risk for Infection: risk factors may include broken skin/traumatized tissue, stasis of body fluids, immunosuppression, invasive procedures, nutritional deficits, and chronic disease.*

CH

risk for ineffective Coping/compromised family Coping: risk factors may include situational crises, family disorganization and role changes, prolonged disease exhausting supportive capacity of SO(s)/family, therapeutic restrictions/long-term therapy needs.*

Respiratory distress syndrome · PED
(premature infant)

(Also refer to Neonatal, premature newborn)

impaired Gas Exchange may be related to alveolar/capillary membrane changes (inadequate surfactant levels), altered O_2 supply (tracheobronchial obstruction, atelectasis), altered blood flow (immaturity of pulmonary arteriole musculature), altered O_2-carrying capacity of blood (anemia), and cold stress, possibly evidenced by tachypnea, use of accessory muscles/retractions, expiratory grunting, pallor, or cyanosis, abnormal ABGs, and tachycardia.

impaired spontaneous Ventilation may be related to respiratory muscle fatigue and metabolic factors, possibly evidenced by dyspnea,

---

*A risk diagnosis is not evidenced by signs and symptoms, as the problem has not occurred and nursing interventions are directed at prevention.

increased metabolic rate, restlessness, use of accessory muscles, and abnormal ABGs.

risk for Infection: risk factors may include inadequate primary defenses (decreased ciliary action, stasis of body fluids, traumatized tissues), inadequate secondary defenses (deficiency of neutrophils and specific immunoglobulins), invasive procedures, and malnutrition (absence of nutrient stores, increased metabolic demands).*

risk for ineffective gastrointestinal Tissue Perfusion: risk factors may include persistent fetal circulation and exchange problems.*

risk for impaired parent/infant Attachment: risk factors may include premature/ill infant who is unable to effectively initiate parental contact (altered behavioral organization), separation, physical barriers, anxiety associated with the parental role/demands of infant.*

Retinal detachment   CH

disturbed visual Sensory Perception related to decreased sensory reception, possibly evidenced by visual distortions, decreased visual field, and changes in visual acuity.

deficient Knowledge [Learning Need] regarding therapy, prognosis, and self-care needs may be related to lack of information/misconceptions, possibly evidenced by statements of concern and questions.

risk for impaired Home Maintenance: risk factors may include visual limitations activity restrictions.*

Reye's syndrome   PED

deficient Fluid Volume [isotonic] may be related to failure of regulatory mechanism (diabetes insipidus), excessive gastric losses (pernicious vomiting), and altered intake, possibly evidenced by increased/dilute urine output, sudden weight loss, decreased venous filling, dry mucous membranes, decreased skin turgor, hypotension, and tachycardia.

ineffective cerebral Tissue Perfusion may be related to diminished arterial/venous blood flow and hypovolemia, possibly evidenced by memory loss, altered consciousness, and restlessness/agitation.

risk for Trauma: risk factors may include generalized weakness, reduced coordination, and cognitive deficits.*

ineffective Breathing Pattern may be related to decreased energy and fatigue, cognitive impairment, tracheobronchial obstruction, and inflammatory process (aspiration pneumonia), possibly evidenced by tachypnea, abnormal ABGs, cough, and use of accessory muscles.

Rheumatic fever   PED

acute Pain may be related to migratory inflammation of joints, possibly evidenced by verbal reports, guarding/distraction behaviors, self-focus, and autonomic responses (changes in vital signs).

Hyperthermia may be related to inflammatory process/hypermetabolic state, possibly evidenced by increased body temperature, warm/flushed skin, and tachycardia.

Activity Intolerance may be related to generalized weakness, joint pain, and medical restrictions/bedrest, possibly evidenced by reports of

R

---

*A risk diagnosis is not evidenced by signs and symptoms, as the problem has not occurred and nursing interventions are directed at prevention.

fatigue, exertional discomfort, and abnormal heart rate in response to activity.

risk for decreased Cardiac Output: risk factors may include cardiac inflammation/enlargement and altered contractility.*

Rickets (osteomalacia) PED

delayed Growth and Development may be related to dietary deficiencies/indiscretions, malabsorption syndrome, and lack of exposure to sunlight, possibly evidenced by altered physical growth and delay or difficulty in performing motor skills typical for age.

deficient Knowledge [Learning Need] regarding cause, pathophysiology, therapy needs, and prevention may be related to lack of information, possibly evidenced by statements of concern, questions, misconceptions, and inaccurate follow-through of instructions.

Ringworm, tinea CH
(Also refer to Athlete's Foot)

impaired Skin Integrity may be related to fungal infection of the dermis, possibly evidenced by disruption of skin surfaces/presence of lesions.

deficient Knowledge [Learning Need] regarding infectious nature, therapy, and self-care needs may be related to lack of information/misinformation, possibly evidenced by statements of concern, questions, and recurrence/spread.

Rubella PED/CH

acute Pain[/Discomfort] may be related to inflammatory effects of viral infection and presence of desquamating rash, possibly evidenced by verbal reports, distraction behaviors/restlessness.

deficient Knowledge [Learning Need] regarding contagious nature, possible complications, and self-care needs may be related to lack of information/misinterpretations, possibly evidenced by statements of concern, questions, and inaccurate follow-through of instructions.

Scabies CH

impaired Skin Integrity may be related to presence of invasive parasite and development of pruritus, possibly evidenced by disruption of skin surface and inflammation.

deficient Knowledge [Learning Need] regarding communicable nature, possible complications, therapy, and self-care needs may be related to lack of information/misinterpretation, possibly evidenced by questions and statements of concern about spread to others.

Scarlet fever PED

Hyperthermia may be related to effects of circulating toxins, possibly evidenced by increased body temperature, warm/flushed skin, and tachycardia.

acute Pain[/Discomfort] may be related to inflammation of mucous membranes and effects of circulating toxins (malaise, fever), possibly evidenced by verbal reports, distraction behaviors, guarding (decreased swallowing), and self-focus.

---

*A risk diagnosis is not evidenced by signs and symptoms, as the problem has not occurred and nursing interventions are directed at prevention.

risk for deficient Fluid Volume: risk factors may include hypermetabolic state (hyperthermia) and reduced intake.*

Schizophrenia (schizophrenic disorders)   PSY/CH

disturbed Thought Processes may be related to disintegration of thinking processes, impaired judgment, presence of psychological conflicts, disintegrated ego-boundaries, sleep disturbance, ambivalence and concomitant dependence, possibly evidenced by impaired ability to reason/problem solve, inappropriate affect, presence of delusional system, command hallucinations, obsessions, ideas of reference, cognitive dissonance.

Social Isolation may be related to alterations in mental status, mistrust of others/delusional thinking, unacceptable social behaviors, inadequate personal resources, and inability to engage in satisfying personal relationships, possibly evidenced by difficulty in establishing relationships with others, dull affect, uncommunicative/withdrawn behavior, seeking to be alone, inadequate/absent significant purpose in life, and expression of feelings of rejection.

ineffective Health Maintenance/impaired Home Maintenance may be related to impaired cognitive/emotional functioning, altered ability to make deliberate and thoughtful judgments, altered communication, and lack/inappropriate use of material resources, possibly evidenced by inability to take responsibility for meeting basic health practices in any or all functional areas and demonstrated lack of adaptive behaviors to internal or external environmental changes, disorderly surroundings, accumulation of dirt/unwashed clothes, repeated hygienic disorders.

risk for self-/other-directed Violence: risk factors may include disturbances of thinking/feeling (depression, paranoia, suicidal ideation), lack of development of trust and appropriate interpersonal relationships, catatonic/manic excitement, toxic reactions to drugs (alcohol).*

ineffective Coping may be related to personal vulnerability, inadequate support system(s), unrealistic perceptions, inadequate coping methods, and disintegration of thought processes, possibly evidenced by impaired judgment/cognition and perception, diminished problem-solving/decision-making capacities, poor self-concept, chronic anxiety, depression, inability to perform role expectations, and alteration in social participation.

interrupted Family Processes/disabled family Coping may be related to ambivalent family system/relationships, change of roles, and difficulty of family member in coping effectively with client's maladaptive behaviors, possibly evidenced by deterioration in family functioning, ineffective family decision-making process, difficulty relating to each other, client's expressions of despair at family's lack of reaction/involvement, neglectful relationships with client, extreme distortion regarding client's health problem including denial about its existence/severity or prolonged overconcern.

Self-Care Deficit [specify] may be related to perceptual and cognitive impairment, immobility (withdrawal/isolation and decreased

---

*A risk diagnosis is not evidenced by signs and symptoms, as the problem has not occurred and nursing interventions are directed at prevention.

psychomotor activity), and side effects of psychotropic medications, possibly evidenced by inability or difficulty in areas of feeding self, keeping body clean, dressing appropriately, toileting self, and/or changes in bowel/bladder elimination.

Sciatica   CH
acute/chronic Pain may be related to peripheral nerve root compression, possibly evidenced by verbal reports, guarding/distraction behaviors, and self-focus.

impaired physical Mobility may be related to neurological pain and muscular involvement, possibly evidenced by reluctance to attempt movement and decreased muscle strength/mass.

Scleroderma   CH
(Also refer to Lupus erythematosus, systemic—SLE)

impaired physical Mobility may be related to musculoskeletal impairment and associated pain, possibly evidenced by decreased strength, decreased range of motion, and reluctance to attempt movement.

ineffective Tissue Perfusion (specify) may be related to reduced arterial blood flow (arteriolar vasoconstriction), possibly evidenced by changes in skin temperature/color, ulcer formation, and changes in organ function (cardiopulmonary, GI, renal).

imbalanced Nutrition: less than body requirements may be related to inability to ingest/digest/absorb adequate nutrients (sclerosis of the tissues rendering mouth immobile, decreased peristalsis of esophagus/small intestine, atrophy of smooth muscle of colon), possibly evidenced by weight loss, decreased intake/food, and reported/observed difficulty swallowing.

risk-prone health Behavior may be related to disability requiring change in lifestyle, inadequate support systems, assault to self-concept, and altered locus of control, possibly evidenced by verbalization of nonacceptance of health status change and lack of movement toward independence/future-oriented thinking.

disturbed Body Image may be related to skin changes with induration, atrophy, and fibrosis, loss of hair, and skin and muscle contractures, possibly evidenced by verbalization of negative feelings about body, focus on past strength/function or appearance, fear of rejection/reaction by others, hiding body part, and change in social involvement.

Scoliosis   PED
disturbed Body Image may be related to altered body structure, use of therapeutic device(s), and activity restrictions, possibly evidenced by negative feelings about body, change in social involvement, and preoccupation with situation or refusal to acknowledge problem.

deficient Knowledge [Learning Need] regarding pathophysiology of condition, therapy needs, and possible outcomes may be related to lack of information/misinterpretation, possibly evidenced by statements of concern, questions, misconceptions, and inaccurate follow-through of instructions.

risk-prone health Behavior may be related to lack of comprehension of long-term consequences of behavior, possibly evidenced by minimizes health status change, failure to take action, and evidence of failure to improve.

Seizure disorder   CH

deficient Knowledge [Learning Need] regarding condition and medication control may be related to lack of information/misinterpretations, scarce financial resources, possibly evidenced by questions, statements of concern/misconceptions, incorrect use of anticonvulsant medication, recurrent episodes/uncontrolled seizures.

chronic low Self-Esteem/disturbed personal Identity may be related to perceived neurological functional change/weakness, perception of being out of control, stigma associated with condition, possibly evidenced by negative feelings about "brain"/self, change in social involvement, feelings of helplessness, and preoccupation with perceived change or loss.

impaired Social Interaction may be related to unpredictable nature of condition and self-concept disturbance, possibly evidenced by decreased self-assurance, verbalization of concern, discomfort in social situations, inability to receive/communicate a satisfying sense of belonging/caring, and withdrawal from social contacts/activities.

risk for Trauma/Suffocation: risk factors may include weakness, balancing difficulties, cognitive limitations/altered consciousness, loss of large or small-muscle coordination (during seizure).*

Sepsis, puerperal   OB

(Also refer to Septicemia)

risk for Infection [spread/septic shock]: risk factors may include presence of infection, broken skin, and/or traumatized tissues, rupture of amniotic membranes, high vascularity of involved area, stasis of body fluids, invasive procedures, and/or increased environmental exposure, chronic disease (e.g., diabetes, anemia, malnutrition), altered immune response, and untoward effect of medications (e.g., opportunistic/secondary infection).*

Hyperthermia may be related to inflammatory process/hypermetabolic state, possibly evidenced by increase in body temperature, warm/flushed skin, and tachycardia.

risk for impaired parent/infant Attachment: risk factors may include interruption in bonding process, physical illness, perceived threat to own survival.*

risk for ineffective peripheral Tissue Perfusion: risk factors may include interruption/reduction of blood flow (presence of infectious thrombi).*

Septicemia   MS

(Also refer to Sepsis, puerperal)

ineffective Tissue Perfusion (specify) may be related to changes in arterial/venous blood flow (selective vasoconstriction, presence of

---

*A risk diagnosis is not evidenced by signs and symptoms, as the problem has not occurred and nursing interventions are directed at prevention.

microemboli) and hypovolemia, possibly evidenced by changes in skin temperature/color, changes in blood/pulse pressure, changes in sensorium, and decreased urinary output.

risk for deficient Fluid Volume: risk factors may include marked increase in vascular compartment/massive vasodilation, vascular shifts to interstitial space, and reduced intake.*

risk for decreased Cardiac Output: risk factors may include decreased preload (venous return and circulating volume), altered afterload (increased SVR), negative inotropic effects of hypoxia, complement activation, and lysosomal hydrolase.*

Serum sickness CH

acute Pain may be related to inflammation of the joints and skin eruptions, possibly evidenced by verbal reports, guarding/distraction behaviors, and self-focus.

deficient Knowledge [Learning Need] regarding nature of condition, treatment needs, potential complications, and prevention of recurrence may be related to lack of information/misinterpretation, possibly evidenced by statements of concern, questions, misconceptions, and inaccurate follow-through of instructions.

Sexually transmitted disease (STD) GYN/CH

risk for Infection [transmission]: risk factors may include contagious nature of infecting agent and insufficient knowledge to avoid exposure to/transmission of pathogens.*

impaired Skin/Tissue Integrity may be related to invasion of/irritation by pathogenic organism(s), possibly evidenced by disruptions of skin/tissue and inflammation of mucous membranes.

deficient Knowledge [Learning Need] regarding condition, prognosis/ complications, therapy needs, and transmission may be related to lack of information/misinterpretation, lack of interest in learning, possibly evidenced by statements of concern, questions, misconceptions; inaccurate follow-through of instructions; and development of preventable complications.

Shock MS

(Also refer to Shock, cardiogenic; Shock, hypovolemic/hemorrhagic)

ineffective Tissue Perfusion (specify) may be related to changes in circulating volume and/or vascular tone, possibly evidenced by changes in skin color/temperature and pulse pressure, reduced blood pressure, changes in mentation, and decreased urinary output.

Anxiety [specify level] may be related to change in health status and threat of death, possibly evidenced by increased tension, apprehension, sympathetic stimulation, restlessness, and expressions of concern.

Shock, cardiogenic MS

(Also refer to Shock)

decreased Cardiac Output may be related to structural damage, decreased myocardial contractility, and presence of dysrhythmias, possibly evidenced by ECG changes, variations in hemodynamic

---

*A risk diagnosis is not evidenced by signs and symptoms, as the problem has not occurred and nursing interventions are directed at prevention.

readings, jugular vein distention, cold/clammy skin, diminished peripheral pulses, and decreased urinary output.

risk for impaired Gas Exchange: risk factors may include ventilation perfusion imbalance, alveolar-capillary membrane changes.*

Shock, hypovolemic/hemorrhagic   MS
(Also refer to Shock)

deficient Fluid Volume [isotonic] may be related to excessive vascular loss, inadequate intake/replacement, possibly evidenced by hypotension, tachycardia, decreased pulse volume and pressure, change in mentation, and decreased/concentrated urine.

Shock, septic   MS
(Refer to Septicemia)

Sick sinus syndrome   MS
(Also refer to Dysrhythmia, cardiac)

decreased Cardiac Output may be related to alterations in rate, rhythm, and electrical conduction, possibly evidenced by ECG evidence of dysrhythmias, reports of palpitations/weakness, changes in mentation/consciousness, and syncope.

risk for Trauma: risk factors may include changes in cerebral perfusion with altered consciousness/loss of balance.[4]

SLE   CH
(Refer to Lupus erythematosus, systemic)

Smallpox   MS

risk of Infection [spread]: risk factors may include contagious nature of organism, inadequate acquired immunity, presence of chronic disease, immunosuppression.*

deficient Fluid Volume may be related to hypermetabolic state, decreased intake (pharyngeal lesions, nausea), increased losses (vomiting), fluid shifts from vascular bed, possibly evidenced by reports of thirst, decreased BP, venous filling and urinary output; dry mucous membranes, decreased skin turgor, change in mental state, elevated Hct.

impaired Tissue Integrity may be related to immunological deficit, possibly evidenced by disruption of skin surface, cornea, mucous membranes.

Anxiety [specify level]/Fear may be related to threat of death, interpersonal transmission/contagion, separation from support system, possibly evidenced by expressed concerns, apprehension, restlessness, focus on self.

          CH

interrupted Family Processes may be related to temporary family disorganization, situational crisis, change in health status of family member, possibly evidenced by changes in satisfaction with family, stress-reduction behaviors, mutual support; expression of isolation from community resources.

---

*A risk diagnosis is not evidenced by signs and symptoms, as the problem has not occurred and nursing interventions are directed at prevention.

ineffective community Coping may be related to human-made disaster (bioterrorism), inadequate resources for problem solving, possibly evidenced by deficits of community participation, high illness rate, excessive community conflicts, expressed vulnerability/powerlessness.

Snow blindness   CH
disturbed visual Sensory Perception may be related to altered status of sense organ (irritation of the conjunctiva, hyperemia), possibly evidenced by intolerance to light (photophobia) and decreased/loss of visual acuity.

acute Pain may be related to irritation/vascular congestion of the conjunctiva, possibly evidenced by verbal reports, guarding/distraction behaviors, and self-focus.

Anxiety [specify level] may be related to situational crisis and threat to/change in health status, possibly evidenced by increased tension, apprehension, uncertainty, worry, restlessness, and focus on self.

Somatoform disorders   PSY
ineffective Coping may be related to severe level of anxiety that is repressed, personal vulnerability, unmet dependency needs, fixation in earlier level of development, retarded ego development, and inadequate coping skills, possibly evidenced by verbalized inability to cope/problem solve, high illness rate, multiple somatic complaints of several years' duration, decreased functioning in social/occupational settings, narcissistic tendencies with total focus on self/physical symptoms, demanding behaviors, history of "doctor shopping," and refusal to attend therapeutic activities.

chronic Pain may be related to severe level of repressed anxiety, low self-concept, unmet dependency needs, history of self or loved one having experienced a serious illness, possibly evidenced by verbal reports of severe/prolonged pain, guarded movement/protective behaviors, facial mask of pain, fear of reinjury, altered ability to continue previous activities, social withdrawal, demands for therapy/medication.

disturbed Sensory Perception (specify) may be related to psychological stress (narrowed perceptual fields, expression of stress as physical problems/deficits), poor quality of sleep, presence of chronic pain, possibly evidenced by reported change in voluntary motor or sensory function (paralysis, anosmia, aphonia, deafness, blindness, loss of touch or pain sensation), *la belle indifférence* (lack of concern over functional loss).

impaired Social Interaction may be related to inability to engage in satisfying personal relationships, preoccupation with self and physical symptoms, altered state of wellness, chronic pain, and rejection by others, possibly evidenced by preoccupation with own thoughts, sad/dull affect, absence of supportive SO(s), uncommunicative/withdrawn behavior, lack of eye contact, and seeking to be alone.

Spinal cord injury (SCI)   MS/CH
(Refer to Paraplegia; Quadriplegia)

Sprain of ankle or foot   CH

acute Pain may be related to trauma to/swelling in joint, possibly evidenced by verbal reports, guarding/distraction behaviors, self-focusing, and autonomic responses (changes in vital signs).

impaired Walking may be related to musculoskeletal injury, pain, and therapeutic restrictions, possibly evidenced by reluctance to attempt movement, inability to move about environment easily.

Stapedectomy   MS

risk for Trauma: risk factors may include increased middle-ear pressure with displacement of prosthesis and balancing difficulties/dizziness.*

risk for Infection: risk factors may include surgically traumatized tissue, invasive procedures, and environmental exposure to upper respiratory infections.*

acute Pain may be related to surgical trauma, edema formation, and presence of packing, possibly evidenced by verbal reports, guarding/distraction behaviors, and self-focus.

STD   CH

(refer to Sexually transmitted disease)

Substance dependence/abuse   PSY/CH
rehabilitation

(following acute detoxification)

ineffective Denial/Coping may be related to personal vulnerability, difficulty handling new situations, learned response patterns, cultural factors, personal/family value systems, possibly evidenced by lack of acceptance that drug use is causing the present situation, use of manipulation to avoid responsibility for self, altered social patterns/participation, impaired adaptive behavior and problem-solving skills, employment difficulties, financial affairs in disarray, and decreased ability to handle stress of recent events.

Powerlessness may be related to substance addiction with/without periods of abstinence, episodic compulsive indulgence, attempts at recovery, and lifestyle of helplessness, possibly evidenced by ineffective recovery attempts, statements of inability to stop behavior/requests for help, continuous/constant thinking about drug and/or obtaining drug, alteration in personal/occupational and social life.

imbalanced Nutrition: less than body requirements may be related to insufficient dietary intake to meet metabolic needs for psychological/physiological/economic reasons, possibly evidenced by weight less than normal for height/body build, decreased subcutaneous fat/muscle mass, reported altered taste sensation, lack of interest in food, poor muscle tone, sore/inflamed buccal cavity, laboratory evidence of protein/vitamin deficiencies.

Sexual Dysfunction may be related to altered body function (neurological damage and debilitating effects of drug use), changes in appearance, possibly evidenced by progressive interference with sexual functioning, a significant degree of testicular atrophy, gynecomastia,

---

*A risk diagnosis is not evidenced by signs and symptoms, as the problem has not occurred and nursing interventions are directed at prevention.

impotence/decreased sperm counts in men; and loss of body hair, thin/soft skin, spider angiomas, and amenorrhea/increase in miscarriages in women.

dysfunctional Family Processes: alcoholism [substance abuse] may be related to abuse/history of alcoholism/drug use, inadequate coping skills/lack of problem-solving skills, genetic predisposition/biochemical influences, possibly evidenced by feelings of anger/frustration/responsibility for alcoholic's behavior, suppressed rage, shame/embarrassment, repressed emotions, guilt, vulnerability, disturbed family dynamics/deterioration in family relationships, family denial/rationalization, closed communication systems, triangulating family relationships, manipulation, blaming, enabling to maintain substance use, inability to accept/receive help.

OB

risk for fetal Injury: risk factors may include drug/alcohol use, exposure to teratogens.*

deficient Knowledge [Learning Need] regarding condition/pregnancy, prognosis, treatment needs may be related to lack/misinterpretation of information, lack of recall, cognitive limitations/interference with learning, possibly evidenced by statements of concern, questions/misconceptions, inaccurate follow-through of instructions, development of preventable complications, continued use in spite of complications.

Surgery, general   MS
(Also refer to Postoperative recovery period)

deficient Knowledge [Learning Need] regarding surgical procedure/expectation, postoperative routines/therapy, and self-care needs may be related to lack of information/misinterpretation, possibly evidenced by statements of concern, questions, and misconceptions.

Anxiety [specify level]/Fear may be related to situational crisis, unfamiliarity with environment, change in health status/threat of death and separation from usual support systems, possibly evidenced by increased tension, apprehension, decreased self-assurance, fear of unspecific consequences, focus on self, sympathetic stimulation, and restlessness.

risk for perioperative-positioning Injury: risk factors may include disorientation, immobilization, muscle weakness, obesity/edema.*

risk for ineffective Breathing Pattern: risk factors may include chemically induced muscular relaxation, perception/cognitive impairment, decreased energy.*

risk for deficient Fluid Volume: risk factors may include preoperative fluid deprivation, blood loss, and excessive GI losses (vomiting/gastric suction).*

Synovitis (knee)   CH
acute Pain may be related to inflammation of synovial membrane of the joint with effusion, possibly evidenced by verbal reports, guarding/

---

*A risk diagnosis is not evidenced by signs and symptoms, as the problem has not occurred and nursing interventions are directed at prevention.

distraction behaviors, self-focus, and autonomic responses (changes in vital signs).

impaired Walking may be related to pain and decreased strength of joint, possibly evidenced by reluctance to attempt movement, inability to move about environment as desired.

Syphilis, congenital   PED
(Also refer to Sexually transmitted disease—STD)

acute Pain may be related to inflammatory process, edema formation, and development of skin lesions, possibly evidenced by irritability/crying that may be increased with movement of extremities and autonomic responses (changes in vital signs).

impaired Skin/Tissue Integrity may be related to exposure to pathogens during vaginal delivery, possibly evidenced by disruption of skin surfaces and rhinitis.

delayed Growth and Development may be related to effect of infectious process, possibly evidenced by altered physical growth and delay or difficulty performing skills typical of age group.

deficient Knowledge [Learning Need] regarding pathophysiology of condition, transmissibility, therapy needs, expected outcomes, and potential complications may be related to caretaker/parental lack of information, misinterpretation, possibly evidenced by statements of concern, questions, and misconceptions.

Syringomyelia   MS

disturbed Sensory Perception (specify) may be related to altered sensory perception (neurological lesion), possibly evidenced by change in usual response to stimuli and motor incoordination.

Anxiety [specify level]/Fear may be related to change in health status, threat of change in role functioning and socioeconomic status, and threat to self-concept, possibly evidenced by increased tension, apprehension, uncertainty, focus on self, and expressed concerns.

impaired physical Mobility may be related to neuromuscular and sensory impairment, possibly evidenced by decreased muscle strength, control, and mass; and impaired coordination.

Self-Care Deficit [specify] may be related to neuromuscular and sensory impairments, possibly evidenced by statement of inability to perform care tasks.

Tay-Sachs disease   PED

delayed Growth and Development may be related to effects of physical condition, possibly evidenced by altered physical growth, loss of/failure to acquire skills typical of age, flat affect, and decreased responses.

disturbed visual Sensory Perception may be related to neurological deterioration of optic nerve, possibly evidenced by loss of visual acuity.

                                                                  CH

[family] Grieving may be related to expected eventual loss of infant/child, possibly evidenced by expressions of distress, denial, guilt, anger, and sorrow; choked feelings; changes in sleep/eating habits; and altered libido.

[family] Powerlessness may be related to absence of therapeutic interventions for progressive/fatal disease, possibly evidenced by verbal expressions of having no control over situation/outcome and depression over physical/mental deterioration.

risk for Spiritual Distress: risk factors may include challenged belief and value system by presence of fatal condition with racial/religious connotations and intense suffering.*

compromised family Coping may be related to situational crisis, temporary preoccupation with managing emotional conflicts and personal suffering, family disorganization, and prolonged/progressive disease, possibly evidenced by preoccupations with personal reactions, expressed concern about reactions of other family members, inadequate support of one another, and altered communication patterns.

Thrombophlebitis   CH/MS/OB

ineffective peripheral Tissue Perfusion may be related to interruption of venous blood flow, venous stasis, possibly evidenced by changes in skin color/temperature over affected area, development of edema, pain, diminished peripheral pulses, slow capillary refill.

acute Pain[/Discomfort] may be related to vascular inflammation/irritation and edema formation (accumulation of lactic acid), possibly evidenced by verbal reports, guarding/distraction behaviors, restlessness, and self-focus.

risk for impaired physical Mobility: risk factors may include pain and discomfort and restrictive therapies/safety precautions.*

deficient Knowledge [Learning Need] regarding pathophysiology of condition, therapy/self-care needs, and risk of embolization may be related to lack of information/misinterpretation, possibly evidenced by statements of concern, questions, inaccurate follow-through of instructions, and development of preventable complications.

Thrombosis, venous   MS
(Refer to Thrombophlebitis)

Thrush   CH
impaired Oral Mucous Membrane may be related to presence of infection as evidenced by white patches/plaques, oral discomfort, mucosal irritation, bleeding.

Thyroidectomy   MS
(Also refer to Hyperthyroidism; Hypoparathyroidism; Hypothyroidism)
risk for ineffective Airway Clearance: risk factors may include hematoma/edema formation with tracheal obstruction, laryngeal spasms.*

impaired verbal Communication may be related to tissue edema, pain/discomfort, and vocal cord injury/laryngeal nerve damage, possibly evidenced by impaired articulation, does not/cannot speak, and use of nonverbal cues/gestures.

---

*A risk diagnosis is not evidenced by signs and symptoms, as the problem has not occurred and nursing interventions are directed at prevention.

risk for Injury [tetany]: risk factors may include chemical imbalance/ excessive CNS stimulation.*

risk for head/neck Trauma: risk factors may include loss of muscle control/support and position of suture line.*

acute Pain may be related to presence of surgical incision/manipulation of tissues/muscles, postoperative edema, possibly evidenced by verbal reports, guarding/distraction behaviors, narrowed focus, and autonomic responses (changes in vital signs).

Thyrotoxicosis   MS
(Also refer to Hyperthyroidism)

risk for decreased Cardiac Output: risk factors may include uncontrolled hypermetabolic state increasing cardiac workload, changes in venous return and SVR, and alterations in rate, rhythm, and electrical conduction.*

Anxiety [specific level] may be related to physiological factors/CNS stimulation (hypermetabolic state and pseudocatecholamine effect of thyroid hormones), possibly evidenced by increased feelings of apprehension, shakiness, loss of control, panic, changes in cognition, distortion of environmental stimuli, extraneous movements, restlessness, and tremors.

risk for disturbed Thought Processes: risk factors may include physiological changes (increased CNS stimulation/accelerated mental activity) and altered sleep patterns.*

deficient Knowledge [Learning Needs] regarding condition, treatment needs, and potential for complications/crisis situation may be related to lack of information/recall, misinterpretation, possibly evidenced by statements of concern, questions, misconceptions; and inaccurate follow-through of instructions.

TIA (Transient ischemic attack)   CH

ineffective cerebral Tissue Perfusion may be related to interruption of blood flow (e.g., vasospasm), possibly evidenced by altered mental status, behavioral changes, language deficit, change in motor/sensory response.

Anxiety/Fear may be related to change in health status, threat to self-concept, situational crisis, interpersonal contagion, possibly evidenced by expressed concerns, apprehension, restlessness, irritability.

risk for ineffective Denial: risk factors may include change in health status requiring change in lifestyle, fear of consequences, lack of motivation.

Tic douloureux   CH
(Refer to Neuralgia, trigeminal)

Tonsillectomy   PED/MS
(Refer to Adenoidectomy)

Tonsillitis   PED

acute Pain may be related to inflammation of tonsils and effects of circulating toxins, possibly evidenced by verbal reports, guarding/

---

*A risk diagnosis is not evidenced by signs and symptoms, as the problem has not occurred and nursing interventions are directed at prevention.

distraction behaviors, reluctance/refusal to swallow, self-focus, and autonomic responses (changes in vital signs).

Hyperthermia may be related to presence of inflammatory process/hypermetabolic state and dehydration, possibly evidenced by increased body temperature, warm/flushed skin, and tachycardia.

deficient Knowledge [Learning Need] regarding cause/transmission, treatment needs, and potential complications may be related to lack of information/misinterpretation, possibly evidenced by statements of concern, questions, inaccurate follow-through of instructions, and recurrence of condition.

Total joint replacement   MS

risk for Infection: risk factors may include inadequate primary defenses (broken skin, exposure of joint), inadequate secondary defenses/immunosuppression (long-term corticosteroid use), invasive procedures/surgical manipulation, implantation of foreign body, and decreased mobility.*

impaired physical Mobility may be related to pain and discomfort, musculoskeletal impairment, and surgery/restrictive therapies, possibly evidenced by reluctance to attempt movement, difficulty purposefully moving within the physical environment, reports of pain/discomfort on movement, limited range of motion, and decreased muscle strength/control.

risk for ineffective peripheral Tissue Perfusion: risk factors may include reduced arterial/venous blood flow, direct trauma to blood vessels, tissue edema, improper location/dislocation of prosthesis, and hypovolemia.*

acute Pain may be related to physical agents (traumatized tissues/surgical intervention, degeneration of joints, muscle spasms) and psychological factors (anxiety, advanced age), possibly evidenced by verbal reports, guarding/distraction behaviors, self-focus, and autonomic responses (changes in vital signs).

Toxemia of pregnancy   OB
(Refer to Pregnancy-induced hypertension)

Toxic shock syndrome   MS
(Also refer to Septicemia)

Hyperthermia may be related to inflammatory process/hypermetabolic state and dehydration, possibly evidenced by increased body temperature, warm/flushed skin, and tachycardia.

deficient Fluid Volume [isotonic] may be related to increased gastric losses (diarrhea, vomiting), fever/hypermetabolic state, and decreased intake, possibly evidenced by dry mucous membranes, increased pulse, hypotension, delayed venous filling, decreased/concentrated urine, and hemoconcentration.

acute Pain may be related to inflammatory process, effects of circulating toxins, and skin disruptions, possibly evidenced by verbal reports, guarding/distraction behaviors, self-focus, and autonomic responses (changes in vital signs).

---

*A risk diagnosis is not evidenced by signs and symptoms, as the problem has not occurred and nursing interventions are directed at prevention.

impaired Skin/Tissue Integrity may be related to effects of circulating toxins and dehydration, possibly evidenced by development of desquamating rash, hyperemia, and inflammation of mucous membranes.

Traction   MS
(Also refer to Casts; Fractures)

acute Pain may be related to direct trauma to tissue/bone, muscle spasms, movement of bone fragments, edema, injury to soft tissue, traction/immobility device, anxiety, possibly evidenced by verbal reports, guarding/distraction behaviors, self-focus, alteration in muscle tone, and autonomic responses (changes in vital signs).

impaired physical Mobility may be related to neuromuscular/skeletal impairment, pain, psychological immobility, and therapeutic restrictions of movement, possibly evidenced by limited range of motion, inability to move purposefully in environment, reluctance to attempt movement, and decreased muscle strength/control.

risk for Infection: risk factors may include invasive procedures (including insertion of foreign body through skin/bone), presence of traumatized tissue, and reduced activity with stasis of body fluids.*

deficient Diversional Activity may be related to length of hospitalization/therapeutic intervention and environmental lack of usual activity, possibly evidenced by statements of boredom, restlessness, and irritability.

Transfusion reaction, blood   MS
(Also refer to Anaphylaxis)

risk for imbalanced Body Temperature: risk factors may include infusion of cold blood products, systemic response to toxins.*

Anxiety [specify level] may be related to change in health status and threat of death, exposure to toxins, possibly evidenced by increased tension, apprehension, sympathetic stimulation, restlessness, and expressions of concern.

risk for impaired Skin Integrity: risk factors may include immunological response.*

Trichinosis   CH

acute Pain may be related to parasitic invasion of muscle tissues, edema of upper eyelids, small localized hemorrhages, and development of urticaria, possibly evidenced by verbal reports, guarding/distraction behaviors (restlessness), and autonomic responses (changes in vital signs).

deficient Fluid Volume [isotonic] may be related to hypermetabolic state (fever, diaphoresis), excessive gastric losses (vomiting, diarrhea), and decreased intake/difficulty swallowing, possibly evidenced by dry mucous membranes, decreased skin turgor, hypotension, decreased venous filling, decreased/concentrated urine, and hemoconcentration.

ineffective Breathing Pattern may be related to myositis of the diaphragm and intercostal muscles, possibly evidenced by resulting

---

*A risk diagnosis is not evidenced by signs and symptoms, as the problem has not occurred and nursing interventions are directed at prevention.

changes in respiratory depth, tachypnea, dyspnea, and abnormal ABGs.

deficient Knowledge [Learning Need] regarding cause/prevention of condition, therapy needs, and possible complications may be related to lack of information, misinterpretation, possibly evidenced by statements of concern, questions, and misconceptions.

Tuberculosis (pulmonary)   CH

risk for Infection [spread/reactivation]: risk factors may include inadequate primary defenses (decreased ciliary action/stasis of secretions, tissue destruction/extension of infection), lowered resistance/suppressed inflammatory response, malnutrition, environmental exposure, insufficient knowledge to avoid exposure to pathogens, or inadequate therapeutic intervention.*

ineffective Airway Clearance may be related to thick, viscous, or bloody secretions; fatigue/poor cough effort, and tracheal/pharyngeal edema, possibly evidenced by abnormal respiratory rate, rhythm, and depth; adventitious breath sounds (rhonchi, wheezes), stridor, and dyspnea.

risk for impaired Gas Exchange: risk factors may include decrease in effective lung surface, atelectasis, destruction of alveolar-capillary membrane, bronchial edema, thick, viscous secretions.*

Activity Intolerance may be related to imbalance between O_2 supply and demand, possibly evidenced by reports of fatigue, weakness, and exertional dyspnea.

imbalanced Nutrition: less than body requirements may be related to inability to ingest adequate nutrients (anorexia, effects of drug therapy, fatigue, insufficient financial resources), possibly evidenced by weight loss, reported lack of interest in food/altered taste sensation, and poor muscle tone.

risk for ineffective Therapeutic Regimen Management: risk factors may include complexity of therapeutic regimen, economic difficulties, family patterns of healthcare, perceived seriousness/benefits (especially during remission), side effects of therapy.*

Tympanoplasty   MS
(Refer to Stapedectomy)

Typhus (tick-borne/Rocky   CH/MS
Mountain spotted fever)

Hyperthermia may be related to generalized inflammatory process (vasculitis), possibly evidenced by increased body temperature, warm/flushed skin, and tachycardia.

acute Pain may be related to generalized vasculitis and edema formation, possibly evidenced by verbal reports, guarding/distraction behaviors, self-focus, and autonomic responses (changes in vital signs).

ineffective Tissue Perfusion (specify) may be related to reduction/interruption of blood flow (generalized vasculitis/thrombi formation),

---

*A risk diagnosis is not evidenced by signs and symptoms, as the problem has not occurred and nursing interventions are directed at prevention.

possibly evidenced by reports of headache/abdominal pain, changes in mentation, and areas of peripheral ulceration/necrosis.

Ulcer, decubitus   CH/MS

impaired Skin/Tissue Integrity may be related to altered circulation, nutritional deficit, fluid imbalance, impaired physical mobility, irritation of body excretions/secretions, and sensory impairments, evidenced by tissue damage/destruction.

acute Pain may be related to destruction of protective skin layers and exposure of nerves, possibly evidenced by verbal reports, distraction behaviors, and self-focus.

risk for Infection: risk factors may include broken/traumatized tissue, increased environmental exposure, and nutritional deficits.*

Ulcer, peptic (acute)   MS/CH

deficient Fluid Volume [isotonic] may be related to vascular losses (hemorrhage), possibly evidenced by hypotension, tachycardia, delayed capillary refill, changes in mentation, restlessness, concentrated/decreased urine, pallor, diaphoresis, and hemoconcentration.

risk for ineffective Tissue Perfusion (specify): risk factors may include hypovolemia.*

Fear/Anxiety [specify level] may be related to change in health status and threat of death, possibly evidenced by increased tension, restlessness, irritability, fearfulness, trembling, tachycardia, diaphoresis, lack of eye contact, focus on self, verbalization of concerns, withdrawal, and panic or attack behavior.

acute Pain may be related to caustic irritation/destruction of gastric tissues, possibly evidenced by verbal reports, distraction behaviors, self-focus, and autonomic responses (changes in vital signs).

deficient Knowledge [Learning Need] regarding condition, therapy/ self-care needs, and potential complications may be related to lack of information/recall, misinterpretation, possibly evidenced by statements of concern, questions, misconceptions; inaccurate follow-through of instructions; and development of preventable complications/recurrence of condition.

Unconsciousness (coma)   MS

risk for Suffocation: risk factors may include cognitive impairment/loss of protective reflexes and purposeful movement.*

risk for deficient Fluid Volume/imbalanced Nutrition: less than body requirements: risk factors may include inability to ingest food/fluids, increased needs/hypermetabolic state.*

total Self-Care Deficit may be related to cognitive impairment and absence of purposeful activity, evidenced by inability to perform ADLs.

risk for ineffective cerebral Tissue Perfusion: risk factors may include reduced or interrupted arterial/venous blood flow (direct injury, edema formation, space-occupying lesions), metabolic alterations, effects of drug/alcohol overdose, hypoxia/anoxia.*

U

*A risk diagnosis is not evidenced by signs and symptoms, as the problem has not occurred and nursing interventions are directed at prevention.

risk for Infection: risk factors may include stasis of body fluids (oral, pulmonary, urinary), invasive procedures, and nutritional deficits.*

Urinary diversion   MS/CH
risk for impaired Skin Integrity: risk factors may include absence of sphincter at stoma, character/flow of urine from stoma, reaction to product/chemicals, and improperly fitting appliance or removal of adhesive.*

disturbed Body Image: related factors may include biophysical factors (presence of stoma, loss of control of urine flow), and psychosocial factors (altered body structure, disease process/associated treatment regimen, such as cancer), possibly evidenced by verbalization of change in body image, fear of rejection/reaction of others, negative feelings about body, not touching/looking at stoma, refusal to participate in care.

acute Pain may be related to physical factors (disruption of skin/tissues, presence of incisions/drains), biological factors (activity of disease process, such as cancer, trauma), and psychological factors (fear, anxiety), possibly evidenced by verbal reports, self-focusing, guarding/distraction behaviors, restlessness, and autonomic responses (changes in vital signs).

impaired Urinary Elimination may be related to surgical diversion, tissue trauma, and postoperative edema, possibly evidenced by loss of continence, changes in amount and character of urine, and urinary retention.

Urolithiasis   MS/CH
(Refer to Calculi, urinary)

Uterine bleeding, abnormal   GYN/MS
Anxiety [specify level] may be related to perceived change in health status and unknown etiology, possibly evidenced by apprehension, uncertainty, fear of unspecified consequences, expressed concerns, and focus on self.

Activity Intolerance may be related to imbalance between O_2 supply and demand/decreased O_2-carrying capacity of blood (anemia), possibly evidenced by reports of fatigue/weakness.

Uterus, rupture of, in pregnancy   OB
deficient Fluid Volume [isotonic] may be related to excessive vascular losses, possibly evidenced by hypotension, increased pulse rate, decreased venous filling, and decreased urine output.

decreased Cardiac Output may be related to decreased preload (hypovolemia), possibly evidenced by cold/clammy skin, decreased peripheral pulses, variations in hemodynamic readings, tachycardia, and cyanosis.

acute Pain may be related to tissue trauma and irritation of accumulating blood, possibly evidenced by verbal reports, guarding/distraction behaviors, self-focus, and autonomic responses (changes in vital signs).

---

*A risk diagnosis is not evidenced by signs and symptoms, as the problem has not occurred and nursing interventions are directed at prevention.

Anxiety [specify level] may be related to threat of death of self/fetus, interpersonal contagion, physiological response (release of catecholamines), possibly evidenced by fearful/scared affect, sympathetic stimulation, stated fear of unspecified consequences, and expressed concerns.

Vaginismus   GYN/CH

acute Pain may be related to muscle spasm and hyperesthesia of the nerve supply to vaginal mucous membrane, possibly evidenced by verbal reports, distraction behaviors, and self-focus.

Sexual Dysfunction may be related to physical and/or psychological alteration in function (severe spasms of vaginal muscles), possibly evidenced by verbalization of problem, inability to achieve desired satisfaction, and alteration in relationship with SO.

Vaginitis   GYN/CH

impaired Tissue Integrity may be related to irritation/inflammation and mechanical trauma (scratching) of sensitive tissues, possibly evidenced by damaged/destroyed tissue, presence of lesions.

acute Pain may be related to localized inflammation and tissue trauma, possibly evidenced by verbal reports, distraction behaviors, and self-focus.

deficient Knowledge [Learning Need] regarding hygienic/therapy needs and sexual behaviors/transmission of organisms may be related to lack of information/misinterpretation, possibly evidenced by statements of concern, questions, and misconceptions.

Varices, esophageal   MS
(Also refer to Ulcer, peptic [acute])

deficient Fluid Volume [isotonic] may be related to excessive vascular loss, reduced intake, and gastric losses (vomiting), possibly evidenced by hypotension, tachycardia, decreased venous filling, and decreased/concentrated urine.

Anxiety [specify level]/Fear may be related to change in health status and threat of death, possibly evidenced by increased tension/apprehension, sympathetic stimulation, restlessness, focus on self, and expressed concerns.

Varicose veins   CH

chronic Pain may be related to venous insufficiency and stasis, possibly evidenced by verbal reports.

disturbed Body Image may be related to change in structure (presence of enlarged, discolored tortuous superficial leg veins), possibly evidenced by hiding affected parts and negative feelings about body.

risk for impaired Skin/Tissue Integrity: risk factors may include altered circulation/venous stasis and edema formation.*

V

Venereal disease   CH
(Refer to Sexually transmitted disease—STD)

*A risk diagnosis is not evidenced by signs and symptoms, as the problem has not occurred and nursing interventions are directed at prevention.

Ventricular fibrillation   MS
(Refer to Dysrhythmias)

Ventricular tachycardia   MS
(Refer to Dysrhythmias)

West Nile fever   CH/MS
Hyperthermia may be related to infectious process, possibly evidenced by elevated body temperature, skin flushed/warm to touch, tachycardia, increased respiratory rate.

acute Pain may be related to infectious process/circulating toxins, possibly evidenced by reports of headache, myalgia, eye pain, abdominal discomfort.

risk for deficient Fluid Volume: risk factors may include hypermetabolic state, decreased intake, anorexia, nausea, losses from normal routes (vomiting, diarrhea).*

risk for impaired Skin Integrity: risk factors may include hyperthermia, decreased fluid intake, alterations in skin turgor, bedrest, circulating toxins.*

Wilms' tumor   PED
(Also refer to Cancer; Chemotherapy)
Anxiety [specify level]/Fear may be related to change in environment and interaction patterns with family members and threat of death with family transmission and contagion of concerns, possibly evidenced by fearful/scared affect, distress, crying, insomnia, and sympathetic stimulation.

risk for Injury: risk factors may include nature of tumor (vascular, mushy with very thin covering) with increased danger of metastasis when manipulated.*

interrupted Family Processes may be related to situational crisis of life-threatening illness, possibly evidenced by a family system that has difficulty meeting physical, emotional, and spiritual needs of its members, and inability to deal with traumatic experience effectively.

deficient Diversional Activity may be related to environmental lack of age-appropriate activity (including activity restrictions) and length of hospitalization/treatment, possibly evidenced by restlessness, crying, lethargy, and acting-out behavior.

Wound, gunshot   MS
(Depends on site and speed/character of bullet)
risk for deficient Fluid Volume: risk factors may include excessive vascular losses, altered intake/restrictions.*

acute Pain may be related to destruction of tissue (including organ and musculoskeletal), surgical repair, and therapeutic interventions, possibly evidenced by verbal reports, guarding/distraction behaviors, self-focus, and autonomic responses (changes in vital signs).

impaired Tissue Integrity may be related to mechanical factors (yaw of projectile and muzzle blast), possibly evidenced by damaged or destroyed tissue.

---

*A risk diagnosis is not evidenced by signs and symptoms, as the problem has not occurred and nursing interventions are directed at prevention.

risk for Infection: risk factors may include tissue destruction and increased environmental exposure, invasive procedures, and decreased hemoglobin.*

CH

risk for Post-Trauma Syndrome: risk factors may include nature of incident (catastrophic accident, assault, suicide attempt) and possibly injury/death of other(s) involved.*

W

---

*A risk diagnosis is not evidenced by signs and symptoms, as the problem has not occurred and nursing interventions are directed at prevention.

NANDA-I's Taxonomy II

The 13 domains and their classes are:

Domain 1 Health Promotion: The awareness of well-being or normality of function and the strategies used to maintain control of and enhance that well-being or normality of function

Class 1 Health Awareness: Recognition of normal function and well-being

Class 2 Health Management: Identifying, controlling, performing, and integrating activities to maintain health and well-being

Domain 2 Nutrition: The activities of taking in, assimilating, and using nutrients for the purposes of tissue maintenance, tissue repair, and the production of energy

Class 1 Ingestion: Taking food or nutrients into the body

Class 2 Digestion: The physical and chemical activities that convert foodstuffs into substances suitable for absorption and assimilation

Class 3 Absorption: The act of taking up nutrients through body tissues

Class 4 Metabolism: The chemical and physical processes occurring in living organisms and cells for the development and use of protoplasm, production of waste and energy, with the release of energy for all vital processes

Class 5 Hydration: The taking in and absorption of fluids and electrolytes

Domain 3 Elimination: Secretion and excretion of waste products from the body

Class 1 Urinary Function: The process of secretion, reabsorption, and excretion of urine

Class 2 Gastrointestinal Function: The process of absorption and excretion of the end products of digestion

Class 3 Integumentary Function: The process of secretion and excretion through the skin

Class 4 Respiratory Function: The process of exchange of gases and removal of the end products of metabolism

Domain 4 Activity/Rest: The production, conservation, expenditure, or balance of energy resources

Class 1 Sleep/Rest: Slumber, repose, ease, or inactivity

Class 2 Activity/Exercise: Moving parts of the body (mobility), doing work, or performing actions often (but not always) against resistance

Class 3 Energy Balance: A dynamic state of harmony between intake and expenditure of resources

Class 4 Cardiovascular/Pulmonary Responses: Cardiopulmonary mechanisms that support activity/rest

Class 5 Self-Care: Ability to perform activities to care for one's body and bodily functions

Domain 5 Perception/Cognition: The human information processing system including attention, orientation, sensation, perception, cognition, and communication

Class 1 Attention: Mental readiness to notice or observe

Class 2 Orientation: Awareness of time, place, and person

Class 3 Sensation/Perception: Receiving information through the senses of touch, taste, smell, vision, hearing, and kinesthesia and the comprehension of sense data resulting in naming, associating, and/or pattern recognition

Class 4 Cognition: Use of memory, learning, thinking, problem solving, abstraction, judgment, insight, intellectual capacity, calculation, and language

Class 5 Communication: Sending and receiving verbal and nonverbal information

Domain 6 Self-Perception: Awareness about the self

Class 1 Self-Concept: The perception(s) about the total self

Class 2 Self-Esteem: Assessment of one's own worth, capability, significance, and success

Class 3 Body Image: A mental image of one's own body

Domain 7 Role Relationships: The positive and negative connections or associations between people or groups of people and the means by which those connections are demonstrated

Class 1 Caregiving Roles: Socially expected behavior patterns by people providing care who are not healthcare professionals

Class 2 Family Relationships: Associations of people who are biologically related or related by choice

Class 3 Role Performance: Quality of functioning in socially expected behavior patterns

Domain 8 Sexuality: Sexual identity, sexual function, and reproduction

Class 1 Sexual Identity: The state of being a specific person in regard to sexuality and/or gender

Class 2 Sexual Function: The capacity or ability to participate in sexual activities

Class 3 Reproduction: Any process by which human beings are produced

Domain 9 Coping/Stress Tolerance: Contending with life events/ life processes

Class 1 Post-Trauma Responses: Reactions occurring after physical or psychological trauma

Class 2 Coping Responses: The process of managing environmental stress

Class 3 Neurobehavioral Stress: Behavioral responses reflecting nerve and brain function

Domain 10 Life Principles: Principles underlying conduct, thought, and behavior about acts, customs, or institutions viewed as being true or having intrinsic worth

Class 1 Values: The identification and ranking of preferred mode of conduct or end states

Class 2 Beliefs: Opinions, expectations, or judgments about acts, customs, or institutions viewed as being true or having intrinsic worth

Class 3 Value/Belief/Action Congruence: The correspondence or balance achieved between values, beliefs, and actions

Domain 11 Safety/Protection: Freedom from danger, physical injury, or immune system damage; preservation from loss; and protection of safety and security

Class 1 Infection: Host responses following pathogenic invasion

Class 2 Physical Injury: Bodily harm or hurt

Class 3 Violence: The exertion of excessive force or power so as to cause injury or abuse

Class 4 Environmental Hazards: Sources of danger in the surroundings

Class 5 Defensive Processes: The processes by which the self protects itself from the non-self

Class 6 Thermoregulation: The physiological process of regulating heat and energy within the body for purposes of protecting the organism

Domain 12 Comfort: Sense of mental, physical, or social well-being or ease

Class 1 Physical Comfort: Sense of well-being or ease and/or freedom from pain

Class 2 Environmental Comfort: Sense of well-being or ease in/with one's environment

Class 3 Social Comfort: Sense of well-being or ease with one's social situations

Domain 13 Growth/Development: Age-appropriate increases in physical dimensions, maturation of organ systems, and/or progression through the developmental milestone[s]

Class 1 Growth: Increases in physical dimensions or maturity of organ systems

Class 2 Development: Progression or regression through a sequence of recognized milestones in life

Definitions of Taxonomy II Axes

Axis 1 The Diagnostic Concept: Defined as the principal element or the fundamental and essential part, the root, of the diagnostic statement describing the "human response" and consisting of one or more nouns, or an adjective with a noun.

Axis 2 Subject of the Diagnosis: Defined as the person(s) for whom a diagnosis is determined. Values are:

> *Individual:* A single human being distinct from others, a person
> *Family:* Two or more people having continuous or sustained relationships, perceiving reciprocal obligations, sensing common meaning, and sharing certain obligations toward others; related by blood and/or choice
> *Group:* A number of people with shared characteristics
> *Community:* A group of people living in the same locale under the same governance (e.g., neighborhoods and cities)
> When the subject of the diagnosis is not explicitly stated, it becomes the individual by default

Axis 3 Judgment: Defined as a descriptor or modifier that limits or specifies the meaning of a nursing diagnostic concept. Values are:

> *Anticipatory:* Realize beforehand, foresee
> *Compromised:* Damaged, made vulnerable
> *Decreased:* Lessened (in size, amount, or degree)
> *Defensive:* Used or intended to defend or protect
> *Deficient:* Insufficient, inadequate
> *Delayed:* Late, slow, or postponed
> *Disabled:* Limited, handicapped
> *Disorganized:* Not properly arranged or controlled
> *Disproportionate:* Too large or too small in comparison with norm
> *Disturbed:* Agitated, interrupted, interfered with
> *Dysfunctional:* Not operating normally
> *Effective:* Producing the intended or desired effect

Enhanced: Improved in quality, value, or extent
Excessive: Greater than necessary or desirable
Imbalanced: Out of proportion or balance
Impaired: Damaged, weakened
Ineffective: Not producing the intended or desired effect
Interrupted: Having its continuity broken
Low: Below the norm
Organized: Properly arranged or controlled
Perceived: Observed through the senses
Readiness for: In a suitable state for an activity or situation
Situational: Related to particular circumstance(s)

Axis 4 Location: Refers to the parts/regions of the body and/or their related functions—all tissues, organs, anatomical sites, or structures. Values are:

Auditory	*Intracranial*	*Peripheral*
Bladder	*Kinesthetic*	*vascular*
Cardiopulmonary	*Mucous membranes*	*Renal*
Cerebral	*Oral*	*Skin*
Gastrointestinal	*Olfactory*	*Tactile*
Gustatory	*Peripheral*	*Visual*
	neurovascular	

Axis 5 Age: Defined as the age of the person who is the subject of diagnosis.
Values are:

Fetus	*School-age child*
Neonate	*Adolescent*
Infant	*Adult*
Toddler	*Older adult*
Preschool child	

Axis 6 Time: Defined as the duration of a period or interval.
Acute: Lasting less than 6 months
Chronic: Lasting more than 6 months
Intermittent: Stopping or starting again at intervals; periodic, cyclic
Continuous: Uninterrupted, going on without stops

Axis 7 Status of Diagnosis: Defined as the actuality or potentiality of the problem or to the categorization of the diagnosis as a wellness/health promotion diagnosis. Values are:
Actual: Existing in fact or reality, existing at the present time
Health Promotion: Behavior motivated by the desire to increase well-being and actualize human health potential

Risk: Vulnerability, especially as a result of exposure to factors that increase the chance of injury or loss

Wellness: The quality or state of being healthy

NANDA-I: Nursing Diagnoses: Definitions & Classification 2007–2008, Philadelphia, 2007.

Bibliography

Books

Aacovou, I: The Role of the Nurse in the Rehabilitation of Patients with Radical Changes in Body Image Due to Burn Injuries. Psychiatric Department, Makarios Hospital, Nicosia, Cyprus, 2004.

Ackley, BJ, and Ladwig, GB: Nursing Diagnosis Handbook: A Guide to Planning Care, 7th ed. Mosby Elsevier. St. Louis, 2006.

Acute Pain Management: Operative or Medical Procedures and Trauma: Clinical Practice Guideline. US Department of Health and Human Services, Public Health Service Agency for Health Care Policy and Research, Rockville, MD, Feb 1992.

Adams, L: Be Your Best, (Rev. ed.). Perigee Trade, 1989.

Alberte, R, and Emmons, M: Your Perfect Right. San Luis Obispo, CA, Impact, 1970.

American Nurses Association: Nursing's Social Policy Statement. Washington, DC, 1995.

American Nurses Association: Nursing's Social Policy Statement, 2nd ed. Washington, DC, 2003:6.

American Nurses Association: Social Policy Statement. Kansas City, MO, 1980.

American Nurses Association: Standards of Clinical Nursing Practice. Kansas City, MO, 1991.

Androwich, I, Burkhart, L, and Gettrust, KV: Community and Home Health Nursing. Delmar, Albany, NY, 1996.

Asp, AA: Diabetes mellitus. In Copstead, LC, and Banasik, JL (Eds.): Pathophysiology, 3rd ed. Elsevier Saunders, Philadelphia, 2005.

Banasik, JL, and Copstead, LEC. (Eds.): Pathophysiology, 3rd ed. Elsevier, Saunders, St. Louis, 2005.

Beers, MH, and Berkow, R: The Merck Manual of Diagnosis and Therapy, 17th ed. Merck Research Laboratories, Whitehouse Station, NJ, 1999.

Bellis, TJ: When the Brain Can't Hear: Unraveling the Mystery of Auditory Processing Disorder. Atria Books, New York, 2002.

Branden, N: The Six Pillars of Self-Esteem. Bantam Books, New York, 1995.

Carey, CF, Lee, HH, and Woeltje, KF (Eds.): The Washington Manual of Medical Therapeutics, 29th ed. Lippincott-Raven, Philadelphia, 1998.

Cassileth, BR: The Alternative Medicine Handbook: The Complete Reference Guide to Alternative and Complementary Therapies. WW Norton & Co, New York, 1998.

Cataract in Adults: Management of Functional Impairment. AHCPR Pub 93–0542, US Department of Health and Human Services, Public Health Agency for Health Care Policy and Research, Rockville, MD, 1993.

Condon, RE, and Nyhus, LM (Eds.): Manual of Surgical Therapeutics, 9th ed. Little, Brown & Co., Boston, 1996.

Cox, H, Saidaromont, K, King, M, et al: Clinical Applications of Nursing Diagnosis: Adult, Child, Women's Psychiatric, Gerontic, and Home Health Considerations, 4th ed. F.A. Davis, Philadelphia, 2002.

Cummings, B: Managing Stress: Coping with Life's Challenges. In Health: The Basics, 5th ed. Pearson Education, 2003.

Deglin, JH, and Vallerand, AH: Davis's Drug Guide for Nurses, 9th ed. F.A. Davis, Philadelphia, 2005.

Depression in Primary Care, Vol. 1, Detection and Diagnosis. AHCPR Pub 93–0550, US Department of Health and Human Services, Public Health Service Agency for Health Care Policy and Research, Rockville, MD, April 1993.

Depression in Primary Care, Vol. 2, Treatment of Major Depression. AHCPR Pub 93–0551, US Department of Health and Human Services, Public Health Service Agency for Health Care Policy and Research, Rockville, MD, April 1993.

Doenges, M, Moorhouse, M, and Murr, A: Nursing Care Plans Across the Life Span, 7th ed. F.A. Davis, Philadelphia, 2006.

Doenges, M, Moorhouse, M, and Murr, A: Nursing Diagnosis Manual: Planning, Individualizing, and Documenting Client Care. F.A. Davis, Philadelphia, 2005.

Doenges, M, Townsend, M, and Moorhouse, M: Psychiatric Care Plans: Guidelines for Planning and Documenting Client Care, 3rd ed. F.A. Davis, Philadelphia, 1999.

Early Identification of Alzheimer's Disease and Related Dementias: Clinical Practice Guideline, US Department of Health and Human Services, Public Health Service Agency for Health Care Policy and Research, Rockville, MD, November 1996.

Engel, J: Pocket Guide to Pediatric Assessment, 4th ed. Mosby, St. Louis, 2002.

Goleman, D: Emotional Intelligence: Why It Matters More than IQ (10th Anniversary ed). Bantam, New York, 2006.

Gordon, M: Manual of Nursing Diagnosis. Mosby, St. Louis, 1997.

Gordon, T: Family Effectiveness Training. Gordon Training International, 1997.

Gordon, T: Parent Effectiveness Training. Three Rivers Press, New York, 2000.

Gordon, T: Teaching Children Self-Discipline: At Home and At School. Random House, New York, 1989.

Gorman, L, Sultan, D, and Raines, M: Davis's Manual of Psychosocial Nursing for General Patient Care. F.A. Davis, Philadelphia, 1996.

Harkulich, JT, et al: Teacher's Guide: A Manual for Caregivers of Alzheimer's Disease in Long-Term Care. Embassy Printing, Cleveland Heights, OH, Copyright pending.

Higgs, ZR, and Gustafson, DD: Community as a Client: Assessment and Diagnosis. F.A. Davis, Philadelphia, 1985.

Ignatavicius, DD, and Workman, ML. (Eds.): Medical-Surgical Nursing: Critical Thinking for Collaborative Care. Elsevier Saunders, St. Louis, 2006.

Jaffe, MS, and McVan, BF: Laboratory and Diagnostic Test Handbook. F.A. Davis, Philadelphia, 1997.

King, L: Toward a Theory for Nursing: General Concepts of Human Behavior. Wiley, New York, 1971.

Kuhn, MA: Pharmacotherapeutics: A Nursing Process Approach, 4th ed. F.A. Davis, Philadelphia, 1998.

Lampe, S: Focus Charting, 7th ed. Creative Healthcare Management, Inc., Minneapolis, 1997.

Lee, D, Barrett, C, and Ignatavicius, D: Fluids and Electrolytes: A Practical Approach, 4th ed. F.A. Davis, Philadelphia, 1996.

Leiniger, MM: Transcultural Nursing: Theories, Research and Practices, 3rd ed. McGraw-Hill, Hilliard, OH, 1996.

Lipson, JG, Dibble, S, and Minarik, P (Eds.), Culture and Nursing Care: A Pocket Guide. UCSF Nursing Press, University of California, San Francisco, 1996.

Management of Cancer Pain. AHCPR Pub 93–0592, US Department of Health and Human Services, Public Health Agency for Health Care Policy and Research, Rockville, MD, 1994.

McCance, KL, and Huether, SE: Pathophysiology: The Biologic Basis for Disease in Adults and Children, 3rd ed. Mosby, St. Louis, 1997.

McCloskey, JC, and Bulechek, GM (Eds.): Nursing Interventions Classification, 3rd ed. Mosby, St. Louis, 2000.

McLeod, ME: Interventions for Clients with Diabetes Mellitus. In Ignatavicius, DD, and Workman, ML.(Eds.): Medical-Surgical Nursing: Critical Thinking for Collaborative Care, 5th ed. Elsevier Saunders, Philadelphia, 2006.

Mentgen, J, and Bulbrook, MJT: Healing Touch, Level I Notebook. Healing Touch, Lakewood, CO, 1994.

Moorehead, S, Johnson, M, and Maas, M: Nursing Outcomes Classification (NOC), 2nd ed. Mosby, St. Louis, 2000.

NANDA Nursing Diagnoses: Definitions and Classification 2005–2006. NANDA International, Philadelphia, 2005.

Olds, SB, London, ML, Ladewig, PW: Maternity-Newborn Nursing: A Family-Centered Approach, 6th ed. Prentice Hall, Upper Saddle River, NJ, 1999.

Peplau, HE: Interpersonal Relations in Nursing: A Conceptual Frame of Reference for Psychodynamic Nursing. Putnam, New York, 1952.

Phillips, CR: Family-Centered Maternity and Newborn Care, 4th ed. Mosby, St. Louis, 1996.

Post-Stroke Rehabilitation: Assessment, Referral, and Patient Management. AHCPR Pub 95–0663, US Department of Health and Human Services, Public Health Service Agency for Health Care Policy and Research, Rockville, MD, 1995.

Pressure Ulcers in Adults: Prediction and Prevention. AHCPR Pub 92–0047, US Department of Health and Human Services, Public Health Service Agency for Health Care Policy and Research, Rockville, MD, 1992.

Purnell, LD, and Paulanka, BJ: Transcultural Health Care: A Culturally Competent Approach, 2nd ed. F.A. Davis, Philadelphia, 2003.

Rimmer, JH: Aging, Mental Retardation and Physical Fitness. Center on Health Promotion Research for Persons with Disabilities. University of Illinois at Chicago, 1996.

Seligman, M, Reivich, K, Jaycox, LH, and Gillham, J: The Optimistic Child. Houghton Mifflin, New York, 1995.

Shore, LS: Nursing Diagnosis: What It Is and How to Do It: A Programmed Text. Medical College of Virginia Hospitals, Richmond, VA, 1988.

Sickle Cell Disease: Screening, Diagnosis, Management, and Counseling in Newborns and Infants. AHCPR Pub 93–0562, US Department of

Health and Human Services, Public Health Service Agency for Health Care Policy and Research, Rockville, MD, April 1993.

Singer Kaplan, H: Sexual Desire Disorders Dysfunctional Regulation of Sexual Motivation. Routledge, London, 1995.

Sommers, MS, and Johnson, SA: Diseases and Disorders: A Nursing Therapeutics Manual, 2nd ed. F.A. Davis, Philadelphia, 2002.

Sparks, SM, and Taylor, CM: Nursing Diagnoses Reference Manual, 5th ed. Springhouse Corporation, Springhouse, PA, 2001.

Stanley, M, Blair, KA, and Beare, PG: Gerontological Nursing: Promoting Successful Aging with Older Adults, 3rd ed. F.A. Davis, Philadelphia, 2005.

Ten Great Things Exercise Can Do for You. Chapter in MCormack, BN, and Yorkey, M. Wiley Pub Inx. American Media, Inc, New York, 2005.

Townsend, M: Nursing Diagnoses in Psychiatric Nursing: Care Plans and Psychotropic Medications, 6th ed. F.A. Davis, Philadelphia, 2004.

Townsend, M: Psychiatric Mental Health Nursing: Concepts of Care, 4th ed. F.A. Davis, Philadelphia, 2003.

Traumatic Brain Injury Medical Treatment Guidelines. State of Colorado Labor and Employment, Division of Worker's Compensation, Denver, March 15, 1998.

Urinary Incontinence in Adults: Clinical Practice Guideline. AHCPR Pub 92–0038, US Department of Health and Human Services, Public Health Service Agency for Health Care Policy and Research, Rockville, MD, March 1992.

Venes, D (Ed.): Taber's Cyclopedic Medical Dictionary, 20th ed. F.A. Davis, Philadelphia, 2005.

Yura, H, and Walsh, MB: The Nursing Process: Assessing, Planning, Implementing, Evaluating, 5th ed. Appleton & Lange, Norwalk, CT, 1988.

Articles

Ackerman, MH, and Mick, DJ: Instillation of normal saline before suctioning patients with pulmonary infections: A prospective randomized controlled trial. Am J Crit Care 7(4):261, 1998.

Acute Confusion/Delirium. Research Dissemination Core, University of Iowa Gerontological Nursing Interventions Research Center (GNIRC). Iowa City, IA, 1998.

Albert, N: Heart failure: The physiologic basis for current therapeutic concepts. Crit Care Nurse (Suppl), June, 1999.

Allen, LA: Treating agitation without drugs. Am J Nurs 99(4):36, 1999.

American Academy of Pediatrics, Task Force on Sleep Position and SIDS: Changing concepts of sudden infant death syndrome: Implications for infant sleeping environment and sleep position. Pediatrics 105:650, 2000.

Anderson, NR: The role of the home healthcare nurse in smoking cessation: Guidelines for successful intervention. Home Healthcare Nurse 24(7):424, 2006.

Angelucci, PA: Caring for patients with benign prostatic hyperplasia. Nursing 27(11):34, 1997.

AORN latex guideline: 2004 standards, recommended practices, and guidelines. AORN J 79(3):653–72, 2004.

Armstrong, ML, and Murphy, KP: A look at adolescent tattooing. School Health Reporter, Summer, 1999.

Astle, SM: Restoring electrolyte balance. RN 68(5):31–4, 2005.

Augustus, LJ: Nutritional care for patients with HIV. Am J Nurs 97(10):62, 1997.

Baldwin, K: Stroke: It's a knock-out punch. Nursing Made Incredibly Easy! 4(2):10–23, 2006.

Baranoski, S: Skin tears: Staying on guard against the enemy of frail skin. Nursing 2003, 33(10) Suppl-Travel Nursing: 14–20, 2003.

Barry, J, McQuade, C, and Livingstone, T: Using nurse case management to promote self-efficiency in individuals with rheumatoid arthritis. Rehabil Nurs 23(6):300, 1998.

Bartley, MK: Keep venous thromboembolism at bay. Nursing 36(10):36–41, 2006.

Barton-Burke, M: Cancer-related fatigue and sleep disturbances: Further research on the prevalence of these two symptoms in long-term cancer survivors can inform education, policy, and clinical practice. AJN 106(3)Suppl:72–7, 2006.

Bates, B, Choi, JY, Duncan, PW, et al: Veterans Affairs/Department of Defense clinical practice guidelines for the management of adult stroke rehabilitation care: An executive summary. Stroke 36(9): 2049–56, 2005.

Bauer, J, and Steinhauer, R: A readied response: The emergency plan. RN 65(6):40, 2002.

Bauldoff, GS, and Diaz, PT: Improving outcomes for COPD patients. The Nurse Practitioner: The American Journal of Primary Care, 31(8):26–43, 2006.

Beattie, S: In from the cold. RN 69(11):22–7, 2006.

Beatty, GE: Shedding light on Alzheimer's. The Nurse Practitioner: The American J of Primary Health Care 31(9):32–43, 2006.

Beauchamp-Johnson, BM: Scale down bariatric surgery risks, Nursing Management 37(9):27–32, 2006.

Becker, B: To stand or not to stand. Rehab Management 18(2):28–34, 2005.

Belza, B: The impact of fatigue on exercise performance. Arthritis Care and Research 7(4), 176–180, 1994.

Bergen, AF: Heads up: A 20–year tale in several parts. Team Rehabilitation Report 9(9):45, 1998.

Berkowitz, C: Epidural pain control: Your job, too. RN 60(8):22, 1997.

Bermingham, J: Discharge planning: Charting patient progress. Contin Care 16(1):13, 1997.

Bernardi, L, Saviolo, R, Sodick, DH, et al: Do hemodynamic responses to the Valsalva maneuver reflect myocardial dysfunction? Chest, May 1, 1989.

Birkett, DP: What is the relationship between stroke and depression? Harv Ment Health Lett 14(12):8, 1998.

Blank, CA, and Reid, PC: Taking the tension out of traumatic pneumothoraxes. Nursing 29(4):41, 1999.

Blann, LE: Early intervention for children and families with special needs. MCN, The American J of Maternal/Child Nursing 30(4):263–7, 2005.

Boesch, C, Myers, J, Habersaat, A, et al: Maintenance of exercise capacity and physical activity patterns after cardiac rehabilitation. J Cardiopulm Rehab 25(1):14-21, 2005.

Bone, LA: Restoring electrolyte balance: Calcium and phosphorus. RN 59(3):47, 1996.

Bonner, SM: TKO knee pain with total knee replacement. Nursing Made Incredibly Easy! 5(2):30–9, 2007.

Boon, T: Don't forget the hospice option. RN 61(2):32, 1998.

Borbasi, S, Jones, J, Lockwood, C, et al: Health professionals' perspective of providing care to people with dementia in the acute setting: Toward better practice. Geriatric Nursing 27(5):300–8, 2006.

Borton, D: Isolation precautions: Clearing up the confusion. Nursing 27(1):49, 1997.

Boucher, MA: When laryngectomy complicates care. RN 59(88):40, 1996.

Bowman, A, Breiner, JE, Doerschug, KC, et al: Implementation of an evidence-based feeding protocol and aspiration risk reduction algorithm. Crit Care Nurse Quarterly 28(4):424–333, 2005.

Bradley, M, and Pupiales, M: Essential elements of ostomy care. Am J Nurs 97(7):38, 1997.

Branski, SH: Delirium in hospitalized geriatric patients. Am J Nurs 97(1):161, 1998.

Bray, B, Van Sell, SL, and Miller-Anderson, M: Stress incontinence: It's no laughing matter. RN 70(4):25–9, 2007.

Breakey, JW: Body image: The inner mirror. Journal of Prosthetics and Orthotics 9(3):107, 1997.

Bright, L: Strategies to improve the patient safety outcome imdicator: Preventing or reducing falls. Home Healthcare Nurse 23(1):29–36, 2005.

Brown, KA: Malignant hyperthermia. Am J Nurs 97(10):33, 1997.

Buckle, J: Alternative/complementary therapies. Crit Care Nurse 18(5):54, 1998.

Burgio, KL, et al: Behavioral training for post-prostatectomy urinary incontinence. J Urol 141(2):303, 1989.

Burkhart, I, and Solari-Twadell, PA. Spirituality and religiousness: Differentiating the diagnosis through a review of the nursing literature. Nurs Diag Int J Nurs Lang Class 12:45–54, 2001.

Burns, SM: Mechanical ventilation of patients with acute respiratory distress syndrome and patents requiring weaning: The evidence guiding practice. Crit Care Nurse 25(4):14–24, 2005.

Burt, S: What you need to know about latex allergy. Nursing 28(10):33, 1998.

Butcher, HK, and McGonigal-Kenney, M: Depression and dispiritedness in later life. AJN 105(12):52–61, 2005.

Calcium in kidney stones. Harv Health Lett 22(8):8, 1997.

Canales, MAP: Asthma management, putting your patient on the team. Nursing 27(12):33, 1997.

Capili, B, and Anastasi, JK: A symptom review: Nausea and vomiting in HIV. JANAC 9(6):47, 1998.

Carbone, IM: An interdisciplinary approach to the rehabilitation of open-heart surgical patients. Rehab Nurs 24(2):55, 1999.

Carlson, EV, Kemp, MG, and Short, S: Predicting the risk of pressure ulcers in critically ill patients. Am J Crit Care 8(4):262, 1999.

Carroll, P: Closing in on safer suctioning. RN 61(5):22, 1998.

Carroll, P: Preventing nosocomial pneumonia. RN 61(6):44, 1998.

Carroll, P: Pulse oximetry: At your fingertips. RN 60(2):22, 1997.

Cataldo, R: Decoding the mystery: Evaluating complementary and alternative medicine. Rehab Manag 12(2):42, 1999.

Catania, K, Huang, C, James, P, and Ohr, M: PUPPI: The pressure ulcer prevention protocol interventions. AJN 107(4):44–51, 2007.

Cavendish, R: Clinical snapshot: Periodontal disease. Am J Nurs 99(3): 36, 1999.

Centers for Disease Control and Prevention: Recommended immunization schedules for persons aged 0–18 years—United States. MMWR 55 (51–52):Q1–Q4, 2006.

Chatters, IM, Taylor, RJ, and Lincoln, KD: Advances in the measurement of religiosity among older African Americans: Implications for health and mental health researchers. J Ment Health Aging 8(1): 181–200, 2001.

Chatterton, R, McTaggart, P, Baum, K, et al: Suicides in an Australian inpatient environment. J Psychosoc Nurs Ment Health Serv 37(6):34, 1999.

Cheever, KH: An overview of pulmonary arterial hypertension: Risks, pathogenesis, clinical manifestations, and management. J Cardiovascular Nursing 20(2):108–116, 2005.

Chilton, BA: Recognizing spirituality. Image J Nurs Sch 30(4):400, 1998.

Cirolia, B: Understanding edema: When fluid balance fails. Nursing 26(2):66, 1996.

Clark, CC: Posttraumatic stress disorder: How to support healing. Am J Nurs 97(8):26, 1996.

Cohen, D: Optional but necessary. Rehab Management 18(10):26–9, 2005.

Consult Stat: Chest tubes: When you don't need a seal. RN 61(3):67, 1998.

Cook, L: The value of lab values. Am J Nurs 99(5):66, 1999.

Cormier, M: The role of Hepatitis C support groups. Gastroenterology Nursing 28 (3 Suppl):S4–S9, 2005.

Creswell, C, and Chalder, T: Defensive coping styles in chronic fatigue syndrome. J Psychosomatic Research 51(4):607–610, 2001.

Crigger, N, and Forbes, W: Assessing neurologic function in older patients. Am J Nurs 97(3):37, 1997.

Crow, S: Combating infection: Your guide to gloves. Nursing 27(3):26, 1997.

Dahlin, C: Oral complications at the end of life. AJN 104(7):40–7, 2004.

D'Arcy, Y: Conquering PAIN: Have you tried these new techniques? Nursing 35(3):36–41, 2005.

D'Arcy, Y: Eye on capnography. Men in Nursing 2(2):25–9, 2007.

D'Arcy, Y: Managing pain in a patient who's drug-dependent. Nursing 37(3):36–40, 2007.

DeJong, MJ: Emergency! Hyponatremia. Am J Nurs 98(12):36, 1998.

Denison, B: Touch the pain away: New research on therapeutic touch and persons with fibromyalgia syndrome. Holist-Nurs-Pract 18(3): 142–51, 2004.

Dennison, RD: Nurse's guide to common postoperative complications. Nursing 27(11):56, 1997.

Diel-Oplinger, L, and Kaminski, MF: Choosing the right fluid to counter hypovolemic shock. Nursing 34(3):52–4, 2004.

diMaria-Ghalili, RA, and Amelia, E: Nutrition in older adults: Interventions and assessment can help curb the growing threat of malnutrition. AJN 105(3):40–50, 2005.

Dionne, M: This bed is just right. Rehab Management 18(1):32–9, 2005.

Dossey, BM: Holistic modalities and healing moments. Am J Nurs 98(6):44, 1998.

Dossey, BM, and Dossey, L: Body-Mind-Spirit: Attending to holistic care. Am J Nurs 98(8):35, 1998.

Drugs that bring erections down. Sex & Health Institute, p. 5, May 1998.

Ducharme, S: Autonomic dysreflexia (sexuality and SCI). Paraplegia News, November 1, 2006.

Dunn, D: Age-smart care: Preventing perioperative complications in older adults. Nursing 4(3):30–9, 2006.

Dunn, D: Preventing perioperative complicatons in special populations. Nursing 35(11):36–43, 2005.

Dunne, D: Common questions about ileoanal reservoirs. Am J Nurs 97(11):67, 1997.

Durston, S: What you need to know about viral hepatitis. Nursing 35(8):36–41, 2005.

Dworak, PA, and Levy, A: Strolling along. Rehab Management 18(9):26–31, 2005.

Edmond, M: Combating infection. Tackling disease transmission. Nursing 27(7):65, 1997.

Edwards-Beckett, J, and King, H: The impact of spinal pathology on bowel control in children. Rehabil Nurs 21(6):292, 1996.

Eisenhauer, C: Media review: The new glucose revolution: The authoritative guide to the glycemic index—the dietary solution for lifelong health. Family & Community Health 30(1):86, 2007.

Elgart, HN, Johnson, KL, and Munro, N: Assessment of fluids and electrolytes. AACN Advanced Critical Care 15(4):607–21, 2004.

Elpern, EH, Covert, B, and Kleinpell, R: Moral distress of staff nurses in a medical intensive care unit. Am J of Critical Care 14:523–539, 2005.

Epps, CK: The delicate business of ostomy care. RN 5(11):32, 1996.

Epstein, CD, and Peerless, JR: Weaning readiness and fluid balance in older critcially ill surgical patients. Am J of Crit Care 15(1):54–64, 2006.

Erickson, EH: Reflections on the dissent of contemporary youth. International Journal of Psychoanalysis 51:11–22, 1970.

Faries, J: Easing your patient's postoperative pain. Nursing 28(6):58, 1998.

Feldman, R, Eidelman, AI, Sirota, L, and Weller, A: Comparison of skin-to-skin (Kangaroo) and traditional care: Parenting outcomes and preterm infant development. Pediatrics 110(1):16–26, 2002.

Ferrin, MS: Restoring electrolyte balance: Magnesium. RN 59(5):31, 1996.

Fish, KB: Suicide awareness at the elementary school level. J Psychosoc Nurs Ment Health Serv 38(7):20, 2000.

Fishman, TD, Freedline, AD, and Kahn, D: Putting the best foot forward. Nursing 26(1):58, 1996.

Flannery, J: Using the levels of cognitive functioning assessment scale with traumatic brain injury in an acute care setting. Rehab Nurs 23(2):88, 1998.

Focazio, B: Clinical snapshot: Mucositis. Am J Nurs 97(12):48, 1997.

Frost, KL, and Topp, R: A physical activity RX for the hypertensive patient. The Nurse Practitioner: The American J of Primary Health Care 31(4):29–37, 2006.

Fry, VS: The creative approach to nursing. Am J Nurs 53:301, 1953.

Galea, S, Nandi, A, and Vlahov, D: The epidemiology of post-traumatic stress disorders after disasters. Epidemiologic Reviews 27(1):78–91, 2005.

Gance-Cleveland, B: Motivational interviewing as a strategy to increase families' adherence to treatment regimens. Journal for Specialists in Pediatric Nursing 10(3):151–155, 2005.

Garnett, LR: Is obesity all in the genes? Harv Health Lett 21(6):1, 1996.

Giasson, M, and Bouchard, L: Effect of therapeutic touch on the well-being of persons with terminal cancer. J of Holistic Nursing 16(3): 383–98, 1998.

Gibbons, S, Lauder, W, and Ludwick, R: Self-neglect: A proposed new NANDA diagnosis. International J Nursing Terminologies and Classifications 17(1):10–18, 2006.

Goertz, S: Eye of diagnostics: Gauging fluid balance with osmolality. Nursing 36(10):70–1, 2006.

Goldrich, G: Understanding the 12–lead ECG, part I. Nursing 36(11):36–41, 2006.

Goldrick, BA, and Goetz, AM: 'Tis the season for influenza. The Nurse Practitioner 31(12):24–33.

Goldstein, LB: Cough and aspiration of food and liquids due to oral-pharyngeal dysphagia: AACP evidence-based clinical practice guidelines. Chest, January 1, 2006.

Good, KK, Verble, JA, Secrest, J, et al: Postoperative hypothermia—The chilling consequences. AORN 83(5):1055–66, 2006.

Goshorn, J: Clinical snapshot: Kidney stones. Am J Nurs 96(9):40, 1996.

Graf, C: Functional decline in hospitalized older adults. AJN 106(1): 58–67, 2006.

Grandjean, CK, and Gibbons, SW: Assessing ambulatory geriatric sleep complaints. Nurse Pract 25(9):25, 2000.

Gray, M: Assessment and management of urinary incontinence. The Nurse Pract 30(7):32–43, 2005.

Gray, M: Overactive bladder: An overview. Journal of Wound, Ostomy and Continence Nursing 32(3) Suppl: 1–5, 2005.

Gray, M, Bliss, DZ, Doughty, DB, et al: Incontinence-associated dermatitis: A consensus. J Wound, Ostomy and Continence Nursing 34(1):45–54, 2007.

Gregory, CM: Caring for caregivers: Proactive planning eases burdens on caregivers. Lifelines 1(2):51, 1997.

Greifzu, S: Fighting cancer fatigue. RN 61(8):41, 1998.

Gritter, M: The latex threat. Am J Nurs 98(9):26, 1998.

Grzankowski, JA: Altered thought processes related to traumatic brain injury and their nursing implications. Rehabil Nurs 22(1):24, 1997.

Hahn, J: Cueing in to client language. Reflections 25(1):8–11, 1999.

Halpin-Landry, JE, and Goldsmith, S: Feet first: Diabetes care. Am J Nurs 99(2):26, 1999.

Hankins, J: The role of albumin in fluid and electrolyte balance. J of Infusion Nursing 29(5):260–5, 2006.

Hanley, C: Delirium in the acute care setting: Med Surg Nurs 13(4):217–25, 2004.

Hanneman, SK, and Gusick, M: Frequency of oral care and positioning of patients in critical care: A replication study. Am. J Crit Care 14(5):378–386, 2005.

Hanson, MJS: Caring for a patient with COPD. Nursing 27(12):39, 1997.

Harvey, C, Dixon, M, and Padberg, N: Support group for families of trauma patients: A unique approach. Crit Care Nurse 15(4):59, 1995.

Hayes, DD: Bradycardia. Keeping the current flowing. Nursing 27(6):50, 1997.

Hayn, MA, and Fisher, TR: Stroke rehabilitation: Salvaging ability after the storm. Nursing 27(3):40, 1997.

Hernandez, D: Microvascular complications of diabetes: Nursing assessment and interventions. Am J Nurs 98(6):16, 1998.

Herson, L, Hart, K, Gordon, M, et al: Identifying and overcoming barriers to providing sexuality information in the clinical setting. Rehabil Nurs 24(4):148, 1999.

Hess, CT: Caring for a diabetic ulcer. Nursing 29(5):70, 1999.

Hess, CT: Wound care. Nursing 28(3):18, 1998.

Hoffman, J: Tuning in to the power of music. RN 60(6):52, 1997.

Holcomb, SS: Understanding the ins and outs of diuretic therapy. Nursing 27(2):34, 1997.

Holm, K, and Foreman, M: Analysis of measures of functional and cognitive ability for aging adults with cardiac and vascular disease. J of Cardiovascular Nursing 21(5–Suppl):40–5, 2006.

Houghton, D: HAI prevention: The power is in your hands. Nursing Management 37(5): Suppl: 1–7, 2006.

Hughes, L. Physical and psychological variables that influence pain in patients with fibromyalgia. Orthopaedic Nursing 25(2):112–19, 2006.

Hunt, R: Community-based nursing. Am J Nurs 98(10):44, 1998.

Hunter, A, Denman-Vitale, S, and Garzon, L: Global infections: Recognition, management, and prevention. The Nurse Practitioner 32(2):34–41, 2007.

Huston, CJ: Emergency! Dental luxation and avulsion. Am J Nurs 97(9):48, 1997.

Hutchison, CP: Healing touch: An energetic approach. Am J Nurs 99(4):43, 1999.

Isaacs, A: Depression and your patient. Am J Nurs 98(7):26, 1998.

Iscoc, KE, Campbell, JE, Jamnik, V, et al: Efficacy of continuous real-time blood glucose monitoring during and after prolonged high-intensity cycling exercise: Spinning with a continuous glucose monitoring system. Diabetes Technology and Therapeutic 8(6):627–35, 2006.

It's probably not Alzheimer's: New insights on memory loss. Focus on Healthy Aging 2(7):1, 1999.

Iyasu, S, Randall, L, Welty, K, et al: Risk factors for sudden infant death syndrome among Northern Plains Indians. JAMA 288(21):2717, 2002.

Jaempf, G, and Goralski, VJ: Monitoring postop patients. RN 59(7):30, 1996.

Jennings, LM: Latex allergy: Another real Y2K issue. Rehab Nurs 24(4):140, 1999.

Jirovec, MM, Wyman, JF, and Wells, TJ: Addressing urinary incontinence with educational continence-care competencies. Image J Nurs Sch 30(4):375, 1998.

Johnson, CV, and Hayes, JA: Troubled spirits: Prevalence and predictors of religious and spiritual concerns among university students and counseling center clients. J of Counseling Psychology 50:409–419, 2003.

Johnson, J, Pearson, V, and McDivitt, L: Stroke rehabilitation: Assessing stroke survivors' long-term learning needs. Rehab Nurs 22(5):243, 1997.

Kachourbos, MJ: Relief at last: An implanted bladder control system helps people control their bodily functions. Team Rehab Rep, p. 31, August, 1997.

Kanachki, L: How to guide ventilator-dependent patients from hospital to home. Am J Nurs 97(2):37, 1997.

Kania, DS, and Scott, CM: Postexposure prophylaxis considerations for occupational and nonoccupational exposures. Advanced Emergency Nursing Journal 29(1):20–32, 2007.

Kaplow, R: AACN synergy model for patient care: A framework to optimize outcomes. Crit Care Nurse Suppl (Feb): 27–30, 2003.

Kearney, PM, and Griffin, T: Between joy and sorrow: Being a parent of a child with a developmental disability. Journal of Advanced Nursing 34:582–592, 2001.

Keegan, L: Getting comfortable with alternative and complementary therapies. Nursing 28(4):50, 1998.

Kersting, K: A new approach to complicated grief. Monitor on Psychology 35(10): 51, 2004.

King, B: Preserving renal function. RN 60(8):34, 1997.

Kinloch, D: Instillation of normal saline during endotracheal suctioning: Effects on mixed venous oxygen saturation. Am J Crit Care 8(4):231, 1999.

Kirshblum, S, and O'Connor, K: The problem of pain: A common condition of people with SCI. Team Rehab Rep, p. 15, August, 1997.

Kirton, C: The HIV/AIDS epidemic: A case of good news/bad news. Nursing Made Incredibly Easy! 3(2):28–40, 2005.

Klonowski, EI, and Masodi, JE: The patient with Crohn's disease. RN 62(3):32, 1999.

Klotter, J: Latex allergy prevention. Townsend Letter for Doctors and Patients, May 1, 2006.

Kolcaba, K, and DiMarco, MA: Comfort theory and its application to pediatric nursing. Pediatr Nurse 31(3):187–194, 2005.

Kolcaba, KY, and Fisher, EM: A holistic perspective on comfort care as an advance directive. Crit Care Nurs Quarterly 18(4):66–7, 1996.

Kopala, B, and Burkhart, L: Ethical dilemma and moral distress: Proposed new NANDA diagnoses. International Journal of Nursing Terminologies and Classifications 16(1):3–13, 2005.

Korinko, A, and Yurick, A: Maintaining skin integrity during radiation therapy. Am J Nurs 97(2):40, 1997.

Kouch, M: Managing symptoms for a "good death." Nursing 36(11): 58–63, 2006.

Kumasaka, L, and Miles, A: "My pain is God's will." Am J Nurs 96(6):45, 1996.

Kurtz, MJ, Van Zandt, DK, and Sapp, LR: A new technique in independent intermittent catheterization: The Mitrofanoff catheterizable channel. Rehab Nurs 21(6):311, 1996.

Lai, SC, and Cohen, MN: Promoting lifestyle changes. Am J Nurs 99(4):63, 1999.

Larden, CN, Palmer, ML, and Janssen, P: Efficacy of therapeutic touch in treating pregnant inpatients who have a chemical dependency. J Holist-Nurs 22(4): 320–32, 2004.

Lark, S: The 21-day arthritis and pain miracle. Article for the Lark Letter: A Woman's Guide to Optimal Health and Balance, Special Report, 2005.

Larsen, LS: Effectiveness of a counseling intervention to assist family caregivers of chronically ill relatives. J Psychosoc Nurs Ment Health Serv 36(8):26, 1998.

Laskowski-Jones, L: Responding to trauma: Your priorities in the first hour. Nursing 36(9):52–8, 2006.

Lewis, ML, and Dehn, DS: Violence against nurses in outpatient mental health settings. J Psychosoc Nurs Ment Health Serv 37(6):28, 1999.

Linch, SH: Elder abuse: What to look for, how to intervene. Am J Nurs 97(1):26, 1997.

Livneh, H, and Antonak, RF: Psychosocial adaptation to chronic illness and disability: A primer for counselors (practice & theory). J of Counseling and Development 83(1):12–20, 2005.

Loeb, JL: Pain management in long-term care. Am J Nurs 99(2):48, 1999.

Lorente, L, Lecuona, M, Jimenez, A, Mora, ML, and Sierra, A: Ventilator-associated pneumonia using a heated humidifier or a heat and moisture exchanger: A randomized controlled trial. Crit Care 10: 4, 2006.

Lorio, AK: Transfer dependent. Rehab Management 18(7):22–6, 2005.

Loughrey, L: Taking a sensitive approach to urinary incontinence. Nursing 29(5):60, 1999.

MacNeill, D, and Weis, T: Case study: Coordinating care. Contin Care 17(4):78, 1998.

Malinowski, A, and Stamler, LL: Comfort: Exploration of the concept in nursing. JAN, the Journal of Advanced Nursing 39(6):599–606, 2002.

Mann, AR: Manage the power of pain. Men in Nursing 1(4):20–8, 2006.

Manoguerra, AS, and Cobaugh, DJ: Guideline on the use of ipecac syrup im the out-of-hospital management of ingested poisons. Clin Toxicol 43(1):1–10, 2005.

Matthews, PJ: Ventilator-associated infections. I. Reducing the risks. Nursing 27(2):59, 1997.

Mauk, KL: Medications for management of overactive bladder. ARN Network. June/July, pp. 3–7, 2005.

McAllister, M: Promoting physiologic-physical adaptation in chronic obstructive pulmonary disease: Pharmacotherapeutic evidence-based research and guidelines. Home Healthcare Nurse 23(8): 523–31, 2005.

McCaffery, M: Pain management handbook. Nursing 27(4):42, 1997.

McCaffery, M, and Ferrell, BR: Opioids and pain management: What do nurses know? Nursing 29(3):48, 1999.

McCaffrey, R, and Rozzano, L: The effect of music on pain and acute confusion in older adults undergoing hip and knee surgery. Holistic Nursing Practice 20(5):218–224, 2006.

McCain, D, and Sutherland, S: Nursing essentials: Skin grafts for patients with burns. Am J Nurs 98(7):34, 1998.

McClave, SA, Lukan, JK, Lowen, JA, et al: Poor validity of residual volumes as a marker for risk of aspiration in critically ill patients. Crit Care Medicine 33(2):324–330, 2005.

McClave, SA, et al: Are patients fed appropriately according to their caloric requirements? JPEN 22(6):375, 1998.

McConnel, E: Preventing transient increases in intracranial pressure. Nursing 28(4):66, 1998.

McCool, FD, and Rosen, MJ: Nonpharmacologic airway clearance therapies. Chest 129:(250S–259S), 2006.

McCullagh, MC: Home modification. AJN 106(10):54–63, 2006.

McHale, JM, Phipps, MA, Horvath, K, et al: Expert nursing knowledge in the care of patients at risk of impaired swallowing. Image J Nurs Sch 30(2):137, 1998.

McKinley, LL, and Zasler, CP: Weaving a plan of care. Contin Care 17(7):38, 1998.

McLean, SE, Jensen, LA, Schroeder, DG, et al: Improving adherence to a mechanical ventialtion weaning protocol for critically ill adults: Outcomes after an implementation program. Am J Crit Care 15(3): 299–309, 2006.

Mendez-Eastman, S: When wounds won't heal. RN 51(1):20, 1998.

Metheny, NA: Preventing aspiration in older adults with dysphagia. (Try this: Best Practices in Nursing Care to Older Adults). MedSurg Nursing, April, 2006.

Metheny, N, et al: Testing feeding tube placement: Auscultation vs pH method. Am J Nurs 98(5):37, 1998.

Michael, KM, Allen, JK, and Macko, RE: Fatigue after stroke: Relationship to mobility, fitness, ambulatory activity, social support, and falls efficacy. Rehabilitation Nursing 31(5):210–217, 2006.

Miller, CK, Ulbrecht, JS, Lyons, J, et al: A reduced-carbohydrate diet improves outcomes in patients with metabolic syndrome: A translational study. Topics in Clinical Nutrition 22(1):82–91, 2007.

Milne, JL, and Krissovich, M: Behavioral therapies at the primary care level: The current state of knowledge. Journal of Wound, Ostomy and Continence Nursing 31(6):367–76, 2004.

Mintz, TG: Relocation stress syndrome in older adults. Social Work Today 5(6):38, 2005.

Mohr, WK: Cross-ethnic variations in the care of psychiatric patients: A review of contributing factors and practice considerations. J Psychosoc Nurs Ment Health Serv 36(5):16, 1998.

Moshang, J: The growing problem of type 2 diabetes. LPN2005,1(3): 26–34, 2005.

Mosocco, D: Clipboard: Childhood vaccines. Home Healthcare Nurse 25(1):7–8, 2007.

Murphy, K: Anxiety: When is it too much? Nursing Made Incredibly Easy! 3(5):22–31, 2005.

Murray-Swank, A, et al: Religiosity, psychosocial adjustment, and subjective burden of persons who care for those with mental illness. Psychiatric Services 57:361–65, 2006.

Nadolski, M: Getting a good night's sleep: Diagnosing and treating insomnia. Plastic Surgical Nursing 25(4):167–73, 2005.

Naylor, MD, Stephens, C, Bowles, KH, et al: Cognitively impaired older adults. AJN 105(2):52–61, 2005.

Newman, DK: Assessment of the patient with an overactive bladder. Journal of Wound, Ostomy and Continence Nursing 32(3, Suppl):5–10, 2005.

Nieves, J, and Capone-Swearer, D: The clot that changes lives. Nursing Critical Care 1(3):18–28, 2006.

No author listed: Changing concepts of sudden infant death syndrome: Implications for infant sleeping environment and sleep position. Task Force on Infant Sleep Position and Sudden Infant Death Syndrome. Pediatr 105(3):650–6, 2000.

No author listed: Defensive Functioning Scale, Brandeis University Psychological Counseling Center, Waltham, MA, 2002.

No author listed: Smog—Who does it hurt? What you need to know about ozone and your health. Public information brochure. United States Environmental Protection Agency, Washington DC, 1999.

No author listed: Taking Control of Stress. Harvard Health Publications Big Sandy, TX, Special Supplement, 2007.

No author listed: The changing concept of sudden infant death syndrome: Diagnostic coding shifts, controversies regarding the sleeping environment, and new variations to consider in reducing risk. Pediatrics 116(5):1245–55, 2005.

No author listed: Understanding transcultural nursing. Nursing 35(1): 14–23, Supplement Career Directory, 2005.

Nunnelee, JD: Healing venous ulcers. RN 60(11):38, 1997.

Oddy, WH, Li, J, Landsborough, L, Kendall, GE, Henderson, S, and Downie, J: The association of maternal overweight and obesity with breastfeeding duration. Journal of Pediatrics 149(2):185–191, 2006.

Odom-Forren, J: Preventing surgical site infections. Nursing 36(6): 59–63, 2006.

O'Donnell, M: Addisonian crisis. Am J Nurs 97(3):41, 1997.

O'Donnell, RP, Rosenbaum, P, Walter, BJ, et al: The health and well-being of caregivers of children with cerebral palsy. Pediatrics 115(6):e626–36, 2005.

Okan, K, Woo, K, Ayello, EA et al: The role of moisture balance in wound healing. Advances for Skin & Wound Care. The J for Prevention and Healing 20(1):39–53, 2007.

Olansky, S: Chronic sorrow: A response to having a mentally defective child. Social Casework 43:190–193, 1962.

O'Neil, C, Avila, JR, and Fetrow, CW: Herbal medicines, getting beyond the hype. Nursing 29(4):58, 1999.

Parkman, CA, and Calfee, BE: Advance directives, honoring your patient's end-of-life wishes. Nursing 27(4):48, 1997.

Parsons, KS, Galinsky, TL, and Waters, T: Suggestions for preventing musculoskeletal disorders in home healthcare workers, Part 1: Lift and transfer assistance for partially weight-bearing home care patients. Home Healthcare Nurse 24(3):158–64, 2006.

Parsons, KS, Galinsky, TL, and Waters, T: Suggestions for preventing musculoskeletal disorders in home healthcare workers, Part 2: Lift and transfer assistance for non-weight-bearing home care patients. Home Healthcare Nurse 24(4):227–33, 2006.

Pasero, C, and McCaffrey, M: No self-report means no pain-intensity rating. AJN 105(10):50–3, 2005.

Pearsen, OR, Busse, ME, van Deuresn, RWM, et al: Quantification of walking mobility in neurological disorders. QJM: An International J of Medicine 97:463–75, 2004.

Perry, A: Quality of life. Rehab Management 18(7):18–21, 2005.

Phillips, JK: Actionstat: Wound dehiscence. Nursing 28(3):33, 1998.

Pickhardt, Carl: (2002) Role Conflict of the Single Parent. Adoption Media, LLC.

Pieper, B, Sieggreen, M, Freeland, B, et al: Discharge information needs of patients after surgery. J Wound, Ostomy and Continence Nursing 33(3):281–90, 2006.

Pierce, LL: Barriers to access: Frustrations of people who use a wheelchair for full-time mobility. Rehab Nurs 23(3):120, 1998.

Pignone, MP, Ammerman, A, Fernandez, L, et al: Counseling to promote a healthy diet in adults: A summary of the evidence for the US Preventive Services Task Force. Am J Prev Med 24(1):75, 2003.

Poe, SS, Cvach, MM, Gartrell, DG, et al: An evidence-based approach to fall risk assessment, prevention, and management: Lessons learned. Journal of Nursing Care Quality 20(2):107–116, 2005.

Powers, J, and Bennett, SJ: Measurement of dyspnea in patients treated with mechanical ventilation. Am J Crit Care 8(4):254, 1999.

Pringle-Specht, JK: Nine myths of incontinence in older adults. AJN 105(6):58–68, 2005.

Pronitis-Ruotolo, D: Surviving the night shift: Making Zeitgeber work for you. Am J Nurs 101(7):63, 2001.

Pruitt, B: Weaning patients from mechanical ventilation. Nursing 36(9):36–41, 2006.

Purgason, K: Broken hearts: Differentiating stress-induced cardiomyopathy from acute myocardial infarction in the patient presenting with acute coronary syndrome. Dimensions in Crit Care Nursing 25(6):247–253, 2006.

Rawsky, E: Review of the literature on falls among the elderly. Image J Nurs Sch 30(1):47, 1998.

Reddy, L: Heads up on cerebral bleeds. Nursing 3(5), Suppl, ED Insider: 4–9, 2006.

Ried, S, and Dassen, T: Chronic confusion, dementia, and impaired environmental interpretation syndrome: A concept comparison. Nursing Diagnosis 11(2):45–59, 2000.

Riggs, JM: Manage heart failure. Nursing Critical Care 1(4):18–28, 2006.

Robertson, RG, and Montagnini, M: Geriatric failure to thrive. Am Fam Physician 70(2):343–50, 2004.

Robinson, AW: Getting to the heart of denial. Am J Nurs 99(5):38, 1999.

Rogers, S, Ryan, M, and Slepoy, L: Successful ventilator weaning: A collaborative effort. Rehab Nurs 23(5):265, 1998.

Romero, DV, Treston, J, and O'Sullivan, AL: Hand-to-hand combat: Preventing MRSA infection. Advances in Skin & Wound Care: The J for Prevention and Healing 19(6):328–33, 2006.

Rosen, L: Sit on it. Rehab Management 18(2):36–41, 2005.

Rosenthal, K: Guarding against vascular site infection. Nursing Management 37(4):54–66, 2006.

Sallis, JF: The role of behavioral science in improving health through physical activity. Summary of presentation. Science Writers Briefing. Sponsored by OBSSR and the American Psychological Association, December, 1996.

Salmon, DA, Moulton, LH, Omer, SB, et al: Factors associated with refusal of childhood vaccines among parents of school-aged children: A case-control. Arch Pediatr Adolesc Med 159(5):470–6, 2005.

Samarel, N, Fawcett, J, Davis, MM, and Ryan, FM: Effects of dialogue and therapeutic touch on preoperative and postoperative experiences of breast cancer surgery: An exploratory study. Oncology Nursing Forum 25(8):1369–76, 1998.

Sampselle, CM: Behavioral interventions in young and middle-age women. Am J Nurs 103(3):9, 2003. (Suppl) State of the Science on Urinary Incontinence.

Sauerbeck, LR: Primary stroke prevention. AJN 106(11):40–9, 2006.

Scanlon, C: Defining standards for end-of-life care. Am J Nurs 97(11):58, 1997.

Schaffer, DB: Closed suction wound drainage. Nursing 27(11):62, 1997.

Scharer, K, and Brooks, G: Mothers of chronically ill neonates and primary nurses in the NICU: Transfer of care. Neonatal Network, 13(5):37–46, 1994.

Scheck, A: Therapists on the team: Diabetic wound prevention is everybody's business. Rehab Nurs 16(7):18, 1999.

Schiffman, RF: Drug and subtance use in Adolescents MCN, The American J of Maternal/Child Nursing 29(1):21–7, 2004.

Schiweiger, JL, and Huey, RA: Alzheimer's disease. Nursing 29(6):34, 1999.

Schmelling, S: Home, adapted home. Rehab Management 18(6):12–19, 2005.

Schraeder, C, et al: Community nursing organizations: A new frontier. Am J Nurs 97(1):63, 1997.

Schulman, A: Staff Working Paper. The Presidents' Council on Bioethics. Bioethics and Human Dignity, 2005.

Schulmeister, L: Pacemakers and environmental safety: What your patient needs to know. Nursing 28(7):58, 1998.

Schumacher, K, Beck, CA, and Marren, JM: Family caregivers: Caring for older adults, working with their families. AJN 106(8):40–49, 2006.

Schwebel, DC, and Barton, BK: Contributions of multiple risk factors to child injury. J of Pediatr Psychol 30(7):553–61, 2005.

Short stature and growth hormone: A delicate balance. Practice Update (newsletter). The Children's Hospital, Denver, Summer, 1999.

Sieggreen, M: A contemporary approach to peripheral arterial disease. The Health Practitioner: The American J of Primary Health Care 31(7):14–25, 2006.

Sieggreen, MY: Getting a leg up on managing venous ulcers. Nursing Made Incredibly Easy! 4(6):52–60, 2006.

Sinacore, DR: Managing the diabetic foot. Rehab Manag 11(4):60, 1998.

Smatlak, P, and Knebel, AR: Clinical evaluation of noninvasive monitoring of oxygen saturation in critically ill patients. Am J Crit Care 7(5):370, 1998.

Smith, AM, and Schwirian, PM: The relationship between caregiver burden and TBI survivors' cognition and functional ability after discharge. Rehab Nurs 23(5):252, 1998.

Smith, DH: Managing acute acetaminophen toxicity. Nursing 37(1):58–63, 2007.

Smith, DW, Arnstein, P, Rosa, KC, and Wells-Federman, C: Effects of integrating therapeutic touch into a cognitive behavioral pain treatment program. Report of a pilot clinical trial. J Holist Nurs 20(4):367–87, 2002.

Smochek, MR, Oblaczynsk, C, Lauck, DL, et al: Interventions for risk for suicide and risk for violence. Nurs Diagn. Int J Nurs Lang Class 11(2):60, April–June 2000.

Sommer, KD, and Sommer, NW: When your patient is hearing impaired. RN 65(12):28–32, 2002.

Spurlock, WR: Spiritual well-being and caregiver burden in Alzheimer's caregivers. Geriatr Nurs 26(3):154–161, 2005.

Stabin, MG, and Breitz, H: Breast milk secretion of radiopharmaceuticals: Mechanisms, findings, and radiation dosimetry. J Nuclear Med 41(5):863–873, 2000.

Stegeman, CA: Oral manifestations of diabetes. Home Healthcare Nurse 23(4):233–40, 2005.

Stockert, PA: Getting UTI patients back on track. RN 62(3):49, 1999.

Strimike, CL, Wojcik, JM, and Stark, BA: Incision care that really cuts it. RN 60(7):22, 1997.

Sullivan, CS, Logan, J, and Kolasa, KM: Medical nutrition therapy for the bariatric patient. Nutrition Today 41(5):207–12, 2006.

Summer, CH: Recognizing and responding to spiritual distress. Am J Nurs 98(1):26, 1998.

Szymanski, L, and King, B: Practice parameters for the assessment and treatment of children, adolescents, and adults with mental retardation and comorbid mental disorders. J Am Acad Child Adolesc Psychiatry Dec 38 (12 Suppl): 1999.

Tablan, OC, Anderson, LJ, Besser, R, Bridges, C, and Hajjeh, R: Guidelines for preventing health-care associated pneumonia, 2003—Recommendations of CDC and Healthcare Infection Control Practices Advisory Committee. MMWR, March 26, 53(RRO3): 1–36, 2004.

Travers, PL: Autonomic dysreflexia: A clinical rehabilitation problem. Rehab Nurs 24(1):19, 1997.

Travers, PL: Poststroke dysphagia: Implications for nurses. Rehab Nurs 24(2):69, 1999.

Travis, S: "Caring for you, caring for me": A ten-year caregiver educational initiative of the Rosalynn Carter Institute for Human Development, Health and Social Work, May 1, 2006.

Trendall, J: Concept analysis: Chronic fatigue. J of Advanced Nursing 32(5):1126–31, 2005.

Turkowski, BB: Managing insomnia. Orthopaedic Nursing 25(5): 339–45, 2006.

Ufema, J: Reflections on death and dying. Nursing 29(6):96, 1999.

Vigilance pays off in preventing falls. Harv Health Lett 24(6):1, 1999.

Walker, BL: Preventing falls. RN 61(5):40, 1998.

Walker, D: Back to basics: Choosing the correct wound dressing. Am J Nurs 96(9):35, 1996.

Wallhagen, MI, Pettengill, E, and Whiteside, M: Sensory impairment in older adults part 1: Hearing loss. AJN 106(10):40–49, 2006.

Wallston, BS, and Wallston, KA: Locus of control and health: A review of the literature. Health Eduction Monographs, University of South Florida, Spring, 1978, 107–117, (Revised January 11, 1999).

Warms, CA, Marshal, JM, Hoffman, AJ, et al: There are a few things you did not ask about my pain: Writing in the margins of a survey questionaire. Rehabilitation Nursing 30(6):248–56, 2006.

Watson, R, Modeste, N, Catolico, O, et al: The relationship between caregiver burden and self-care deficits in former rehabilitation patients. Rehab Nurs 23(5):258, 1998.

Waugh, KG: Measuring the right angle. Rehab Management 18(1):40–7, 2005.

Weeks, SM: Caring for patients with heart failure. Nursing 26(3):52, 1996.

Wehling-Weepie, AK, and MCarthy, A: A healthy lifestyle program: Promoting child health in schools. J School Nurs 18(6):322, 2002.

Weiss, B: When a family member requires your care. RN 68(4):63–5, 2005.

Wheeler, MS: Pain assessment and management in the patient with mild to moderate cogntive impairement. Home Healthcare Nurse 24(6): 354–9, 2006.

Wheeler, SL, and Houston, K: The role of diversional activities in the general medical hospital setting. Holistic Nursing Practice 19(?): 67–9, 2005.

Whetstone, L, and Morrissey, S: Children at risk: The association between perceived weight status and suicidal thoughts and attempts in middle school youth. J School Health 77(2):59–66, 2007.

Whiteman, K, and McCormick, C: When your patient is in liver failure. Nursing 35(4):58–63, 2005.

Whiteside, MM, Wallhagen, MI, and Pettengill, E: Sensory impairment in older adults: Part 2: Vision loss. AJN 106(11):52–61, 2006.

Whitfield, W: Research in religion and mental health. Naming of parts—Some reflections. Int J Psychiatr Nurs Res 8(1):891–896, 2002.

Whittle, H, et al: Nursing management of pressure ulcers using a hydrogel dressing protocol: Four case studies. Rehab Nurs 21(5):237, 1996.

Williams, AM, and Deaton, SB: Phantom limb pain: Elusive, yet real. Rehab Nurs 22(2):73, 1997.

Woods, DL, Craven, RF, and Whitney, J: The effect of therapeutic touch on behavioral symptoms of persons with dementia. Altern-Ther-Health-Med 11(1):66–74, 2005.

Woods, DL, and Dimond, M: The effect of therapeutic touch on agitated behavior and cortisol in persons with Alzheimer's disease. Biol Res Nurs 4(2):104–14, 2002.

Wooten, JM: OTC laxatives aren't all the same. RN 69(9):78, 2006.

Wyman, JF: Behavioral interventions for the patient with overactive bladder. Journal of Wound, Ostomy and Continence Nursing 32(3) Suppl: 11–15, 2005.

Wyman, JF: Treatment of urinary incontinence in men and older women. Am J Nurs 103(3):26, 2003. (Suppl) State of the Science on Urinary Incontinence.

Wyman, JF, Fantl, JA, McClish, DK, et al: Comparative efficacy of behavioral interventions in the management of female urinary incontinence. Am J Obstet Gynecol 179(4):999, 1998.

Zink, EK, and McQuillan, K: Managing traumatic brain injury. Nursing 35(9):36–43, 2005.

Electronic Resources

Aazer, SA. (2005). Constipation in adults. Retrieved January 2007, at http://www.emedicinehealth/com.

Adams, L: Working together: Climate—The emotional one that is (Dec. 2006). Retrieved March 2007, at http://www.gordontraining.com/pdf/wt-200612–climate-the-emotional-one-that-is.pdf

Adams, L: Working together: Paying attention to children. Retrieved April 2007, at http://www.gordontraining.com/pdf/wt-200603–paying-attention-to-children.pdf

Adams, L: Working together: The language of love. Retrieved April 2007, at http://www.gordontraining.com/pdf/wt-200702–the-language-of-love.pdf

Adams, L: Working together: The power of P.E.T. Retrieved April 2007, at http://www.gordontraining.com/pdf/wt-200607–the-power-of-pet.pdf

Albo, M, and Richter, HE. (2006). Urodynamic testing. Fact sheet for National Kidney and Urologic Diseases Information Clearinghouse. Retrieved May 2007, at http://kidney.niddk.nih.gov/kudiseases/pubs/urodynamic/index.htm

Allergy testing. Retrieved February 2007, at http://www.labtestsonline.com

American Academy of Clinical Toxicology: Position statement—Ipecac syrup. Retrieved April 2007, at http://www.clintox.org/Pos_Statements/Ipecac.html

American Academy of Family Physicians: Breastfeeding (Position paper). Accessed Feb 2007, at http://www.aafp.org/online/en/home/policy/policies/b/breastfeedingpositionpaper.html

American Academy of Pediatrics: Ten steps to support parents' choice to breastfeed their baby. Revised May 2003. Accessed Feb 2007, at http://www.aap.org/breastfeeding/tenSteps.pdf

American Geriatrics Society Foundation for Health in Aging. (2004): Incontinence. In Eldercare at Home, Chapter 10. Retrieved May 2007, at http://healthinaging.org/public_education/eldercare/10.xml

American Society of Health-System Pharmacists Fact Sheet (no date listed). Medicatons and you. Retrieved Jan 2007, at http://www.safemedication.com

Amitai, A, and Sinert, D. (2006). Ventilator management. Retrieved May 2007, at http://www.emedicine.com/emerg/topic788.htm

Arnold, JL. (2006). Personal protective equipment. Article for patient education, eMedicineHealth website. Retrieved February 2007, at http://www.emedicinehealth.com

Assertiveness Training. Retrieved April 2007, at http://www.csusm.edu/caps/Assertiveness.html

Ballas, P: Sexual problems overview, 2006. Retrieved May 2007, at MedlinePlus: http://www.nlm.nih.gov/medlineplus/ency/article/001951.htm

Barclay, L, and Lie, D. (2007). New guidelines issued for family support in patient-centered ICU. CME/CE for Medscape website. Retrieved February 2007, at http://www.medscape/viewarticle/551738

Bates, B: Simple questions can help uncover urinary incontinence. Family Practice News, Feb 15, 2007. Retrieved May 2007, at http://www.highbeam.com

Beckett, C: Family theory as a framework for assessment. (2000). Retrieved April 2007, at http://jan.ucc.nau.edu/~nur350–c/class/2_family/theory/lesson2–1–3.html

Behrman, AJ, and Howarth, M. (2005). Latex allergy. Retrieved February 2007, at http://www.emedicime.com/emerg/topic814.htm

Beland, N: Special report: The pursuit of happiness. Women's Health, April/May 2005. Retrieved April 2007, at http://womenshealthmag.com/article/0,6176,s1–3–72–111–2,00.html

Boyles, S. (2005). Hope for people stuck in grief. Article for WebMD. Retrieved March 2007, at http://www.webmd.com/ depression/news/20050531/

Boyles, S. (2005). Spouse caregivers most likely to be abusive. Retrieved February 2007, at http://www.webmd.com/content/Article/100/105831.htm

Brain basics: Understanding sleep, National Institute of Neurological Disorders and Stroke (NINDS). Retrieved August 2003, at http://www.ninds.nih.gov

Brandler, ES, Sinert, R, and Hostetler, MA. (2006). Shock, cardiogenic. Retrieved January 2007, at http://www.emedicine.com/emerg/topic 530.htm

Breastfeeding guidelines following radiopharmaceutical administration. Retrieved Feb 2007, at http://nuclearpharmacy.uams.edu/resources/breastfeeding.asp

Breazeale, Tami. (2001). Attachment Parenting: A Practical Approach for the Reduction of Attachment Disorders and the Promotion of Emotionally Secure Children. A Master's Thesis Submitted to the Faculty of Beth-el College. Retrieved Feb 2007, at http://www.visi.com/~jib/thesis.html

Bridges, LJ, and Moore, KA. (September 2002). Religious Involvement and Children's Well-Being: What Research Tells Us (And What It Doesn't), Child Trends Research Brief. Washington DC. Child Trends Data Bank http://www.childstrendsdatabank.org/Files/religiositiyRB.pdf

Buse, JB. (2003). Normal A1C but unstable blood glucose. Article for Medscape Diabetes and Endocrinology site. Retrieved January 2007, at http://www.medscape.com/viewarticle/46302

Callen, J, and Pinelli, J: A review of the literature examining the benefits and challenges, incidence and duration, and barriers to breastfeeding in preterm infants. Adv Neonatal Care 5(2):72–88, 2005. Retrieved Feb 2007, at http://www.medscape. com/ viewarticle/502591

Calver, P, Braungardt, T, Kupchik, N, et al: The big chill: Improving the odds after cardiac arrest, 2005. CE Home Study Program for RNweb. Retrieved March 2007, at http://www.rnweb.com

Campagnolo, DI. (2006). Autonomic dysreflexia in spinal cord injury. Retrieved January 2007, at http://www. emedicine.com

Carls, C: The prevalence of stress urinary incontinence in high school and college-age female athletes in the Midwest: Implications for education and prevention. Urol Nurs 27(1):21–24, 39, 2007. Retrieved May 2007, at http://www.medscape.com/viewarticle/555700? src=mp

Center for Disease Control and Prevention. (2007). Adult immunization schedule. Fact sheet for National Immunization Program. Retrieved March 2007, at http://www.cdc.gov/nip

Center for Disease Control and Prevention. (2003). What would happen if we stopped vaccinations? Fact sheet for National Immunization Program. Retrieved March 2007, at http://www.cdc.gov/nip

Centers for Disease Control and Prevention: When should a mother avoid breastfeeding. Aug 2006. Retrieved Feb 2007, at http://www.cdc.gov/breastfeeding/disease/contraindicators.htm

Champion Aspirations for Human Dignity. The White House. Retrieved March 2007, at http://www.whitehouse.gov/nsc/nss2.html

Cheshire, Jr., WP: Grey matters when eloquences is inarticulate. An article for Ethics & Medicine: An International Journal of Bioethics 22(3), 2007. Retrieved March 2007, at The Center for Bioethics Human Dignity http://www.cbhd.org/resources/neuroethics/cheshire_2007–01–26.htm

Child Trends Data Bank: Religiosity. Retrieved November 2005, at http://www.childrtrendsdatabank.org

Children's Hospital Boston Fact sheet (no date listed). Poisons. Retrieved April 2007, at http://www.childrenshospital.org/az/Site868

Clinical Manual for Management of the HIV-Infected Adult, 2006 edition. Section 3: Antiretroviral therapy adherence, pp. 3–11. Retrieved April 2007, at http://www.aidsetc.org/aetc/pdf/AETC-CM_092206.pdf

Cody, T, and Zieroff, V. (2005). Autonomic dysreflexia. Fact Sheet for Northeast Rehabilitation Health Network. Retrieved January 2007, at http://www.northeatrehab.com.

Connecticut Poison Control Center. Fact Sheet (no date listed). About Poisons. Retrieved March 2007, at http://www.poisoncontrol.uchc.edu/poisons/medications.htm

Cooper, S: Sylvia's inquiry into violence and the brain. Retrieved May 2007, at http://serendip.brynmawr.edu/local/suminst/bbi01/projects/cooper/

Coping with Anxiety and Phobias. Harvard Medical School. 2007. Retrieved January 2007, at http://www.health.harvard.edu/special_health_reports/Coping_with_Anxiety_an_Phobias.htm

Coping with Breastfeeding Challenges. US Department of Health & Human Services-womenshealth.gov, August, 2005. Retrieved Feb 2007, at http://www.4woman.gov/Breastfeeding/index.cfm?page=229

Cultural Awareness Self Concept. Retrieved April 2007, at http://academic.cuesta.edu/atorrey/culture.pdf

Darby, F, and Brown, D: Nice work if you can get it. (2003). Retrieved April 2007, at http://www.pocket-stress.com/articles/nice% 20work.php

Davis, JL. (2006) New Type 2 diabetes treatment options. Retrieved January 2007 at http://www.webmd.com/content/Article/129/117304.htm

Davis, N. (2003). (Short online summaries from): Multi-Sensory Trauma Processing, A Manual for Understanding and Treating PTSD and Job-Related Trauma. Retrieved April 2007, at http://www.rescue-workers.com/1.htm

dbS Productions. (2000–2007). Alzheimer's disease and related disorders SAR research: Wandering overview. Excerpt from book in progress available at Source of Search & Rescue Research, Publications and Training. http://www.dbs-sar.com/SAR_Research/wandering.htm

DeNoon, D. (2006). *C. Diff:* New threat from old bug: Epidemic gut infection causeing rapid rise in life-threatening disease. Retrieved February 2007, at http://www.medicinenet.com

Diego, R. (2003). Man in denial. Retrieved February 2007, at http://www.insmkt.com/myhome.htm

Dion, R. (2005). Overcoming relocation stress. Article provided by Military OneSource, PTSD Support Services. Retrieved April 2007, at http://www.ptsdsupport.net/relocation_ stress.html

Dire, DJ. (2005). Biological warfare. Article for patient education, eMedicineHealth website. Retrieved February 2007, at http://www.emedicinehealth.com

Diskin, A. (2006). Gastroenteritis. Retrived February 2007, at http://www.emedicine.com/emerg/topic213.htm

Diversional therapy, 2006. Article for the Diversional Therapy Association of New South Wales. Retrieved February 2007, at http://www/diversionaltherapy.com.au

Doheny, K. (2006). Adults with children at home consume more fat, study shows. Article for WebMD Medical News. Retrieved January 2007, at http://www.webmd.com/content/Article/131/117923.htm

Dowshen, S. (2005). Kids and dangerous "suffocation games." Article for KidsHealth website. Retrieved April 2007, at http://www.kidshealth.org/research/suffocation.html

Dunai, J. (2003). Assessment of unilateral neglect. (Update). (Patient behavior pattern after stroke). Article for HighBeam Research. Retrieved December 2006, at http://www.highbeam.com

Eby, N, and Car, M: Violence and brain injuries: Quality matters, Spring 2004. Retrieved May 2007, at Brain Injury Association of Montana: http://www.biamt.org/publications/violence.htm

Editorial staff. (2006). Fitness at any age. Article for MedicineNet website. Retrieved March 2007, at http://www.medicincnct.com

Effective and Ineffective Coping: The Process of Stress. Texas Medical Association. Retrieved March 2007, at http://www.texmed.org/Template.aspx?id=4479

Enslein, J, et al. (2002). Evidence-based protocol. Interpreter facilitation for persons with limited English proficiency. University of Iowa Gerontological Nursing Interventions Research Center. Retrieved from National Guidelines Clearinghouse, June 2003, at http://www.guideline.gov.

Ethical Decision Making. (2000). Providence Health System. Retrieved February 2007, at http://www.providence.org/phs/ethics/resources/decision_managers.htm

Evans, M: Loneliness, Self-Help Information Counseling and Testing Center, University of Oregon Counseling Center. Retrieved March 2007, at http://darkwing.uoregon.edu/~counsel/loneliness.htm

Female sexual dysfunction. Retrieved May 2007, at womenshealthchannel: http://www.womenshealthchannel.com/ fsd/index.shtml

Ferry, RJ, and Shim, M. (2006). Gigantism and acromegaly. Retrieved March 2007, at http://www.emedicine.com/ ped/topic2634.htm

Finch, A. (2007). Fed up with feeling alone? Self-esteem eZine "Touching Half the World," Retrieved February 2007, at www.selfesteem4women.com

Focus Adolescent Services: Self-Injury, 2000. Retrieved April 2007, at http://www.focusas.com/SelfInjury.html

Fong, T. (2002). Acetaminopen (Tylenol) liver damage. Retrieved December 2006, at http://www.medicinenet.com

Forrette, TL. (2006). Transitioning from mechanical ventilation. CE article for Medscape website. Retrieved May 2007, at http://www.medscape.com/viewprogram/5230_pnt

Frey, R: Self-mutilation. Gale Encyclopedia of Medicine, December, 2006. Retrieved April 2007, at http://www.healthatoz.com/healthatoz/Atoz/common/standard/transform.jsp?requestURI=/healthatoz/Atoz/ency/self-mutilation.jsp

Gardner, BM. (2002). Current approaches to type 2 diabetes mellitus. Article for Medscape CME. American Academy of Family Physicians (AAFP) 2002 Annual Scientific Assembly Common Clinical Problem Update and Family Medicine Research. Retrieved December 2006, at http://www.medscape.com/viewarticle/444348

Gettinger-Dinner, L: Suicide risk assessment: What providers need to know, April 30, 2007. Retrieved May 2007, at http://news.nurse.com/apps/pbcs.dll/article?AID=/20070430/CA09/304300012&SearchID=73281745058190

Gladwell, Malcoln: (2006). Blink, snap decision making. Retrieved february 2007, at www.talentsmart.com

Goleman, Daniel: Early violence leaves its mark on the brain. The New York Times, Tuesday, October 3, 1995. Retrieved May 2007, at http://www.cirp.org/library/psych/goleman/

"Gordon Training International." Retrieved April 2007, at newsletter@gordontraining.com

Gore, TA, and Richards-Reid, GM. (2006). Posttraumatic stress disorder. Retrieved April 2007, at http://www.emedicine. com/med/topic1900 .htm

Grenz, K, Bynum, G, Pine, D, et al. (update verson 2005). Preventive services for children and adolescents. Institute for Clinical Systems Improvement [ICSI]. Article for National Guideline Clearinghouse.website. Retrieved February 2007, at http://www.guideline .gov

Haines, C. (2006). Diabetes: Treating diabetes with insulin. Retrieved January 2007, at http://www.webmd.com/content/Article/46/1667_50931.htm

Haines, C. (2006). Digestive diseases: Swallowing problems. Retrieved April 2007, at Medicinenet: http://www.medicinetnet.com/swallowing/

Haines, C. (2005). Heart failure: Recognizing caregiver burnout. Retrieved February 2007, at http://www.webmd.com/content/Article/51/40695.htm

Haines, C. (2006). Learning about allergies to latex. Retrieved February 2007, at http://www.webmd.com/content/pages/10/1625.htm

Hallenbeck, J, and Weissman, D: Treatment of nausea and vomiting (2007). Retrieved April 2007, at http://www.jasonprogram.org/nausea_treatment.htm

Headsets911. Retrieved March 2007, at http://www.headsets911.com/activecoping.htm

Health Sciences Centre. (2007). Suffocation. Fact sheet for IMPACT website. Retrieved April 2007, at http://www.hsc.mb.ca/impact/suffocation.htm

Hertz, G, and Cataletto, ME. (2006). Sleep dysfunction in women. Retrieved December 2006, at http://www.emedicine.com/med/topic656.htm

Hingley, AT: Preventing accidental poisoning (2007). Article for Pregnacy Weekly website. Retrieved April 2007, at http://www.pregnancy-weekly.com

Hobdell, E: Chronic sorrow and depression in parents of children with neural tube defects. J Neurosci Nurs 36(2):82–88, 94, 2004. Retrieved May 2007, at http://www.medscape.com/ viewarticle/474596_1

Holson, D, and Gathers, S. (2006). Constipation. Retrieved January 2007, at http://www.emedicine.com/emerg/topic111.htm

Homeir, BP. (2004). Household safety: Preventing suffocation. Article for KidsHealth website. Retrieved April 2007, at http://www.kidshealth.org/parent/positive/family/safety_suffocation.html

Hope for Today Al-Anon Group. Retrieved March 2007, at http://health.groups.yahoo.com/group/HopeForTodayGroup/

Hoppe, J, and Sinert, R. (2006). Heat exhaustion and heatstroke. Retrieved March 2007, at http://www.emedicine.com/emert/topic236.htm

Hospital and Palliative Nurses Association: Spiritual Distress-Patient/Family Teaching Sheets, 2005. Retrieved May 2007, at http://www.hpna.org/pdf/PatientSheet_SpiritualDistress.pdf

House, J: Social Isolation Kills, But How and Why? Psychosomatic Medicine 63:273–274, 2001. Retrieved May 2007, at http://www.psychosomaticmedicine.org/cgi/content/full/63/2/273

Hubbynet, Coping with Stress. 2000 Retrieved March 2007, at http://www.hubbynet.com/stresscoping.htm

Human Medication Noncompliance. Retrieved April 2007, at http://www.alrt.com/humnonc.html

Hyman, SE: Thinking about violence in our schools, Discussion at the White House, August 3, 1998. National Institute of Mental Health. Retrieved May 2007, at http://www.medhelp.org/NIHlib/GF-376.html

International Lactation Consultant Association: Evidenced-based guidelines for breastfeeding management during the first fourteen days. April 1999. Retrieved Feb 2007, at http://www.ilca.org/pubs/ebg.pdf

Issues and Answers: Fact Sheet on Sexuality Education, 2004. Seicus Report, 29(6), 2001. Retrieved May 2007, at http://www.siecus.org/pubs/fact/fact0007.html

Jacobs, DH. (2005). Aphasia. Retrieved February 2007, at http://www.emedicine.com/NEURO/topic437.htm

Jacobs, DH. (2006). Confusional states and acute memory disorders. Retrieved January 2007, at http://www.emedicine.com/neuro/topic435.htm

Jagminas, L. (2005). CBRN—Evaluation of a biological warfare victim. Retrieved February 2007, at http://www.emedicime.com/emerg/topic891.htm

Jagminas, L, and Erdman, DP. (2006). CBRNE—Chemical decontamination. Retrieved February 2007, at http://www.emedicime.com/emerg/topic893.htm

Kalvemark, S, Hoglund, AAT, Hansson, MG, Westerholm, P, and Arnetz, B: Living with conflicts-ethical dilemmas and moral distress in the health care system. Soc Sci Med 58(6):1075–84, 2004. Dept of Public Health and Caring Sciences, Uppsala University, Sweden. Retrieved March 2007, at sofia.kalvermark@apoteket.se

Kater, K. (2006). Building healthy body esteem in a body toxic world. Retrieved April 2007, at http://www.BodyImageHealth.org

Kearney, P: (updated 2006) Chronic Grief (Or Is It Periodic Grief?) Grief in a Family Context. Retrieved May 2007, at http://www.indiana.edu/~famlygrf/units/chronic.html

Keepnews, D, and Mitchell, PH. (2003). Health Systems' Accountability for patient safety. Online J of Issues in Nursing 8(2). Manuscript 2. Retrieved March 2007, at http://nursingworld.org/ojin/topic22/tpc22_2.htm

Keim, SM, and Kent, M: Nausea and vomiting (2005). Retrieved April 2007, at http://www.emedicinehealth.com/vomiting_and_nausea/article_em.htm

Kemp, S, and Gungor, N. (2005). Growth failure. Retrieved March 2007, at http://www.emedicine.com/ped/topic 902.htm

Klimes, R. (2007). Managing stress: Living without stress overload. CE offering for Learn.Well.org website. Retrieved April 2007, http://www.learnwell.org/stress.htm

Kolcaba, K. (2006). FAQs (frequently asked questions). On the comfort line. Website devoted to the Concept of Comfort in Nursing. Retrieved February 2007, at http://www.thecomfortline.com/FAQ.htm

Kreal's Guide to the Sociology of the Family. Retrieved April 2007, at http://www.trinity.edu/~mkearl/family.html

Lafreniere, R, Berguer, R, Seifert, PC, et al. (2005). Preparation of the operating room. Retrieved March 2007, at http://www.medscape.com/viewarticle/503004

Lamemeh,T, Shah, AM, and Hsu, K. (2006). Anxiety. Retrieved January 2007, at http://www.emedicine.com/emerg/topic35.htm

Lashley, FR. (2006). Emerging infectious dieases at the beginning of the 21st century. The Online Journal of Issues in Nursing 11(1). Retrieved March 2007, at http://www.nursingworld.org.ojin/topic29_1.htm

Lauer, T: Rape trauma. American Association for Marriage and Family Therapy. Retrieved April 2007, at http://www.aamft.org/ families/Consumer_Updates/RapeTrauma.asp

Lawrence, S. (2005). When health fears are overblown. Article for WebMD Health and Balance Feature Stories. Retrieved February 2007, at http://www.webmd.com/balance/features

Lehrer, JK. (2006). Bowel incontinence. Article for MedlinePlus, a service of National Library of Medicine and National Institutes of Health. Retrieved January 2007, at http://www.nlm.nih.gov/medlineplus.

Li, J, and Decker, W. (2005). Hypothermia. Retrieved March 2007, at http://www.emedicine.com/emerg/topic279.htm

Lien, CA. (no date listed). Thermoregulation in the elderly. Syllubus on Geriatric Anesthesiology. American Society of Anesthesologists website. Retrieved January 2007, at http://www.asahq.org/clinical/geriatrics/thermo.htm

Llewelllyn-Thomas, H: Helping patients make health care decisions. Center for the Evaluative Cinical Sciences Dartmouth Medical School. 2004. Retrieved March 2007, at www.dartmouthatlas.org

Lubit, R. (2005). Acute treatment of disaster survivors. Retrieved March 2007, at http://www.emedicine.com/med/topic3540.htm

Lyons, SS, and Specht, JKP. (1999). Prompted voiding for persons with urinary incontinence. Iowa City (IA): University of Iowa Gerontological Nursing Interventions Research Center Web Site. Retrieved from the National Guidelines Clearinghouse [NGC: 950], June 2003, at http://www.guideline.gov

Male Sexual Health, 2005. Retrieved May 2007, at http://www. modern-therapy.com/male/sexual-health.html

Management of breastfeeding for healthy full term infants. National Guideline Clearinghouse (AHRQ), June, 2003. Accessed Feb 2007, at http://www.guideline.gov/summary/summary.aspx?view_id=1&doc_id=3624

Marks, JW. (2006). Constipation. Retrieved January 2007, at http://www.medicinenet.com.

Marks, JW, and Lee, D. (2004). Diarrhea. Retrieved February 2007, at http://www.medicinenet.com

Mathur, R. (2007). Obesity. Retrieved April 2007, at http://www. medicinet.com

Mayo Clinic-Rochester: Mild cognitive impairment prevalent in elderly population: Risk increases as age goes up and education goes down. April 4, 2006. Retrieved January 2007, at http://www.mayoclinic.org/news2006–rst/3306.html

Mayo Clinic Staff. (2005). Alzheimer's: Understand and control wandering. Retrieved May 2007, at http://www.mayoclinic. com/health/alzheimers/HQ00218

Mayo Clinic Staff. (2007). Dehydration. Article for Mayo Clinic website. Retrieved February 2007, at http://www.mayoclinic.com/ health/dehydration/DS0056/DSECTION=1

McElgunn, V. (1990). Environmental hazards and child health and development: Advances in research and policy. Presentation in the Linking Research to Practice: Second Canadian Forum Proceedings Report and published by the Canadian Child Care Federation. Retrieved February 2007, at http://www.cfc-efc.ca/

McPherson, M, Smith-Lovin, L, and Brashears, M: Social isolation in US: Changes in core discussion networks over two decades. American Sociological Review 71(June 353–375), 2006. Retrieved May 2007, at http://www.asanet.org/galleries/default-file/June06ASRFeature.pdf

Meadows, M. (2006). Nutrition: Healthy eating. Retrieved April 2007, at http://www.medicinet.com

Menna, A: Rape trauma syndrome: The journey to healing belongs to everyone. Retrieved April 2007, at http://www.giftfromwithin.org/html/journey.html

Messina, J, and Messina, C: Tools for coping with life's stressors. Retrieved March 2007, at http://www.coping.org/control/manipul.htm

Miller, L, et al. (1999). Religiosity as a protective factor in depressive disorder. Am J Psychiatry 156:808A-809. Retrieved Jan 2007, at http://ajp.psychiatryonline.org

Mills, J: The ontology of religiosity: The oceanic feeling and the value of the lived experience. Humanists, 2006. Retrieved April 2007, at http://www.huumanists.org/rh/mills.html

Morrissey, P. (2005). Noncompliance after transplantation. A newsletter from the transplant team at Rhode Island Hospital. Retrieved March 2007, at http://www.lifespan.org/rih/services/transplant/news/02–07.htm

Muche, JA, and McCarty, S. (2006). Geriatric rehabilitation. Retrieved April 2007, at http://www.emedicine.com/pmr/topic164.htm

Muller, C. (1996). Dealing with the modern crisis of religiosity: Reflections from the Aum Case. http://www.hm.tyg.jp/~acmuller/articles/dayori1.htm

National Ag Safety Database (NASD). (2002). Sleep deprivation: Cause and consequences. Fact sheet for Nebraska Rural Health and Safety Coalition. Retrieved Jan 2007, at http://www.cdc.gov.nasd/

National Coalition for Cancer Survivors: Palliative care and management: Nausea and vomiting. Retrieved April 2007, at http://www.canceradvocacy.org/resources/essential/effects/nausea.aspx

National Comprehensive Cancer Network: Nausea and vomiting: Treatment guidelines for patients with cancer. Vol 3, 2005. Retrieved April 2007, at http://www.cancer.org/downloads/CRI/NCCN_Nasuea.pdf

National Institute of Aging: Exercise can boost cardiac fitness in conditioned and out of shape people. Public Information Article released August 1996. Retrieved July 2005, at http://www.nia.nih.gov

National Institute on Deafness and Other Communication Disorders (NIDCD). (2006). Strategic plan: Plain language version FY 2003–2005. Retrieved April 2007, at NIDCD website http://www.nidcd.nih/

National Institute for Neurological Disorders and Stroke (NINDS): Swallowing disorders information page, 2007. Retrieved April 2007, at http://www.ninds.nih.gov/

National Women's Health Resource Center Fact Sheet. (2005). Medication safety. Retrieved April 2007, at http://www. healthywomen.org

Newman, DK. (2006). Using the BladderScan® for bladder volume assessment. Retrieved May 2007, at http://www.seekwellness.com/incontinence/using_the_bladderscan.htm

Newton, E. (2005). Hyperventilation syndrome. Retrieved January 2007, at http://www.emedicine.com/emerg/topic270.htm

No author or pub date listed. Anticipatory grief. Featured Columns under Life Topics/Grief & Loss for Psychologist 4therapy website. Retrieved March 2007, at http://www.4therapy.com

No author listed. (April 1, 1990). Bag the brown bag paper bag. (Bag rebreathing as a treatment for hyperventilation). Newsletter-People's Medical Society, Inc. Retrieved January 2007, at http://www.highbeam.com/doc/1G1–9094801.html

No author listed. (1999). Chemical toxins safety. Fact sheet for Resources for Child Care Givers. All Family Resources website. Retrieved February 2007, at http://familymanagement. com/childcare/facility/chemical.toxins.safety.html

No author listed. Diabetes and healthy eating. Better Health Channel Fact Sheet. (2000–2004). Victoria, Australia. Retrieved January 2007, at http://www.betterhealth.vic.gov.au

No author or pub date listed. Health maintenance evaluation: Replacing the "annual physical." Fact sheet for Palo Alto Medical Foundation website. Retrieved March 2007, at http://www.pamf.org/children/maintenance/healtheval.html

No author listed. (2005). Hyperthermia: Too hot for your health. Article for National Institute on Aging website. Retrieved March 2007, at http://www.niapublications/org/agepages/hyperther.asp

No author listed. (2005). Liver blood enzymes. Retrieved December 2006, at http://www.medicinenet.com

No author listed. Monitoring diabetes control. Diabetes Manual. Royal Children's Hospital. Retrieved January 2007, at http://www.rch.org.au/diabetesmanual.cfm

No author listed. (2006). Oral cancer. Retrieved April 2007, at http://www.medicinenet.com

No author listed. (2007). Preventing leading causes of premature death, disease and disability. Fact sheet of the World Health Organization

(WHO). Retrieved March 2007, at http://www.who.int/school_ youth_health/en/

No author or pub date listed. Sometimes grief becomes complicated, unresolved or stuck. Featured Columns under Life Topics/Grief & Loss for Psychologist 4therapy website. Retrieved March 2007, at http://www.4therapy.com

No author listed. (2007). The causes, effects and dangers of sleep deprivation. Article for Sleep Deprivation website. Retrieved April 2007, at http://www.sleep-deprivation.com/

No author or pub date listed. The Development of Social Skills. Retrieved May 2007, at http://www.incrediblehorizons.com/social-skills.htm

No author or pub date listed. Symptom: Walking symptoms. Retrieved May 2007, at http://wrongdiagnosis.com/sym/walking_symptoms. htm

No author listed. (1995–2007). Urinary incontinence. The Merck Manual of Health & Aging (online), Section 3, Ch 57. Retrieved May 2007, at http://www.merck.com/pubs/mmanual_ha/sec3/ch57/ch57a.html

No author listed. (2002). World Health Report. Reducing risks, promoting healthy life. Report of the World Health Organization (WHO). Retrieved March 2007, at http://www.who.int/whr/2002/en/whr02 _en.pdf

Noise. Information Sheet. American Speech-Language-Hearing Association (ASHA). Retrieved, June 2003, at www.asha.org

Null, J. (2007). Hyperythermia deaths of children in vehicles. Fact sheet for San Fransisco State University department of Geosiences website. Retrieved March 2007, at http://ggweather.com/heat/

Olade, R, Safi, A, and Kesari, S. (2006). Cardiac catheterization (left heart). Retrieved January 2007, at http://www.emedicine.com/emerg/ topic2958,htm

Older Americans Month. Food & Nutrition Information. American Dietetic Association Web site. Retrieved June 2003, at http://www .eatright.org/Public/Nutritioninformation/92_12402. cfm

Oommen, K. (2006). Neurological history and physical examination. Retrieved April 2007, at http://www.emedicine.com/neuro/topic632 .htm

Organizational Development & Training Tip Sheet. (2002). Tufts University. Retrieved March 2007, at http://www.tufts.edu/hr/tips/assert.html

Owens, TA. (2005). Medical Encyclopedia: Delayed growth. Retrieved March 2007, at http://nim.nih.gov/medlineplus/ency/article/ 003021.htm

Palmer, RM. (2006). Management of common clinical disorders in geriatric patients: Delerium. Retrieved May 2007, at http://www.medscape.com/viewarticle/53466

Panzera, AK: Interstitial cystitis/painful bladder syndrome. Urol Nurs 27(1):13–19, 2007. Retrieved May 2007, at http://www.medscape. com/viewarticle/555699?src=mp

Paula, R. (2006). Compertment syndrome, abdominal. Retrieved April 2007, at http://www.emedicine.com/emerg/topic935.htm

Personal identity. (2007). Stanford Encyclopeida of Philosophy. Retrieved March 2007, at http://plato.stanford.edu/entries/identity-personal/

Pisacane, A, Continisio, G, et al: A controlled trial of the father's role in breastfeeding promotion. Pediatrics, 116(4):e494–e498, 2005. Retrieved Feb 2007, at http://www.sidsalliance.org/research/ Fathers%20Role%20in%20Successful% 20Breastfeeding. pdf

Planned Parenthood: Sexual health-sexuality, 2006. Retrieved May 2007, at http://plannedparenthood.org/sexual-health/sexual-health-relationship/sexuality.htm

Policastro, MA, Sinert, R, and Guerrero, P: Urinary obstruction, (2007). Retrieved May 2007, at http://www.emedicine.com/emerg/topic624.htm

Questions/Answers about Voice Problems. Information Sheet. American Speech-Language-Hearing Association (ASHA). Retrieved June 2003, at www.asha.org

Rackley, R, and Vasavada, SP. (2006). Incontinence, urinary: Nonsurgical therapies. Retrieved May 2007, at http://www.emedicine.com/med/topic3085.htm

Rajen, M. (2006). Toxins everywhere. Article for New Straits Times on HighBeam Research website. Retrieved February 2007, at http://www.highbeam.com

Rasul, AT. (2005). Compartment Syndrome. Retrieved May 2007, at http://www.emedicine.com/pmr/topic33.htm

Reasoner, R: The true meaning of self-esteem. National Association for Self-Esteem. Retrieved April 2007, at http://www.self-esteem-nase.org/whatisselfesteem.shtml

Rehabilitation Institute of Chicago–Spinal Cord Injury Team. (2006). Complications: Autonomic dysreflexia. Rehabilitation Institute of Chicago Life Center website. Retrieved January 2007, at http://lifecenter.ric.org.

Renter, TA. (no pub date listed). Upper extremity positioning injuries during operative/other invasive procedures. Article for Anesthesia Consulting website. Retrieved March 2007, at http://www.anesthesia-consulting.com

Robert, P: Sleeplessness clouds moral choices. American Academy of Sleep Medicine, March, 2007. Retrieved March 2007, at http://www.healthday.com/printer.asp?AID=602367

Robinson, K. (2007). Counseling Services, University of New York at Buffalo. Retrieved March 2007, at http://ub-counseling.buffalo.edu/loneliness.shtml

Saglimbeni, AJ. (2005). Exercise-induced asthma. Retrieved January 2007, at http://www.emedicine.com

Salinas, P, and Hanbali, F. (2006). Closed head trauma. Retrieved March 2007, at http://www.emedicine.com/med/ topic3403.htm

Santos, A, and Hunt, M. (2005). Managing incontinence: Once a cause of isolation and embarrassment, incontinence does not have to limit quality of life. Paraplegia News 59(11), 2005. Available from http://www.pvamagazines.com/pnnews/magazine/article.php?art=1687

Savrock, J. (2006). Counseling distressed students may be improved by religious discussion. Retrieved May 2007, at http://www.ed.psu.edu/news/spiritual.asp

Scheinfeld, NS, and Mokashi, A. (2007). Protein-energy malnutrition. Retrieved April 2007, at http://www.emedicine.com/derm/topic797.htm

Schoenborn, C: Marital Status and Health: United States, 1999–2002. Advance Data from Vital and Health Statistics, no 351. Retrieved March 2007, at http://www.cdc.gov/nchs/data/ad/ad351.pdf

Schuman, W: Keeping your sunny side up. Retrieved April 2007, at http://www.beliefnet.com/story/147/story_14745_1.html

Scott-Conner, CEH, and Ballinger, B: Abdominal angina (2005). Retrieved May 2007, at http://www.emedicine.com/med/ topic2 .htm

Searle, J: Eating and swallowing. Fact sheet regarding Hunington's disease, (no date listed). Retrieved April 2007, at http://www.kumc.edu/ hosp/huningtons/swallowing.htm

Seepersad, Sean: Critical Analysis Paper. Understanding loneliness using attachment and systems theories & developing an applied intervention. Retrieved March 2007, at http://www.webofloneliness .com/publications/critical/pubintro.htm

Self-help Brochures, Assertiveness, UIUC. Retrieved April 2007, at http://www.couns.uiuc.edu/Brochures/assertiv.htm

Sharma, S, and Hayes, JA. (2006). Hypoventilation syndromes. Retrieved May 2007, at http://www.emedicine.com/emerg/topic3470.htm

Sharma, VP. (1996). Normal mourning and "complicated grief." Article for Mind Publications website. Retrieved March 2007, at http://www .Mindpub.com/art045.htm

Sherman, C: Antisuicidal effect of psychotropics remains uncertain. Clin Psychiatry News 30(8), 2002. Retrieved May 2007, at http://www .namiscc.org/Research/2002/AntipsychoticSuicideRisk.htm

Simon, JH. (2004). Schizophrenia. CME article for Hardin Memorial Hospital website. Retrieved May 2007, at http://www.hmh.net/ adam/patientreports/000047.htm

Singleton, JK. (no date listed). Nurses' perspectives of encouraging client's care-of-self in a short-term rehabiltiation unit within a long-term care facility. CE offering for ARN website. Retrieved April 2007, at http://www.rehabnurse.org/ce/ 010200/010200_a.htm

Society for Neuroscience: What is Neuroscience. (2007). Retrieved May 2007, at http://www.sfn.org/index.cfm?pagename=whatIsNeuroscience

Spader, C: Post MI cooldown, 2006. Article for Nursing Spectrum website. Retrieved March 2007, at http://www.community.nursingspectrum.com

Speech for Clients with Tracheostomies or Ventilators. Information Sheet. American Speech-Language-Hearing Association (ASHA). Retrieved June 2003, at www.asha.org

Stotts, NA, Wipke-Tevis, DD, and Hopf, HW. (2007). Cofactors in impaired wound healing (excerpts). In Chronic Wound Care 4th Edition Excerpts. Retrieved Feb 2007, at http://www.chronicwoundcarebook.com/

Swan, L. (2001). Unilateral spatial neglect. Article for HighBeam Research. Retrieved December 2006, at http://www.highbeam.com/

The Center for Ethics and Advocacy in Healthcare. Retrieved March 2007, at http://www.healthcare-ethics.org/about/

The Rape, Abuse, & Incest National Network (RAINN): Prevention. Retrieved April 2007, at http://www.rainn.org/

Tooth decay: Prevention. (2005). Article for WebMD health topics website. Retrieved February 2007, at http://www.webmd.com/hw/dental/hw/172611.asp

Vij, S, and Gentili, A. (2005). Sleep disorder, geriatric. Retrieved December 2006, at http://www.emedicine.com/med/topic3179.htm

Vinik, AI, Freeman, R, and Erbas, T. (2004). Diabetic autnomic neuropathy. Retrieved April 2007, at http://www.medscape.com/ viewarticle/43205

Von Wager, K: Identity crisis—Theory and research. Retrieved March 2007, at http://psyschology.about.com/od/ theoriesofpersonality/a/identitycrisis.htm

Weiss, BD: Diagnostic evaluation of urinary incontinence in geriatric patients. American Family Physician 57(11), 1998. Retrieved May 2007, at http://www.aafp.org/afp/980600ap/weiss.html

What is language? What is speech? Information Sheet. American Speech-Language-Hearing Association (ASHA). Retrieved August 2003, at http://www.asha.org/public/speech/development

What is SIDS? Public information of the National SIDS/Infant Death Resource Center. Health Resources, Services Administration (HRSA) Maternal, and Child Health Bureau website. Retrieved February 2007, at http://www.hrsa.gov

Wilson, L, and Kolcaba, K. (2004). Practical application of comfort theory in the perianesthesia setting. J of Perianesthesia Nursing Online. Retrieved February 2007, at http://www.aspan.org/JOPAN/comfot_theory.htm

terWolbeek, M, vanDoormen, LJ, Kavelaars, A, et al: Severe fatigue in adolescents: A common phenomenon? Pediatrics 117(6):e1078–86, 2006. Retrieved February 2007, at http://pediatrics.aappublications.org/cgi/content/abstract/117/6/e1078

Woolston, C. (2006). Stress and aging. Article for Caremark Health Resources. Retrieved April 2007, at http://www.healthresources.caremark.com

World Health Organization (WHO). (2007). Sedentary lifestyle: A global public health problem. "Move for health" information sheet. Retrieved from WHO website March 2007, at http://www.who.int

Zuger, Abigail. (2001). Adherence by any measure still matters. Journal Watch. Retrieved April 2007, at http://aids-clinical-care.jwatch.org/cgi/content/full/2001/701/1

Index